Schatzberg's Manual of Clinical Psychopharmacology

Tenth Edition

T0293465

Schatzberg's Manual of Clinical Psychopharmacology

Tenth Edition

Charles DeBattista, D.M.H., M.D.

Director, Depression Research Clinic
Director of Medical Student Education in Psychiatry
Professor of Psychiatry and Behavioral Sciences
Stanford University School of Medicine, Stanford, California

Alan F. Schatzberg, M.D.

Kenneth T. Norris, Jr., Professor
Department of Psychiatry and Behavioral Sciences
Stanford University School of Medicine, Stanford, California

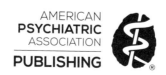
AMERICAN
PSYCHIATRIC
ASSOCIATION
PUBLISHING

Contents

List of Tables

List of Figures

Preface

This is the tenth edition of our *Manual of Clinical Psychopharmacology*, the first edition of which appeared in 1986. As with that original edition and all subsequent editions, our intention has been to provide a readable, up-to-date guide to clinical psychopharmacology. Reader response generally has indicated that the manual has met the original goal. However, the ever-expanding number of available agents with widening indications understandably led to ever-larger editions of the manual. In the past few editions, we began to eliminate or shorten sections on agents that had become less commonly used (e.g., barbiturates) to allow us to present information regarding a number of new agents that have been approved (e.g., vesicular monoamine transporter type 2 inhibitors for tardive dyskinesia, new antipsychotics such as pimavanserin and cariprazine) or recently released or that are in late-stage review (e.g., novel antidepressants such as brexanolone, esketamine, buprenorphine/samidorphan) by the FDA. In addition, we added a chapter on pharmacogenomic testing and other commercially available tests that purport to help clinicians choose the right medication for the right patient. All the while, we have attempted to maintain the collegial, reader-friendly style that has characterized the manual through all its editions. In this regard, we continue to provide summary tables with key information on classes of psychotropics to serve as quick-reference guides.

The manual reflects our most up-to-date thinking about specific agents—efficacy, dosing, side effects, and so forth. Material is largely evidence based, with an intermingling of our personal experiences. These experiences are offered as guides for the reader's own practice. We encourage the reader to cross-check recommendations (particularly doses) with other standard references and texts, particularly the latest edition of the *Physicians' Desk Reference*.

Sadly, Jonathan Cole died in mid-2009 around the time of our seventh edition. The field lost one of the original pioneers in psychopharmacology, a man of great intelligence and humanism.

The American Psychiatric Association (APA) graciously renamed the ninth edition as *Schatzberg's Manual of Psychopharmacology*, and for the tenth edition we have decided to change the order of the authors, with Charles DeBattista becoming the lead author and Alan Schatzberg being listed second. We have enjoyed updating this edition—as we have with those that preceded it—and we look forward to future editions as well.

There are so many people to thank in writing this type of book. Our families have been patient and understanding of our need to spend time on this project. And we thank them as always.

Robert Chew made numerous editorial suggestions that were of invaluable help. The editorial staff at APA Publishing, including Erika Parker, Greg Kuny, Tammy Cordova, and Judy Castagna, deserve a great deal of credit for their support, critical reading, and technical know-how. Greg Kuny retired in 2022 and will be missed. The APA Publishing leadership—Laura Roberts as editor-in-chief and John McDuffie as publisher, who also retired in 2022—have had unwavering confidence in us as authors, and we are eternally grateful to them. We are delighted that Simone Taylor has taken over from John McDuffie at the helm, and we look forward to continuing to work with her. We are also appreciative of our colleagues and trainees at Stanford University. Our experiences have been enriched by their insights. Last, we are indebted to the many patients we have treated over the past decades. They have taught us much about drug treatment.

We hope the reader will find this tenth edition of the manual even more informative and helpful than the first nine, and we look forward to your feedback as we plan for future editions.

Charles DeBattista, D.M.H., M.D.

Alan F. Schatzberg, M.D.

June 2023

Disclosure of Competing Interests

Charles DeBattista, D.M.H., M.D.—*Grant support*: Relmada, Compass, Beckley Scientific, Sage, Janssen. *Consultant*: Corcept, Sage, Abbott.

Alan F. Schatzberg, M.D.—*Consultant*: Alkermes, Avanir, Bracket, GLG, Jazz, McKinsey, Myriad Genetics, Neuronetics, Owl, Sage, Sunovion, Xhale; *Equity*: Corcept (co-founder), Delpor, Epiodyne, Gilead, Incyte Genetics, Madrigal, Merck, Owl, Seattle Genetics, Titan, Xhale. *Research*: Janssen Pharmaceuticals. *Intellectual property*: Named inventor on pharmacogenetic use patents on prediction of antidepressant response and on glucocorticoid antagonists in psychotic major depression.

1

General Principles of Psychopharmacological Treatment

Over two decades beginning largely in the 1970s, psychiatry experienced a rapid metamorphosis in its methods of treatment. The move from a largely psychoanalytic orientation toward a more biological stance radically changed not only its basic approaches to patients but also the professional identities of psychiatrists. For most older psychiatrists, the transformation in the 1980s and 1990s was not easy. At first, keeping up with ever-expanding information on biological theories, new laboratory tests, computerization, new medications, and new, additional uses for old medications was in itself a full-time occupation—one that often allowed little time or energy for integrating current information into daily practice. Moreover, the proliferation of biological and psychopharmacological information occurred so rapidly that the task of integrating biological and psychotherapeutic approaches became ever more difficult. However, the transition has now passed, and over the past two or more decades, a cadre of psychiatrists well versed in psychopharmacology has been trained.

For many academics and practitioners, biological and psychopharmacological approaches have become the essence of psychiatry, whereas for many years, others insisted that these drugs merely masked underlying diseases, worked against conflict resolution, interfered with therapy, and so forth. During the transition, most practitioners developed more balanced, practical approaches, combining elements of both psychotherapy and psychopharmacology. In an odd way, academic psychiatry, with its sometimes hypertrophied and polarized approaches, lagged behind clinical practice, where a practical blending is needed. Indeed, we believe intuitively that psychiatry as a medical subspecialty is incorporating aspects of psychosocial, psychobiological, and psychopharmacological theories to form a truly new psychiatry, although residency training experiences, particularly with exceedingly short lengths of stay and undue reliance on applying DSM criteria, may not be preparing residents optimally.

One major reason for needing a blended approach is that although psychotropic drugs exert profound and beneficial effects on cognition, mood, and behavior, they often do not change the underlying disease process, which is frequently highly sensitive to intrapsychic, interpersonal, and psychosocial stressors. As a rule, beneficial outcomes can be achieved only by simultaneously reducing symptoms and promoting the capacity of the individual to adapt to the exigencies of their life. Strikingly, some practitioners of internal medicine have embraced psychosocial principles to help treat illnesses such as hypertension, rheumatoid arthritis, and juvenile diabetes. Similarly, psychiatrists who embrace psychopharmacology as the be-all and end-all will probably find themselves in the same position as internists who feel that prescribing thiazides is a simple solution to hypertensive illness. Conversely, practitioners of psychoanalysis or other psychotherapies should not expect such an approach to cure or significantly reduce vegetative symptoms in endogenously depressed patients. Rather, they need to realize the potential benefits of alternative treatments—particularly psychotropic medication.

For practitioners without extensive experience, the transition to a more pharmacological practice was not without difficulties. A favorable clinical outcome after prescribing a psychotropic drug does reinforce confidence in psychopharmacological approaches. Practically speaking, because favorable outcomes often can be effected more quickly with a psychopharmacological approach than with psychotherapy, confidence in psychopharmacology can be achieved more readily. The selective serotonin reuptake inhibitors (SSRIs), with their ease of use and wide therapeutic effects, helped practitioners become effective pharmacological treaters.

Although this book is primarily a guide to psychopharmacology, it should not lead the reader to conclude that understanding how to select and prescribe psychotropic medications obviates the basic need to comprehensively evaluate and understand psychiatric patients. Our primary purpose is to provide the reader-practitioner with basic and practical information regarding the many classes of psychiatric medications. This book is written as a practical, usable clinical guide to the selection and prescription of appropriate drug therapies for individual patients, drawing on our own clinical experience as well as on the scientific literature. It is not a series of meticulously documented review papers; therefore, not all statements in the text are individually referenced. Rather, references are provided for key statements, and each chapter is followed by a list of selected relevant articles and books for readers who want to go beyond the material presented here. We believe this makes for a more reader-friendly book. For each new edition, we have made changes in response to reviewers' and readers' feedback, and we hope the reader will find this edition as useful as—if not even more useful than—previous ones.

General Advice

Today, younger psychiatrists generally are more formally trained in psychopharmacology than many of their older colleagues had been. In the past, we advised clinicians to concentrate on one or two members per class of agents to become comfortable with prescribing. Although that is still reasonable advice today, there are growing concerns that as pharmaceutical companies cut back on educational program support and academic institutions move away from allowing detailing, clinicians may not obtain sufficient information on the newest agents to be able to prescribe them with comfort. This is unfortunate, because for some patients a new agent may prove to be lifesaving. One would hope that over time, a more rational and balanced approach to dealing with the industry can be developed. What should practitioners do to keep up? Clearly, following the literature and attending continuing medical education programs can be helpful, but they may not provide timely information on new agents. One potential source of useful current information is pharmacology newsletters. These can be supplemented with some key resource materials, such as textbooks on psychopharmacology and the *Physicians' Desk Reference* (PDR). (Some helpful titles are found in the appendix at the end of this manual.) For the "modern agers," downloading a product like Epocrates onto your computer or phone is very handy and essentially provides you with an electronic PDR.

Moreover, practitioners should be familiar with a number of books directed at the lay audience that can help supplement information provided to patients (see appendix at the end of this manual). It is also a good idea to identify local psychopharmacological consultants who can provide second opinions when needed—for example, if patients fail to respond or if they experience severe side effects.

In this book, we provide practical information regarding many different psychotropic drugs. Information regarding dosages is for adult patients (ages 18–65 years) unless otherwise noted. We have included information derived from our reading of the psychiatric literature as well as from our own clinical practice. We attempt to indicate, whenever possible, the uses that have not been approved officially by the FDA for marketing purposes, but we also attempt to provide readers with sufficient data to aid them in deciding whether or how they may want to prescribe specific drugs. In so doing, we are not endorsing the use of these specific drugs; rather, we are realistically attempting to place a drug in its proper perspective. We believe real-world psychiatric practice dictates that we give the practitioner information based either on the scientific literature or on common clinical use, even though a drug's indications may not yet have been changed or—perhaps because of economic reasons—may never be changed. Information about specific agents should be checked against the PDR and package inserts to ensure accuracy before prescribing for specific patients.

Practice Guidelines

Since the early 1990s, practice guidelines have been developed by professional societies, academic leaders, and public payers. Such guidelines can be helpful because they are generally based on evidence in the literature. Unfortunately, overreliance on these guidelines imposes limitations. First, guidelines may quickly become out of date with the reporting of evidence or new indications or new treatments. Second, available evidence in the published literature may be for agents that are not the most effective for treating patients with more atypical or comorbid conditions. Third, evidence often breaks down when the practitioner encounters a lack of response to the initial therapy, leaving them to fall back once again on clinical experience or judgment. Fourth, recommendations often are based on the consensus opinions of experts. These opinions are helpful but are not necessarily accurate. Last, guidelines may be most helpful for nonspecialist practitioners and less helpful for more experienced treaters of patients with refractory conditions. In the end, there is still a need for considerable art in the practice of medicine.

Legal, Ethical, and Economic Issues

It seems prudent to discuss briefly a number of legal, ethical, and economic issues that arise in psychopharmacology. Because a comprehensive discussion of all these issues is beyond the scope of this manual, the reader is referred elsewhere for specific information (see appendix at the end of this manual). An excellent review of work in this area by Hoop et al. (2009) is available.

Informed Consent

Informed consent has become an increasingly important issue in medicine. Standard medical practice has long called for informing patients of the benefits versus the risks of various surgical and medical procedures. In the past decade, greater attention has been paid to the question of informed consent; for psychiatry, however, several key problems quickly arise. For one, psychiatrists must wrestle with the problem of evaluating the patient's capacity either to understand fully the benefits and risks of the medication prescribed or to interpret the provided information in a reflective and beneficial way. Obviously, this issue is particularly pressing with psychotic patients, and legal guardianship may be required at times to effect adequate informed consent. Fortunately, these patients represent a minority of the average practitioner's patient population.

Paranoid but competent patients present practical problems that are best overcome by creating a solid working relationship. Such patients are less commonly encountered than highly anxious, obsessive, or agitated patients, who are prone to a phobic approach to medication. The practitioner at first glance may view informed consent in such cases as an insurmountable obstacle. Practically speaking, however, such patients will be anxious even if the practitioner does not inform them of side effects. Indeed, disclosing the facts often relieves their anxiety. It also connotes a respect for the severity of their illness and the need to assume some risks mutually.

Should the physician inform the patient of every side effect listed in the PDR or merely highlight the most common ones? Some courts have judged that physicians may be liable if they do not tell the patient of every side effect. Practically speaking, most clinicians do not do so—for several reasons, including the time involved and concern for unduly frightening the patient. The latter is particularly relevant when one reflects on the fact that package insert information lists virtually all side effects ever reported in drug trials, even if they were not due to the drug, plus side effects observed only or mainly with similar drugs. Still, patients now have access to the latest information about every possible drug at their fingertips. They have to look no further than their cell phones to view online information from sources of varying reliability. Some drug information from sources such as Epocrates, WebMD, and PDR.net is quite reliable. In a sense, patient access to online information can help obviate the issue of physician liability. Nevertheless, physicians need to enter into an open dialogue with all patients regarding the benefits and side effects of medication, even (or particularly) patients who are self-taught. We also have an important role in helping patients interpret the information they have learned online and disabusing patients of inaccurate information. Patients who read the PDR need to be informed of the relative probability of the occurrence of one or another side effect. For example, patients should be made to realize that a dry mouth as the result of taking a tricyclic antidepressant (TCA) is to be expected, but agranulocytosis or anaphylaxis is extremely rare. Our experience is that patients are reassured by the physician's belief (and hope) that these side effects will not be encountered. Today, package inserts often include tables comparing side effects in patients treated with a given drug with those observed with a placebo. This places the issues in a much better perspective. Some physicians routinely give patients written materials (often a separate sheet for each medication) that spell out the medication's relative risks. This works well, but only if the practitioner feels comfortable with this approach and it becomes truly routine in their practice.

For many years, until the introduction of atypical antipsychotics, a particularly difficult problem revolved around informed consent regarding the risk of developing tardive dyskinesia, an unfortunate side effect generally due to long-term treatment with the more typical antipsychotic medications (see Chapter 4, "Antipsychotic Drugs"). It was shown to affect some 14% of patients receiving maintenance therapy with standard neuroleptic medication for 3 or more years, and it may have been more common in patients with affective disorders than in those with schizophrenia. Thus, practitioners had to be particularly conservative in administering neuroleptics to patients who did not demonstrate frequent or chronic psychotic episodes. However, because chronic psychotic disorders do unfortunately exist, even prudent practice with first-line antipsychotics could not eliminate the risk of tardive dyskinesia. Newer antipsychotics offer greater promise for reducing the risk of this problem, although the risk has not been completely eliminated. Indeed, as these drugs have been used more chronically, we have seen the emergence of tardive dyskinesia. Fortunately, the introduction of valbenazine to treat tardive dyskinesia offers much hope for patients. Tardive dyskinesia is less of a real risk in psychiatric practice today.

What should the physician tell the patient about tardive dyskinesia, and when? Here, a variety of approaches have been developed. One is to inform the patient and/or the family of the risk of tardive dyskinesia before prescribing typical neuroleptics. This may be too anxiety provoking and impractical, particularly for acutely psychotic patients, because tardive dyskinesia is generally a long-term side effect and there is a pressing need to help the patient quickly. Another approach is to broach the subject of the risk of tardive dyskinesia after approximately 4–6 weeks of treatment with an antipsychotic, before embarking on long-term or maintenance therapy. This seems more prudent to us. The risk with second-generation antipsychotics is relatively low but does exist.

Should one obtain written verification of informed consent? Here, too, different approaches have emerged. Some institutions and practitioners have adopted formal, written informed consent. Others have followed traditional verbal informed consent procedures and have placed written documentation of the interchange in the patient's record. Still others have routinely provided the patient with additional written information (beyond that provided in the PDR) regarding the risks of tardive dyskinesia or other side effects but have not asked the patient to provide written informed consent. Each of these approaches has its advantages and its proponents. Currently, we recommend that 1) practitioners and institutions adopt some formal, documented disclosure of the risk of tardive dyskinesia with first-generation antipsychotics; 2) they combine this disclosure with conservative administration of first-generation antipsychotics (in terms of both time and dosage); and 3) they and the patient cooperate in monitoring the patient for the emergence of dyskinetic movements. Much of this issue is less relevant today because initiation of long-term therapy with typical antipsychotics is relatively uncommon in the United States.

With the release of clozapine, psychiatrists needed to seriously consider adopting a standard documented informed consent procedure for this potentially lethal but therapeutically unique drug. Patients who are incompetent to give informed consent should have a guardian who provides the consent. Second-generation agents such as olanzapine, which do not have the apparent risks for agranulocytosis, have largely obviated the problem, but some patients with refractory conditions may still require clozapine therapy.

Although the second-generation antipsychotics are safer in some ways than were first-generation agents, weight gain, insulin resistance (metabolic syndrome), and diabetes are major worries with some of these agents, particularly olanzapine and clozapine. Diabetic ketoacidosis is a rare but serious side effect that has garnered a great deal of attention. More common, however, is the weight gain seen with several of the newer compounds, with a possible loss of insulin sensitivity. Patients who begin taking these agents should be monitored closely for both weight gain and insulin resistance. Patients should be particularly warned about such side effects if the agent is thought to have an increased risk (e.g., clozapine, olanzapine). As indicated in Chapter 4, the offending agent may need to be discontinued.

Off-Label and Other Nonapproved Uses

Since the early 1990s, physicians have been increasingly faced with the dilemma of prescribing standard drugs for indications that have not been approved by the FDA or at doses that are higher than those recommended in the PDR. In some instances when this practice is followed, drugs can be misprescribed, and this obviously can be dangerous. In many other instances, considerable clinical or research data have emerged that point to potentially great benefits for many patients, but package insert information may not have been changed because of economic or regulatory factors. For example, imipramine had for many years been commonly prescribed to both outpatients and inpatients at a dosage of 300 mg/day. Still, the package insert stated that outpatients should not receive more than 225 mg/day. In part, this reflected the fact that approved dosage regimens were determined on the basis of data generated many years ago, when a greater proportion of seriously depressed patients had been treated as inpatients and before plasma levels were applied (see Chapter 3, "Antidepressants"). The package insert was never changed. In many cases, additional studies designed to document further the efficacy and safety of higher dosages would be too costly for drug manufacturers, who can no longer hope to recoup the costs of such study because the patents for the drug have long since expired. One pharmaceutical manufacturer several years ago applied for and was granted FDA approval to raise the maximum daily dosage of its nortriptyline compound (Pamelor) from 100 mg/day to 150 mg/day. A manufacturer of an identical nortriptyline compound, Aventyl, did not apply, and that product called for only a 100-mg maximum daily dose. Thus, we had on the U.S. market two identical nortriptylines with different maximum daily doses. Aventyl is now off the U.S. market.

Examples of so-called nonapproved uses described in previous editions of this manual include the use of imipramine and phenelzine in treating agoraphobia or panic disorder and, for many years, the use of carbamazepine in treating bipolar disorder. Over the years, many other such uses emerged, including valproic acid for maintenance therapy in bipolar disorder, SSRIs in treating body dysmorphic disorder and related disorders, bupropion in treating ADHD, lamotrigine for treating major depression, and trazodone for sleep problems. A reasonable body of data supports the effectiveness of these drugs for some of these indications, but market conditions and regulatory guidelines may result in some, or even all, of these drugs not being granted official new indications.

One generally nonapproved indication for SSRIs has been in adolescent depression. The FDA had warned that efficacy data for this class and for venlafaxine are limited and that these agents carry a risk for increasing suicidal behavior. Fluoxetine was an exception on both counts and is approved for children and adolescents ages 8–18 years (March et al. 2004). Escitalopram is also FDA approved for children (Carandang et al. 2011). We thus recommend initially using fluoxetine or escitalopram in adolescents with depression. Should the patient not respond, alternatives can be considered, and if an alternative agent is used, the practitioner should provide clear documentation. The risks and benefits of these agents need to be discussed with young patients and their parents whenever possible. After the FDA instituted a black box warning about the potential risk of using antidepressants in adolescents and children, prescription rates by pediatricians dropped by approximately 20% (Nemeroff et al. 2007). Since that time, suicide rates among the young have risen. A report by Gibbons (2006) pointed to a significant rise in suicide rates in younger male adolescents (about age 15 years) in the Netherlands after institution of the warning. Likewise, there was a 22% increase in overdose attempts among adolescents and young adults in the United States in the second year after the FDA warning (Lu et al. 2014). These data indicate that discussion of side effects without discussing potential benefits can have unfortunate results.

Is the practitioner at legal risk when prescribing drugs for nonapproved indications? Generally, the American Medical Association and the FDA have taken the position that the use of any marketed drug for nonapproved indications or at higher dosages for individual patients is within the purview of the clinician. PDR is not an official textbook of medical practice but rather a compendium of drug information for marketing purposes. It sets limitations on what pharmaceutical companies can claim for their products. Malpractice is based on failure to practice within community norms. Still, many clinicians will not easily accept the risk of being sued—even if such a suit may have little merit—by a patient who experiences an untoward reaction to a standard drug used for a nonapproved indication or to a dose of a drug that is higher than the recommended maximum dose. Another issue is that some insurance companies will not pay for medications when they are prescribed outside the approved dosage ranges. Here, the practitioner can try to provide a clinical rationale and published reports on higher-than-usual doses for nonresponders (see, e.g., Ninan et al. 2006).

What are the solutions? Until various forces (both patients and physicians) come to the fore to effect a change in the system for widening indications or for redefining maximum doses, each clinician must decide whether to assume the risk. However, although clinicians may attempt a conservative approach, they will at some point encounter patients who will require alternative treatments. One possible aid is to acquire outside consultation from more expert psychopharmacologists or from other practitioners in the community. Another is to explain the scope of the problem to patients, providing them with available published reports on positive benefits of the treatment and documenting these actions in their records. Some physicians ask for written documentation that the patient has been informed. In the end, there are no simple solutions, and the physician will at some point be faced with this problem.

Obtaining Medications Outside the United States or Online

Another issue faces psychiatrists who treat patients with treatment-resistant conditions. Many additional antidepressant and antipsychotic drugs are available in Canada or in European countries. Before clomipramine received FDA approval in 1989, Canadian drugstores regularly mailed the drug to the United States after receiving a prescription and a check from the patient. With the growth of pressure from patients with AIDS, the FDA and the U.S. Customs Service appeared to view favorably (or at least passively) the importation of a 3-month supply of drugs not available in the United States for the treatment of an individual patient. Well-established drugs such as mianserin, older monoamine oxidase inhibitors (iproniazid, nialamide), and newer drugs such as agomelatine and tianeptine are available in Canada or Europe, and psychiatrists or patients may be able to obtain them through pharmacies, colleagues, friends, or relatives there.

Many patients received Canadian clomipramine for years without our ever hearing of a malpractice suit. Nevertheless, the possibility existed. State laws have varied as to whether such use is or was appropriate. Psychiatrists who want to treat patients with imported drugs not approved in the United States should consider the risks to themselves as well as to their patients. We recommend having the patient sign an informed consent document if a foreign medication is to be used. Information on the issue can be obtained from the FDA website (www.fda.gov). King (1998) discusses these issues and outlines the procedures for obtaining FDA and investigational new drug application approval, primarily for investigational agents.

As with other aspects of documentation, it is particularly important to document various steps taken in the course of treatment, including differential diagnosis, drug selection rationale, dosages selected and/or administered, other medications used, informed consent, and so forth. Practical tips have been articulated in a paper by Lamb (2001).

A somewhat related issue has emerged over the past few years with the internet. Some patients have ordered medications online, often from abroad, and we have suspected that many of the preparations are not legitimate. One recent patient entirely lost her positive response to aripiprazole augmentation after she reordered the medication over the Web. The preparation from India did not produce any effect. She recaptured the benefit when she went back to taking the U.S. proprietary preparation.

Medical Insurance and Cost Containment Issues

Managed care has had a tremendous impact on psychiatric practice. Building on the initial success of psychopharmacology, it has in a sense reshaped psychiatric practice, primarily along pharmacological lines. By providing limited benefits, it has forced psychiatrists to emphasize drug treatment. This has been a somewhat shortsighted approach, resulting in many patients receiving limited care. Moreover, the limited sessions and the avoidance of hospitalization lead at times to unrealistic expectations by patients and their families and inordinate pressure on providers. Although psychopharmacological approaches imply ease of care for a large caseload of patients, providers must keep in mind that responses to treatment are gradual at best and that any short-term successes must be followed by the continuation and maintenance phases of treatment.

Cost containment has led many health plans to prefer generic compounds over proprietary drugs. We are frequently asked about the advisability of prescribing generic compounds. For many years, the FDA has required only that a manufacturer demonstrate that a given dose of a compound will produce blood levels within 20%–30% of those produced by the proprietary form. Obviously, for some medications (e.g., TCAs) this standard can prove problematic. Lower blood levels of a TCA may result in the patient's not achieving therapeutic levels when treated with traditional doses. Moreover, switching to an equivalent dose of a generic compound in patients who have responded to a given dosage of a standard antidepressant may result in loss of therapeutic effect. In August 2001, fluoxetine was the first SSRI to become available in a generic formulation. Fluoxetine produces relatively high concentrations in blood and brain, and generic forms did not prove to be problematic. Similarly, we did not hear of problems with generic paroxetine. In previous editions of this book, we noted it is conceivable that in the future, efficacy will need to be demonstrated for generic formulations, and, indeed, there had been problems with a generic formulation of bupropion. A few years ago, this issue came to the fore again with the concern that some generic cardiac medications may not have offered efficacy equal to that seen with the brand product. Differences between generic and proprietary forms can go in both directions, with use of the generic form leading to higher, potentially toxic blood levels.

More than 20 years ago, the FDA ordered that a number of generic benzodiazepine compounds be removed from the market because they had fallen below minimum standards. Thus, quality control of the manufacturing of generic compounds may not necessarily meet acceptable standards. However, there may be significant variability between different batches of the same proprietary drug as well, and large pharmaceutical companies have had other problems with the manufacturing of proprietary compounds. In recent years, generic compounds in general have appeared closer in equivalency to their proprietary counterparts.

In early editions, we recommended that physicians start their patients on proprietary compounds (particularly in the case of TCAs) and adjust dosages until therapeutic benefit is achieved and side effects are limited. Generic compounds can then be used for maintenance therapy. Blood levels for the specific medication, if available, can be obtained while the patient is still being treated with the proprietary compound—before switching to the generic—and rechecked while the patient is taking the equivalent dose of the generic if the patient loses therapeutic benefit or experiences side effects. Over the years we have come to feel less staunchly about this, in part because a good deal of practice today is with generic medication and the TCA class is used much less commonly. Also, we do not have good data on therapeutic blood levels of the second-generation compounds, and blood levels are less readily available. Still, as noted above, issues can arise on occasion.

Another consequence of cost containment is health plans' insistence that patients obtain 3-month supplies of medications, generally during maintenance therapy. Obviously, for patients with a history of abuse of medications or suicidal behavior or with medications with narrow safety margins, this requirement can prove problematic. We recommend using good clinical sense in deciding how many pills or capsules to prescribe. Frequently, local pharmacies will work with physicians and patients to come to a clinically and economically sound compromise (e.g., agreeing to hold supplies in patients' names but dispensing in 1- to 2-week quantities). However, this practice is a problem with mail-order drugs that are made available through health insurance plans. Again, newer medications tend to have wide safety margins, and the problem has been obviated to a large extent.

There has been controversy about the propriety of states and municipal governments condoning the large-scale importation of pharmaceuticals approved in the United States from Canada and other countries. The FDA has opposed this attempt to reduce costs in part because the origin, safety, and efficacy of medications imported from Canada cannot be verified (for further information, see www.fda.gov/importeddrugs). At the time of the writing of this edition, the issue is unresolved. However, the availability of medications approved in the United States for psychiatric or other uses at a much lower cost in Canada has encouraged physician ordering of medications from specific Canadian pharmacies. This approach has seemed better than possibly unreliable internet ordering by patients, although there may be unresolved regulatory issues here.

Technology and Psychopharmacology

Over the past decade, technology has begun to have an impact on psychiatric practice, including psychopharmacology. Two examples are pharmacogenetics (Zeier et al. 2018; Zubenko et al. 2018) and brain stimulation therapies (Cole et al. 2022). Pharmacogenetic algorithm predictors of antidepressant treatment response in particular have become available through commercial purveyors, but these have been the subject of considerable debate (see, e.g., Moran 2018; Zeier et al. 2018; Zubenko et al. 2018). Many clinicians have found them helpful, although these algorithms largely help to identify relative risk for intolerance, on the basis of both pharmacogenetically and pharmacodynamically related markers. A number of studies point to specific genetic markers that can predict responses to specific antidepressants (Schatzberg et al. 2015; Uhr et al. 2008) and that could be incorporated into such algorithms in the future. We now have included material on pharmacogenetics in this manual.

Suggested Readings

Applebaum PS: Legal and ethical aspects of psychopharmacologic practice, in Clinical Psychopharmacology, 2nd Edition. Edited by Bernstein JC. Boston, MA, Wright PSG, 1984, pp 13–28

Archer JD: The FDA does not approve uses of drugs. JAMA 252(8):1054–1055, 1984 6748212

Erickson SH, Bergman JJ, Schneeweiss R, Cherkin DC: The use of drugs for unlabeled indications. JAMA 243(15):1543–1546, 1980 7359738

Gutheil TG: Liability issues and malpractice prevention, in Handbook of Clinical Psychopharmacology. Edited by Tupin JP, Shader RI, Harnett DS. Northvale, NJ, Jason Aronson, 1988, pp 439–453

Gutheil TG: Reflections on ethical issues in psychopharmacology: an American perspective. Int J Law Psychiatry 35(5–6):387–391, 2012 23063110

Nonapproved uses of FDA-approved drugs. JAMA 211:1705, 1970

Slovenko R: Update on legal issues associated with tardive dyskinesia. J Clin Psychiatry 61(Suppl 4):45–57, 2000 10739331

Strous RD: Ethical considerations in clinical training, care and research in psychopharmacology. Int J Neuropsychopharmacol 14(3):413–424, 2011 20860879

Use of approved drugs for unlabeled indications. FDA Drug Bull 12(1):4–5, 1982 7075926

Use of drugs for unapproved indications: your legal responsibility. Eye Ear Nose Throat Mon 51(12):493–495, 1972

References

Carandang C, Jabbal R, Macbride A, Elbe D: A review of escitalopram and citalopram in child and adolescent depression. J Can Acad Child Adolesc Psychiatry 20(4):315–324, 2011 22114615

Cole EJ, Phillips AL, Bentzley BS, et al: Stanford neuromodulation therapy (SNT): a double-blind randomized controlled trial. Am J Psychiatry 179(2):132–141, 2022 34711062

Gibbons RD: Efficacy and safety of antidepressants for depression and suicide risk in youth and adults: results of new analyses. Neuropsychopharmacology 31(Suppl 1):S50, 2006

Hoop JG, Layde JB, Roberts LW: Ethical considerations in psychopharmacological treatment and research, in The American Psychiatric Publishing Textbook of Psychopharmacology, 4th Edition. Edited by Schatzberg AF, Nemeroff CB. Washington, DC, American Psychiatric Publishing, 2009, pp 1477–1495

King SM: Legal and risk management concerns relating to the use of non-FDA approved drugs in the practice of psychiatry. Rx for Risk 6(2):1–7, 1998

Lamb K: Risk management and medication prescribing/administering. Rx for Risk 9(1):1–3, 2001

Lu CY, Zhang F, Lakoma MD, et al: Changes in antidepressant use by young people and suicidal behavior after FDA warnings and media coverage: quasi-experimental study. BMJ 348:g3596, 2014

March J, Silva S, Petrycki S, et al: Fluoxetine, cognitive-behavioral therapy, and their combination for adolescents with depression: Treatment for Adolescents With Depression Study (TADS) randomized controlled trial. JAMA 292(7):807–820, 2004 15315995

Moran M: Task force on gene testing for antidepressant efficacy concludes tests not yet ready for widespread use. Psychiatr News July 19, 2018

Nemeroff CB, Kalali A, Keller MB, et al: Impact of publicity concerning pediatric suicidality data on physician practice patterns in the United States. Arch Gen Psychiatry 64(4):466–472, 2007 17404123

Ninan PT, Koran LM, Kiev A, et al: High-dose sertraline strategy for nonresponders to acute treatment for obsessive-compulsive disorder: a multicenter double-blind trial. J Clin Psychiatry 67(1):15–22, 2006 16426083

Schatzberg AF, DeBattista C, Lazzeroni LC, et al: ABCB1 genetic effects on antidepressant outcomes: a report from the iSPOT-D trial. Am J Psychiatry 172(8):751–759, 2015 25815420

Uhr M, Tontsch A, Namendorf C, et al: Polymorphisms in the drug transporter gene ABCB1 predict antidepressant treatment response in depression. Neuron 57(2):203–209, 2008 18215618

Zeier Z, Carpenter LL, Kalin NH, et al: clinical implementation of pharmacogenetic decision support tools for antidepressant drug prescribing. Am J Psychiatry 175(9):873–886, 2018 29690793

Zubenko GS, Sommer BR, Cohen BM: On the marketing and use of pharmacogenetic tests for psychiatric treatment. JAMA Psychiatry 75(8):769–770, 2018 29799933

2

Diagnosis and Classification

Since the late 1970s, psychiatry has paid greater attention to rigorous diagnosis and classification, as evidenced by the 1980 publication of the then forward-thinking DSM-III (American Psychiatric Association 1980). Unlike earlier editions, DSM-III provided detailed diagnostic criteria and descriptive diagnoses. Subsequent editions, including DSM-III-R (American Psychiatric Association 1987), DSM-IV (American Psychiatric Association 1994) (the text revision of which, DSM-IV-TR, was published in 2000; American Psychiatric Association 2000), and most recently DSM-5 (American Psychiatric Association 2013) and the DSM-5 Text Revision (DSM-5-TR; American Psychiatric Association 2022), refined these diagnostic criteria. They have made changes primarily on the basis of new empirical data and the results of field trials. Over the years, much of the attention to more rigorous nosology had been sparked by advances in the biology and treatment of various psychiatric disorders, making precise diagnosis seemingly ever more important. For example, the response to lithium carbonate of many patients diagnosed as having bipolar (formerly manic-depressive) illness fostered diligent efforts to discriminate between manic-depressive illness and schizophrenia, which resulted in a change

17

of diagnosis for many patients and alterations in their treatment. However, diagnostic precision does not always lead to clear and effective treatment.

Approaches to psychopharmacological treatment are often based on trying to match a given treatment or a combination of treatments with a specific diagnosis. Although this approach represents the ideal, it is effective in only approximately 60% of patients because

- Many patients have a disorder not easily classified into one particular syndrome
- Many patients have comorbid disorders
- Some patients with a seemingly classic disorder may not respond to a traditional drug

Various drugs (e.g., anticonvulsants) have increasingly been shown to exert wider actions than their drug class eponym suggests. For example, when first used in bipolar disorder, anticonvulsants were not approved for the syndrome. Controlled clinical trials did eventually lead to FDA approval for valproate, lamotrigine, carbamazepine, and oxcarbazepine in treating this disorder. Today, except for clozapine, second-generation antipsychotics are approved in the treatment of acute mania, with several (olanzapine, aripiprazole, and quetiapine) having indications in the maintenance treatment of bipolar disorder.

For many years, clinicians had to combine the "ideal" paradigm with a more flexible approach—one in which the clinician attempted to match a given treatment with various clusters of symptoms rather than with an overall syndrome. The danger of this approach is that if carried too far, it can result in overly innovative treatment or even unhealthy polypharmacy. Obviously, the clinician must attempt to develop a general strategy for matching a range of specific treatments to patients with particular diagnoses or symptoms. It is best to do the following:

- Ascertain whether the patient meets symptom criteria for a disorder (e.g., major depressive disorder with or without melancholia)
- Determine the class of drug (e.g., tricyclic antidepressants [TCAs] or selective serotonin reuptake inhibitors [SSRIs]) or treatment that is commonly thought to be effective in treating that disorder
- Prescribe classic representatives of the given drug class (e.g., imipramine, citalopram)

- Shift to less traditional medications or to combinations of medications if initial trials do not prove effective

Such an approach is sound overall; however, clinicians must be aware that diagnostic classifications have inherent limitations that can make diagnoses misleading. For example, early on, many patients who had DSM-III major depression that did not respond to antidepressant drugs often required some form of psychotherapy (e.g., interpersonal psychotherapy or cognitive therapy). In part, this was due to the limited number and type of symptoms required for a disorder to be diagnosed as major depression. Indeed, although major depression is commonly mistaken as representing an endogenous type of depressive illness, in fact—historically and practically speaking—endogenous depression, which is classically believed to respond to TCAs, is only a subtype of major depression. DSM-IV-TR and DSM-5-TR criteria for major depressive disorder are somewhat tighter than they were in DSM-III—a change that obviated the problem to some degree.

Another reason that a match of medication with diagnosis is not working may have to do with specific symptoms predicting poor response, as in anxiety being a poor predictor of medication response (Fava et al. 2008). In those situations, alternative strategies that may involve combinations of antidepressants with anxiolytics may be required. DSM-5 has introduced measures of key dimensions (e.g., anxiety and depression) across diagnostic categories to better describe patients' disorders. How well these will work is open to question given practitioners' busy schedules and time constraints.

Although comprehensive discussion of psychiatric classification is beyond the scope of this manual, it is still useful to review the current (DSM-5-TR) system and the prevalence rates for major categories of adult psychiatric disorders and to highlight which types of psychopharmacological agents often prove most beneficial in each category. Prevalence rates provided in this chapter are based primarily on reports from the Epidemiologic Catchment Area (ECA) study and the National Comorbidity Survey (NCS).

Overall Organization of DSM-5-TR

DSM has been reorganized such that in DSM-5-TR there is a more formal ordering of sections, in part to imply shared features (Table 2–1). For example,

Table 2–1.   DSM-5-TR Section II mental disorders

Neurodevelopmental disorders

Schizophrenia spectrum and other psychotic disorders

Bipolar and related disorders

Depressive disorders

Anxiety disorders

Obsessive-compulsive and related disorders

Trauma- and stressor-related disorders

Dissociative disorders

Somatic symptom and related disorders

Feeding and eating disorders

Elimination disorders

Sleep-wake disorders

Sexual dysfunctions

Gender dysphoria

Disruptive, impulse-control, and conduct disorders

Substance-related and addictive disorders

Neurocognitive disorders

Personality disorders

Paraphilic disorders

Other mental disorders

Medication-induced movement disorders and other adverse effects of medication

Other conditions that may be a focus of clinical attention

the initial section includes the neurodevelopmental disorders (e.g., autism spectrum disorder, ADHD), and contiguous to them are the psychotic disorders (e.g., schizophrenia). Bipolar disorder then follows to indicate shared features with schizophrenia, followed by the depressive disorders, which share features with bipolar disorder. The DSM-IV anxiety disorders have been broken up, with PTSD and obsessive-compulsive disorder being grouped with the trauma- and stressor-related disorders and the obsessive-compulsive and related disorders, respectively. The chapter structure continues through sleep-wake disorders and neurocognitive disorders, among others (see Table 2–1).

Although DSM-5-TR is not radically different from DSM-IV, it is worthwhile to mention a number of the changes and the implications for medication treatment. One change is that the childhood disorders are now sprinkled throughout the other 22 diagnostic categories. For example, a new childhood disorder—disruptive mood dysregulation disorder—is included in the depressive disorders chapter. Separation anxiety disorder is listed under anxiety disorders. Of importance is that some disorders that were characterized as childhood disorders, such as ADHD, are now conceptualized to allow for adult patients receiving the diagnosis. Often a criterion is included regarding whether the symptoms are expected for the level of development—for example, separation anxiety in younger children—to avoid pathologizing normal behavior.

Neurodevelopmental Disorders

The autism disorders have been consolidated under the rubric of *autism spectrum disorder*. The diagnosis emphasizes both social communication deficits and behavioral problems. The prevalence rate is approximately 1%. There is no indication for a medication therapy for the overall treatment of autism spectrum disorder, but risperidone does have an FDA-approved indication for the treatment of the agitation seen in the disorder, and a number of other medications are commonly used for other features, although they are often used off-label. In addition, a number of agents are being studied for features of autism (e.g., intranasally administered oxytocin for social affinity). ADHD is also listed under neurodevelopmental disorders. The prevalence rates of ADHD are estimated to be 5% in children and 2.5% in adults (American Psychiatric Association 2013). Typically, patients with the disorder are treated with methylphenidate, amphetamine, or atomoxetine. Classically, whereas ADHD has its onset in childhood, an adult form almost certainly exists (usually in patients who were hyperactive as children.)

Schizophrenia Spectrum and Other Psychotic Disorders

The psychotic disorders have changed in two major ways. First, under the schizophrenia rubric, the various subtypes (e.g., paranoid, disorganized) have been consolidated into a single categorical diagnosis. The criteria for schizophrenia have been altered to not allow for making the diagnosis without a classic psychotic symptom such as a hallucination or delusion. Thus, a thought disorder alone without a so-called positive symptom no longer suffices.

The course of the illness is chronic (at least 6 months) and often deteriorating, and the patient commonly shows social isolation and withdrawal. Six-month and lifetime prevalence rates of schizophrenic disorders in the ECA study were 0.8% and 1.3%, respectively, although DSM-5-TR lists the lifetime prevalence rate as 0.3%–0.7%.

Primary treatments are the second-generation antipsychotics (e.g., olanzapine, risperidone, quetiapine), as well as the first-generation, neuroleptic antipsychotics, which include phenothiazines, butyrophenones, and thioxanthenes. Acute management may include the addition of valproate to the second-generation antipsychotic agent. Some investigators have also reported limited benefit with lithium. The efficacy of TCAs and SSRIs for some anergic, depressed patients with schizophrenia has also been demonstrated—interestingly, with a relatively low incidence of worsening of psychosis.

Schizophreniform disorder, which is included in the schizophrenia spectrum disorders (Table 2–2), was previously thought to differ from schizophrenia only in the duration of illness, lasting from 4 weeks to 6 months. Schizophreniform disorder is a rare disorder, with 6-month and lifetime prevalence rates of 0.1%. Acute treatment for this condition generally involves antipsychotic agents. The term *schizoaffective disorder* is used to describe patients with chronic symptoms of schizophrenia that also meet the criteria for mania, hypomania, or depression in the course of the illness. In schizoaffective disorder, the psychotic symptoms are not limited to the concurrent affective episodes. For example, some patients with an episodic mood disorder and a significant thought disorder as seen in schizophrenia would receive this diagnosis. Furthermore, patients with residual evidence of psychosis when their mood symptoms are largely in remission may also receive this diagnosis. The major change in diagnostic criteria for the disorder is that the diagnosis is made on the basis of the lifetime pattern of psychotic and mood symptoms rather than cross sectionally during any one episode. Patients with the disorder often receive the most complex drug regimen in a valiant effort to control a mix of affective, schizophrenic, and even anxiety symptoms.

Table 2–2.   DSM-5-TR schizophrenia spectrum and other psychotic disorders

Schizotypal (personality) disorder

Delusional disorder

Brief psychotic disorder

Schizophreniform disorder

Schizophrenia

Schizoaffective disorder

Substance/medication-induced psychotic disorder

Psychotic disorder due to another medical condition

Catatonia associated with another mental disorder (catatonia specifier)

Catatonic disorder due to another medical condition

Unspecified catatonia

Other specified schizophrenia spectrum and other psychotic disorder

Unspecified schizophrenia spectrum and other psychotic disorder

Mood Disorders

Mood disorders, by definition, are pathological affective states. In DSM-III-R, these disorders were divided into bipolar and depressive disorders, which were then further subdivided into distinct entities. In addition, the severity of the disorder and the degree of psychosocial precipitants and seasonal pattern were specified. From DSM-IV through DSM-5-TR, this classification was largely retained (Table 2–3). Revisions included the elimination of organic mood disorder and the addition of bipolar II disorder, an atypical depression qualifier, substance/medication-induced bipolar and related disorder, and mood disorder due to a medical condition. In DSM-5-TR, bipolar disorder is viewed as its own category and is listed contiguous to the depressive disorders.

Bipolar and Related Disorders

Bipolar disorders are subdivided into bipolar I disorder (manic, hypomanic, depressed, or unspecified), bipolar II disorder, cyclothymic disorder, bipolar and related disorder due to another medical condition, other specified/unspecified bipolar and related disorder, and unspecified mood disorder. To re-

Table 2–3.   DSM-5-TR mood disorders

Bipolar and related disorders

Bipolar I disorder

   Current or most recent episode manic

   Current or most recent episode hypomanic

   Current or most recent episode depressed

   Current or most recent episode unspecified

Bipolar II disorder

   Current or most recent episode hypomanic

   Current or most recent episode depressed

Cyclothymic disorder

Substance/medication-induced bipolar and related disorder

Bipolar and related disorder due to another medical condition

Other specified bipolar and related disorder

Unspecified bipolar and related disorder

Unspecified mood disorder

Depressive disorders

Disruptive mood dysregulation disorder

Major depressive disorder

   Specifiers: anxious distress, mixed, melancholic, atypical, psychotic (mood-congruent and mood-incongruent), catatonia, peripartum onset, seasonal

   Single episode

   Recurrent episode

Persistent depressive disorder

Premenstrual dysphoric disorder

Substance/medication-induced depressive disorder

Depressive disorder due to another medical condition

Other specified depressive disorder

Unspecified depressive disorder

ceive a diagnosis of bipolar disorder (formerly manic-depressive illness), the patient must currently meet criteria for hypomania or mania or must have had a prior episode that met the criteria for either of these syndromes. The current episode is further categorized according to whether the patient has manic symptoms, is depressed, or is experiencing a mixed-affect state.

The DSM-5-TR core criteria for a manic episode of bipolar I disorder are pretty much identical to the DSM-IV criteria and include a distinct period of persistently elevated or irritable mood sufficient to cause harm or to result in hospitalization. At least three of seven symptoms need to be included (four if only irritability is present): inflated self-esteem, decreased need for sleep, increased speaking, flight of ideas, distractibility, increase in goal-directed activity, and overinvolvement in high-risk activities (e.g., spending sprees, reckless driving). As in previous editions, the current criteria indicate that symptoms must persist at least 7 days, or for any duration if the symptoms require hospitalization. However, if the symptoms last for fewer than 7 but more than 4 days and do not severely affect functioning or require hospitalization, the episode meets the criteria for hypomania, and bipolar II disorder is diagnosed. Any previous episode that met the criteria for mania would make the diagnosis bipolar I disorder, regardless of whether the current episode is hypomanic. One change to bipolar I disorder in DSM-5-TR is that the mixed episode category with depression has been supplanted by a specifier of mixed features. In the ECA study data, the 6-month and lifetime prevalence rates of mania in the general population were approximately 0.5% and 0.8%, respectively; prevalence data were slightly higher in the NCS. Bipolar I and bipolar II disorders have combined prevalence rates of approximately 1.5%. In DSM-5-TR, 12-month prevalence rates are estimated to be 0.6% for bipolar I and 0.8% for bipolar II disorders.

The classic psychopharmacological treatment approach for overall mood stabilization of these disorders has involved lithium carbonate or lithium citrate. Carbamazepine, oxcarbazepine, valproic acid, some benzodiazepines, and atypical antipsychotics have also been shown to have mood-stabilizing effects, most prominently in acute mania (see Chapter 5, "Mood Stabilizers"). Treatment of acute hypomania or mania includes the mood-stabilizing drugs noted above as well as antipsychotics and sedative-hypnotics for sleep. Treatment of bipolar depression often requires combining lithium or valproate with treatments used for major depression (see subsection "Depressive Disorders" in this chapter). Three agents are approved for bipolar depression: olanzapine-fluoxetine combination, quetiapine, and lurasidone. Lamotrigine is approved for the prevention of depressive episodes. At one time, mixed states were more responsive to anticonvulsants than to lithium, but this is no longer clear.

The major strides made toward a wider redefinition of bipolar manic states have undoubtedly resulted in more patients receiving mood stabilizers.

The potential benefit to many patients in this broadening of diagnoses must be weighed against a procrustean tendency to overdiagnose the disorder in order to justify lithium or other thymoleptic treatment. Not uncommonly, clinicians see patients who have a chronic disorder that was once termed schizophrenia but has been rediagnosed as either a bipolar manic-depressive illness or a schizoaffective illness. Likewise, the affective instability and impulsivity of borderline personality disorder are sometimes mistaken for symptoms of bipolar II disorder. Unfortunately, many such patients do not respond to mood stabilizers; this points to certain inherent limitations in overbroadening this category.

Cyclothymic disorder is a more chronic and less severe illness than bipolar disorder. For the criteria for this disorder to be met, a minimum of 2 years of repeated episodes of mild mood cycles is required. Patients with cyclothymic disorder may develop superimposed bipolar I or II disorder. Many investigators claim that lithium carbonate is of benefit to some patients with cyclothymic disorder.

Depressive Disorders

DSM-5-TR criteria for a major depressive episode are essentially unchanged from DSM-IV. By definition, major depressive disorder is a unipolar disorder if the patient does not have a history of hypomania or mania (i.e., a bipolar disorder). Six-month and lifetime prevalence rates for major depressive episode in the ECA study were 3% and 6%, respectively, and women are twice as commonly affected as men. The 12-month and lifetime prevalence rates for major depressive disorder in the NCS were much higher: 10.3% and 17.1%, respectively.

Criteria for a major depressive episode consist of a variety of signs and symptoms, including appetite disturbance, sleep disturbance, psychomotor retardation or agitation, suicidality, decreased interest in life, and guilt. Obviously, some of these symptoms are those that European and American investigators have used to describe endogenous depression. However, a patient may meet criteria for a major depressive episode without demonstrating much in the way of endogenous depression symptoms. In DSM-III-R, only four symptoms were required to meet the diagnosis of major depressive episode; DSM-IV and DSM-5 require five symptoms. However, in both systems, only a 2-week duration of symptoms is needed in order for the criteria to be fulfilled. Major depressive disorder has been shown to respond to many different types of antidepressants, including the TCAs, SSRIs, serotonin-norepinephrine reuptake inhibitors (SNRIs), monoamine oxidase inhibitors (MAOIs), and other available agents.

A subtype of major depressive disorder, *with melancholic features*, more closely resembles endogenous depression. In DSM-IV and DSM-5, the criteria for this subtype had been modified from DSM-III and DSM-III-R criteria. The current diagnosis still requires anhedonia or lack of pleasure from enjoyable stimuli. In addition, three of the following six symptoms must be present: distinct quality of depressed mood, diurnal variation, early morning awakening, marked psychomotor retardation or agitation, significant anorexia or weight loss, and excessive or inappropriate guilt. Biological abnormalities such as dexamethasone nonsuppression and hyperadrenocorticism are thought to be more common in major depressive disorder with melancholic features than in less severe forms of depression, but these abnormalities are not included in the current criteria. It is still not clear whether major depressive disorder with melancholic features fully approximates endogenous depression. The criteria include brief time periods similar to those for major depressive disorder but, at present, do not include earlier criteria for good past response to biological therapies. The disorder responds to all of the antidepressants, although there continues to be considerable debate as to whether the SSRIs are less effective than the TCAs or SNRIs in the treatment of melancholia. Further research will, it is hoped, lead to even better phenomenological definition of this disorder.

DSM-IV, DSM-5, and DSM-5-TR include a specifier to indicate a subtype of major depressive disorder that has been described for many years in the psychiatric literature: *with atypical features*. This subtype, unlike melancholia, is characterized by significant reactivity of mood to pleasurable stimuli, in addition to at least two of four other symptoms: significant weight gain or increase in appetite, excessive sleeping, heaviness in the limbs, and sensitivity to interpersonal rejection. This subtype appears to be less responsive to TCAs but more responsive to MAOIs and possibly to SSRIs.

Another specifier included in DSM-IV and continued in DSM-5-TR relates to *peripartum onset*. Women have increased vulnerability to a variety of mood disorders, including depression and mania, in the postpartum period. This specifier may be used when mood symptoms develop during pregnancy or within 4 weeks of giving birth.

DSM-IV (and DSM-IV-TR) also included *mixed anxiety-depressive disorder* in Appendix B as a criteria set provided for further study. For DSM-5, field trials were conducted for a syndrome that included two or three criteria from major depressive episode and generalized anxiety disorder, but the syndrome had poor reliability and was not included in DSM-5. DSM-5 did not include a separate syndrome for presentations that meet full criteria for both disorders. Anxiety can be measured using dimensional scales in DSM-5-TR, and this may help identify patients with significant anxiety, whose depressive symptoms are often more poorly responsive to antidepressant monotherapy. A patient's depressive disorder can be also designated as having mixed features (i.e., mania or hypomania) in parallel with the designation for bipolar disorder.

One change to the criteria for major depressive disorder in DSM-5 was the elimination of the bereavement exclusion. This change reflects the overwhelming data that point to prolonged and severe symptoms of depression in the context of a loss being similar to depression occurring outside a loss (Zisook et al. 2012). The criteria for bereavement include persistent or recurrent dysphoric mood for at least 1 month, with symptoms including worry, irritability, fatigue, sleep disturbance, and difficulty concentrating. Some data suggest that the SSRIs and other antidepressants may be useful for this condition. Recent data suggest that this is a relatively rare disorder.

Finally, a very important, and generally severe, subtype of major depressive episode—*major depressive episode with psychotic features*—by definition involves delusional thinking, evidenced by guilty or nihilistic delusions, hallucinations, and even communicative incompetence. This subtype represents 15%–19% of all major depressions, with a current prevalence of approximately 0.4% (Ohayon and Schatzberg 2003). In DSM-IV, the presentation of patients with this disorder was classified along the severity dimension as severe with psychotic features. In DSM-5-TR, psychosis is designated by its own independent level of severity. This change reflected a number of studies that reported that severity of depression was somewhat independent of psychosis (Keller et al. 2007; Maj et al. 2007; Ohayon and Schatzberg 2003). Typically, depression with psychotic features is much less responsive to monotherapy with antidepressants. Treatment of this disorder typically requires the addition of an antipsychotic or of electroconvulsive therapy. Some data suggest that glucocorticoid antagonists may be effective in the treatment of this disorder (Block et al. 2018; DeBattista et al. 2006; Flores et al. 2006). (The authors of this book do have a conflict of interest with a company attempting to develop these agents for this use; see "Disclosure of Competing Interests" at the beginning of this manual.)

In earlier editions of DSM, dysthymic disorder was a more chronic condition, and its symptoms by definition were not severe enough to meet the criteria for major depressive disorder. In DSM-5-TR, dysthymia has been combined with chronic major depression (i.e., duration of at least 2 years) to form *persistent depressive disorder*. In DSM-III, the criteria for dysthymic disorder were broad, and a number of the symptom criteria (e.g., anxiety, irritability, obsessionality) were not specifically those of depression. The current nomenclature requires two of the following six depressive symptoms: appetite disturbance, sleep disturbance, fatigue, decreased self-esteem, poor concentration or indecisiveness, and hopelessness. DSM-IV dropped the distinction between primary and secondary dysthymic disorder because of lack of evidence for the validity of this distinction. Lifetime prevalence rates for dysthymic disorder were approximately 3% in the ECA study and 6.4% in the NCS. SSRIs are useful in treating this disorder. Older evidence suggested that dysthymic disorder preferentially responded to MAOIs over TCAs. The data on the utility of antidepressants for dysthymic disorder, historically, were sketchy, but studies on the SSRIs have clarified this issue.

Disruptive mood dysregulation disorder was added to DSM-5 to deal with the growing use of a bipolar disorder diagnosis in children and the related increase in use of atypical antipsychotics. The disorder emphasizes verbal or behavioral temper outbursts that are out of proportion to the situation. The differential diagnosis often includes oppositional defiant disorder. Previously, children with temper outbursts would often be given a bipolar diagnosis.

Premenstrual dysphoric disorder refers to symptoms in the last week before menses, including marked affective lability, irritability, depressed mood, and anxiety. In DSM-5, the 1-year prevalence of the disorder is estimated to range between 1.8% and 5.8%. The syndrome is typically treated with SSRIs.

Last, DSM-5 encourages the use of dimensional measures such as anxiety or depressive symptoms across disorders. In addition, for depressive disorders, a number of specifiers can be used to describe patients' disorders (e.g., with anxious distress, with mixed features, with melancholic features).

Anxiety Disorders

The classification of anxiety disorders has evolved over the previous editions of DSM. The DSM-III classification of anxiety disorders was radically different from that of its predecessor, DSM-II (American Psychiatric Association 1968), and the more recent editions and revisions have elaborated further on this approach. Anxiety in DSM-III was divided into two main categories: phobias and anxiety states. Since then, the broad distinction between anxiety states and phobias was dropped. In DSM-IV (and DSM-IV-TR), the anxiety disorders were divided into 12 subtypes, including panic disorder (with and without agoraphobia), specific phobia (formerly called simple phobia, such as phobia of heights or of snakes), agoraphobia (fear of being in places where escape options are limited), generalized anxiety disorder (GAD), obsessive-compulsive disorder (OCD), and anxiety disorder due to a general medical condition or related to substance abuse. In addition, DSM-IV (and DSM-IV-TR) anxiety disorders included posttraumatic stress disorder (PTSD) and incorporated a new, related diagnosis: acute stress disorder. This diagnosis was added to describe a reaction to a traumatic stressor occurring within 1 month of the stressor and lasting 2 days to 4 weeks.

Although considerable progress in classifying anxiety was reflected in the previous editions and revisions of DSM, a great deal of confusion and debate still remained. This was particularly evident in the lingering questions of how to subdivide the group of disorders included under agoraphobia, agoraphobia with panic attacks, panic disorder, social phobia, and GAD; whether and how PTSD is related to these disorders; and where OCD fits in.

DSM-5-TR anxiety disorders include separation anxiety disorder, selective mutism, specific phobia, social anxiety disorder, panic disorder, agoraphobia, GAD, substance/medication-induced anxiety disorder, anxiety disorder due to another medical condition, other specified anxiety disorder, and unspecified anxiety disorder (Table 2–4). OCD has been moved from the anxiety disorders to a new diagnostic category, obsessive-compulsive and related disorders, and PTSD is now included in the trauma- and stressor-related disorders. The close relationships between these disorders are reflected in the grouping together of these chapters in DSM-5-TR.

The specific phobias include encapsulated fears and avoidance of specific stimuli (e.g., heights, animals, enclosed spaces). Animal phobias are almost

Table 2–4. DSM-5-TR anxiety disorders

Separation anxiety disorder
Selective mutism
Specific phobia
Social anxiety disorder
Panic disorder
Agoraphobia
Generalized anxiety disorder
Substance/medication-induced anxiety disorder
Anxiety disorder due to another medical condition
Other specified anxiety disorder
Unspecified anxiety disorder

exclusively found in females and generally begin in childhood. The 6-month and lifetime prevalence rates of simple phobias are extremely high: approximately 8% and 13%, respectively, in both the ECA study and the NCS. In DSM-5-TR, the 12-month rate is estimated to be 7%–9%. These conditions are generally treated with behavior therapy.

Social phobias involve intense and undue fears and avoidance of interpersonal interactions, urinating in public bathrooms, and other events. They occur in both sexes and begin in late adolescence and early adulthood. Social phobia in adolescence may be a prodrome of major depression in adulthood. MAOIs, SSRIs, and SNRIs are effective in treating patients with this disorder. The 12-month prevalence in DSM-5-TR is 7%.

Agoraphobia—the fear of being in places where escape may be difficult or embarrassing (e.g., supermarkets, shopping malls)—attracted considerable attention in the 1980s, particularly reflected in the numerous psychopharmacological and psychotherapeutic studies on DSM-III-defined agoraphobia with panic attacks. As indicated, panic disorder may occur with or without agoraphobia. When frank panic attacks are not present, a diagnosis of agoraphobia without panic is made. Patients with this presentation may experience partial panic attacks (*limited symptom attacks*). Some investigators have argued that agoraphobia does not occur without significant limited symptom or panic attacks; however, analysis of ECA study data indicates that agoraphobia without frank panic attacks is far more common than was once thought. Agoraphobia is far more common in women than in men, and the mean age at onset is the late 20s. The lifetime prevalence rate of agoraphobia is approximately 4%. In DSM-5-TR, the annual rate is given as 1%–1.7%. The disorder can be disabling because patients may markedly constrict their daily activities. The phobic aspects may be treated via behavior therapy or psychotherapy. Acute symptomatic relief may be best effected with benzodiazepines.

The criteria for panic disorder in DSM-IV through DSM-5-TR are somewhat broader than they were in DSM-III-R. Panic disorder is characterized by recurrent, unexpected panic—acute, almost incapacitating anxiety—followed by persistent fear (lasting at least 1 month) of having another attack. (This criterion contrasts with the DSM-III-R criterion requiring four attacks in 4 weeks.) The attacks are characterized by at least 4 of 13 symptoms, including palpitations, sweating, dyspnea, chest discomfort, hot or cold flashes, and lightheadedness or feeling faint. If the symptoms are associated with agoraphobia, a diagnosis of panic disorder with agoraphobia is made. The 6-month and lifetime prevalence rates of panic disorder in the ECA study were found to be approximately 0.8% and 1.1%, respectively, whereas the lifetime prevalence in the NCS was 3.5%. In DSM-5-TR, the 12-month prevalence is estimated to be 2%–3%. Women have panic disorder about twice as commonly as men. Because panic attacks are commonly seen in a variety of disorders, a well-defined panic attack specifier has now been added in DSM-5-TR.

Panic disorder with and without agoraphobia may be responsive to a variety of agents, including many TCAs, MAOIs, SSRIs, SNRIs, reboxetine (not available in the United States), alprazolam, and clonazepam. There is some indication that agoraphobia also may be responsive to these agents even if panic symptoms are not evident.

The criteria for GAD in DSM-5-TR are generally similar to those in DSM-IV. In DSM-III, GAD was characterized by persistent anxiety with at least a 1-month duration. The more recent editions and revisions of DSM reflected that GAD is chronic, lasting at least 6 months. DSM-IV simplified the 18-symptom checklist in DSM-III-R by clustering symptoms in six areas: restlessness, fatigue, difficulty concentrating, irritability, muscle tension (shakiness, tension, trembling), and sleep disturbance (usually initial insomnia). DSM-IV, in its criteria for panic disorder, severely limited the use of this diagnosis by designating patients with one panic attack followed by GAD symptoms as having panic disorder. Earlier studies pointed to prevalence rates ranging between 2% and 6%. In the NCS and the ECA study, 1-year prevalence of GAD as defined by DSM-III-R criteria was estimated to be 3%, and lifetime prevalence was estimated to be about 5%. In DSM-5-TR, the 12-month adult prevalence is given as 2.9%.

Various drug classes may be effective in treating GAD; these include benzodiazepines, buspirone, and antihistamines. However, of these medications, benzodiazepines have been overwhelmingly the most commonly prescribed. The TCAs have also been shown to be effective in treating this disorder, as has trazodone. Other antidepressants, including the SSRIs and venlafaxine, have also proved effective in the treatment of GAD and now have FDA-approved indications. Pregabalin has been reported to be effective in several double-blind studies (Baldwin et al. 2015) but as of this writing has not received an indication from the FDA for treatment of GAD.

Obsessive-Compulsive and Related Disorders

In DSM-5-TR, a variety of disorders are characterized in the diagnostic class of obsessive-compulsive and related disorders: OCD, body dysmorphic disorder, hoarding disorder, trichotillomania (hair-pulling disorder), excoriation (skin-picking) disorder, substance/medication-induced obsessive-compulsive and related disorder, obsessive-compulsive and related disorder due to another medical condition, other specified obsessive-compulsive and related disorder, and unspecified obsessive-compulsive and related disorder (Table 2–5).

OCD is characterized by obsessions and compulsions producing significant distress. DSM-IV (and DSM-IV-TR) attempted to clarify the distinction between obsessions and compulsions. By DSM-III-R criteria, a counting ritual could be either an obsession or a compulsion; however, in DSM-IV, an obsession was an idea, thought, or impulse that is experienced as being intrusive or inappropriate and that provokes anxiety. A compulsion, on the other hand, was a repetitive behavior or mental image that serves the function of avoiding or relieving anxiety. Thus, in DSM-IV (and DSM-IV-TR), most counting rituals were compulsions, even though they are repetitive thoughts, as opposed to actions. This was continued in DSM-5-TR. The disorder is more common in women than in men, and 6-month and lifetime prevalence rates were 1.5% and 2.5%, respectively, in the ECA study. In DSM-5, the 12-month prevalence

Table 2–5.   DSM-5-TR obsessive-compulsive and related disorders

Obsessive-compulsive disorder
Body dysmorphic disorder
Hoarding disorder
Trichotillomania (hair-pulling disorder)
Excoriation (skin-picking) disorder
Substance/medication-induced obsessive-compulsive and related disorder
Obsessive-compulsive and related disorder due to another medical condition
Other specified obsessive-compulsive and related disorder
Unspecified obsessive-compulsive and related disorder

rate is listed as 1.2%. Often, patients with pronounced obsessive-compulsive symptoms are, on closer inspection, found to meet the criteria for major depressive disorder. In Europe, OCD is commonly regarded as a mood disorder rather than an anxiety disorder. Many studies have found that clomipramine, a TCA with pronounced serotonin reuptake–blocking properties, is effective, and it is FDA approved for OCD. The SSRIs have also been demonstrated to be effective for this condition, and fluoxetine, fluvoxamine, sertraline, and paroxetine have received FDA approval for the treatment of OCD. In limited studies, other TCAs and MAOIs have been found to be much less effective.

Disorders such as trichotillomania, kleptomania, and body dysmorphic disorder appear to be closely related to OCD. Trichotillomania is characterized by a recurrent pulling out of one's hair. The hair pulling has a compulsive quality in that it is ego-dystonic but relieves tension. Likewise, kleptomania is characterized by compulsive stealing without an agenda of monetary gain. Body dysmorphic disorder includes both obsessions and compulsive behaviors and, according to DSM-5-TR, has a point prevalence of 2.4%. However, in DSM-IV (and DSM-IV-TR), trichotillomania and kleptomania were listed as impulse-control disorders, and body dysmorphic disorder was listed under somatoform disorders; they were not considered anxiety disorders or variants of OCD. In DSM-5-TR, trichotillomania and body dysmorphic disorder are now included with the obsessive-compulsive and related disorders, whereas kleptomania remains with the disruptive, impulse-control, and conduct disorders. Interestingly, the SSRIs have proved to be very useful in treating most patients with trichotillomania and in treating some patients with kleptomania or body dysmorphic disorder.

Trauma- and Stressor-Related Disorders

This diagnostic class includes reactive attachment disorder, disinhibited social engagement disorder, PTSD, acute stress disorder, adjustment disorders, prolonged grief disorder, other specified trauma- and stressor-related disorder, and unspecified trauma- and stressor-related disorder (Table 2–6). PTSD has come under increased attention since the Vietnam War, and the interest has continued through our recent wars, with civilian trauma also garnering considerable attention as well. The disorder is characterized by the existence of a recognizable stressor that is likely to evoke distress in most individuals. Previous trauma is reexperienced via recurrent recollections or dreams of the event or a sudden sense that the event is recurring. Often, patients with this disorder demonstrate decreased responsiveness to or involvement with the external world. In civilian PTSD, rape, assault, and car accidents are common stressors. Common symptoms include startle responses, memory or concentration problems, sleep disturbance, guilt about surviving, avoidance of stimuli that mimic or simulate the event, and recrudescence of symptoms on exposure to such stimuli. One key difference between DSM-IV and DSM-5 PTSD is that emotional reactions to the traumatic event (e.g., fear, helplessness) are no longer included in Criterion A. These symptoms were not found to occur in men or women. Although the disorder has achieved wide popular interest because of the political aspects of the Vietnam War, similar disorders, such as traumatic war neurosis in World War II pilots, have long been reported in the literature. The prevalence of PTSD appears to be higher in DSM-5 than in previous DSM editions, with a lifetime prevalence rate of 8.7% and a 12-month rate of 3.5%.

Psychopharmacological treatment for PTSD was for many years not well studied. A number of earlier studies suggested that phenelzine (an MAOI) and imipramine could reduce specific symptoms but had limited overall effect. Likewise, carbamazepine was shown to have some utility for treating the reexperiencing of traumatic events that characterizes the disorder. Adrenergic receptor agents such as propranolol and clonidine have been used to decrease the autonomic hyperarousal of PTSD. One agent, prazosin, has been shown to be effective in reducing nightmares as well as other symptoms in veterans

Table 2–6. DSM-5-TR trauma- and stressor-related disorders

Reactive attachment disorder
Disinhibited social engagement disorder
Posttraumatic stress disorder
Acute stress disorder
Adjustment disorders
Prolonged grief disorder
Other specified trauma- and stressor-related disorder
Unspecified trauma- and stressor-related disorder

with PTSD (Raskind et al. 2013). The SSRIs paroxetine and sertraline are effective in the treatment of PTSD, and they have received FDA approval for the disorder. Other SSRIs and SNRIs are likely to be effective as well.

DSM-IV (and DSM-IV-TR) included the then-new diagnosis *acute stress disorder*. This term describes the acute reaction to a traumatic stressor in the period immediately after the stressful event. The disorder is characterized by the same trauma that may precipitate PTSD, but the diagnosis focuses on anxiety symptoms that begin or worsen after an extreme stressor. The diagnosis requires at least nine symptoms from the following categories: intrusion, negative mood, dissociation, avoidance, and arousal. It is expected that the development of an acute stress disorder may predict a typically more chronic disorder such as PTSD. At this time, there are no reliable studies on the pharmacological treatment of acute stress disorder. However, it is expected that antianxiety agents such as benzodiazepines are likely to be effective in the treatment of this disorder.

Somatic Symptom and Related Disorders

Somatic symptom and related disorders are a new diagnostic class in DSM-5 and DSM-5-TR that includes somatic symptom disorder, illness anxiety disorder, functional neurological symptom disorder (conversion disorder), psychological factors affecting other medical conditions, factitious disorder, other specified somatic symptom and related disorder, and unspecified somatic symptom and related disorder. In DSM-III and DSM-IV, somatoform disorders represented a class of disorders involving physical complaints that are without objective medical basis. The five major illnesses in this group were somatization disorder, conversion disorder, pain disorder, hypochondriasis, and body dysmorphic disorder. The prevalence rate of this group of disorders was approximately 0.1% in the ECA study, and the disorders were predominantly found in women. However, the prevalence rates of the disorders as defined in DSM-5-TR are not well known. Patients with somatization disorder are overly preoccupied with physical symptoms that usually do not have an organic basis. The earlier somatoform pain disorder has been reported to respond to antidepressant therapy. The other disorders have not been shown to be particularly responsive to older psychopharmacological therapies, but in some cases individuals who worry about their health and whose symptoms meet the criteria for somatic symptom disorder have been effectively treated with SSRIs. Of interest is the observation that the SNRIs venlafaxine and duloxetine are both effective in diabetic neuropathic pain. Duloxetine has received FDA approval for use in that disorder, as well as in back pain and fibromyalgia. Pregabalin, an analog of gabapentin, is also approved in diabetic neuropathic pain and fibromyalgia. Duloxetine also appears to reduce pain in patients with major depressive disorder. Several studies, in both clinic and community samples, now point to chronic pain being commonly comorbid with major depressive disorder (Ohayon and Schatzberg 2003, 2010).

Personality Disorders

Prior to DSM-5 (e.g., DSM-IV), personality disorder diagnoses were made on Axis II. In DSM-5, the axial diagnostic system was dropped, and personality disorders now fall under the old Axis I rubric. In the deliberations on how to best subdivide personality disorders, considerable debate emerged, with some people advocating a more unitary approach similar to what was done with schizophrenia, and others arguing to maintain the subtypes. The latter was decided, and the classification in DSM-5 and DSM-5-TR is essentially as it was in the previous edition. An alternative classification is included in Section III of DSM-5 and DSM-5-TR for further study. Generally, these disorders have not been found to respond robustly to psychopharmacological treatment; however, medication may reduce certain symptoms.

Three personality disorders are of particular note for this manual: borderline personality disorder, paranoid personality disorder, and antisocial personality disorder. Borderline personality disorder, which has attracted great interest and study in recent years, is characterized by unstable and intense interpersonal relationships, identity disturbances, impulsivity, self-destructive physical acts, affective instability, a chronic sense of emptiness, and inappropriate and intense anger. In addition, transient, stress-related paranoid ideation or severe dissociative symptoms were added in DSM-IV. Patients with borderline personality disorder (or variants of the disorder) may respond to mood-stabilizing agents (initially for emotionally unstable character), phenelzine (for hysteroid dysphoria), and typical and atypical antipsychotics. SSRIs have proved to be of significant utility in treating the dysphoria, aggression, and impulsivity common in borderline personality disorder, and valproate has been shown to be effective in decreasing aggressive outbursts.

Paranoid personality disorder is characterized by pervasive, unwarranted suspiciousness, hypersensitivity, and restricted affectivity. By definition, the paranoia is not due to schizophrenia or paranoid disorder. Although the somatic treatment of paranoid personality has not been well studied, trials of atypical antipsychotics or lithium carbonate may prove useful in this disorder.

Antisocial personality disorder is characterized by chronic antisocial behavior, with onset before age 15. This personality disorder is characterized by repeated unlawful acts and lying, impulsivity, disregard of the safety of others, irresponsibility, and lack of remorse over misdeeds. DSM-IV also added the requirement of evidence of a conduct disorder before age 15 years. This disorder is three times more common in men than in women. Six-month and lifetime ECA study prevalence rates for the disorder are approximately 0.8% and 2.5%, respectively. In DSM-5-TR, the 12-month rate is reported as varying between 0.2% and 3.3%. Pharmacotherapy has not proved particularly helpful in the treatment of this disorder. However, mood-stabilizing agents have been somewhat useful in treating impulsive, repetitive violent outbursts in some patients.

Substance-Related and Addictive Disorders

Historically, prior to DSM-5, DSM-III-R and DSM-IV differentiated between substance abuse and dependence. *Abuse* reflected pathological use of a substance or impairment in social and occupational performance secondary to substance use. *Dependence* included a psychological need for continuing a substance as well as abuse of, tolerance of, or characteristic symptoms on withdrawal from the particular substance. In DSM-5 and DSM-5-TR, the differentiation has been eliminated, with abuse seen as an early stage of dependence and the two together representing an overall use disorder.

The prevalence of substance use disorders is, unfortunately, high in the United States. Six-month and lifetime prevalence rates for alcohol abuse/dependence were approximately 5% and 13%, respectively, in the ECA study, and these rates are similar to those in the NCS. In DSM-5-TR, the 12-month rates are 4.6% in adolescents and 8.5% in adults. Alcohol abuse/dependence is five times more common in men than in women. Drug abuse/dependence is somewhat less common: 6-month and lifetime prevalence rates are 2% and 6%, respectively. Drug abuse/dependence is only slightly more common in men than in women. In DSM-5-TR, substance use disorders are listed for each class of drug of abuse (e.g., opioids).

In disorders involving substance use or abuse, pharmacological treatment is generally aimed at ameliorating symptoms of withdrawal or at promoting abstinence, either by producing physical discomfort in the face of intoxication (e.g., disulfiram for alcohol abuse) or by blocking drug-induced euphoria (e.g., methadone, naltrexone). Acamprosate has been approved for promoting abstinence in alcoholic patients postwithdrawal. Smoking cessation can be helped via the administration of bupropion and varenicline. Recent reports have indicated that gabapentin is helpful in treating patients who abuse alcohol or marijuana (Mason et al. 2012, 2014), although it is not FDA approved for those uses. Also, mifepristone appears to reduce alcohol intake in alcohol-dependent subjects who are not necessarily interested in stopping their drinking (Vendruscolo et al. 2015). When the substance has been abused in the context of another disorder (such as major depressive disorder), treatment of the underlying disorder (e.g., with an SSRI) is warranted.

Feeding and Eating Disorders

As indicated earlier in the section "Overall Organization of DSM-5-TR," the childhood disorders have generally been combined with adult disorders under the various diagnostic classes. This is evident in the feeding and eating disorders, which include pica, rumination disorder, avoidant/restrictive food intake disorder, anorexia nervosa, bulimia nervosa, binge-eating disorder, other specified feeding or eating disorder, and unspecified feeding or eating disorder. One disorder that in DSM-IV (and DSM-IV-TR) was categorized as a disorder with onset in childhood or adolescence illustrates the change and deserves mention. Bulimia nervosa, characterized by intense eating binges and purges, occurs in both adolescents and adults and has been thought by some investigators to be related to depression or affective disease. In DSM-IV, it was confusing for clinicians to list some disorders as being of childhood. As with other classes of disorders, adult and childhood forms are included under the same rubric. Although there is some debate as to the nature of the possible relationship, it is clear that for many patients, their bulimia responds to treatment with antidepressants, including TCAs and SSRIs. Some bulimic patients also report positive responses to behavior therapy.

In DSM-5 and DSM-5-TR, binge-eating disorder is a new disorder to describe patients who binge but do not purge. Binge-eating disorder appears to be different from bulimia nervosa in a number of features beyond purging. The disorder may respond to a specific preparation of amphetamine.

FDA Approval of Symptom Reduction Strategies

For many years, the FDA's position was to approve specific medications for specific disorders (e.g., fluoxetine for major depressive disorder or OCD). Recently, the FDA has begun to approve indications for symptom reduction in multiple disorders. For example, intramuscular olanzapine has been approved for acute relief of agitation, and various atypical antipsychotics are being studied for the relief of psychosis or behavioral disinhibition in Alzheimer's disease. It is likely we will have a host of adjunctive medications approved for components of multiple disorders.

DSM-5-TR and Genetics

In the previous edition of this book, we noted that DSM-5 would attempt to incorporate data from recent studies on biology (e.g., genetics) into a new nomenclature. That unfortunately has not happened. We also noted that there would be efforts to deal more reasonably with the common comorbidities seen in practice. Dimensions were to have been developed to capture key characteristics such as psychosis, cognitive dysfunction, severity, anxiety, and depression. A report by Regier et al. (2009) highlighted the approach being used.

In the future, genetics is likely to help with both classification and treatment. The Human Genome Project has provided us with a great deal of data on our own genetic building blocks. This information will, it is hoped, provide us with allelic variations of genes related to specific syndromes or symptoms. Such data will ultimately help clarify the relationship of many disorders that often occur comorbidly, such as childhood ADHD and bipolar disorder, GAD and major depressive disorder, and schizophrenia and bipolar disorder. We had hoped that this would occur to some extent in DSM-5, but the field is not ready for that type of approach. It is not unlikely that genetic information, particularly that regarding symptoms, could lead to a new classification system with newly defined syndromes based on a combination of biological, genetic, and clinical data. The DSM-5-TR dimensions and the National Institute of Mental Health's efforts on Research Domain Criteria (Insel 2014) may help that process greatly.

DSM-5-TR and Drug Side Effects

One area of improvement for DSM-5-TR is a chapter on the description and classification of major drug side effects (e.g., drug discontinuation, tardive dyskinesia). The new chapter, "Medication-Induced Movement Disorders and Other Adverse Effects of Medication," reviews the new terms for both the movement disorders and other adverse events as well as for the involved drug classes (e.g., atypical antipsychotics are now second-generation antipsychotics). This chapter is germane both to this new edition of the manual and to clinical practice writ large.

Summary

Accurate diagnosis and classification provide clues for developing psychopharmacological strategies. However, the clinician should not expect to find complete correlations between the types of patients encountered in practice and the classic prototypes in the literature. This caveat may prove particularly important when the clinician follows a patient over many years. In such a case, a flexible approach needs to be developed—one that includes routine and regular reassessment of the patient's condition and consideration of the need for changes in medication. These issues are discussed in more detail in subsequent chapters of this manual.

Suggested Readings

Bauer MS, Dunner DL: Validity of seasonal pattern as a modifier for recurrent mood disorders for DSM-IV. Compr Psychiatry 34(3):159–170, 1993 8339533

Bourdon KH, Boyd JH, Rae DS, et al: Gender differences in phobias: results of the ECA community survey. J Anxiety Disord 2:227–241, 1988

Boyd JH, Burke JD Jr, Gruenberg E, et al: Exclusion criteria of DSM-III: a study of co-occurrence of hierarchy-free syndromes. Arch Gen Psychiatry 41(10):983–989, 1984 6477056

Fink M: Catatonia in DSM-IV. Biol Psychiatry 36(7):431–433, 19947811838

Frances A, Mack AH, First MB, et al: DMS-IV meets philosophy. J Med Philos 19(3):207–218, 1994 7964208

Gelenberg AJ, Lydiard RB, Rudolph RL, et al: Efficacy of venlafaxine extended-release capsules in nondepressed outpatients with generalized anxiety disorder: a 6-month randomized controlled trial. JAMA 283(23):3082–3088, 2000 10865302

Kessler RC, McGonagle KA, Zhao S, et al: Lifetime and 12-month prevalence of DSM-III-R psychiatric disorders in the United States: results from the National Comorbidity Survey. Arch Gen Psychiatry 51(1):8–19, 1994 8279933

Liebowitz MR: Mixed anxiety and depression: should it be included in DSM-IV? J Clin Psychiatry 54(suppl):4–7, discussion 17–20, 1993 8509357

Marks I, Lader M: Anxiety states (anxiety neurosis): a review. J Nerv Ment Dis 156(1):3–18, 1973 4570384

Myers JK, Weissman MM, Tischler GL, et al: Six-month prevalence of psychiatric disorders in three communities 1980 to 1982. Arch Gen Psychiatry 41(10):959–967, 1984 6332591

Nathan PE: DSM-IV: empirical, accessible, not yet ideal. J Clin Psychol 50(1):103–110, 1994 8150989

Ohayon MM, Schatzberg AF: Prevalence of depressive episodes with psychotic features in the general population. Am J Psychiatry 159(11):1855–1861, 2002 12411219

Pope HG Jr, Lipinski JF Jr: Diagnosis in schizophrenia and manic-depressive illness: a reassessment of the specificity of 'schizophrenic' symptoms in the light of current research. Arch Gen Psychiatry 35(7):811–828, 1978 354552

Regier DA, Boyd JH, Burke JD Jr, et al: One-month prevalence of mental disorders in the United States: based on five Epidemiologic Catchment Area sites. Arch Gen Psychiatry 45(11):977–986, 1988 3263101

Robins LN, Helzer JE, Weissman MM, et al: Lifetime prevalence of specific psychiatric disorders in three sites. Arch Gen Psychiatry 41(10):949–958, 1984 6332590

Rush AJ, Weissenburger JE: Melancholic symptom features and DSM-IV. Am J Psychiatry 151(4):489–498, 1994 8147445

Sadler JZ, Hulgus YF, Agich GJ: On values in recent American psychiatric classification. J Med Philos 19(3):261–277, 1994 7964211

Schatzberg AF: Classification of affective disorders, in The Brain, Biochemistry, and Behavior (Proceedings of the Sixth Arnold O. Beckman Conference in Clinical Chemistry). Edited by Habig RL. Washington, DC, American Association for Clinical Chemistry, 1984, pp 29–46

Schatzberg AF, Rothschild AJ: Psychotic (delusional) major depression: should it be included as a distinct syndrome in DSM-IV? Am J Psychiatry 149(6):733–745, 1992 1590491

Schatzberg AF, Kremer C, Rodrigues HE, Murphy GM Jr; Mirtazapine vs. Paroxetine Study Group: Double-blind, randomized comparison of mirtazapine and paroxetine in elderly depressed patients. Am J Geriatr Psychiatry 10(5):541–550, 2002 12213688

Sheehan DV, Sheehan KH: The classification of anxiety and hysterical states part I: historical review and empirical delineation. J Clin Psychopharmacol 2(4):235–244, 1982 6749908

Sheehan DV, Sheehan KH: The classification of anxiety and hysterical states part II: toward a more heuristic classification. J Clin Psychopharmacol 2(6):386–393, 1982 7174861

Smeraldi E, Zanardi R, Benedetti F, et al: Polymorphism within the promoter of the serotonin transporter gene and antidepressant efficacy of fluvoxamine. Mol Psychiatry 3(6):508–511, 1998 9857976

Stein MB, Fyer AJ, Davidson JR, et al: Fluvoxamine treatment of social phobia (social anxiety disorder): a double-blind, placebo-controlled study. Am J Psychiatry 156(5):756–760, 1999 10327910

Woody G, Schuckit M, Weinrieb R, Yu E: A review of the substance use disorders section of the DSM-IV. Psychiatr Clin North Am 16(1):21–32, 1993 8456046

Zanarini MC, Schulz SC, Detke HC, et al: A dose comparison of olanzapine for the treatment of borderline personality disorder: a 12-week randomized, double-blind, placebo-controlled study. J Clin Psychiatry 72(10):1353–1362, 2011 21535995

References

American Psychiatric Association: Diagnostic and Statistical Manual of Mental Disorders, 2nd Edition. Washington, DC, American Psychiatric Association, 1968

American Psychiatric Association: Diagnostic and Statistical Manual of Mental Disorders, 3rd Edition. Washington, DC, American Psychiatric Association, 1980

American Psychiatric Association: Diagnostic and Statistical Manual of Mental Disorders, 3rd Edition, Revised. Washington, DC, American Psychiatric Association, 1987

American Psychiatric Association: Diagnostic and Statistical Manual of Mental Disorders, 4th Edition. Washington, DC, American Psychiatric Association, 1994

American Psychiatric Association: Diagnostic and Statistical Manual of Mental Disorders, 4th Edition, Text Revision. Washington, DC, American Psychiatric Association, 2000

American Psychiatric Association: Diagnostic and Statistical Manual of Mental Disorders, 5th Edition. Arlington, VA, American Psychiatric Association, 2013

American Psychiatric Association: Diagnostic and Statistical Manual of Mental Disorders, 5th edition, Text Revision. Washington, DC, American Psychiatric Association, 2022

Baldwin DS, den Boer JA, Lyndon G, et al: Efficacy and safety of pregabalin in generalised anxiety disorder: a critical review of the literature. J Psychopharmacol 29(10):1047–1060, 2015 26259772

Block TS, Kushner H, Kalin N, et al: Combined analysis of mifepristone for psychotic depression: plasma levels associated with clinical response. Biol Psychiatry 84(1):46–54, 2018 29523415

DeBattista C, Belanoff J, Glass S, et al: Mifepristone versus placebo in the treatment of psychosis in patients with psychotic major depression. Biol Psychiatry 60(12):1343–1349, 2006 16889757

Fava M, Rush AJ, Alpert JE, et al: Difference in treatment outcome in outpatients with anxious versus nonanxious depression: a STAR*D report. Am J Psychiatry 165(3):342–351, 2008 18172020

Flores BH, Kenna H, Keller J, et al: Clinical and biological effects of mifepristone treatment for psychotic depression. Neuropsychopharmacology 31(3):628–636, 2006 16160710

Insel TR: The NIMH Research Domain Criteria (RDoC) project: precision medicine for psychiatry. Am J Psychiatry 171(4):395–397, 2014 24687194

Keller J, Schatzberg AF, Maj M: Current issues in the classification of psychotic major depression. Schizophr Bull 33(4):877–885, 2007 17548842

Maj M, Pirozzi R, Magliano L, et al: Phenomenology and prognostic significance of delusions in major depressive disorder: a 10-year prospective follow-up study. J Clin Psychiatry 68(9):1411–1417, 2007 17915981

Mason BJ, Crean R, Goodell V, et al: A proof-of-concept randomized controlled study of gabapentin: effects on cannabis use, withdrawal and executive function deficits in cannabis-dependent adults. Neuropsychopharmacology 37(7):1689–1698, 2012 22373942

Mason BJ, Quello S, Goodell V, et al: Gabapentin treatment for alcohol dependence: a randomized clinical trial. JAMA Intern Med 174(1):70–77, 2014 24190578

Ohayon MM, Schatzberg AF: Using chronic pain to predict depressive morbidity in the general population. Arch Gen Psychiatry 60(1):39–47, 2003 12511171

Ohayon MM, Schatzberg AF: Chronic pain and major depressive disorder in the general population. J Psychiatr Res 44(7):454–461, 2010 20149391

Raskind MA, Peterson K, Williams T, et al: A trial of prazosin for combat trauma PTSD with nightmares in active-duty soldiers returned from Iraq and Afghanistan. Am J Psychiatry 170(9):1003–1010, 2013 23846759

Regier DA, Narrow WE, Kuhl EA, Kupfer DJ: The conceptual development of DSM-V. Am J Psychiatry 166(6):645–650, 2009 19487400

Vendruscolo LF, Estey D, Goodell V, et al: Glucocorticoid receptor antagonism decreases alcohol seeking in alcohol-dependent individuals. J Clin Invest 125(8):3193–3197, 2015 26121746

Zisook S, Corruble E, Duan N, et al: The bereavement exclusion and DSM-5. Depress Anxiety 29(5):425–443, 2012 22495967

3

Antidepressants

According to the Centers for Disease Control and Prevention 2017 report "Antidepressant Use Among Persons Aged 12 and Over: United States, 2011–2014," 12.7% of the American population were taking a prescribed antidepressant in the past month (Pratt et al. 2017). The wisdom of such a widespread use of this class of medications is debated in the literature and the popular press. However, what is not debatable is that clinicians have felt increasingly comfortable in prescribing these medications over the past 30 years. The continued popularity of antidepressants rests on a number of factors, including their efficacy in the treatment of depression, broad spectrum of activity, relative safety, and ease of use. Factors such as marketing also have played a role in the widespread adoption of antidepressants in clinical practice.

The utility of antidepressants in the treatment of major depression has been established in a half century of randomized clinical trials. Relative to placebo, antidepressants generally appear to be effective in reducing the different symptom domains of major depression, effecting a 50% improvement in overall symptoms from baseline, achieving higher rates of remission of symptoms, and preventing relapse in patients with recurrent major depression. Advantages over placebo are most evident in more severe forms of depression. However, the placebo response rate has grown steadily in clinical trials, and many trials are no longer adequately powered to show a difference from placebo. There is some recent stabilization at 35%–50% (Furukawa et al. 2016).

Some researchers have come to the conclusion that when negative trials, including unpublished studies, are included in meta-analyses evaluating the efficacy of antidepressants, the advantages of antidepressants are small and may not outweigh the potential disadvantages. This conclusion is probably incorrect. First of all, the placebo in depression trials is not simply the administration of a sugar pill in a vacuum. Clinical depression trials include many nonspecific effects that would be difficult to replicate outside the research setting. These include extensive contact over weeks or months with highly devoted research personnel and physicians. The placebo might be administered in an inpatient setting with all the attendant therapeutic effects a hospitalization might provide. The increase in placebo response rates also means that many studies may be underpowered to show a difference now, in contrast to years ago. Underpowering of sample sizes in depression trials contributes to more trials failing to show a separation from placebo. Finally, studies that have demonstrated only minor benefits of antidepressants over placebo have tended to focus on change from baseline scores on a standardized rating scale such as the Hamilton Depression Rating Scale (HDRS). Antidepressants are known to have benefits to patients that might not be adequately captured by evaluating mean differences in scores on a depression scale. We know that antidepressants may have an impact on a whole variety of symptoms that are not adequately captured on a scale such as the HDRS, including pain, different dimensions of anxiety, work productivity, and cognition. These nondepression effects of antidepressants are very important in determining patient well-being but are not fully assessed by evaluating symptom dimensions of antidepressant effects.

The popularity of antidepressants stems in no small part from the broad spectrum of uses these agents possess. In addition to their use in the treatment of major depression, antidepressants emerged in the 1990s as a viable treatment for most anxiety disorders. Many of the selective serotonin reuptake inhibitors (SSRIs) and serotonin-norepinephrine reuptake inhibitors (SNRIs) have received FDA indications for treatment of generalized anxiety disorder (GAD). Compared with other treatments for GAD, such as benzodiazepines, the antidepressants appear to be at least as effective, although slower acting.

However, the antidepressants lack the risk of dependence more common to benzodiazepines. The SSRIs have also been approved for the treatment of panic disorder, PTSD, social anxiety disorder, and OCD and are now first-line treatments for these conditions. The efficacy of antidepressants in treating anxiety disorders such social anxiety disorder is often greater than that seen in the treatment of major depression.

Although the treatment of major depression and anxiety disorders constitutes the major uses of antidepressants, these medications are used to treat a variety of psychiatric conditions. Fluoxetine and sertraline are approved to treat bulimia and premenstrual dysphoric disorder (PMDD). Off-label uses have included the treatment of negative symptoms of schizophrenia, agitation in dementia, impulse-control disorders, and borderline personality disorder.

FDA-approved nonpsychiatric uses of antidepressants include treatment of pain conditions such as neuropathic pain, musculoskeletal pain, and fibromyalgia (duloxetine); vasomotor symptoms of menopause (paroxetine); smoking cessation and weight loss (bupropion); and enuresis (imipramine). Off-label uses have included migraine prophylaxis and treatment of premature ejaculation.

The popularity of newer antidepressants such as the SSRIs, SNRIs, bupropion, and mirtazapine, relative to the older tricyclic antidepressants (TCAs) and monoamine oxidase inhibitors (MAOIs), also arises from their relative ease of use and safety. Most of the newer antidepressants are administered once daily, and the starting dose is often the therapeutic dose. Although all antidepressants have side effects that limit their use, newer agents tend to be considerably better tolerated than either the TCAs or the MAOIs. In addition, most newer antidepressants are relatively safe in overdose, whereas an overdose of a TCA or MAOI is commonly lethal.

Most of the newer antidepressants and all of the older antidepressants are now quite inexpensive since going off patent and becoming available in generic form. In fact, as of this writing, a 90-day supply of most antidepressants costs $10 at one major pharmacy chain. Only the most recently available agents (vortioxetine, levomilnacipran, milnacipran, vilazodone, esketamine, brexanolone, and bupropion/dextromethorphan) do not have generic equivalents as of this writing.

Limitations of the antidepressants include side effects, slow onset of action, and lack of efficacy in many patients. In the past few years, there has been research on a wave of novel, non-monoamine antidepressants that may address some of the shortcomings of currently available antidepressants, but these medications carry their own challenges. For example, intravenous ketamine and intranasal esketamine often show efficacy within hours of a single administration as opposed to the many weeks that may be required with conventional oral antidepressants. However, repeated administration is required to maintain response, and long-term administration in the treatment of depression is not well studied. Another intravenous antidepressant, brexanolone, approved for the treatment of postpartum depression, shows more sustained benefits after a single 60-hour intravenous administration but needs to be administered in a hospital or overnight medical facility because of the risks of excessive sedation. Zuranolone, an orally active agent with a similar mechanism to brexanolone, is currently under review for the treatment of depression. Opioid-like agents such as esmethadone also appear to act quickly and may be effective in treating some patients not treatable with current medications. Esmethadone appears to have a favorable side effect profile, and testing is under way to determine its long-term efficacy and safety.

In addition, a number of psychedelics, including psilocybin, have shown preliminary benefit in controlled trials in treatment-resistant depression (TRD) with a single administration combined with psychedelic psychotherapy. However, most psychedelics are currently Schedule I drugs and carry a certain amount of historical baggage that would need to be overcome for these medications to be adopted. Still, the growing availability of novel antidepressants portends hope to the many patients who have been unable to tolerate or respond to more traditional antidepressant treatment.

History

The modern antidepressants were discovered serendipitously. In the early 1950s, investigators noted that tuberculosis patients showed prolonged elevation of mood when treated with iproniazid (Marsilid), an MAOI thought to be an antitubercular agent. Iproniazid proved ineffective for tuberculosis, but its impact on mood led to some of the earliest double-blind studies in psychopharmacology, demonstrating that MAOIs were effective antidepressant agents. The biological and pharmacological observations that MAOIs were antidepressants and that monoamine oxidase degraded norepinephrine and serotonin (5-HT) became cornerstones of the so-called biogenic amine theories of depression. Iproniazid was taken off the U.S. market in the 1960s because of associated hepatic necrosis. For many years the use of other MAOIs declined, partly because of the introduction of TCAs and partly because of the occurrence of significant hypertensive crises in patients.

The TCAs were also discovered serendipitously. The first reports on TCA efficacy in depression came in Switzerland from Professor Roland Kuhn (1958), who astutely noted that a three-ringed compound, imipramine, which was being investigated as a treatment for schizophrenia, appeared to elevate mood even though it did not relieve psychosis. The drug was similar in structure to the phenothiazines, but a simple substitution of nitrogen for sulfur in the central ring appeared to confer unique antidepressant properties.

Two antidepressants with a four-ringed structure, maprotiline and amoxapine, have pharmacological effects similar to those of the more traditional TCAs. These effects are not unexpected because the development of many of the earlier antidepressant compounds was based on the similarity of their activity in certain animal models to that of prototypical TCAs—a similarity that led some people to call them *me-too drugs*. However, there are both subtle and pronounced differences among many of the so-called me-too drugs. For example, amoxapine is a potent $5\text{-HT}_2/5\text{-HT}_3$ antagonist. Another four-ringed antidepressant, mirtazapine, has a very different profile than that of the TCAs. Mirtazapine appears to increase norepinephrine release by blocking presynaptic α_2 receptors. This release also appears to, in turn, stimulate serotonin release. Like many TCAs, mirtazapine is very antihistaminic but lacks the antimuscarinic effects seen in the TCAs.

The success of traditional antidepressants in treating depression led to a search in the pharmaceutical industry for compounds that would have the efficacy of the TCAs without many of the adverse effects, such as cardiotoxicity. In 1972, a research team composed of Bryan Malloy, Dave Wong, and Ray Fuller synthesized an agent at Eli Lilly labeled LY86032 that possessed these properties. This compound was altered somewhat to produce fluoxetine hydrochloride (Prozac). After an initial release in Belgium and South Africa, fluoxetine was released to the U.S. market in 1988. The first serotonergic agent, trazodone, which is mainly a 5-HT_2 antagonist, had been released in 1981, but it did not have nearly the impact of fluoxetine. No other drug in the history of psychiatry has received as much attention, both positive and negative, as has fluoxetine. In any case, fluoxetine offered an alternative to traditional agents because it retained the efficacy of traditional antidepressants but did not have many of their side effects. In addition, fluoxetine appeared safe in overdose. As a result, fluoxetine and related antidepressants have supplanted the TCAs as the first-line agents in the treatment of major depression. Sales for fluoxetine alone topped $2 billion in 2000 in the United States. (Fluoxetine went off patent in mid-2001.) This success prompted other pharmaceutical companies to investigate agents that selectively enhance 5-HT function, and several other new agents were later released.

Venlafaxine, which is a selective SNRI, appears to possess much of the efficacy of TCAs without the degree of overdose risk and the myriad side effects of the TCAs. Its metabolite desvenlafaxine appears to be a more balanced serotonin-norepinephrine drug than its parent. Likewise, duloxetine, levomilnacipran, and milnacipran are all more noradrenergic than venlafaxine. Selegiline, a selective monoamine oxidase B (MAO-B) agent at low oral doses, circumvents some of the problems of traditional MAOIs when given transdermally or, for that matter, sublingually. Reversible inhibitors of monoamine oxidase A (RIMAs) represent another attempt to render difficult-to-tolerate MAOIs in a more manageable form. Vortioxetine is a multimodal agent with serotonin reuptake–blocking properties as well as effects on many different serotonin receptors. It may offer some advantages over some other antidepressants in possessing relatively low rates of sexual side effects, weight gain, and sedation. Likewise, vilazodone may have lower rates of sexual side effects compared with SSRIs.

Despite the tremendous success of the newer classes of antidepressants in enhancing safety and tolerability, the delayed onset of action and lack of adequate efficacy for up to 30%–50% of patients taking monoamine antidepressants has led to the search for agents with novel mechanisms. In the early 2000s, Zarate and colleagues at the National Institute of Mental Health (NIMH) showed that ketamine, which appears to act on multiple receptors, including N-methyl-D-aspartate (NMDA) and μ opioid receptors, often worked quickly and effectively in patients with treatment-resistant mood disorders (Zarate et al. 2006). These findings led to Janssen doing studies on intranasal esketamine (Canuso et al. 2018), which then led to its approval in the adjunctive treatment of resistant depression in 2019. Meanwhile, studies in postpartum depression identified a role of specific hormonal factors in the etiology of this condition. A specific neurosteroid, allopregnanolone (brexanolone), was also approved in 2019 for the treatment of postpartum depression. Classic psychedelics, such as psilocybin and lysergic acid diethylamide (LSD), were actively studied for their therapeutic potential in the 1950s and 1960s. Although they are 5-HT$_2$ agonists, they appear to work quite differently than standard antidepressants in their ability to induce rapid changes in plasticity that may have sustained benefits. Research on psychedelics was largely halted by the Drug Abuse Prevention and Control Act of 1970, which outlawed these medications. However, limited studies in the 1990s at Johns Hopkins University and in the United Kingdom led to a resurgence of interest in the therapeutic potential of psychedelics. Currently, psilocybin for the treatment of resistant depression and 3,4-methylenedioxymethamphetamine (MDMA) for the treatment of PTSD have received a breakthrough designation from the FDA. Both have positive trial data and reasonable safety data (Goodwin et al. 2022; Mitchell et al. 2023; Raison et al. 2023) and MDMA has filed for FDA approval.

General Principles of Antidepressant Use

Although the antidepressants vary considerably in their mechanisms of action, toxicity, dosing, and potential for drug interactions, some clinical decisions apply to the use of all antidepressants. These include the criteria for choosing an antidepressant, deciding what dose is adequate, and determining the optimal duration of treatment.

Choosing an Antidepressant

As the number of antidepressants available has steadily increased, choosing an agent has become somewhat more difficult. Although side effect profile is generally mentioned as the primary factor in choosing an antidepressant, optimally matching an antidepressant to a specific patient is as much art as science. Patient parameters, including depression subtype, age, sex, and medical status, are matched with drug parameters such as side effects, safety, and cost. The general wisdom is that all antidepressants on the market are equally efficacious in the treatment of depression. This is unlikely. Depression is much too heterogeneous to suggest that agents with diverse actions all work equally well for all types of depression.

The notion that antidepressants are equally efficacious is based on the fact that it has not been possible to show that any antidepressant is reliably more than 50%–70% effective in a given clinical trial. In contrast, placebos tend to be about 30% effective in outpatient trials. Efficacy is usually defined as a 50% improvement on a standard depression rating scale such as the HDRS. When remission, rather than more general improvement, is the criterion for efficacy, differences between antidepressants may begin to emerge. Even a 5% difference between classes of antidepressants in the ability to achieve remission would be clinically meaningful. However, adequately powering a study to show such a difference might take a sample size of several thousand subjects. The funding necessary to do such a trial is often prohibitive. Thus, a meta-analysis of similar studies is often employed to increase power and detect smaller differences. There had been some speculation that antidepressants with more complex neurotransmitter effects, such as the TCAs, venlafaxine, duloxetine, mirtazapine, and MAOIs, are more likely to achieve remissions than are SSRIs—a hypothesis that has been investigated. Some studies, such as the meta-analysis by Thase et al. (2001), indicated that venlafaxine was significantly more likely to effect a remission than were the SSRIs with which it was compared. However, this area is controversial. The FDA chided pharmaceutical company Wyeth for using the Thase study in their marketing, pointing out that venlafaxine's superiority may be inferred only in comparison to fluoxetine. Indeed, more recent meta-analyses by Nemeroff et al. (2003) and Weinmann et al. (2008) failed to show a clear advantage of venlafaxine over SSRIs overall. One major problem is that the original venlafaxine studies were not designed to compare maximum doses over time or to treat to remission.

In a review of randomized clinical trials, Montgomery et al. 2007 concluded that there is evidence of probable superiority of some antidepressants over others. This review found that three antidepressants—clomipramine, venlafaxine, and escitalopram—tended to show superiority in efficacy in comparison studies. The review relied more on direct comparisons than meta-analyses to come to this conclusion. Indeed, many psychiatrists would concur that clomipramine, venlafaxine, and escitalopram may offer efficacy advantages over other agents. However, the advantages are relatively modest and may be outweighed by disadvantages for many patients, including side effects.

When subtypes of depression such as atypical, melancholic, and psychotic depression are evaluated, differences between antidepressant classes appear. Atypical depression, which is characterized by mood reactivity along with reverse vegetative symptoms such as increased sleep and appetite, have long been shown to respond better to MAOIs than to TCAs. Because atypical depression may also respond well to SSRIs and bupropion, these agents still would be first-line agents in the treatment of this subtype. However, it may be quite reasonable to consider an MAOI for a patient with TRD with atypical features. Transdermal selegiline, with its favorable side-effect profile and lack of dietary restrictions, should probably now be the first MAOI that is considered in either atypical depression or TRD.

Debate continues as to whether melancholic or psychotic depression responds better to TCAs or SNRIs than to SSRIs. Although most studies of antidepressant efficacy in these subtypes have involved TCAs, prospective, head-to-head comparisons have never been done, and the literature remains inconclusive. Melancholic depression clearly appears to respond to TCAs, and it may be more reasonable to start with venlafaxine or mirtazapine, which are TCA-like in their dual actions, than with an SSRI. Likewise, psychotic depression has responded to electroconvulsive therapy (ECT); amoxapine, which is a tetracyclic agent; or the combination of a TCA and an antipsychotic. There are controlled data showing that the combination of fluoxetine and olanzapine is also effective, and this would be the recommended first-line strategy because of safety and ease of use.

The age of the patient is an important consideration in antidepressant choice. In geriatric patients, toxicity is more likely because of the number of concurrent medications they are taking, increased fat-to-muscle ratios, and reduced hepatic function and renal clearance. Among the SSRIs, escitalopram, citalopram, and sertraline appear to be among the best tolerated and the least likely to have serious pharmacokinetic interactions. Likewise, venlafaxine and mirtazapine have a low risk of interactions in geriatric patients. However, there has been some concern about the safety of venlafaxine in frail nursing home patients (Oslin et al. 2003). TCAs and MAOIs tend to be more poorly tolerated in geriatric patients and would be second- or third-line agents in this population, although some geriatricians still emphasize nortriptyline for elderly melancholic patients, and isocarboxazid was well tolerated in geriatric studies done some years ago.

Sex is also an important factor in tolerability and efficacy of a given antidepressant class. Substantial evidence suggests that men may respond to and tolerate the TCAs better than do women. Conversely, premenopausal women appear to do better with serotonergic agents than do men. Thus, men may be better treated with venlafaxine, duloxetine, or a TCA, and women may be better treated with an SSRI or a 5-HT$_2$ antagonist. Although clinicians would generally be advised not to start with a TCA because of safety concerns, it may be better to start male patients with a more noradrenergic agent than with an SSRI. Again, head-to-head comparison studies are needed before clearer recommendations can be made, and this area is still controversial.

The medical status of the patient is an important consideration in choosing an antidepressant. Patients with pain conditions may do better with duloxetine, venlafaxine, or a TCA than with other agents. There is some evidence that the SNRIs and TCAs may be effective in treating both depression and some types of pain conditions. Patients with a history of a seizure disorder, stroke, or head trauma are more safely treated with an SSRI or venlafaxine than with a TCA or bupropion. Likewise, patients with a history of arrhythmia or coronary artery disease are more safely treated with serotonergic agents than with TCAs or MAOIs. Caution should be used in prescribing nefazodone for AIDS patients who are taking protease inhibitors because it may increase toxicity of the protease inhibitors through pharmacokinetic interactions.

The primary drug parameters in choosing an antidepressant are side effects and safety. Most SSRIs are available generically and are quite inexpensive. Older agents such as the TCAs and MAOIs usually require more visits and monitoring, and this may offset the low expense of the drugs. The SSRIs are relatively safe in overdose and better tolerated than the TCAs and MAOIs for most patients. In 2011 the FDA issued a warning about the risk of QT prolongation with doses higher than 40 mg/day of citalopram and modified the warning in 2012. Theoretically, at least, citalopram might be more likely than other SSRIs to induce a lethal arrhythmia in overdose. However, few data exist to suggest a higher lethality of citalopram compared with other SSRIs. The SNRI venlafaxine may also be less safe in overdose than are the SSRIs but is safer than the TCAs. From a safety standpoint alone, it is difficult to justify using a TCA or an MAOI as a first treatment option. Most of the SSRIs are given once per day, and the starting dose is sometimes the therapeutic dose. Thus, the SSRIs are also among the easiest agents to use. A few years ago, the National Institute for Health and Care Excellence, the British advisory group, noted that overdoses with venlafaxine were more likely to be lethal than overdoses with SSRIs. For a while, it advised against first-line use of the drug and recommended routine electrocardiogram (ECG) monitoring but eventually changed its position. The FDA has not agreed to that warning. Side effects differ considerably from class to class. Among the more important long-term side effects that influence compliance are weight gain and sexual dysfunction. TCAs, MAOIs, and mirtazapine are probably the most problematic agents for weight gain, whereas fluoxetine and bupropion may be the least problematic. Sexual dysfunction is common to most antidepressants, especially the MAOIs, clomipramine, and the SSRIs. A number of agents are less likely to cause sexual side effects; these include nefazodone, bupropion, and mirtazapine. In addition, transdermal selegiline also appears to have low risk for sexual side effects. It has been suggested that more noradrenergic SNRIs, such as duloxetine, may also have lower rates of sexual side effects than do the SSRIs, but data from well-designed prospective studies are not available.

Another common approach to choosing an antidepressant is to target specific symptoms of a depressive episode. For example, a patient with depression characterized by insomnia might benefit from a sedating agent such as mirtazapine or a tertiary-amine tricyclic. Patients with significant anxiety tend to be treated with an SSRI or SNRI. Sequenced Treatment Alternatives for Resistant Depression (STAR*D) demonstrated that patients with comorbid anxiety did more poorly while taking citalopram and other antidepressants than did nonanxious patients (Fava et al. 2008). Similar data were reported in the international Study to Predict Optimized Treatment in Depression (iSPOT-D) study for escitalopram, venlafaxine, and sertraline (Arnow et al. 2015; Saveanu et al. 2015). Patients with insomnia or anxiety may also be treated with the combination of an SSRI or SNRI and a hypnotic, benzodiazepine, or sedating atypical antipsychotic such as quetiapine. Recent data indicate that the neurosteroid zuranolone is effective in major depression with anxiety (Parikh et al. 2023). Alternatively, many clinicians will choose a more stimulating antidepressant such as bupropion or transdermal selegiline in treating patients who are experiencing hypersomnia and fatigue. Patients with significant cognitive deficits or executive functioning problems might be treated with vortioxetine or duloxetine, for which positive prospective data are available (McIntyre et al. 2014; Raskin et al. 2007). This targeted approach to the treatment of depression is intuitively sound and is supported by empirical data.

In many areas of medicine, laboratory studies help guide the clinician in choosing a medication for a specific condition. For example, a bacterial culture helps in the selection of a specific antibiotic or sensitivity in internal medicine, and genotyping is increasingly guiding treatment in gynecology. At this time, psychiatry lacks a biological assay that might help us choose a specific treatment. Some very preliminary data suggest that a number of approaches might help clinicians in making antidepressant choices in the future. For example, functional MRI and PET have shown some promise in early detection of whether an antidepressant might be effective or not by imaging early changes in limbic mood-generating areas and connectivity to cortical regions. In some studies, quantitative electroencephalography (QEEG) has shown benefit in predicting subsequent response to a specific antidepressant through changes in prefrontal brain wave activity in the first week. Other small and very preliminary studies have found that QEEG might predict specific classes of agents to which a patient is most likely to respond on the basis of comparisons with a referenced database of responders. Pharmacogenomics may also play an important role in determining the best choice of an antidepressant (see Chapter 13, "Laboratory-Guided Pharmacotherapy"). Furthermore, neuropsychological deficits, particularly in the elderly, may predict poor antidepressant response in that population. It seems likely that in the coming decades, genomics, functional imaging, psychometric testing, and tools such as QEEG will provide additional data on which to make a clinical decision about the choice of an antidepressant, and this would be most welcome. Until then, clinical judgment remains the only viable option in terms of antidepressant choice.

Dosage and Administration

The optimal dose of an antidepressant is the lowest efficacious dose that has the least side effects. The decision about how much to push the dose of an antidepressant always comes down to balancing efficacy and side effects. If, with a given dose of antidepressant, there are no signs of improving symptoms after 4 weeks, the chances are very small that that dose will ever be effective (Quitkin et al. 1996). Likewise, older patients with depression who do not achieve at least 30% improvement by week 4 have only a 17% chance of achieving a remission by week 12 (Sackeim et al. 2005). On the other hand, partial response in the first 4 weeks predicts more complete response over the next 8 weeks, even if the dose is held constant. If a given dose is tolerated and not producing partial benefits at 4 weeks, the dose should be increased rather than the medication switched. Generally, increasing the dose every 2 weeks gives some opportunity for the clinician to assess the benefits and side effects of a given dose. If the increase in dose is tolerated and less than complete remission is observed, the dose should be gradually increased to the maximum recommended dose.

Duration of Treatment

Although standard antidepressant trials in the 1960s and 1970s were often 4 weeks, 6- to 12-week trials are the current standard. It is difficult to assess the efficacy of an antidepressant in less than 4 weeks. Furthermore, it is unlikely that 4 weeks will be adequate to assess higher doses in a tolerant patient. Quitkin et al. (1984), in reviewing a large series of depressed patients who were treated with traditional TCAs, concluded that relatively few patients demonstrated significant improvement after only 2 weeks of therapy and that many required as long as 6 weeks to respond. Years ago, our group (Schatzberg et al. 1981) reported that patients with slow response to maprotiline and those with rapid response could be identified biologically by their pretreatment urinary levels of 3-methoxy-4-hydroxyphenylglycol (MHPG), which are indicative of norepinephrine function. Patients with low MHPG levels demonstrated rapid responses (in less than 14 days), and those with very high MHPG levels needed 4–6 weeks of treatment. More recent reviews by Nierenberg et al. (1995, 2000) have also suggested that a lack of improvement while taking a given dose of fluoxetine for 4 weeks predicts lack of response at 8 and 12 weeks.

All patients who respond to a given dose of an antidepressant should be maintained at that dose for at least 6–12 months. The continuation of all antidepressants studied to date appears to substantially reduce the risk of relapse. In a major NIMH collaborative study (Prien et al. 1984), imipramine was generally more effective than placebo or lithium in preventing relapse of major depression over a 2-year maintenance period. In contrast to that study, two earlier major studies, one in the United States and the other in the United Kingdom, found lithium to be as effective as TCAs in preventing relapses in patients with unipolar depression. In the U.S. study by Prien et al. (1984), the overall relapse rate in the unipolar group was relatively high (64%; 49% in the imipramine group), and the authors argued for the need to develop newer, alternative strategies, perhaps with drugs other than TCAs. (For further discussion of maintenance therapy in affective disorders, see Chapter 4, "Antipsychotic

Drugs.") In the first edition of this manual, we indicated that after receiving maintenance therapy for some 3–4 months at the doses at which they responded, many patients can be maintained at lower doses (one-half to three-quarters that of the original dose) for the remaining months. However, the results of Frank et al. (1990) suggest that full doses are needed for successful maintenance therapy. These investigators found that 80% of patients with recurrent depression were free from relapse or recurrence for 3 years when full doses of imipramine (average of 200 mg/day) were maintained. We second the recommendations of Frank and colleagues that patients be maintained at their therapeutic dosage levels unless pronounced side effects are present. More recent studies examining the maintenance efficacy of venlafaxine demonstrated that patients are about twice as likely to stay well during treatment over the course of 2 years as patients randomly assigned to a placebo during the same period. In a maintenance venlafaxine study, patients continued on their acute dose unless side effects required a dosage decrease (Kornstein 2008). Because depression recurs in some 87% of patients within 15 years of the index episode, long-term maintenance therapy should certainly be considered for anyone who has had three or more serious depressive episodes or two episodes in the past 5 years.

However, emerging data on the neurobiology of depression put into question whether it is always wise to wait until the second or third episode to consider long-term or lifetime maintenance treatment. Some studies have now suggested that depression could be associated with a progressive loss of volume in the hippocampus and perhaps other brain areas, including anterior cingulate and medial orbital frontal cortex. Furthermore, these changes may progress as a function of duration of depressive illness and the number of recurrences a patient experiences (Maletic et al. 2007). These morphological changes may be difficult to overcome or could perhaps become permanent. In addition, the cumulative alterations in brain morphology are consistent with the progressive nature of depression in many patients. Subsequent recurrence may be more resistant to treatment, more chronic, more severe, and less related to external stresses. Recurrences may also be associated with an accumulation of cognitive deficits, especially memory loss, that is consistent with the observation of progressive loss in the hippocampus (Gorwood et al. 2008). In fact, Gorwood and colleagues (2008) estimated a permanent loss of 2%–3% in memory performance for each of the first four episodes of depression a patient experiences. Thus, it may be advisable for some patients to consider long-term maintenance treatment even after one initial serious depressive episode.

Long-term treatment with antidepressants can represent a challenge for the patient in adhering to the prescribed regimen. Most patients are not enamored by the idea of continuing to take antidepressants for long periods of time. Stigma, side effects, cost, and inconvenience all contribute to nonadherence to maintenance antidepressant treatment. Several interventions can increase compliance. It is helpful to educate the patient and family about the course of depressive illness, the length of time it takes for antidepressants to work, and the need to continue treatment when the patient is feeling better. We increasingly educate patients about the potential for depression-associated progressive brain changes and long-term cognitive deficits that have been increasingly reported in the literature. Reviewing potential side effects is also helpful. Asking for feedback and answering any questions the patient may have allows the clinician to check the patient's understanding of the prescribed treatment. Instructing the patient not to change the dosage or discontinue the medication without consulting their physician is often helpful as well.

Selective Serotonin Reuptake Inhibitors

Although the TCAs were the dominant class of antidepressants worldwide for more than 30 years, the SSRIs overtook them in popularity by the mid-1990s. This class includes fluoxetine, paroxetine, sertraline, fluvoxamine, citalopram, and escitalopram (Figure 3–1). Fluvoxamine does not have an FDA-approved indication for the treatment of depression but received an approval for social anxiety in 2008 in addition to its long-standing indication for OCD. Furthermore, fluvoxamine is marketed in many countries as an antidepressant. Unlike the TCAs or any other group of prescribed psychotropic agents, the SSRIs, particularly fluoxetine, have had tremendous exposure in the nonscientific literature.

The SSRIs have been both vilified and praised in the lay press, but the popularity of these drugs among patients and physicians has remained quite consistent. This popularity is due in no small part to their favorable safety and side-effect profile relative to the MAOIs and the TCAs. The SSRIs have also proven to have a broad spectrum of activity in a variety of psychiatric disorders, and they have an additional advantage in that it is easier to attain the op-

Selective serotonin reuptake inhibitors (SSRIs): overview	
Efficacy	First-line treatment in the following: MDD (FDA approved for all except fluvoxamine), persistent depressive disorder Panic disorder (FDA approved for fluoxetine, paroxetine, and sertraline) OCD (FDA approved for all except citalopram and escitalopram) Social anxiety disorder (FDA approved for sertraline and paroxetine) PTSD (FDA approved for sertraline and paroxetine) Bulimia (FDA approved for fluoxetine) GAD (FDA approved for paroxetine and escitalopram) PMDD (FDA approved for fluoxetine [Sarafem only], paroxetine [controlled release only], and sertraline)
Side effects	Gastrointestinal side effects (nausea, diarrhea, heartburn) Sexual dysfunction (↓ libido, delayed orgasm) Headache Insomnia/somnolence
Safety in overdose	Generally safe in overdose to 30–90 days' supply; manage with vital sign support, lavage Seizures/status epilepticus (rare)
Dosage and administration	Citalopram, paroxetine, fluoxetine: once daily dosing, starting at 10–20 mg, increasing to a maximum of 40 mg (citalopram), 50 mg (paroxetine), and 80 mg (fluoxetine). Escitalopram: once daily dosing, starting at 10 mg, increasing to 20 mg after minimum of 1 week. Sertraline: start at 25–50 mg and increase, as needed, to 200 mg maximum.
	Full benefits in 4–8 weeks
Discontinuation	Paroxetine, fluvoxamine, sertraline: discontinuation associated with parasthesias, nausea, headaches, flulike symptoms 1–7 days after sudden discontinuation
Drug interactions	MAOI (**contraindicated**): serotonin syndrome ↑ Tricyclic antidepressant levels (paroxetine, fluoxetine) ↑ Carbamazepine, phenobarbital, phenytoin levels ↑ Haloperidol, clozapine levels (fluvoxamine) ↑ Theophylline levels (fluvoxamine) ↑ Encainide, flecainide levels (**avoid**)

Note.   GAD=generalized anxiety disorder; MAOI=monoamine oxidase inhibitor; MDD= major depressive disorder; PMDD=premenstrual dysphoric disorder.

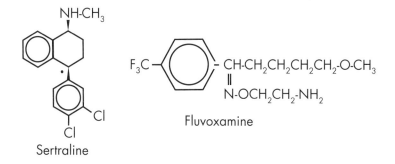

Figure 3–1. Chemical structures of selective serotonin reuptake inhibitors.

timal therapeutic dose. In addition, all the SSRIs are now generic and quite inexpensive. In 2018, a major pharmacy chain was selling most of the SSRIs for about 5–10 dollars for a month's supply. However, not all patients tolerate or respond to the SSRIs, and, as suggested earlier (see "Choosing an Antidepressant" subsection earlier in this chapter), they may not be as effective as other antidepressants for some types of depression and some specific symptoms, such as pain.

Pharmacological Effects

As the name of this class of antidepressants indicates, the SSRIs selectively block the reuptake of 5-HT through their inhibiting effects on the Na^+/K^+ adenosine triphosphatase–dependent serotonin transporter in presynaptic neurons. Compared with a standard TCA such as amitriptyline, which has about an equal tendency to block neuronal reuptake of 5-HT and norepinephrine, fluoxetine is 200 times more selective in blocking the reuptake of 5-HT than of norepinephrine. Fluoxetine is approximately 4 times as potent a 5-HT reuptake inhibitor in vitro as is amitriptyline, and paroxetine is approximately 80 times as potent an inhibitor as amitriptyline. Of the five currently available SSRIs, paroxetine and citalopram appear to be the most potent 5-HT uptake blockers.

However, selectivity is a relative term. Although the SSRIs are more selective than, say, the TCAs, all the SSRIs impact other neurotransmitter systems, at least modestly. For example, there is in vitro evidence that paroxetine at high dosages (>40 mg/day) may be as much, if not more, of a norepinephrine reuptake blocker as is venlafaxine. Sertraline also appears to block the reuptake of dopamine and may be more potent in this regard than bupropion. Likewise, paroxetine may have as strong of an anticholinergic effect as desipramine.

The reuptake-blocking properties of the SSRIs enhance general serotonergic tone in at least two distinct steps. Initially, the SSRIs contribute to a significant increase in the availability of 5-HT in the synaptic cleft. However, it is unlikely that this effect has any bearing on antidepressant efficacy because the SSRIs share the delayed onset of action typical of all antidepressants. With recurrent administration of the drugs, however, there is a reduction in the sensitivity of the somatodendritic and terminal 5-HT_{1A} autoreceptors, and the time course of this effect is associated more closely with antidepressant response. In addition, blockade of the serotonin transporter by chronic administration of SSRIs is associated with an increase in neurotrophin expression.

SSRIs enhance transcription of neurotrophic factors, including brain-derived neurotrophic factor (BDNF). The increase in antidepressant-induced BDNF is associated with an increase in synaptogenesis, neurogenesis, and neuronal resilience. These increases appear to be an important consequence of long-term administration of SSRIs and other effective antidepressant classes.

Unlike the TCAs, the SSRIs have relatively little affinity for histaminic (H_1, H_2), muscarinic, or α_1-adrenergic receptors. Although sertraline may have 25% of the in vitro affinity for α_1-adrenergic receptors that imipramine has, this finding is of little clinical relevance. On the other hand, paroxetine has weak but somewhat clinically meaningful antimuscarinic activity. The anticholinergic affinity for paroxetine is roughly equivalent to that for desipramine. In general, however, the selective nature of the SSRIs results in the very favorable side-effect profile and the large therapeutic index of these drugs.

The SSRIs are extensively metabolized by hepatic isoenzymes, especially the cytochrome P450 (CYP) 2D6 enzyme (Table 3–1). Sertraline is also metabolized via the CYP3A3/4 enzyme. Only fluoxetine and sertraline have pharmacologically active metabolites (Table 3–2). Fluoxetine is demethylated to norfluoxetine, and sertraline is metabolized to N-desmethylsertraline and a hydroxyketone. As a result, the functional half-lives of fluoxetine and sertraline are considerably longer than those of paroxetine and fluvoxamine. Fluoxetine has a half-life of about 34 hours; the half-life of norfluoxetine is at least 1 week. Sertraline has a half-life of about 26 hours, and the half-lives of its metabolites tend to range from 48 to 72 hours. Both paroxetine and fluvoxamine have half-lives that average under 20 hours, whereas citalopram has a half-life of around 35 hours. With repeated administration of the drugs, the half-lives of all of the SSRIs, but particularly paroxetine and fluoxetine, increase substantially because the drugs appear to inhibit their own metabolism. Thus, the functional half-lives of fluoxetine and norfluoxetine, with continued use, are closer to 2–3 weeks. Plasma level monitoring of the SSRIs has not proved clinically useful. The variability of SSRI plasma levels among individuals is so great that it has been nearly impossible to correlate efficacy or toxicity with plasma levels.

Indications

The SSRIs are indicated primarily for the treatment of major depression, and numerous studies have supported this use. Many double-blind, placebo-controlled studies have established that the SSRIs are useful in the treatment of mild to

Table 3–1. Inhibition of cytochrome P450 enzymes by antidepressants

Enzyme	Drugs metabolized	Antidepressant inhibitors
2D6	TCAs (hydroxylation) Bupropion/bupropion + dextromethorphan Venlafaxine Thioridazine Class 1C antiarrhythmics β-blockers Paroxetine Risperidone Codeine Haloperidol Clozapine Benztropine Perphenazine	Fluoxetine (norfluoxetine) Sertraline (desmethylsertraline) Paroxetine Fluvoxamine and citalopram (weakest) Bupropion
1A2	Caffeine Theophylline Phenacetin TCAs (demethylation) Clozapine Diazepam	Fluvoxamine
3A3/4	Alprazolam Triazolam TCAs (demethylation) Terfenadine Astemizole Carbamazepine Erythromycin Dexamethasone Citalopram Escitalopram Cyclosporine Indinavir Nelfinavir Ritonavir	Fluoxetine Sertraline Fluvoxamine Nefazodone
2C19	TCAs (demethylation) Warfarin Tolbutamide	Fluoxetine Fluvoxamine Sertraline

Table 3–1. Inhibition of cytochrome P450 enzymes by antidepressants *(continued)*

Enzyme	Drugs metabolized	Antidepressant inhibitors
2C19 *(continued)*	Phenytoin	
	Diazepam	
	Omeprazole	
	Esomeprazole	

Note. TCA = tricyclic antidepressant.

Table 3–2. Pharmacokinetics of selective serotonin reuptake inhibitors (SSRIs)

SSRI	Half-life (hours)	Metabolite and its half-life	Peak plasma level (hours)	% Protein bound
Fluoxetine	24–72 96–144[a]	Norfluoxetine, 7–14 days	6–8	94
Sertraline	26	*N*-desmethylsertraline, 2–3 days	4.5–8.4	98
Paroxetine	<20	NA	2–8	95
Fluvoxamine	15	NA	2–8	80
Citalopram	35	NA	4–6	80
Escitalopram	32	*S*-desmethylcitalopram	5	56

Note. NA = not applicable.
[a]During chronic administration.

moderate major depression in outpatients (Rickels and Schweizer 1990). Some studies also suggest that the SSRIs are also efficacious in the treatment of more severe depression, although there has been debate about this over the years (see below). In fact, Montgomery and colleagues (2007) concluded that evidence supporting escitalopram in severe depression may be stronger than evidence for other antidepressants. The SSRIs are effective in atypical depression, in combination with standard antipsychotics in the treatment of psychotic depression, and in the maintenance therapy of recurrent depression in trials lasting 1 year. In addition, SSRIs are also useful in the treatment of chronic major depression with dysthymia. Some clinicians have come to regard these agents as the treatments of choice for these disorders.

However, there is ongoing debate about the role of the SSRIs in more serious forms of depression, including melancholia. Large meta-analyses and randomized controlled trials (RCTs) have failed to show a significant difference in efficacy between SSRIs and TCAs or SNRIs in the treatment of severe depression (Bielski et al. 2004; Hirschfeld 1999). Still, relatively few studies of SSRIs have involved more severely depressed inpatients, and some of the studies that did involve such patients did not directly compare the SSRIs with older agents such as the TCAs. Some studies that made these direct comparisons suggested that paroxetine was inferior to clomipramine in inducing remission in melancholic inpatients (Danish University Antidepressant Group 1990) and that fluoxetine was much less effective than nortriptyline in treating melancholic elderly cardiac patients who were hospitalized for depression (Roose et al. 1994). These studies defined response not as a reduction in overall severity but rather as remission. Other studies have failed to find any difference in efficacy between the SSRIs and SNRIs in any subtype of depression, including melancholic major depression (Arnow et al. 2015). This debate about the efficacy of the SSRIs in more severe depression is likely to continue. The available data suggest that the SSRIs may not be quite as effective in treating some seriously depressed elderly inpatients but that they do have a more favorable side-effect profile than either the TCAs or SNRIs.

The second indication for the SSRIs is the treatment of OCD. The utility of clomipramine (a serotonergic TCA) in the treatment of OCD was first noted in 1968. Since that time, it has become clear that other serotonergic agents are also useful in the treatment of this historically difficult-to-treat disorder (Chouinard et al. 1990; Tollefson et al. 1994). Fluvoxamine, fluoxetine, sertraline, and paroxetine all have an FDA indication for the treatment of OCD, but all the SSRIs have demonstrated efficacy in treating the disorder. SSRI doses for the treatment of OCD are usually higher than those required for the treatment of depression, and the latency to response is usually longer.

A third indication for the SSRIs, and a fairly well studied one, is the treatment of eating disorders, particularly bulimia nervosa. Fluoxetine has been shown to have a positive effect on the binge-purge cycle in some bulimic patients (Fluoxetine Bulimia Nervosa Collaborative Study Group 1992). The SSRIs may also ameliorate the carbohydrate craving and mood disturbance associated with bulimia nervosa and obesity. Fluoxetine and sertraline have been shown to have a modest effect on weight and food intake in obese patients. Unfortunately, most patients who lose weight during therapy with an SSRI gain it back over time. There are few data on the use of the SSRIs to treat classic anorexia nervosa, but one report suggested that fluoxetine may be useful for this condition (Kaye et al. 1991). The largest controlled study to date of fluoxetine in the prevention of relapse in anorexic patients failed to show any benefit for fluoxetine in preventing relapse relative to placebo (Walsh et al. 2006). However, this study involved adults with a more chronic form of the illness, and there may be subsets of anorexic patients who appear to do better while taking an SSRI.

Finally, there appears to be a role for the SSRIs in the treatment of most anxiety disorders, including panic disorder, social anxiety disorder, and GAD, as well as PTSD. Although patients with panic disorder may be sensitive to the activating effects of some SSRIs, most are able to tolerate a slow titration of dosage upward. For example, some reports indicate that although some patients do not tolerate an initial dosage of 20 mg/day of fluoxetine, many patients are able to benefit if the starting dosage is 5 mg/day (Schneier et al. 1990). The SSRIs, including citalopram and fluvoxamine, all appear, based on published data, to be effective in treating panic disorder. Paroxetine, sertraline, and fluoxetine received an FDA-approved indication for the treatment of panic disorder.

In 1999, paroxetine received an FDA-approved indication for treating social anxiety disorder, and preliminary data support the use of other SSRIs in the treatment of this disorder. Several double-blind studies indicate that paroxetine at dosages of 20–50 mg/day is more effective than placebo in alleviating symptoms, including undue fear and avoidance of interpersonal interaction. Further, paroxetine appears to reduce the significant disability associated with more severe forms of this disorder (Stein et al. 1998). Other SSRIs, including escitalopram, have had positive controlled trials in the treatment of social anxiety but have not received approval for this indication. In general, the SSRIs appear at least as efficacious in the treatment of social anxiety as they are in the treatment of major depression. However, whereas social anxiety disorder is among the more common anxiety disorders, it is also less commonly diagnosed and treated than other anxiety disorders.

PTSD is associated with a variety of comorbid conditions, especially depression and substance abuse. SSRIs have been used since the late 1980s to treat some of the symptoms of PTSD, including depression, insomnia, hyper-arousal, and agitation. Substantial evidence exists that fluoxetine, paroxetine, and sertraline help alleviate these symptoms and may even have an impact on comorbid substance use. In 1999, sertraline became the first drug to be approved by the FDA for the treatment of PTSD. Many patients with PTSD who are treated with sertraline appear to require doses above 100 mg/day for maximum effects. With paroxetine, a dosage of 20 mg/day appears to be about as effective as 40 mg/day in treating PTSD.

All of the SSRIs should help with GAD, and paroxetine and escitalopram have received FDA approval for this indication. Paroxetine, at dosages of 20–50 mg/day, was effective in reducing anxiety by 60% on the Hamilton Anxiety Rating Scale. Large-scale studies of escitalopram have also shown benefit in the treatment of generalized anxiety.

PMDD is a very disruptive monthly occurrence for about 3% of the female population. In 1995, in the first large study of fluoxetine in the treatment of PMDD (Steiner et al. 1995), 20- and 60-mg doses were more effective than placebo for treating symptoms over six consecutive menstrual cycles. The effect was seen as early as the first cycle after initiation of the medication. Since then, a number of studies have supported the use of SSRIs, especially fluoxetine and sertraline, in treating this disorder. Both of these drugs have also been used as intermittent treatment in the luteal phase of the cycle and appear to be effective (Jermain et al. 1999). In 1999, fluoxetine (Sarafem) became the first medication approved for the treatment of PMDD.

The most recent FDA approval for an SSRI indication was the approval of paroxetine for vasomotor symptoms in 2014. Paroxetine at dosages of 7.5 mg/day significantly reduced hot flashes in perimenopausal women. Although there is a newer name-brand version of paroxetine, an inexpensive 10-mg dose of generic paroxetine is likely to work just as well.

The list of disorders in which the serotonergic system plays a part is long, and the potential role for the SSRIs is continually expanding. The SSRIs appear to be useful in treating the anger or impulsive aggression associated with some personality disorders (Kavoussi et al. 1994; Rinne et al. 2002) and perhaps certain pain disorders such as diabetic neuropathy and fibromyalgia (Wolfe et al. 1994), although here the mixed norepinephrine-serotonin reuptake blockers appear to be far more effective.

Side Effects

As noted previously, the SSRIs tend to be safer and better tolerated than their pre-decessors. Many overdoses have occurred in clinical practice with the SSRIs, but these have rarely been eventful. In fact, a review of 234 fluoxetine overdose attempts, with doses up to 1,500 mg, revealed no fatalities, and more than half the patients were completely asymptomatic (Borys et al. 1992). Nothing more than supportive care was required for any patient. Moderate overdoses (5–30 times the total daily dose) are rarely serious. Nonetheless, fatal overdoses with SSRIs have occurred. One analysis suggests that as many as 14/1,000 overdoses with SSRIs might be fatal (McKenzie and McFarland 2007). However, many of these overdoses are complicated by the ingestion of additional substances. Still, a rate of 1.4% of SSRI overdoses associated with fatality is a fraction of the rate of lethal TCA overdoses and also lower than the fatal overdoses seen with venlafaxine. The usual cause of death appears to be complications of seizures or status epilepticus and typically involves ingesting thousands of milligrams (Barbey and Roose 1998).

In early clinical studies, approximately twice as many patients were likely to drop out because of adverse effects of TCAs than because of adverse effects of SSRIs. The SSRIs are largely devoid of the anticholinergic side effects that plague the TCAs. Furthermore, orthostatic hypotension does not typically occur with SSRI use. In general, the SSRIs also appear to be better tolerated than are the MAOIs, and the SNRIs as well. That is not to say that all people tolerate the SSRIs better than they do other classes of antidepressants. Some patients who cannot tolerate an SSRI's sexual side effects, for example, might do well with some SNRIs, bupropion, or even transdermal selegiline.

The most common reasons patients discontinue an SSRI early in treatment are gastrointestinal (GI) side effects. These include nausea, diarrhea, cramping, heartburn, and other symptoms of GI distress. The gut is lined with 5-HT receptors, including 5-HT$_3$, which appear to be responsible for SSRI-induced GI distress. Whereas the earliest reports suggested that approximately 20%–30% of patients treated with fluoxetine developed GI side effects, the incidence in clinical practice has been much lower. In early studies, the dosage was often started at 20 mg/day but reached 60 mg/day by the end of the first week. In clinical practice, the starting dosage of 20 mg/day is maintained for 3 weeks, and nausea is both less common and less severe. Further-more, the GI side effects tend to diminish over the first 2–4 weeks of treatment. Several strategies may be useful in reducing SSRI-induced GI distress. The first is a slow titration of the medication. Starting at half, or less than half, of the usual starting dose and moving the dose up slowly in sensitive patients allows adaptation to occur. Another strategy is instructing patients to take their medication with meals. A full stomach appears to mitigate some GI distress. Other $5-HT_3$ antagonists, such as dolasetron (Anzemet) and ondansetron (Zofran), are also clearly helpful but are too expensive to use routinely. Mirtazapine (Remeron) is a potent $5-HT_2$ and $5-HT_3$ antagonist and has been used in combination with SSRIs. In fact, oncologists and anesthesiologists are increasingly using mirtazapine as a less expensive alternative to the traditional $5-HT_3$ antagonists for treating postoperative and chemotherapy-induced nausea (Kast and Foley 2007).

Another group of side effects commonly encountered with SSRIs is related to CNS activation. At least 10%–20% of patients receiving SSRI therapy complain of insomnia, jitteriness, and agitation in the course of treatment. These side effects are not particularly surprising, given the selective, but not specific, effect of SSRIs on CNS serotonergic transmission. That is, the SSRIs affect diffuse serotonergic pathways, and some of these pathways contribute to CNS arousal. For this reason, fluoxetine, which has a reputation for activating properties, should be taken in the morning, when it is less likely to interfere with sleep. Likewise, if patients develop insomnia with other SSRIs, it is often effective to have the patients take the dose earlier in the day. Occasionally, patients require modest doses of a benzodiazepine (e.g., clonazepam 0.5 mg bid, lorazepam 0.5 mg bid, alprazolam 0.25 mg bid) early during therapy to help with agitation and sleep. Trazodone is another commonly used agent shown to be helpful at doses of 50–100 mg at bedtime for SSRI-induced insomnia. A few case reports also suggest that trazodone may augment response to the SSRIs.

Conversely, some patients may become sedated when taking SSRIs. This effect is seen mostly with paroxetine. When sedation occurs, taking the dose at about 8:00 P.M. is useful for matching the peak blood level with the optimal time of sedation (about 2:00 A.M.). Some patients taking other SSRIs experience the emergence of a numbed or anergic feeling in the context of a euthymic mood. Donald Klein has recommended low dosages of bromocriptine (2.5 mg qd or bid) or stimulants to counteract this effect (McGrath et al. 1995).

Modafinil (Provigil) has been applied to counteract antidepressant-induced hypersomnia. Modafinil is a stimulant with low abuse potential and is FDA approved for the treatment of narcolepsy and idiopathic hypersomnia. We have found that doses of 100–200 mg in the morning are helpful in alleviating treatment-emergent somnolence (DeBattista et al. 2003). In addition, modafinil may have a role in helping other dimensions of depression, including fatigue and cognition. Armodafinil, the *R*-enantiomer of modafinil, is longer acting than modafinil but has similar utility in the treatment of antidepressant-induced side effects.

Since the advent of the SSRIs in the 1990s, it has become increasingly clear that treatment-emergent sexual dysfunction is a much bigger problem with SSRI treatment than was previously recognized. Premarketing studies suggested that the incidence of sexual dysfunction—including delayed ejaculation, anorgasmia, impotence, and diminished libido—was less than 4%. However, more recent reports suggested that the incidence may be closer to 30%–40% for all the SSRIs. Although accommodation to sexual side effects does occur in some patients, such improvement may take months or even years. Holding the dose of shorter-acting SSRIs, such as paroxetine and sertraline, for 24 hours prior to anticipated sexual activity has been anecdotally reported to be helpful in some 50% of patients. The long half-life of fluoxetine makes this approach ineffective.

Several interventions to counteract treatment-emergent sexual dysfunction have been described (Table 3–3), but most have not been well studied. Virtually all the reported benefits of adjunctive agents for treatment-emergent sexual side effects are based on case reports or open-label studies. A few controlled studies have been completed, but their findings are not conclusive. In one of the few double-blind studies of sexual dysfunction antidotes to be published, buspirone, a partial agonist of the 5-HT_{1A} receptor, was shown to be useful in treating SSRI-induced sexual dysfunction in some patients at dosages of 20–60 mg/day (Landén et al. 1999). However, another double-blind study of buspirone used in the treatment of SSRI-induced sexual side effects did not find buspirone to be useful in this regard (Michelson et al. 2000). Mirtazapine was also ineffective in a controlled trial, although olanzapine, a $5\text{-HT}_2/\text{D}_2$ antagonist, was significantly more effective than placebo (Michelson et al. 2002). Switching to bupropion (Walker et al. 1993) or adding bupropion at dosages of 75–150 mg/day to the SSRI regimen (Ashton and Rosen 1998;

Table 3–3.   Adjunctive agents for selective serotonin reuptake inhibitor–induced sexual dysfunction

Adjunctive agent	Dosage	Studies
Buspirone	20–60 mg/day	Landén et al. 1999; Norden 1994
Bupropion	75–150 mg/day	Ashton and Rosen 1998; DeBattista et al. 2005; Labbate and Pollack 1994
Sildenafil	50–100 mg prn	Ashton and Bennett 1999; Fava et al. 2006a; Gupta et al. 1999; Nurnberg et al. 1999a, 1999b, 2008
Tadalafil	10–20 mg prn	Segraves et al. 2007
Vardenafil	10–20 mg prn	Rosen et al. 2006
Ginkgo biloba	60–240 mg/day	Wheatley 2004
Amantadine	100–300 mg/day	Balon 1996; Shrivastava et al. 1995
Cyproheptadine	4–12 mg prn	Aizenberg et al. 1995; Keller Ashton et al. 1997
Yohimbine	5.4 mg tid	Jacobsen 1992; Price and Grunhaus 1990

Hirschfeld 1999; Labbate and Pollack 1994) has proved useful in some cases. We completed a double-blind study of bupropion as an add-on therapy and found it helpful for mood but not for sexual performance at a fixed dosage of 150 mg/day (DeBattista et al. 2005). Bupropion was found to be only marginally effective at increasing sexual arousal; however, a dose of 300 mg or more may be needed to improve sexual function. Clayton and colleagues (2004) found that bupropion at a dosage of 150 mg bid improved desire and interest in sexual activity on some measures after 4 weeks.

The use of sildenafil (Viagra) has been reported to be significantly more effective than placebo in men with SSRI-induced sexual dysfunction (Fava et al. 2006a; Nurnberg et al. 2001). The reported utility of sildenafil in countering SSRI-induced sexual side effects is somewhat counterintuitive, because the most common sexual side effects of SSRIs are decreased libido and delayed orgasm rather than erectile problems. However, sildenafil has been reported to increase overall sexual satisfaction in both men and women. In a controlled study in women, we observed sildenafil (50–100 mg/day) to be significantly more effective than placebo in improving global measures of sexual function in patients with purported antidepressant-induced sexual side effects (Nurnberg et al. 2008). Similar agents such as vardenafil also appear to be effective in anti-depressant-associated sexual dysfunction, at least in men (Rosen et al. 2006). Cyproheptadine at dosages of 4–12 mg/day may reverse some of the dysfunction. Unfortunately, cyproheptadine may also reverse the antidepressant or anti-obsessive effects of the SSRIs and is quite sedating. The α-adrenergic agonist yohimbine helps some patients (Jacobsen 1992) but was ineffective in a controlled trial (Michelson et al. 2002). Unfortunately, yohimbine can be quite anxiogenic for some patients, and this effect tends to be counterproductive. Similarly, some case reports have suggested that dopaminergic agents such as amantadine, amphetamine, and bromocriptine may be helpful for some patients. The ancient herb *Ginkgo biloba* has been anecdotally reported to help some patients with SSRI-induced sexual dysfunction. However, beneficial effects may require a higher dosage (e.g., 240 mg/day) for weeks, and such dosages have sometimes been associated with GI side effects, increased bleeding, and confusion in elderly patients. As is often the case, more carefully controlled studies have failed to show a benefit of *Ginkgo biloba* in treating antidepressant-induced sexual dysfunction (Wheatley 2004). Given the lack of evidence supporting ginkgo and the potential for some side effects, we do not encourage patients to try it. Finally, a more recent study has found that a subgroup of women with SSRI-induced sexual side effects who have a polymorphism of the androgen receptor respond to small doses of sublingual testosterone (van Rooij et al. 2015). Testosterone appears important in the libido of both men and women but obviously can have masculinizing effects in women. The FDA had previously rejected a Procter & Gamble application for a testosterone patch for treating low libido in women because of equivocal results and safety risks. Flibanserin, a 5-HT_{1A} agonist and 5-HT_2 antagonist, ultimately was approved in 2015 for treating female hyposexual desire after having been previously rejected. We participated in the studies of flibanserin and did not find it particularly effective in treating low libido in women. Even though we think the risk of a serotonin syndrome is low in combination with an SSRI, flibanserin can interact with CYP3A4 inhibitors and cause severe hypotension. Thus, flibanserin should not be used with nefazodone, protease inhibitors, ketoconazole, and other medications that may put the patient at risk for hypotension.

A number of other adverse effects are associated with the SSRIs, but these occur less consistently. Headaches may occur early in the course of therapy with some patients. On the other hand, the SSRIs have shown some utility in the prophylaxis of migraine when used long-term. Autonomic symptoms such as excessive perspiration and dry mouth are frequently reported. Excessive perspiration is very problematic for some patients. Anecdotal approaches to the treatment of SSRI-induced perspiration, such as the use of β-blockers and anticholinergic agents, are largely untested. α_2-Adrenergic agents may be helpful here. Tremor may develop in a dose-related pattern and is often responsive to propranolol in modest dosages (10 mg tid). Dry mouth is seen in some 20% of patients treated with paroxetine, reflecting the mild anticholinergic effects of this medication.

The question of whether weight gain is associated with chronic use of SSRIs has become a focus of interest. In general, it has been difficult to reliably correlate significant weight gain with SSRI treatment. After a year of treatment, most of the SSRIs are associated with either no weight gain or modest weight increases. Among the SSRIs, paroxetine may be somewhat more associated with weight gain and fluoxetine somewhat less.

Teicher et al. (1990) reported the emergence of intense preoccupation with suicide in six patients early in fluoxetine treatment. This phenomenon may also occur with other antidepressants. Subsequent studies and analyses of data sets have failed to find any greater proclivity for suicide with fluoxetine than with other antidepressants (Beasley et al. 1991). In addition, there has been no association of fluoxetine with suicidality in bulimia (Wheadon et al. 1992) or OCD (Beasley et al. 1992). This suggests that the phenomenon of treatment-emergent suicidal thoughts may be an artifact of the patient's underlying depression rather than a result of the medication. However, fluoxetine is associated with agitation or perhaps akathisia-like side effects, and it is conceivable that some depressed patients may become more suicidal when these effects occur (Rothschild and Locke 1991). Rothschild and Locke (1991) reintroduced fluoxetine in three patients who had previously attempted suicide while taking fluoxetine. They reported that all three patients developed severe akathisia with the reintroduction. In two of the three cases, suicidal distress was relieved by propranolol. Thus, switching to a less activating antidepressant or using a benzodiazepine such as clonazepam or lorazepam or a β-blocker concurrently with the SSRI may be advisable in cases of treatment-emergent suicidal ideation. Some patients who experience this phenomenon while taking a TCA may not experience it with fluoxetine.

Jonathan O. Cole, M.D., the coauthor of our previous editions, was involved in the Teicher et al. (1990) report on obsessive suicidal thoughts associated with fluoxetine and believed he would see rare cases of patients experiencing this phenomenon. Fisher et al. (1993), in a prescription-based survey, found that 0.5% of patients who had recently filled a fluoxetine prescription called an 800 number to report a new suicidal drive; no patients who had filled trazodone prescriptions reported such adverse effects. The rare incidence of treatment-emergent suicidal thoughts is not a justification for avoidance of SSRIs. The controversial FDA review of antidepressants and suicidality in children found an increased risk of about 3% with the antidepressants and 1.5% with placebo. This resulted in a black box warning regarding the risks of all antidepressants used in adolescents and children. However, this increased risk must be balanced with the improvement in suicidal ideation that occurs in many more patients while they are taking antidepressants.

Studies subsequent to the black box warning that have examined the risk of suicidal behavior with antidepressant use have generally failed to find an association (Hammad et al. 2006a, 2006b; Kaizar et al. 2006; Simon et al. 2006; Søndergård et al. 2006a, 2006b). Of note was the study by Simon et al. (2006), in which risk of suicide attempts was highest in the month before initiation of therapy. Likewise, an analysis of suicide rates in real-life samples estimated that compared with treatment without antidepressants, treatment with an antidepressant markedly diminished the risk of completed suicides, regardless of age, biological sex, or parasuicide history (Cougnard et al. 2009). The more recent FDA-initiated study of 100,000 patients in an FDA clinical trial database revealed a 2% risk of emergent suicidal-like behavior in subjects 18–25 years treated with an antidepressant versus 1% in same-age subjects receiving placebo. Older patients appeared to not show such increased risk, and elderly subjects showed a significant decrease. However, as with adults, there may be small subsets of patients at greater risk for suicidal behavior (e.g., young adults) while taking antidepressants. These could include patients with latent bipolar disorder, patients who experience agitation while taking an antidepressant, and patients who become energized enough while taking an antidepressant to act on suicidal impulses before their mood has substantially improved.

We continue to recommend that these drugs be used in both children/adolescents and adults, but with appropriate warning and monitoring. In view of the clustering of adverse reports with paroxetine in children, it does seem wise to use another agent before trying paroxetine in children.

Overdose

The popularity of the SSRIs rests in part on their safety in overdose (Barbey and Roose 1998). Thousands of overdoses have occurred in the past 30 years, but very few fatalities have resulted from overdosing on an SSRI alone. In 2003 there were 55,977 reported SSRI overdoses in the United States. There were 106 fatalities in this group, and many of the fatalities were complicated by ingestion of other substances (McKenzie and McFarland 2007). Fluoxetine, the first SSRI in the United States and the most used, has the most fatalities associated with overdose. Moderate overdoses (at up to 30 times the common daily dose) tend to be associated with minor symptoms. The most common symptoms of large overdoses include vomiting, nausea, tremor, and sedation. At very high doses (more than 75 times the common daily dose), more serious adverse events—cardiovascular events, seizures, and altered or decreased consciousness—have been reported.

The most common causes of death in an SSRI overdose are typically complications of status epilepticus and cardiovascular events such as arrhythmias. Citalopram is known to prolong QT intervals, and there have been rare fatalities attributed to arrhythmias in citalopram overdoses. Most fatalities have involved the co-ingestion of other drugs, particularly alcohol or drugs dependent on the CYP2D6 system, such as the TCAs (Dalfen and Stewart 2001). In general, lavage and supportive care in the emergency department are all that are required in most SSRI overdoses. In severe overdoses or those involving other drugs, cardiac monitoring or interventions for seizure control may be required.

Drug Interactions

The risk of serious drug interactions is fairly limited with SSRIs. However, several types of drug interactions may occur. The most serious of these is the interaction with the MAOIs. Fatalities have been reported from serotonin syndrome when SSRIs were used in close proximity to MAOIs, even if the drugs were not used concurrently. In two of these cases, fluoxetine had been stopped but an MAOI had been started promptly thereafter. Therefore, an adequate washout must occur after an SSRI is discontinued before an MAOI is initiated (see SSRI "Discontinuation" subsection later in this chapter). Serotonin syndrome has proved difficult to treat. The most important interventions in treating this syndrome are stopping the offending agents and initiating medical support, including lowering of body temperature, if needed. Beyond that, cyproheptadine at a dosage of 16 mg/day may be helpful in less severe cases in which myoclonic jerking is present. Dantrolene may also be helpful (see Chapter 10, "Emergency Department Treatment").

Another type of potential drug interaction occurs because of the tendency of the SSRIs to competitively inhibit enzymes of the CYP system (see Table 3–1). The inhibition of the CYP2D6 enzyme by the SSRIs is perhaps the best understood. Many drugs are metabolized by this enzyme, including the TCAs, type 1C antiarrhythmic agents, some β-blockers, benztropine, and many antipsychotic medications. Most of the SSRIs can inhibit the CYP2D6 enzyme, leading to increased plasma levels of other agents. For example, fluoxetine may be associated with up to an eightfold increase in TCA plasma levels when the two drugs are used concurrently. On a molar basis, fluoxetine, paroxetine, and sertraline are fairly equal in their proclivity to competitively inhibit the CYP2D6 enzyme, whereas citalopram (and escitalopram) and fluvoxamine do not significantly inhibit this enzyme. Sheldon Preskorn at the University of Kansas reported that 20 mg of fluoxetine raises desipramine levels several times higher than does 50 mg of sertraline (Preskorn 1993). However, other studies indicate that higher dosages of sertraline (e.g., 150 mg/day) can produce significant increases in desipramine levels. Fluvoxamine is about 10 times less potent a competitive inhibitor of the CYP2D6 enzyme than the other SSRIs, yet it was associated with a twofold increase in amitriptyline levels in two patients and a sevenfold increase in clomipramine levels in a third patient (Bertschy et al. 1991). Fluvoxamine has also been associated anecdotally with significantly increasing clozapine levels, probably through its inhibition of the CYP1A2 enzyme. Thus, caution should be exercised when combining any of the SSRIs with drugs predominantly dependent on the CYP2D6 enzyme because the risk of toxicity from the concurrent drug will be enhanced. For example, it is prudent to monitor TCA serum levels and ECGs when any of the TCAs are used in combination with an SSRI. However, in a geriatric study, Murphy et al. (2003) failed to find a relationship between specific CYP2D6 alleles and the risk of dropping out due to adverse events, even though patients were taking a variety of medical drugs that were known substrates for the CYP2D6 enzyme.

Although the CYP2D6 enzyme is the best characterized of the CYP enzymes, there are many others, and the SSRIs may be associated with the competitive inhibition of some of them as noted above. Fluvoxamine is known to inhibit the CYP1A2 enzyme, which is responsible for the metabolism of theophylline, caffeine, certain benzodiazepines, and haloperidol. It would therefore be prudent to use lower doses of theophylline when treating asthmatic patients with fluvoxamine. In addition, fluoxetine and fluvoxamine can inhibit the CYP3A3/4 enzyme, which degrades such common drugs as triazolo compounds, including alprazolam, triazolam, and trazodone. Increased drowsiness has been reported in patients treated concurrently with SSRIs and alprazolam, but no serious reactions have been reported. However, lower doses of the concomitant drugs may be required. At one point, H_2 blockers were thought to be particularly problematic vis-à-vis untoward interactions, but this has not been borne out.

Among the SSRIs, citalopram and escitalopram currently exhibit the least potential for pharmacokinetic interactions. Citalopram and escitalopram are weak inhibitors of not only CYP2D6 but also CYP3A3/4, CYP1A2, and CYP2C19. With venlafaxine, citalopram shares a low risk of drug interactions, which has made it popular in the treatment of geriatric patients.

Dosage and Administration

Among the factors that have contributed to the enormous popularity of the SSRIs is that the starting dose of the drug is frequently the optimal dose as well (Table 3–4). Given the already lengthy latency of onset of antidepressant action, the SSRIs typically do not require a prolonged titration period in which to achieve a therapeutic dose, as is common with the TCAs and the MAOIs.

Fluoxetine is usually initiated at 20 mg/day, and the maximum recommended dosage is 60 mg/day. A review of the efficacy data from double-blind studies of the use of fluoxetine in the treatment of major depression revealed that fluoxetine produced maximal benefits at 20–40 mg/day, with lesser benefit noted at 60 mg/day. In fact, 60 mg/day appeared to be less effective and to have more side effects than did 20–40 mg/day. Because 20 mg was often effective and the drug has a long half-life, the manufacturer finalized the rec-

Table 3–4. Selective serotonin reuptake inhibitors (SSRIs) and other available antidepressants: names, formulations and strengths, and dosages

Generic name[a]	Brand name[b]	Formulations[c] and strengths	Usual therapeutic dosage (mg/day)[d]
5-HT$_2$ antagonists			
Nefazodone hydrochloride	Nefazodone hydrochloride	Tablets: 50, 100, 150, 200, 250 mg	300–500
Trazodone hydrochloride	Trazodone hydrochloride	Tablets: 50, 100, 150, 300 mg	150–300
MAOIs			
Isocarboxazid	Marplan	Tablets: 10 mg	20–60
Phenelzine sulfate	Nardil	Tablets: 15 mg	
Selegiline	Emsam	Film (extended release): 6, 9, 12 mg/24 hr	6–12
Selegiline hydrochloride	Selegiline hydrochloride	Capsules: 5 mg	5–20
		Tablets: 5 mg	5–20
	Zelapar	Orally disintegrating tablets: 1.25 mg	1.25–5
Tranylcypromine sulfate	Parnate	Tablets: 10 mg	30–60
SNRIs			
Desvenlafaxine	Desvenlafaxine	Tablets (extended release): 50, 100 mg	50–100
Desvenlafaxine succinate	Pristiq	Tablets (extended release): 25, 50, 100 mg	50–100
Duloxetine hydrochloride	Cymbalta	Capsules (delayed release): 20, 30, 60 mg	60–120
	Duloxetine hydrochloride	Capsules (delayed release): 20, 30, 40, 60 mg	60–120
Levomilnacipran hydrochloride	Fetzima	Capsules: 20, 40, 80, 120 mg	40–120
Milnacipran hydrochloride	Savella[f]	Tablets: 12.5, 25, 50, 100 mg	100–200
Venlafaxine besylate	Venlafaxine besylate	Tablets (extended release): 112.5 mg	
Venlafaxine hydrochloride	Effexor XR	Capsules: 37.5, 75, 150 mg	75–375
	Venlafaxine hydrochloride	Tablets (extended release): 37.5, 75, 150, 225 mg	75–375
		Tablets: 25, 37.5, 50, 75, 100 mg	75–375

Table 3–4.   Selective serotonin reuptake inhibitors (SSRIs) and other available antidepressants: names, formulations and strengths, and dosages *(continued)*

Generic name[a]	Brand name[b]	Formulations[c] and strengths	Usual therapeutic dosage (mg/day)[d]
SSRIs			
Citalopram hydrobromide	Celexa	Tablets: 10, 20, 40 mg	20–40
	Citalopram hydrobromide	Capsules: 30 mg	20–40
		Solution: 10 mg/5 mL	
Escitalopram oxalate	Escitalopram oxalate	Solution: 5 mg/5 mL	10–20
	Lexapro	Tablets: 5, 10, 20 mg	10–20
Fluoxetine hydrochloride	Fluoxetine hydrochloride	Capsules (delayed release): 90 mg	20–60
		Solution: 20 mg/5 mL	
		Tablets: 10, 20, 60 mg	
	Prozac	Capsules: 10, 20, 40 mg	
Fluvoxamine maleate	Fluvoxamine maleate	Capsules (extended release): 100, 150 mg	100–200
		Tablets: 25, 50, 100 mg	
Paroxetine hydrochloride	Paxil	Suspension: 10 mg/5 mL	20–50
		Tablets: 10, 20, 30, 40 mg	
	Paxil CR	Tablets: 12.5, 25, 37.5 mg	
Paroxetine mesylate	Brisdelle	Capsules: 7.5 mg	7.5[g]
Sertraline hydrochloride	Sertraline hydrochloride	Capsules: 150, 200 mg	50–200
		Concentrate: 20 mg/mL	
	Zoloft	Tablets: 25, 50, 100 mg	50–200

Table 3–4. Selective serotonin reuptake inhibitors (SSRIs) and other available antidepressants: names, formulations and strengths, and dosages (continued)

Generic name[a]	Brand name[b]	Formulations[c] and strengths	Usual therapeutic dosage (mg/day)[d]
TCAs			
Amitriptyline hydrochloride	Amitriptyline hydrochloride	Tablets: 10, 25, 50, 75, 100 mg	
Clomipramine hydrochloride	Anafranil	Capsules: 25, 50, 75 mg	
Desipramine hydrochloride	Norpramin	Tablets: 10, 25, 50, 75, 100, 150 mg	
Doxepin hydrochloride	Doxepin hydrochloride	Capsules: 10, 25, 50, 75, 100, 150 mg	
		Concentrate: 10 mg/mL	
	Silenor	Tablets: 3, 6 mg	
Imipramine hydrochloride	Imipramine hydrochloride	Tablets: 10, 25, 50 mg	
Imipramine pamoate	Imipramine pamoate	Capsules: 75, 100, 125, 150 mg	
Nortriptyline hydrochloride	Nortriptyline hydrochloride	Solution: 10 mg/5 mL	
	Pamelor	Capsules: 10, 25, 50, 75 mg	
Protriptyline hydrochloride	Protriptyline hydrochloride	Tablets: 5, 10 mg	
Trimipramine maleate	Trimipramine maleate	Capsules: 25, 50, 100 mg	
Other			
Amitriptyline hydrochloride + chlordiazepoxide	Chlordiazepoxide and amitriptyline hydrochloride	Tablets: 5 mg/12.5 mg; 10 mg/25 mg	
Amitriptyline hydrochloride+perphenazine	Perphenazine and amitriptyline hydrochloride	Tablets: 2 mg/10 mg, 2 mg/25 mg, 4 mg/10 mg, 4 mg/25 mg, 4 mg/50 mg	
Brexanolone	Zulresso	Solution: 5 mg/mL	
Bupropion hydrobromide	Aplenzin	Tablets (extended release): 174, 348, 522 mg	

Table 3–4. Selective serotonin reuptake inhibitors (SSRIs) and other available antidepressants: names, formulations and strengths, and dosages *(continued)*

Generic name[a]	Brand name[b]	Formulations[c] and strengths	Usual therapeutic dosage (mg/day)[d]
Bupropion hydrochloride	Bupropion hydrochloride	Tablets: 75, 100 mg	200–450
	Forfivo XL	Tablets: 450 mg	
	Wellbutrin SR	Tablets: 100, 150, 200 mg	
	Wellbutrin XL	Tablets: 150, 300 mg	
Dextromethorphan hydrobromide+bupropion hydrochloride	Auvelity	Tablets (extended release): 45 mg/105 mg	
Esketamine hydrochloride	Spravato	Spray: 28 mg	
Mirtazapine	Mirtazapine	Tablets: 7.5, 15, 30, 45 mg	15–45
	Remeron Soltab	Orally disintegrating tablets: 15, 30, 45 mg	15–45
Olanzapine+fluoxetine hydrochloride	Symbax	Capsules: 3 mg/25 mg, 6 mg/25 mg, 6 mg/25 mg, 6 mg/50 mg, 12 mg/25 mg, 12 mg/50 mg	
Vilazodone hydrochloride	Viibryd	Tablets: 10, 20, 40 mg	40
Vortioxetine hydrobromide	Trintellix	Tablets: 5, 10, 20 mg	10–20

Note. CR=controlled release; 5-HT$_2$=serotonin$_2$ receptor; MAOIs=monoamine oxidase inhibitors; SR=sustained release; TCAs=tricyclic antidepressants; XL=extended release; XR=sustained release.

[a]All the tricyclic and tetracyclic antidepressants shown are available generically. Most of the brand-name drugs listed have been discontinued.

[b]Where the brand name is the same as generic name, the brand-name products may be no longer available.

[c]Injectable formulations not available.

[d]Dosage ranges are approximate. Many patients will respond at relatively low dosages (even dosages below the ranges given). Other patients may require higher dosages.

[e]Available in divided dose formulations.

[f]Approved by the FDA for fibromyalgia; dosages given are recommended for that use.

[g]Dosage for vasomotor symptoms in menopause.

ommended initial dosing at 20 mg/day for 3 weeks, with subsequent increases to 40–80 mg/day if indicated. Patients with significant psychomotor retardation often seem to require at least 40 mg/day. In other patients, 10 mg/day may be effective. The drug is currently available in 10-mg, 20-mg, and 40-mg capsules, as well as in 10- and 20-mg tablets and in a suspension. Dosages as low as 2 mg/day can be obtained with the suspension, and this is particularly useful in patients who cannot initially tolerate higher dosages. Patients who have not responded to a lower dosage (20 mg/day) may subsequently improve if the dosage is increased to 40–60 mg/day (Fava et al. 1994).

Some years ago, a 90-mg, once-weekly form of fluoxetine was introduced. This form was designed to be an alternative to daily treatment with fluoxetine at 20 mg/day and is meant for use in the maintenance phase of treatment only. Some patients prefer taking one capsule weekly rather than daily. Taking one capsule every 3 days appears roughly equivalent to 40 mg/day. Some patients take two capsules per week on the same day to achieve the equivalent of 40 mg/day. (It is unclear, however, whether taking two 90-mg capsules equals 40 mg/day.) Staggering the dose every 3 days decreases side effects. Dosing the weekly form of fluoxetine every 3 days appears to be well tolerated.

Dosing of paroxetine is much like that of fluoxetine, with an initial dosage of 20 mg/day. The immediate-release form of the drug is currently available in 10-mg, 20-mg, 30-mg, and 40-mg tablets. The tablets are scored, and patients intolerant of a full tablet can have the dose reduced to a half tablet for 2–3 weeks. If no response is seen, the dosage may then be increased each week by 10–20 mg/day until a maximum dosage of 50 mg/day is achieved. Data suggest that patients with more serious depression require higher dosages (30–50 mg/day). Controlled-release (CR) paroxetine is currently available in 12.5-mg, 25-mg, and 37.5-mg tablets, which are equivalent to the 10-mg, 20-mg, and 30-mg immediate-release tablets, respectively. (At one point since the previous edition of this manual, the CR formulation was taken off the market because of quality control issues during the manufacturing.)

Citalopram is dosed at 20–40 mg/day. In 2011 the FDA put out a warning about an increase in QT interval with citalopram dosages greater than 40 mg/day. The QT prolongation was modest but enough to result in the FDA warning. Thus, 40 mg/day is the current maximum recommended dosage. The FDA warning has not been extended to escitalopram, and we do not routinely obtain ECGs for patients taking citalopram or escitalopram. Elderly patients and those with a history of arrhythmia may benefit from a baseline and repeat ECG. The side effects of escitalopram at 20 mg/day roughly equal those seen with citalopram at 40 mg/day.

The dosage range for sertraline is somewhat wider than that for fluoxetine, paroxetine, and citalopram. In addition, a more linear dose-response curve separates sertraline from the other SSRIs, which have a relatively flat dose-response curve. Therapy is usually initiated at 50 mg/day, although, as with the other SSRIs, a lower starting dosage is sometimes required. The 50-mg dose may be continued for 2 weeks, and if no response is seen, the dosage may then be increased weekly by 50 mg/day until a maximum dosage of 200 mg/day is achieved. Sertraline is available in 25-mg, 50-mg, and 100-mg tablets as well as a concentrate. The different tablet strengths are priced similarly. Thus, it is typically more economical to prescribe the scored 100-mg tablets and instruct patients to break them in half to achieve a dosage of 50 mg/day.

Fluvoxamine, like sertraline, has a wider dosage range. It is usually initiated at 50–100 mg/day. Because of fluvoxamine's short half-life, dosages higher than 100 mg/day require divided doses in order to optimize drug availability. In premarketing studies, most patients with major depression required dosages in the range of 100–200 mg/day. However, some patients required a dosage as high as 300 mg/day. The recommended starting dosage for fluvoxamine CR is 100 mg/day taken at bedtime. As with the immediate-release form, the maximum dosage for fluvoxamine CR is 300 mg/day, but this formulation can be taken once a day.

Discontinuation

Discontinuation symptoms may be less common with the SSRIs than with the TCAs. However, a number of case reports and double-blind studies do indicate that a discontinuation syndrome may occur with the sudden discontinuation of some SSRIs, especially the shorter-acting agents paroxetine, sertraline, and fluvoxamine.

The most common presentation of an SSRI discontinuation syndrome is a flulike condition with malaise, nausea, and headaches occurring within 2–7 days of stopping an SSRI. Paresthesias, dizziness, agitation, and rebound depression have also been reported when the drugs are suddenly discontinued. The mechanism underlying these symptoms is unclear. Because of paroxetine's greater effect at the serotonin transporter, shorter half-life, and anticholinergic properties, discontinuation symptoms may be more common with this agent than with the other SSRIs. Fluoxetine's very long half-life and citalopram's medium half-life may diminish the risk of discontinuation symptoms with these drugs. Of the SSRIs, fluoxetine may be stopped abruptly without much risk of difficulty. However, for the shorter-acting SSRIs, it may be prudent to taper the drugs over several weeks, particularly if the patient required a prolonged titration upward because of adverse effects. Tapering by 25% of the dose per week for doses greater than 30 mg of paroxetine, 100 mg of sertraline, and 150 mg of fluvoxamine is quite reasonable if it is practical to do so. In trials of 4 weeks or less, faster taper schedules can be tried, and most patients will not require a taper.

If discontinuation symptoms occur, the first step may be to increase the dose to the previous dose and taper more gradually. Often, resuming the previous dose will resolve the discontinuation symptoms within 48 hours. Occasionally, clinicians have substituted a longer-acting agent such as fluoxetine for a shorter-acting agent such as paroxetine in patients with substantial discontinuation symptoms. However, there are no good data on the safety or efficacy of this approach.

When starting an MAOI after discontinuing an SSRI, a safe washout period depends on the half-life of the drug and its metabolites. For fluoxetine, the manufacturer has recommended waiting 5 weeks when changing from fluoxetine to an MAOI. This period is five times the half-life of the active metabolite of fluoxetine, norfluoxetine. It is conceivable that a shorter period (e.g., 3 weeks) may suffice, but no data are available. The other SSRIs are shorter acting than fluoxetine, and a 2-week washout appears adequate. When going from an MAOI to an SSRI, a period of 2 weeks of no MAOI is recommended before starting the SSRI.

A common question in clinical practice is "Does it make sense to switch from one SSRI to another if one is not working?" Although the practice of switching from one SSRI to another is common, very few prospective, controlled data are available to support the practice. Clearly, however, patients who are intolerant of one SSRI may achieve benefit by being switched to another. Brown and Harrison (1995) reported that patients may respond to sertraline after not responding to fluoxetine. The largest study to date to examine the question of switching to another SSRI after not achieving response with the first is STAR*D (Rush et al. 2006). In that study, 727 patients who did not achieve remission while taking citalopram were switched to either sertraline, venlafaxine, or bupropion. The remission and response rates when patients were switched to sertraline were about the same as those for patients who were switched to venlafaxine or bupropion. Although this open study design may contribute to one-comparison agents tending to consistently look similar in outcome, the study does support that switching within the class of SSRIs may be as good as switching outside the class. Thase and colleagues (1997) found that patients who had a poor response to an initial trial of sertraline often achieved a good response when switched to fluoxetine. As many as 50% of patients who have not responded to one SSRI may respond to another. However, melancholic inpatients who have not responded to an adequate trial of an SSRI appear to have a much lower chance of responding to another SSRI. Along the same lines, Sacchetti et al. (1994) found that patients with recurrent major depression were far more likely to respond to the same SSRI they had responded to in a previous episode than they were to respond to a different SSRI. For example, if a patient had responded to fluoxetine in the index depressive episode, they had about a 90% chance of responding to fluoxetine in a subsequent episode but only a 50% chance of responding to fluvoxamine. It is unclear from the report whether patients were blinded to the challenge. It is evident that many patients in clinical practice who start off taking one SSRI will end up taking another agent. In a retrospective review, at least 25% of patients treated with one SSRI subsequently ended up taking another SSRI (Nurnberg et al. 1999c). The authors concluded that the SSRIs are not interchangeable because patients who discontinue one SSRI because of either lack of efficacy or lack of tolerability may do well with another agent. Likewise, in another study, 91% of patients who were intolerant to fluoxetine tolerated sertraline (Brown and Harrison 1995).

Serotonin-Norepinephrine Reuptake Inhibitors

The SNRIs inlcude venlafaxine, desvenlafaxine, duloxetine, levomilnacipran, and milnacipran. Venlafaxine (Effexor) (Figure 3–2) is a phenylethylamine that was released to the U.S. market in 1994. In 1998, it became available in an extended-release form (Effexor XR), which is taken once a day. Along with its FDA indication for the treatment of depression, Effexor XR became the

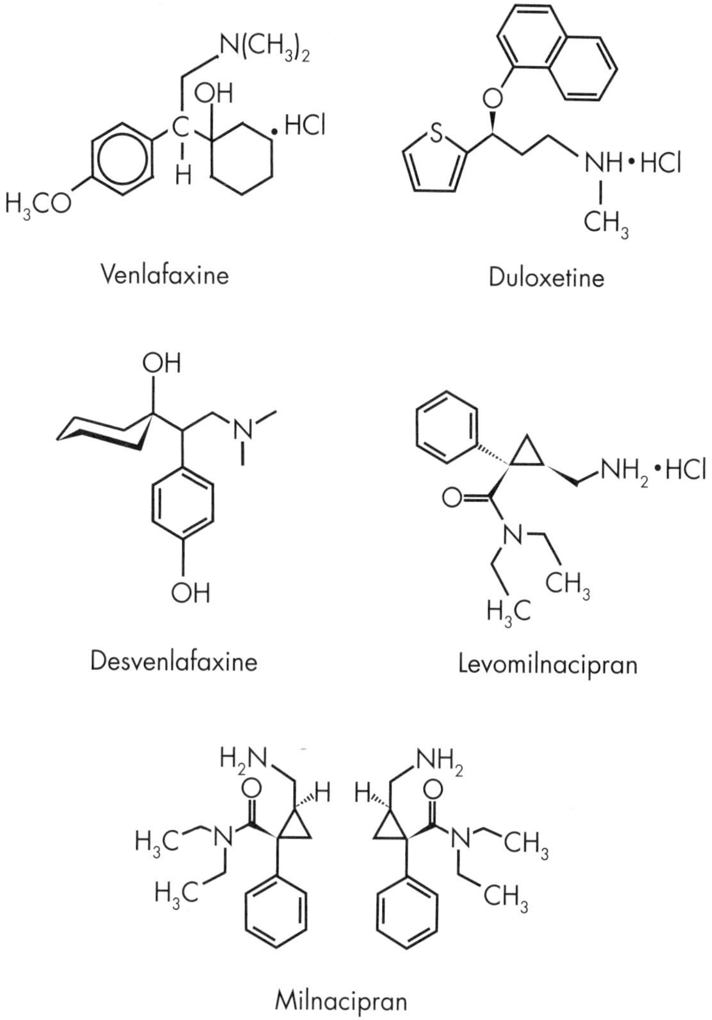

Figure 3–2. Chemical structures of the serotonin-norepinephrine reuptake inhibitors.

first antidepressant approved for the treatment of GAD and has also been approved for the treatment of social anxiety disorder.

Venlafaxine and other SNRIs have grown in popularity as drugs with an efficacy and mechanism of action that may be like those of TCA drugs without the safety or side-effect liability of the TCAs. Venlafaxine's major metabolite, desmethylvenlafaxine, became available in 2008 for the treatment of major depression. Desvenlafaxine is a more potent reuptake inhibitor of norepinephrine than venlafaxine but is less potent an inhibitor than duloxetine.

Duloxetine (Cymbalta) was released in 2004 after a long delay. Like venlafaxine and desvenlafaxine, it has little affinity for other neurotransmitter receptors such as muscarinic or histaminic. However, it is a relatively more potent norepinephrine reuptake inhibitor than is venlafaxine. Whether this increased potency translates into improved efficacy is unclear. Initially, we see duloxetine as an antidepressant that will be a first-line agent in depressed patients who have comorbidities such as pain or stress incontinence. Duloxetine also makes sense as a first-line agent for patients with serious depression, including those with melancholic and psychotic subtypes. We suspect it will have an important role to play in treating resistant depression. Over time, the SNRIs have become first-line agents for less severe depression as well.

A fourth SNRI, milnacipran (Savella), was approved in 2009 in the United States for the treatment of fibromyalgia. Many randomized trials have been completed, mostly overseas, in the treatment of major depression, with mixed results. In 2013 the active enantiomer of milnacipran, levomilnacipran (Fetzima), was approved for the treatment of major depression.

Pharmacological Effects

In contrast to the SSRIs, the potent 5-HT-blocking effects of venlafaxine are complemented by mild norepinephrine transporter (NET) inhibition. Typically, dosages of venlafaxine greater than 150 mg/day are needed to see a clinically significant effect on norepinephrine. In contrast, duloxetine is a potent 5-HT and norepinephrine reuptake inhibitor, whereas desvenlafaxine is a stronger inhibitor of NET than is venlafaxine but a less potent inhibitor of NET than is duloxetine.

Several other pharmacological properties distinguish the SNRIs. For example, the SNRIs promote a rapid downregulation of β-adrenergic receptor–coupled cyclic adenosine monophosphate. This effect may correlate with an earlier onset of action for the SNRIs, as some premarketing studies have suggested. In addition, venlafaxine and desvenlafaxine are more weakly bound to protein (27%) than are other antidepressants; this weaker binding may decrease the likelihood of displacing tightly bound drugs, such as warfarin and phenytoin. Also, both venlafaxine and desvenlafaxine share with citalopram and escitalopram a very low potential for pharmacokinetic drug interactions because they are not potent inhibitors of any CYP hepatic enzymes. However, whereas venlafaxine is a substrate for CYP2D6, desvenlafaxine is not. Therefore, desvenlafaxine's metabolism is not affected by drugs that are inhibitors (e.g., fluoxetine) or inducers (carbamazepine) of CYP2D6. In fact, desvenlafaxine does not undergo much hepatic metabolism at all. Relative to other antidepressants, hepatic metabolism of desvenlafaxine is among the most limited. Likewise, milnacipran undergoes very little hepatic metabolism. Both milnacipran and levomilnacipran have shorter half-lives and lower protein binding than does venlafaxine. In addition, both milnacipran and levomilnacipran are excreted largely unchanged in the urine. Levomilnacipran undergoes demethylation via CYP3A3/4. The two drugs are also well absorbed with oral dosing.

Indications

The SNRIs have proven useful in the treatment of both outpatients with major depression and inpatients with more severe forms of depression. Given the ongoing debate about the utility of the SSRIs for more seriously depressed inpatients, the SNRIs appear to provide a safe and effective alternative to the TCAs in treating melancholic patients. In one study, venlafaxine appeared to be markedly more effective than fluoxetine in the treatment of melancholic inpatients (Clerc et al. 1994). Similar studies have suggested that duloxetine may be more effective than SSRIs in achieving remission, but other studies have not demonstrated this finding (Khan et al. 2011).

Like venlafaxine, duloxetine appears to be an effective antidepressant. Several but not all double-blind studies have now demonstrated the utility of duloxetine, particularly at achieving remission of depressive symptoms relative to placebo. In a 9-week trial, duloxetine 60 mg administered once daily was compared with placebo in treating patients with major depression. By the end of 9 weeks, 44% of 123 duloxetine-treated patients had achieved remission, compared with only 16% of the 122 patients receiving placebo (Detke et al. 2002). In a second trial, 173 patients were randomly assigned to treatment with duloxetine up to 120 mg/day, fluoxetine 20 mg/day, or placebo for 8 weeks. Duloxetine appeared to be more likely to achieve response and remission than either fluoxetine or placebo (Goldstein et al. 2002).

Desvenlafaxine is indicated only in the treatment of major depression. Its efficacy in the treatment of major depression appears comparable to that of other SNRIs. Dosages of 50–400 mg/day have been studied and found to be effective in the treatment of major depressive disorder (MDD). However, the higher dosages were not more effective than lower dosages but were associated with more adverse events. Thus, 50 mg/day is the standard dosage of desvenlafaxine (Lohoff and Rickels 2008).

A second FDA indication for Effexor XR and duloxetine is for the treatment of GAD. All five controlled trials of Effexor XR in the treatment of GAD reported to date have shown superiority to placebo and sometimes to comparison drugs such as buspirone (Davidson et al. 1999; Diaz-Martinez et al. 1998). Some studies indicated that relatively low dosages of Effexor XR (75–150 mg/day) are useful in the treatment of GAD, and most patients obtain some benefit within 2 weeks, with additional improvement often seen over the next 6 weeks of treatment. Studies out to 6 months have reported significantly greater efficacy for Effexor XR over placebo, with many patients continuing to improve beyond their acute responses (Gelenberg et al. 2000). Extended-release venlafaxine is approved for the treatment of social anxiety disorder (Altamura et al. 1999; Lenderking et al. 1999). Likewise, venlafaxine has some demonstrated efficacy in the treatment of PTSD, including PTSD that has not responded to an SSRI (Hamner and Frueh 1998).

Duloxetine's efficacy in the treatment of GAD looks like that of venlafaxine. Three pivotal trials in GAD involving about 800 patients indicated that patients with GAD who were treated with duloxetine were significantly more likely to show improvement, response, and remission on the Hamilton Anxiety Scale than were patients receiving placebo. Duloxetine was effective at dosages of 60–120 mg/day, but higher dosages were not necessarily more effective than lower dosages (Rynn et al. 2008).

Because the mechanism of action of the SNRIs is similar to that of the TCAs, the SNRIs also have utility in treating some pain conditions. Venlafaxine has been studied in the treatment of neuropathic pain, fibromyalgia, and other chronic pain conditions (Davis and Smith 1999; Kiayias et al. 2000; Pernia et al. 2000). Venlafaxine appears to be about as useful as the TCAs and superior to the SSRIs for chronic pain. Dosages higher than 150 mg/day are often required. Duloxetine also appears to be useful in the treatment of some somatic and pain symptoms. In a study by Detke and colleagues (2002), duloxetine-treated patients had not only an improvement in their depression but also a significant reduction in shoulder pain, back pain, and pain that interfered with daily activities. It is likely that, as with the TCAs, the improvement in pain was independent of the improvement in depression. Indeed, studies of duloxetine in the treatment of diabetic neuropathy have shown clear benefit, and duloxetine was approved for the treatment of neuropathy shortly after it was approved for the treatment of depression.

In 2008, duloxetine was also the second drug (after pregabalin) approved for the treatment of fibromyalgia. Two pivotal trials involving about 900 patients demonstrated that duloxetine at dosages of 60 mg/day or 120 mg/day reduced overall pain on the brief pain inventory at 3 months. In one of the studies, sustained benefit in pain was also seen with 6 months of duloxetine treatment of fibromyalgia (Russell et al. 2008). Lilly, the manufacturer of duloxetine, obtained additional approval for the drug in an expanded indication for musculoskeletal pain based on two trials in the treatment of knee pain associated with osteoarthritis and one study in the treatment of chronic back pain. Milnacipran has been used for chronic pain conditions in Europe for some years and received a fibromyalgia indication in the United States in January 2009. Controlled trials with milnacipran show a consistent benefit on the pain component of fibromyalgia but also associated features such as sleep and cognition. The manufacturer of desvenlafaxine is also expected to seek indications for various pain conditions. Early studies suggested a role for desvenlafaxine in the treatment of neuropathic pain, but reportedly this was not confirmed in follow-on studies. Not surprisingly, venlafaxine has also shown benefit in pain conditions, including neuropathic pain associated with diabetes, in controlled trials.

The SNRIs also have been studied for use in other disorders. For example, several studies suggest that venlafaxine may be effective in both childhood and adult ADHD at dosages of 150–300 mg/day. Like other antidepressants that appear useful in ADHD, including desipramine and bupropion, venlafaxine lacks the disadvantages of drugs such as methylphenidate that have some potential for abuse and require Drug Enforcement Administration triplicate forms.

Another condition duloxetine may be valuable in treating is stress urinary incontinence. In fact, duloxetine is approved outside the United States for treating stress urinary incontinence. In a large trial involving 533 women, duloxetine at dosages of 20–80 mg/day was superior to placebo in reducing the frequency of incontinence episodes. Patients treated with duloxetine had up to a 64% decrease in incontinence episodes, whereas patients receiving placebo had a 41% decrease in such episodes (Norton et al. 2002). The differences from placebo were even greater in patients who had a high baseline frequency of incontinence episodes.

Desvenlafaxine, like venlafaxine and paroxetine, appears to be effective in the treatment of vasomotor symptoms associated with menopause. At dosages of 100 mg/day and 150 mg/day, desvenlafaxine reduced the number and intensity of hot flashes associated with menopause in 454 women (Archer et al. 2009), although here, too, there are failed trials. Earlier work with venlafaxine also suggested benefit in the treatment of vasomotor symptoms.

Levomilnacipran is approved in the treatment of major depression, whereas milnacipran currently has an FDA-approved indication only for fibromyalgia. Milnacipran joins only duloxetine and pregabalin as medications approved for fibromyalgia at this writing. However, it might be assumed that all the SNRIs have some utility in the treatment of fibromyalgia and other pain conditions. The relative equipotency of milnacipran on the serotonin transporter and norepinephrine transporter appears to make the drug well suited for the treatment of pain conditions. In contrast, levomilnacipran is a more potent noradrenergic agent. Although levomilnacipran has been well vetted as a treatment for depression, it may be less well tolerated than the other SNRIs in the treatment of anxiety disorders. On the other hand, the noradrenergic properties of levomilnacipran would seem to lend themselves well to the treatment of ADHD. There are some early, yet unpublished, investigations that suggest that levomilnacipran may be effective in the treatment of pediatric ADHD.

Side Effects

SNRIs share many of the side effects of the SSRIs. For example, GI side effects are common with the SNRIs. In fact, the SNRIs may have a somewhat greater propensity for causing nausea than do some of the SSRIs. As with the SSRIs, adaptation to this side effect occurs rapidly, in the first 2–3 weeks of therapy. Some studies suggest that the rate of sexual side effects seen with duloxetine may be lower than the rate seen with SSRIs. However, these have tended not to apply to specific rating instruments. Any potent serotonin reuptake inhibitor can cause sexual side effects, and all three SNRIs are potently serotonergic. Nonetheless, it is possible the noradrenergic effects of duloxetine may mitigate the serotonergic sexual side effects. Venlafaxine and desvenlafaxine, which are less noradrenergic, may have a greater tendency for sexual side effects, but no comparison studies have yet been done to examine this issue.

One side effect of the SNRIs that differs from those of the SSRIs is treatment-emergent hypertension. This noradrenergically mediated side effect occurs in about 5% of patients at dosages of venlafaxine (immediate release) less than 200 mg/day and in 13% of patients at dosages greater than 300 mg/day. The increase in blood pressure is usually modest, with an average increase in diastolic blood pressure of about 5–7 mm Hg with venlafaxine at high doses and about 2 mm Hg with duloxetine. Desvenlafaxine also shows a dose-related increase in blood pressure, with 0.5% of patients showing a sustained increase in diastolic blood pressure of >90 mm Hg and 10 points above baseline, compared with about 2.3% of patients treated at a dosage of 400 mg/day showing this elevation. Duloxetine may also increase blood pressure, but perhaps less so than the other SNRIs. One possible explanation for the lower rates of hypertension in use of duloxetine may be its greater protein binding relative to desvenlafaxine and venlafaxine. Nonetheless, it is important to monitor blood pressure, particularly in the first 2 months of treatment at higher doses of the SNRIs. We have seen some patients with a rise in diastolic blood pressure of 20–30 mm Hg while taking an SNRI. If hypertension occurs, reducing the dose is often helpful. If it is not feasible to do so, then clinicians should consider adding a β-blocker or an α-blocker. The impression is that hypertension has been less problematic with the extended-release formulation, perhaps reflecting lower total daily doses or lack of peak effects.

A related noradrenergic side effect of SNRIs is an increase in heart rate. The average increase with the SNRIs is around 1–4 bpm (beats per minute), but higher doses are clearly associated with greater increases than are lower doses. Some patients, particularly elderly patients with a history of tachyarrhythmias, should be monitored more carefully. An SSRI might be a better choice in these patients.

Hepatotoxicity has been reported with duloxetine in patients with preexisting liver disease, and duloxetine has a hepatic warning in the package insert. Inclusion of the warning was based on a finding of 77 cases of treatment-emergent hepatic events in more than 8,000 treated patients versus 34 cases of treatment-emergent hepatoxicity in more than 6,000 patients with placebo control. The overall rate of hepatic events, such as an increase in liver enzymes to three times the upper limits of normal, is about 0.008%, a rate similar to that seen in SSRIs and many other drugs. It makes clinical sense to monitor liver function in any patient with preexisting liver disease treated with a drug that undergoes extensive hepatic metabolism. It appears that milnacipran also has some association with elevations in liver function test values, particularly in patients with preexisting liver disease. Thus, it carries the same warning as does duloxetine.

The more potent noradrenergic effects of levomilnacipran, milnacipran, duloxetine, and, to a lesser extent, desvenlafaxine also result in a variety of anticholinergic-like side effects, including dry mouth, constipation, and urinary retention. Elderly males might be particularly susceptible to retaining urine and should be monitored.

Overdose

Fatal overdoses with venlafaxine, as with the SSRIs, are rare but are occasionally reported. As with the SSRIs, moderate overdoses of less than 30 times the daily dose tend to be more associated with GI upset than with other symptoms. Gastric lavage is often helpful in these cases of moderate overdose. More substantial overdoses involving 10 g or more have sometimes resulted in seizures (Bhattacharjee et al. 2001; Gittelman and Kirby 1993; Mainie et al. 2001) and a serotonin syndrome (Spiller et al. 1994). In the United Kingdom, there has been considerable concern about the safety margin of venlafaxine in overdoses (Buckley and McManus 2002). A warning about risk for lethality in overdose was added to venlafaxine's package insert there in 2004. However, those warnings were revised in 2006 and no longer require a baseline ECG or a contraindication in patients with electrolyte imbalances. Still, there is some evidence of an increased arrhythmia risk in overdose, although the risk is substantially less than that associated with the TCAs, and caution is warranted in patients with preexisting arrhythmias (Taylor et al. 2013). Fatal overdoses appear more uncommon with duloxetine than with venlafaxine. Overdoses up to 1,200 mg have been treated with lavage and supportive care. Likewise, desvenlafaxine overdoses have generally not been associated with fatalities (Cooper et al. 2017). However, in postmarketing surveillance, desvenlafaxine overdoses in combination with other drugs have sometimes been associated with arrhythmias, serotonin syndrome, rhabdomyolysis, and other life-threatening events. Because these cases were not single-drug overdoses, it is unclear how much desvenlafaxine contributed to the toxicity. Given the additional concern about venlafaxine overdoses relative to SSRIs, it may be prudent also to be more careful about the use of desvenlafaxine in suicidal patients. There have been few cases of milnacipran or levomilnacipran overdoses. In clinical trials, modest overdoses of up to 360 mg of levomilnacipran or 1,000 mg of milnacipran (about a week's supply) were not associated with serious side effects.

Drug Interactions

The SNRIs can precipitate a serotonin syndrome when combined with the MAOIs, and this combination is therefore contraindicated. Therefore, 2 weeks should elapse after stopping an MAOI before starting an SNRI. Because venlafaxine has a short half-life (5 hours for venlafaxine and 11 hours for *O*-desmethylvenlafaxine), a 1-week washout is sufficient before starting an MAOI.

Venlafaxine and duloxetine are weak inhibitors of CYP2D6. Like citalopram and escitalopram, the SNRIs do not appear to be potent inhibitors of other hepatic enzymes. However, both duloxetine and venlafaxine are metabolized by the CYP2D6 enzyme and, to some extent, the CYP1A2 enzyme as well. Therefore, cimetidine, paroxetine, or other drugs that inhibit the metabolism of CYP2D6 could result in a more pronounced increase in blood pressure or other side effects. Venlafaxine can increase haloperidol blood levels, but this is not mediated by an effect on the CYP1A2 or CYP2D6 enzyme. Rather, it may reflect an effect on excretion.

Desvenlafaxine is neither a substrate nor an inhibitor of CYP2D6. Thus, it is less likely to be a problem than other SNRIs in either an individual who is a genetically slow or rapid metabolizer of CYP2D6 or someone who is also taking a CYP2D6 inhibitor or inducer.

Like desvenlafaxine, milnacipran undergoes minimal CYP metabolism, and the majority of the drug is excreted unchanged. It is even less tightly bound to protein (13%) than either desvenlafaxine or venlafaxine. The risk of pharmacokinetic drug interactions appears small with milnacipran. Likewise, the protein binding for levomilnacipran is only about 22%, and this drug is not likely to displace other drugs that are tightly protein bound. Levomilnacipran is a substrate for CYP3A4, and the drug doagse should probably not exceed 80 mg/day in patients who are taking potent inhibitors of CYP3A4 drugs, such as ketoconazole.

Dosage and Administration

The manufacturer recommends that the extended-release formulation of venlafaxine (Effexor XR) be initiated at 37.5 mg. Thereafter, doses can be increased by 37.5 mg every 3 days or 75 mg per week until a dosage of 150 mg/day is reached. Beyond that, increases should be at a rate of 75 mg per week. Although the manufacturer suggests that elderly patients do not require a lower starting dosage, many geriatric psychiatrists have found that a starting dosage of 37.5 mg/day is better tolerated. Increase of dosage should be gradual. For the extended-release formulation of venlafaxine, the maximum recommended dosage is 225 mg/day; for the immediate-release form, it is 375 mg/day. We recommend using the extended-release formulation. Most depressed outpatients appear to respond to dosages in the range of 75–225 mg/day. Therefore, if no response is seen at the starting dosage for 2 weeks, the dosage may be titrated upward in 37.5-mg increments every 3 days or so, as tolerated. In premarketing studies, the dosage was sometimes increased rapidly to the maximum dosage in the first week of treatment. This rapid titration was sometimes associated with a more rapid onset of action, but it also was poorly tolerated in many cases. Venlafaxine does have a linear dose-response curve, and higher dosages are associated with greater response (as well as more prominent side effects). Inpatients with melancholic depression and patients with depression that was refractory to other treatments often require dosages closer to the maximum dosage of 375 mg/day (for the immediate-release form) administered in divided doses. On occasion we have used even higher dosages (450–600 mg/day) without problem.

We have tried a variety of doses of duloxetine in clinical trials. In general, starting the duloxetine at 20 or 30 mg in the morning with food is a reasonable approach. After 3–7 days, we increase the dosage to 60 mg/day. Some patients have less nausea at 30 mg bid, but most patients can manage 60 mg taken once daily. It is reasonable to keep the dosage at 60 mg/day for 4 weeks before going up to 90 mg/day and then 120 mg/day in divided doses. However, dosages above 60 mg/day are not necessarily more effective than 60 mg/day.

One trial compared venlafaxine (immediate release) and duloxetine in the treatment of major depression. Starting dosages were 75 mg/day of venlafaxine and 60 mg/day of duloxetine. Duloxetine was associated with twice as high a rate of dropout due to side effects as venlafaxine. These data suggest that 30 mg of duloxetine is more like 75 mg of venlafaxine from a tolerability standpoint.

The starting dosage of desvenlafaxine is 50 mg/day, although it is not unreasonable to start older patients or those with a history of medication intolerance at 25 mg/day. The registration trials did not demonstrate that higher doses of desvenlafaxine were more efficacious than lower doses. However, the registration trials were not designed or powered to show a difference between different doses. Thus, in a patient who has not responded to 50 mg of desvenlafaxine for 4 weeks, it is not unreasonable to increase the dose to 100 mg. Dosages up to 400 mg/day have been studied. These higher dosages are clearly associated with greater side effects but not necessarily greater efficacy. Therefore, for most patients, the recommended dosage is 50–100 mg/day.

Most of the studies examining the utility of milnacipran in the treatment of depression have started at 50 mg. Nausea has been a problem at these doses. For fibromyalgia, the starting dosage is 12.5 mg/day, with increases to 25 mg/day by day 3 and 50 mg/day by day 7. The target dosage is 100–200 mg/day for fibromyalgia. These dosages have generally been the ones used in antidepressant trials as well. The dosing of levomilnacipran is more straightforward. Levomilnacipran is started at 20 mg/day for 2 days, and the dosage is increased to 40 mg/day thereafter. A dosage of 40 mg/day may be effective in many patients, but, as with other SNRIs, some patients will only respond to higher dosages (up to 120 mg/day). Because the drug undergoes renal clearance, the maximum dosage of levomilnacipran in patients with severe renal insufficiency is probably 40 mg/day. However, even patients with more advanced liver disease seem to be able to tolerate higher doses of levomilnacipran because hepatic clearance of the drug is relatively low.

Discontinuation

The relatively short half-life and low protein binding of venlafaxine, desvenlafaxine, and milnacipran may predispose patients to an increased risk of discontinuation symptoms when the drug is stopped suddenly. At least half of patients taking desvenlafaxine (and one-third of patients receiving placebo) experience discontinuation symptoms when the medication is stopped suddenly, even at 50 mg/day. Significant dizziness has been reported with rapid discontinuation of venlafaxine, as have paresthesias and the typical SSRI withdrawal symptoms. Therefore, the manufacturer advises tapering the dose for any patient who has been taking the drug for longer than 7 days.

For patients taking venlafaxine for more than 2 weeks, a gradual taper over at least a 2-week period is advised, and some patients may require a 4-week taper or longer. Decreasing the dosage by 37.5 mg every 3 days or 75 mg per week circumvents withdrawal symptoms in many patients. The lowest dose of desvenlafaxine is 50 mg, so advising the patient to take the drug every other day for 1 week might be beneficial. Milnacipran may be decreased by 25 mg per week but may require tapering by 12.5-mg increments below 50 mg/day. The dosage of levomilnacipran can be tapered by a rate of 20 mg every 3–7 days in most patients. Switching to sertraline (Luckhaus and Jacob 2001) or supplementing with the antiemetic ondansetron (Raby 1998) may also help. In double-blind studies of duloxetine, rapid discontinuation was associated with expected symptoms. However, duloxetine's longer half-life and higher protein binding may be associated with a lower frequency of discontinuation symptoms compared with venlafaxine. Duloxetine may be safely tapered in most patients by decreasing the total dose by 30 mg per week.

5-HT$_2$ Receptor Antagonists

Medications in another class of antidepressants act as 5-HT$_2$ antagonists (Figure 3–3 and Table 3–5) and have several other direct effects on 5-HT receptors that distinguish these agents from the SSRIs. The class currently includes the phenylpiperazine nefazodone and the triazolopyride trazodone. Trazodone was synthesized in Italy in the mid-1960s and eventually was released to the U.S. market in 1981. It represented the first 5-HT-specific agent in the United States. Nefazodone was synthesized in the 1980s by Bristol-Myers Squibb (BMS) with the specific intent of improving the side-effect profile of trazodone. Nefazodone (Serzone) became available in the United States in 1995. In December 2001, the FDA issued a black box warning about the risk of hepatotoxicity associated with nefazodone. In late 2003, BMS withdrew Serzone from markets in the United States and Canada, but nefazodone is still available generically.

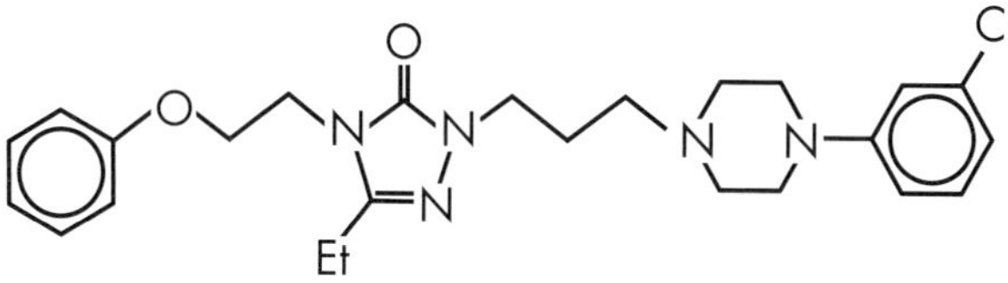

Nefazodone

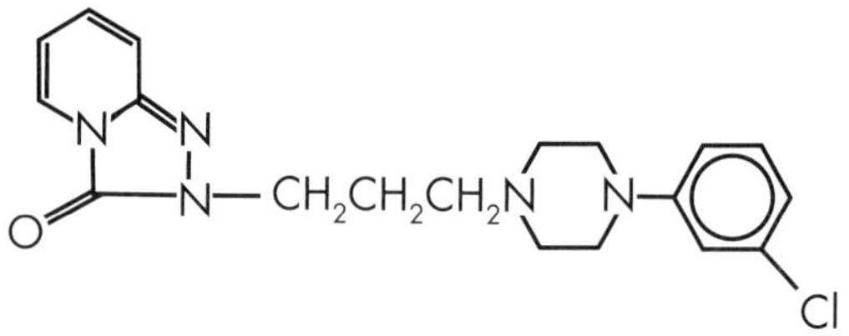

Trazodone

Figure 3–3. Chemical structures of serotonin$_2$ (5-HT$_2$) antagonists.

Table 3–5. Serotonin$_2$ (5-HT$_2$) antagonists

Drug	Starting dosage (mg/day)	Maximum dosage (mg/day)
Trazodone (Desyrel)	50–100	600
Trazodone extended-release (Oleptro)	150, 300	375
Nefazodone (Serzone)	50–100	600

Pharmacological Effects

The pharmacology of the 5-HT$_2$ antagonists is somewhat more complex than the name implies, and questions still remain. The principal effect of both trazodone and nefazodone appears to be antagonism of the postsynaptic 5-HT$_{2A}$ and 5-HT$_{2C}$ receptors. Nefazodone is the more potent antagonist. This antagonism causes a paradoxical downregulation of 5-HT$_2$ sites, which may explain the antidepressant effects of such 5-HT$_2$ antagonism. The 5-HT$_2$ receptor is also linked with other receptors, including the 5-HT$_{1A}$ receptor, which is thought to be important in depression, anxiety, and violent behavior. There is growing evidence that both nefazodone and trazodone stimulate the 5-HT$_{1A}$ site, possibly through antagonizing the 5-HT$_2$ receptor. In addition to their effects as 5-HT$_2$ antagonists, both trazodone and nefazodone block the reuptake of 5-HT to some extent. Although the inhibition of the 5-HT transporter with these two drugs is weak in comparison to that of the SSRIs, it may be clinically significant.

Finally, *m*-chlorophenylpiperazine (m-CPP), a major active metabolite of both nefazodone and trazodone, is a potent direct agonist of 5-HT, mostly at the 5-HT$_{2C}$ receptor, which may contribute both to the efficacy of the drugs and to their side effects.

Indications

The primary indication for both trazodone and nefazodone is major depression. More than two dozen double-blind, placebo-controlled studies of trazodone and at least eight double-blind studies of nefazodone have established the efficacy of these drugs in the treatment of major depression. Most of these studies suggest that trazodone and nefazodone are as effective as comparison drugs, primarily the TCAs, in the treatment of major depression. However, many of the controlled studies have involved outpatients with mild to moderate major depression, and there have been persistent questions about the efficacy of trazodone in the treatment of more severely depressed patients. Some investigators have suggested that trazodone is not particularly helpful for retarded depressions. However, a review of efficacy studies (Schatzberg 1987) found that there appeared to be no difference between TCAs and trazodone in the treatment of depressed inpatients and of those with more classic endogenous features. Interestingly, the studies that reported the poorest results with trazodone used aggressive dosing, with doses that reached a total of 300–450 mg in the first week of treatment. Thus, trazodone may be effective and is better tolerated at lower rather than higher doses, particularly at first. At least one study has also concluded that nefazodone is effective in the treatment of more severely depressed inpatients (Ansseau et al. 1994).

Both trazodone and nefazodone appear to be effective anxiolytic agents. The antianxiety effects of the drugs are often evident earlier than the antidepressant effects. A comparison of low-dose trazodone with chlordiazepoxide for general anxiety suggested that the two agents had equal efficacy (Schwartz and Blendl 1974). Likewise, one study suggested that trazodone compared favorably with imipramine and diazepam in the treatment of GAD (Rickels et al. 1993). In depressed patients, anxiolytic effects of nefazodone were noted at dosages less than 250 mg/day (Fontaine et al. 1994), but trazodone, an antidepressant, has shown significant utility as a hypnotic at doses of 25–100 mg at night. Because trazodone is quite sedating and does not have an addiction potential, it offers a safe alternative to the benzodiazepines. Likewise, trazodone has been used successfully to treat SSRI- and MAOI-induced insomnia.

Next to depression, the best-studied disorder treated with nefazodone is PTSD. Prior to the black box hepatotoxicity warning, nefazodone was among the more common agents prescribed in treating PTSD because of commonly occurring symptoms such as sleep disturbance and agitation, as well as comorbid conditions such as substance abuse and depression. At least six open-label studies of nefazodone in the treatment of PTSD suggested that the drug can help ameliorate nightmares and hyperarousal and decrease anger (Hidalgo et al. 1999). However, concerns about hepatotoxicity have greatly diminished nefazodone prescriptions in general. Dosages ranging from 300 to 600 mg/day appear to be efficacious for the treatment of PTSD.

Nefazodone does not share trazodone's utility as a hypnotic because the former is generally less sedating. However, preliminary data (Armitage et al. 1994) suggested that nefazodone, unlike many psychotropics, may enhance rapid eye movement sleep and therefore may increase restful sleep in some patients.

Case reports suggest a number of other potential roles for nefazodone. Nefazodone has been reported to be useful in the treatment of social phobia, panic disorder, and PMDD and as an adjunctive agent in the treatment of negative symptoms of schizophrenia.

Side Effects

Although the 5-HT$_2$ antagonists are 5-HT-specific agents, they differ from the SSRIs in mechanism of action and thus in side-effect profile as well (Table 3–6). One common side effect of all currently available serotonergic antide-

Table 3–6.   Common or troublesome side effects of trazodone and nefazodone

Gastrointestinal effects
  Nausea
  Dyspepsia
Liver failure (nefazodone—rare)
Adrenergic blockade
  Orthostasis (trazodone >> nefazodone)
  Dizziness
Neurological effects
  Headaches
  Visual trails (nefazodone > trazodone)
CNS depression
  Sedation (trazodone >> nefazodone)
CNS activation
  Restlessness (nefazodone > trazodone)
Sexual effects
  Priapism (trazodone)

Note. >> = much greater than.

pressants is GI upset. The incidence of nausea with trazodone and nefazodone is less than that found with the SSRIs. However, it was still the leading cause for discontinuation of nefazodone in prerelease trials. Higher doses of trazodone, particularly when taken on an empty stomach, may also be correlated with nausea. As with the SSRIs, the GI side effects of these drugs are lessened by taking them with food.

As reported, neither trazodone nor nefazodone has particularly strong anticholinergic effects. They can, however, produce dry mouth because of their α_1-adrenergic receptor blockade. (Salivation is controlled by both the acetylcholine and the noradrenergic systems.) The α_1-adrenergic blockade may also result in significant orthostasis with trazodone, especially in elderly persons. Dizziness and even frank syncope may occur in patients taking large doses of trazodone on an empty stomach, as well as in some elderly patients taking nefazodone. It is therefore useful to monitor blood pressure for orthostasis with vulnerable patients and to encourage proper hydration. Support stockings may also be helpful. The incidence of orthostasis with nefazodone is thought to be lower than with trazodone. However, orthostasis has been reported with higher doses of nefazodone and in vulnerable patients. Trazodone also differs from nefazodone in the amount of sedation it produces. As described, trazodone is very sedating and is useful as a hypnotic at modest doses. Nefazodone may produce daytime somnolence, but this usually occurs at higher doses. Shifting the bulk of the dose to bedtime will mitigate this problem.

CNS activation is generally reported not to be a problem with either drug. However, patients who are deficient in the CYP2D6 enzyme or who are taking SSRIs may experience activation secondary to the effects of the metabolite m-CPP, which is cleared by this enzyme. We have also seen some patients develop dysphoric activation while taking nefazodone, even without recent exposure to the SSRIs. Therefore, starting nefazodone at lower doses appears prudent.

More than 200 cases of priapism have been reported in males treated with trazodone. Although rare, priapism—with an incidence of 1 per 6,000 patients—is very problematic. Risk of trazodone-associated priapism is thought to be higher in younger males with prolonged erections in the morning on awakening or those who can have frequent erections over a relatively short period (several hours). Some patients may require surgical intervention. The acute treatment involves injection of an α-adrenergic receptor agonist (e.g., epinephrine) into the penis. If not treated promptly, priapism may result in permanent erectile dysfunction. Male patients should thus be warned to stop the drug immediately if they experience any symptoms suggestive of priapism (occasional erections are not problematic) and to seek emergency department treatment if the erection persists longer than 1 hour. At least one case of clitoral priapism has also been reported (Pescatori et al. 1993).

Because priapism is mediated via adrenergic pathways, nefazodone is thought to present less of a problem than trazodone in this regard. There have been no reports of nefazodone-induced priapism, but there have been isolated reports of prolonged erections in men and reports of increased nocturnal penile tumescence. A case of clitoral engorgement, but not priapism, with nefazodone has also been reported.

Sexual side effects generally appear to be rare with nefazodone. In fact, it is difficult to demonstrate that the rate of sexual dysfunction with nefazodone treatment is any higher than with placebo treatment. Feiger and colleagues (1996) found that sertraline and nefazodone were comparable in antidepressant efficacy. However, sertraline had negative effects on sexual function, whereas nefazodone had none.

Visual side effects may also occur in up to 12% of patients taking nefazodone. These side effects often take the form of an afterimage during tracking of moving objects. Interestingly, the afterimage during tracking may be a serotonin-enhancing effect because other agonists, such as LSD, also produce this effect. Patients should be told that the visual side effects generally improve with time.

In 1999, there was an isolated report at one center of three patients being treated with nefazodone who sustained liver failure. The patients were all women between the ages of 16 and 57 who were treated with 200–400 mg of nefazodone for a period averaging several months (Aranda-Michel et al. 1999). All patients showed significant hepatocellular damage, and two of the three underwent liver transplants. The third recovered without transplantation. In at least one of the patients, a concomitant medication could have contributed to hepatotoxicity. Since that first report, a number of other cases have emerged that led the FDA to advise BMS that they must include a black box warning in the package insert that alerts the public about the risk of severe liver toxicity. The risk is estimated at about 1/250,000 for every patient-year of treatment with nefazodone. In other words, if a quarter million patients were taking nefazodone for a year, one patient would be expected to develop potentially severe liver damage. Although these odds are very small, this is about three to four times the background rate for severe liver damage, and use of nefazodone dropped dramatically with the black box warning. BMS voluntarily removed Serzone from the market, but nefazodone is still available generically. Many antidepressants, including TCAs, have rarely and idiosyncratically been associated with fulminant hepatic failure. There do not appear to be clear demographic variables that predict hepatic toxicity from a given antidepressant. However, in any patient with a history of hepatic difficulties, it is prudent to obtain baseline liver enzymes and monitor the enzyme levels periodically. Nefazodone should not be prescribed in any patient with a history of liver disease. We are frequently asked whether a patient who has done well while taking nefazodone should continue the medication. We have not routinely taken patients who have responded to the drug off the medication. If there is a reasonable alternative to nefazodone, it should be considered. If alternatives have been unsuccessful or poorly tolerated, it may be particularly reasonable to continue the nefazodone while informing the patient of the known risk. Patients should also be educated about symptoms of liver illness, including jaundice, anorexia, GI disturbance, and malaise, and the drug should be discontinued if the patient has any symptoms suggesting toxicity.

Overdose

Trazodone and nefazodone appear to have a wide safety margin in cases of overdose. Doses as high as 10 g of trazodone have been taken without untoward incidents. The lethal dose in animals averages 500 mg/kg.

Although the risk of fatal overdoses with nefazodone or trazodone is very small, several reports suggest that the combination of trazodone and other CNS depressants, such as alcohol, can be lethal when taken in overdose. The usual cause of death is respiratory depression. Although a trazodone overdose alone can result in a seizure or respiratory arrest, the lethal dose in animals approaches half of body weight, or about 500 mg/kg. Nefazodone has been taken in overdoses of up to 12 g, or 20 times the maximum daily dose, without serious effects.

Drug Interactions

The 5-HT$_2$ antagonists have few drug interactions. Trazodone may potentiate the effects of other CNS depressants and lead to excessive sedation. Similarly, the postural hypotension associated with trazodone is exacerbated by concurrent administration of antihypertensive agents, and such combinations should be monitored with frequent checks of orthostatic blood pressure. Because both of the 5-HT$_2$ antagonist drugs have proserotonergic effects, there is a theoretical risk of precipitating a serotonin syndrome with the MAOIs, particularly at higher doses. However, neither trazodone nor nefazodone is a potent catecholamine reuptake inhibitor (although nefazodone has some reuptake inhibition); therefore, the risk of hypertensive crises with concurrent use of 5-HT$_2$ antagonists and MAOIs is low.

Nefazodone is a potent inhibitor of the CYP3A3/4 enzyme. As stated previously, this enzyme is responsible for the metabolism of such common drugs as the triazolobenzodiazepines alprazolam and triazolam, ketoconazole, erythromycin, and carbamazepine. The combination of nefazodone and anti-arrhythmics, pimozide, or ziprasidone may enhance cardiac toxicity. Concurrent use of nefazodone with these agents may raise serum levels, and clinicians should exercise caution in combining these drugs.

Occasionally, switching from an SSRI to a 5-HT$_2$ antagonist drug, particularly nefazodone, may be problematic. One of the metabolites of nefazodone is m-CPP, which is metabolized via the CYP2D6 enzyme. Increased serum levels of m-CPP have been associated with dysphoric agitation. Thus, simultaneous use of an SSRI and nefazodone, either current or recent (before the washout period has ended), may be poorly tolerated in some patients. Fluoxetine can contribute to elevated levels of m-CPP for 4–5 weeks after it is discontinued, and the other SSRIs may have this effect for 1–2 weeks after they are discontinued. Therefore, it would be useful, ideally, to have a washout period between stopping an SSRI and starting nefazodone. However, an alternative strategy is to allow no washout period but start with smaller dosages of nefazodone (50–100 mg/day) and titrate upward more gradually after discontinuing the SSRI.

Dosage and Administration

The manufacturer recommends starting trazodone at 150 mg/day and then increasing the dosage up to 600 mg/day (see Table 3–5). Our experience has been that the drug is quite sedating, and we begin patients at 50 mg/day and increase the dosage to 150 mg/day by day 7. Thereafter, each week, we increase the daily dosage by 50–75 mg, up to 300 mg/day. In our experience, patients respond at a modal dosage of 150–300 mg/day.

Because of trazodone's short half-life, the optimal dosing for the treatment of depression is in two or three divided doses a day. The bulk of the dose may be taken at bedtime to mitigate daytime somnolence.

Some investigators have proposed that trazodone has a therapeutic window; as with nortriptyline, too-high plasma levels are associated with poor responses. Our experience suggests this may be so, and several studies have supported a correlation between plasma levels and efficacy (Monteleone and Gnocchi 1990; Spar 1987). Steady-state trazodone plasma levels above 650 ng/mL may be ideal for antidepressant response. However, more study is needed to determine whether it is worthwhile to obtain trazodone plasma levels routinely.

The manufacturer's recommended starting dosage of nefazodone is 100 mg bid. However, we recommend starting at 50 mg bid or lower and increasing the dose by 50 mg every 4 days to reach 200 mg/day. Thereafter, each week, the daily dose may be increased by 100 mg until a therapeutic dose is achieved. Minimal therapeutic antidepressant dosage is 300 mg/day, and most patients will require at least 400 mg/day. Thus, it is reasonable to titrate the dosage to

400 mg/day and then maintain this dosage for 3–4 weeks. If a response is not observed, the dosage may then be further increased to a maximum of 600 mg/day. The initial dosage in elderly patients should be 50 mg/day. Some patients may feel too sedated or activated at 100 mg bid, but they are often able to tolerate an initial dosage of 50 mg bid. Therefore, we have recently come to start all patients routinely at 50–100 mg/day. The manufacturer recommends twice daily dosing, but some practitioners prescribe the drug to be administered nightly, and this appears particularly feasible once patients have been on a steady dose for a few weeks. A slow-release formulation is being developed that would allow once-a-day dosing. However, at the time of this writing, a once-a-day formulation is not available.

Discontinuation

Discontinuation syndromes appear uncommon for both trazodone and nefazodone but have been reported. Some case reports suggested that the rapid discontinuation of trazodone may occasionally lead to withdrawal symptoms, particularly rebound insomnia (Otani et al. 1994). As with the SSRIs, there have been reports of paresthesias and dizziness associated with the sudden discontinuation of nefazodone (Benazzi 1998; Kotlyar et al. 1999; Lauber 1999; Markowitz 1999). Therefore, it is generally prudent to taper these medications rather than to stop them suddenly. The total daily dose of nefazodone and trazodone can be decreased by 50–100 mg each week.

Combined Noradrenergic-Dopaminergic Antidepressant Bupropion and Bupropion/Dextromethorphan

Bupropion (Wellbutrin) is a unicyclic antidepressant (Figure 3–4) that was to be released in 1986, but its release was delayed pending an evaluation of its risk of inducing seizures. It was not released until mid-1989, when it became clear that the increased seizure risk was dose related and tended to occur in specific populations. In 1998, bupropion became available in a sustained-release formulation (Wellbutrin SR) that allows twice-a-day administration and also appears to decrease the risk of seizures to about that associated with SSRIs. In 2003, bupropion became available in an extended-release formula-

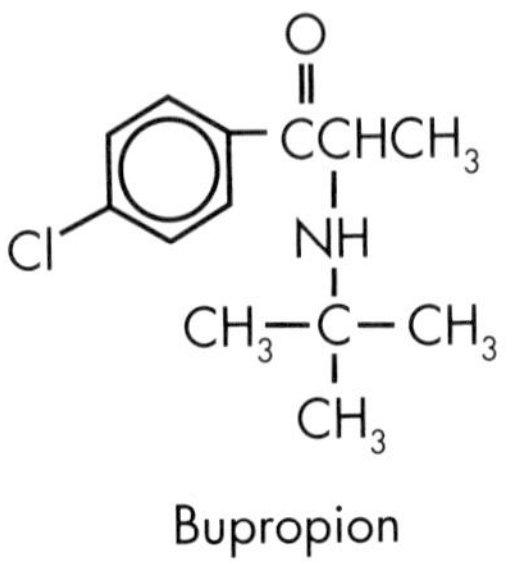

Bupropion

Figure 3–4.   Chemical structure of bupropion.

tion (Wellbutrin XL) for once-a-day dosing. All formulations are now off patent and available generically.

Pharmacological Effects

Bupropion is not a 5-HT reuptake blocker and does not inhibit monoamine oxidase. Its biochemical mode of action is not completely understood. It was hypothesized to act via dopamine reuptake blockade; however, its dopamine-potentiating effects in animals appear to occur at very high dosages and blood levels, well beyond those routinely used in humans. The dopamine reuptake–blocking properties of bupropion are an order of magnitude less than those of sertraline. Activation of the nucleus accumbens, a common consequence of enhanced dopaminergic transmission, is easier to demonstrate in animal studies of bupropion than in human functional imaging studies. Nonetheless, the dopaminergic effects may be important because the plasma levels of homovanillic acid, the primary metabolite of dopamine, decrease in patients who respond to bupropion but not in patients who do not respond (Golden et al. 1988).

Over time, the noradrenergic effects of bupropion have become increasingly evident. The major active metabolite of bupropion, hydroxybupropion, does appear to block the reuptake of norepinephrine in rats. Earlier studies involving mice failed to show an effect on norepinephrine, but this species metabolizes the drug differently. Indirect evidence for an effect on noradrenergic activity also comes from data showing that the drug decreases 24-hour excretion of norepinephrine metabolites.

The combination of bupropion and dextromethorphan (Auvelity) was approved for the treatment of MDD in 2022. Dextromethorphan has a complicated pharmacology that includes NMDA antagonism, σ_1 agonism with some mild serotonin reuptake blocking, and μ opioid properties. Dextromethorphan has been available as an over-the-counter antitussive agent since the 1950s amd has been studied in the treatment of mood disorders since at least 2014. It is rapidly metabolized via the CYP2D6 isoenzyme. Therefore, dextromethorphan has been combined with a CYP2D6 inhibitor, such as quinidine, to slow the metabolism of dextromethorphan. The combination of quinidine and dextromethorphan (Nudexta) was approved in 2010 for the treatment of pseudobulbar affect. In 2014 an open-label study of quinidine plus dextromethorphan for the treatment of major depression showed a 35% remission rate and 45% response rate over 10 weeks of treatment (Murrough et al. 2017). Subsequent studies with the quinidine plus dextromethorphan combination were not consistently effective. However, bupropion is also a CYP2D6 inhibitor and showed substantial benefit when combined with dextromethorphan in a Phase II study (Tabuteau et al. 2022). The combination of bupropion 105 mg plus dextromethorphan 45 mg twice daily was compared with bupropion alone at 105 mg twice daily in 80 patients with MDD. Notably, the combination formula separated from bupropion monotherapy by week, showing a 26% remission at week 2 versus only 3% for bupropion alone. At week 6, the remission rate on the Montgomery-Åsberg Depression Rating Scale (MADRS) was 46% for the combination and 17% for bupropion monotherapy. Bupropion 105 mg twice daily was chosen as the comparator because that was the bupropion dose in the combination tablet. However, the usual therapeutic dosage of bupropion is 300–450 mg/day, and it is unclear whether the combined formulation is comparable with these higher dosages of bupropion. The Phase III program showed consistent superiority of the combination tablet compared with placebo (Iosifescu et al. 2022). Bupropion 105 mg plus dextromethorphan 45 mg twice daily separated from placebo by week 1 and demonstrated a remission rate of 40% at week 6 versus 17% for placebo, similar to the Phase II comparison with bupropion monotherapy. Anxiety was the side effect that led to discontinuation of the combination tablet at higher rates than with placebo and was seen in 2% of patients. Thus, bupropion plus dextromethorphan appears well tolerated.

The question for clinicians is where bupropion plus dextromethorphan fits in the current pharmacopeia of antidepressant monotherapy. From the side-effect profile and efficacy, it would seem like a reasonable option in the same patients who might be candidates for bupropion monotherapy: patients with MDD who have lower anxiety and fewer sleep difficulties (because of the activating nature of bupropion) and those concerned about sexual side effects and weight gain with other agents. However, because bupropion plus dextromethorphan is a branded drug, it is possible that third-party payers will require failed trials of one or more generic medications, including bupropion monotherapy, before allowing the combination tablet. This could be a complicated requirement because a study of the combination in refractory depression failed to demonstrate efficacy (Schatzberg 2022).

Another question is how efficacious over-the-counter (OTC) dextromethorphan is as an add-on alternative to the combination tablet. Dextromethorphan is available as an OTC antitussive in doses of 10–30 mg tablets and is quite inexpensive. The branded formulation is an extended-release formulation. No data are available currently on OTC dextromethorphan as an adjunctive treatment. In addition, some caution should be exercised in those patients with personal or family history of opioid abuse because dextromethorphan, although not scheduled, is abusable at high doses.

Indications

Bupropion appears to be effective in many types of depression. It has demonstrated utility in outpatients with mild to moderate depression as well as in inpatients with more severe depression. The drug appears to be safe in depressed cardiac patients. There have been reports that the drug is less likely to produce mania or rapid cycling, but episodes of mania in patients taking bupropion do occur. Few data exist supporting the use of SSRIs and SNRIs in bipolar depression, so bupropion is a reasonable first-line antidepressant agent in combination with mood stabilizers.

The second FDA indication for bupropion is in smoking cessation. Two controlled clinical trials indicate that the sustained-release formulation of bupropion (which is also marketed under the trade name Zyban) at 300 mg/day aids in smoking cessation (Goldstein 1998). More than 3,000 patients were studied in a clinical trial of the sustained-release formulation of bupropion in the treatment of smoking cessation. As with the treatment of depression, the benefits of bupropion SR are not immediate and take several weeks or longer to be evident. After 7 weeks of treatment, more than twice as many patients taking bupropion 300 mg/day (36%) were abstinent from nicotine as patients administered placebo (17%). At 26-week follow-up, only 19% of bupropion-treated patients and 11% of placebo-administered patients remained abstinent from smoking. These results mirror those commonly seen in smoking cessation studies with nicotine preparations. In a more recent trial, we reported that bupropion was no better than placebo in achieving smoking abstinence in adolescents. However, bupropion appeared to significantly decrease nicotine use (Killen et al. 2004).

Bupropion was studied for appetite suppression in combination with naltrexone (Contrave) and was approved for that use in 2014. It is indicated as an adjunct to a reduced-calorie diet for the management of weight in patients with a BMI >30 or BMI ≥ 27 in the presence of at least one weight-related comorbidity (e,g., hypertension, type 2 diabetes mellitus, dyslipidemia). The extended-release tablet contains 90 mg of bupropion hydrochloride and 8 mg of naltrexone hydrochloride. Dose titration proceeds at one tablet in the morning during the first week, one tablet in the morning and evening during the second week, two tablets in the morning and one in the evening during the third week, and thereafter two tablets in the morning and in the evening. The average weight loss in the three registration trials with Contrave was 5–9 pounds over the course of a year. One of us (A.F.S.) has found it quite useful in antipsychotic-induced and anticonvulsant-induced weight gain.

Bupropion has also been used in the treatment of seasonal affective disorder (SAD). Historically, SAD has been treated with phototherapy, antidepressants, and mood stabilizers. However, no FDA-approved therapy was available for this disorder until the approval of bupropion XL in 2006. Studies indicate that when treatment with bupropion is started while patients are well, the drug appears to prevent relapse and time to onset of depressive symptoms when compared with placebo (Modell et al. 2005). Because some patients with SAD may have illness that falls on the bipolar spectrum, we have found that a mood stabilizer such as lamotrigine or lithium can also be helpful, although there are few empirical data for the use of a mood stabilizer.

Another fairly common use of bupropion is in the treatment of ADHD, where it appears to be effective in both adults and children (Cantwell 1998). However, over the many years that bupropion has been available, few good, controlled trials of bupropion in the treatment of ADHD have been conducted (Verbeeck et al. 2017). Because bupropion is metabolized to a number of amphetamine-like products, it appears to be a safe alternative to stimulants in the treatment of ADHD. In adolescents who have comorbid substance abuse problems, bupropion might be the first-line treatment (Riggs et al. 1998).

Two important uses of bupropion are as an adjunct to SSRI treatment to augment the antidepressant effect and as an adjunct to counteract the sexual side effects of SSRIs. Bupropion does appear to augment SSRI antidepressant effects and is generally less complicated to use than either lithium or thyroid supplements. The STAR*D study found that bupropion added to an SSRI was helpful but that it was no more helpful than a parallel nonrandomized track in which buspirone was added (Trivedi et al. 2006). Bupropion augmentation is discussed in greater detail in Chapter 9, "Augmentation Strategies for Treatment-Resistant Disorders."

Bupropion is unique among the antidepressants in that it is probably not effective in the treatment of anxiety disorders. One pilot study of bupropion in the treatment of panic disorder yielded negative findings (Sheehan et al. 1983). To our knowledge, no recent studies have examined the efficacy of bupropion in the treatment of panic disorder. Many anxious patients find bupropion too activating and prefer other agents.

Bupropion's metabolism is probably dependent on several hepatic enzymes; therefore, interactions with the SSRIs may be less problematic than once thought. Still, there has been at least one case report of a seizure being associated with the combination of fluoxetine and bupropion.

Side Effects

Bupropion has a favorable side-effect profile, in part because of its low affinity for muscarinic, α-adrenergic, and histaminic receptors. The only side effects of bupropion SR that occurred reliably more commonly than with placebo in clinical trials of 100–300 mg/day were insomnia, dry mouth, and tremor. The insomnia is best managed by moving the evening dose to earlier in the afternoon (for the immediate-release and SR formulations of bupropion). A separation of at least 8 hours between the morning and evening doses is advised.

Bupropion does not induce orthostatic hypotension or stimulate appetite. Some investigators have argued that bupropion could be particularly useful in patients who gain weight while taking other agents. There are reports that patients with sexual dysfunction who are taking other antidepressants do better with bupropion, and, again, the drug has been reported to counteract SSRI-induced sexual dysfunction.

Seizures with the immediate-release formulation of bupropion have been reported at the rate of 4 per 1,000 at dosages less than 450 mg/day; this risk increased to 4 per 100 when the dosage was increased above 450 mg/day. The sustained-release formulation, which has largely supplanted the immediate-release formulation, appears to carry a seizure risk of about 1 per 1,000 patients at dosages less than 400 mg/day. This risk is similar to the seizure risk associated with most antidepressants. The risk of seizures appears to be enhanced in patients with a prior history of seizure disorders, head injury, bulimia, and anorexia. Concurrent use of alcohol, stimulants, or cocaine also enhances the risk of seizures. The manufacturer also cautions that single doses of the drug should never exceed 150 mg for the immediate-release formulation and 200 mg for the sustained-release preparation. The extended-release formulation may be taken as a single dose of up to 450 mg.

Overdose

Bupropion has proved relatively safe in overdose. However, there have been cases of completed suicide with bupropion alone (Rohrig and Ray 1992). In some cases, patients who overdosed on bupropion had significant neurological complications, including seizures and status epilepticus (Schmit et al. 2017; Spiller et al. 1994; Storrow 1994). Thus, some caution should be exercised in prescribing large supplies of bupropion for suicidal patients.

Drug Interactions

Serious drug interactions are uncommon with bupropion. Bupropion is metabolized by the CYP2D6 as well as the CYP2B6 enzyme, which is responsible for metabolizing very few drugs (orphenadrine and cyclophosphamide). Thus, potential pharmacokinetic interactions with other antidepressants or general medicines are lower. However, caution should be exercised with potent CYP2D6 inhibitors, particularly with the bupropion plus dextromethorphan combination because both hydroxybupropion (the active metabolite of bupropion) and dextromethorphan are CYP2D6 substrates.

Any drug that lowers the seizure threshold should be used cautiously with bupropion. Thus, drugs such as clozapine, theophylline, and clomipramine should be used cautiously or avoided with bupropion. Likewise, it may be prudent to avoid the use of bupropion in patients who are dependent on alcohol or benzodiazepines because sudden discontinuation of these drugs in the context of concurrent bupropion use can increase seizure risk.

The use of an MAOI with bupropion or with the bupropion plus dextromethorphan combination is contraindicated. There appears to be an enhanced risk of general toxicity with phenelzine and bupropion as well as a greater risk of hypertensive crises.

Dosage and Administration

Bupropion has a relatively wide usual dosage range (200–450 mg/day). The modal optimum dosage range in our experience has been 300–400 mg/day. Bupropion is available in an immediate-release formulation (75-mg and 100-mg tablets); in a sustained-release preparation (Wellbutrin SR; 100-mg, 150-mg, and 200-mg tablets) given twice daily; and in an extended-release once-daily formulation (150-mg and 300-mg tablets).

The combination of bupropion 105 mg plus dextromethorphan 45 mg is started at 1 tablet daily and increased after 3 days to 1 tablet twice daily separated by at least 8 hours. Patients with significant renal or liver disease and slow metabolizers of CYP2D6 should generally be limited to one combination tablet daily.

Mirtazapine

Mirtazapine (Remeron), which was released in the United States in 1996, is chemically related to mianserin, a drug that had been used for a number of years in Europe. Mirtazapine is FDA approved for the treatment of depression but appears to be useful for a variety of other disorders such as insomnia. Although it did not emerge as being among the more popular antidepressants during the late 1990s, mirtazapine has established an important niche in clinical practice. Mirtazapine has been available generically since 2004.

Pharmacological Effects

Mirtazapine has a tetracyclic chemical structure (Figure 3–5) but is unrelated to the TCAs. Its mechanism of action is fairly unusual among the available antidepressants. It appears to be an antagonist of central presynaptic α_2-adrenergic

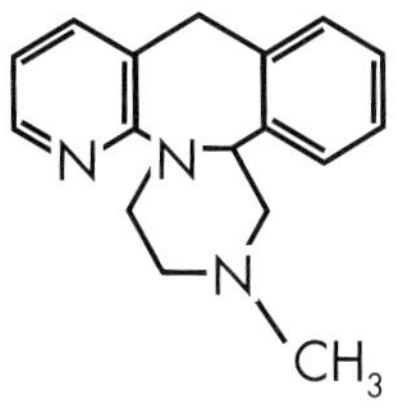

Mirtazapine

Figure 3–5. Chemical structure of mirtazapine.

receptors. As an α_2-adrenergic receptor blocker, mirtazapine acts to increase norepinephrine release. The increased noradrenergic tone results in a rapid increase in synaptic 5-HT levels by mobilizing 5-HT release secondary to stimulation of α_1-adrenergic receptors on 5-HT cell bodies. Mirtazapine also blocks 5-HT$_2$ and 5-HT$_3$ receptors. Mirtazapine is not a specific reuptake blocker of any monoamine neurotransmitter. However, it does appear to be a potent antagonist of H$_1$ receptors—a feature that confers some of the drug's more problematic side effects. Mirtazapine does not have particularly strong anticholinergic effects and does not significantly block postsynaptic α-adrenergic receptors. As a result, postural hypotension is generally not associated with mirtazapine use.

Mirtazapine is available in 7.5-mg, 15-mg, 30-mg, and 45-mg tablets. A quick-dissolving wafer formulation (Remeron SolTabs) has been commonly used in geriatric patients.

Mirtazapine is well absorbed from the GI tract and extensively metabolized to at least four active products. Each of these metabolites, including the most common one, desmethylmirtazapine, is less active than the parent drug. Mirtazapine is metabolized by CYP2D6, CYP3A3/4, and CYP1A2 enzymes but is neither an inducer nor an inhibitor of these hepatic enzymes (Fawcett and Barkin 1998). Thus, it can be taken safely with other psychotropic agents.

Indications

In premarketing trials of mirtazapine, which involved several thousand patients, the drug appeared to be as effective as the TCAs amitriptyline and clomipramine. Both outpatients with milder depression and more severely depressed inpatients respond to mirtazapine. Compared with trazodone, mirtazapine appears to be superior in the treatment of depressed inpatients (van Moffaert et al. 1995). Mirtazapine has also been studied for treatment of brief recurrent depression, which meets all of the DSM-IV (American Psychiatric Association 1994) criteria for major depression except the time criterion. Brief depression lasts less than 2 weeks but tends to recur many times over a year. Mirtazapine at low doses appears, on the basis of case reports, to effectively treat these depressive episodes (Stamenkovic et al. 1998). Other subtypes of depression, including atypical depression and seasonal depression, may also be responsive to mirtazapine (Falkai 1999).

Other studies have directly compared mirtazapine with SSRIs in the treatment of depression (Fava et al. 2001; Leinonen et al. 1999; Quitkin et al. 2001; Wheatley et al. 1998). Mirtazapine was reported to be comparable in efficacy to fluoxetine, paroxetine, and citalopram and in each study was slightly, but not significantly, more effective. Compared with the SSRIs, mirtazapine may have more rapid anxiolytic and antidepressant effects (Thompson 1999). With mirtazapine, in contrast to citalopram and paroxetine, the antidepressant and antianxiety effects are sometimes seen by the second week. A meta-analysis by Thase (2003) found that mirtazapine was significantly more effective than SSRIs. However, another meta-analysis failed to show an efficacy advantage of mirtazapine over the SSRIs (Papakostas et al. 2008). Thus, the advantages of mirtazapine over SSRIs may be more in side-effect profile (fewer sexual side effects, more sedating at night) than in efficacy.

Because mirtazapine, with its greater propensity for sedation and weight gain, is often used after SSRIs have been tried without success, the STAR*D study evaluated the utility of mirtazapine for achieving remission after the failure of two trials (Fava et al. 2006b). Mirtazapine was as effective (or ineffective) as nortriptyline in achieving remission after two failed antidepressant trials. The remission rate for mirtazapine on the HDRS at this late stage of the study was only 8%. Additionally, the dropout rate from adverse effects with mirtazapine appears to be usually similar to that of the SSRIs. We reported on a comparison of paroxetine and mirtazapine in elderly depressed patients (Schatzberg et al. 2002). Mirtazapine was associated with significantly earlier response and fewer dropouts due to adverse events than was paroxetine.

Preliminary data from open-label trials suggest that mirtazapine is useful for most of the anxiety disorders that are responsive to SSRIs or venlafaxine. For example, mirtazapine may be useful in the treatment of panic disorder, with or without concurrent depression (Carpenter et al. 1999b). Patients with depression and comorbid GAD appear to do well when taking mirtazapine at dosages of 15–45 mg/day (Goodnick et al. 1999). Pilot studies of mirtazapine for PTSD also appeared promising (Connor et al. 1999; Williams et al. 2022).

Another potential use for mirtazapine is in augmenting antidepressant effects. Because of its low risk of pharmacokinetic interaction, mirtazapine should be relatively easy to combine with many antidepressants. The drug, with its complex pharmacology, may complement antidepressants that act more specifically. Preliminary data have shown that mirtazapine effectively augments SSRIs (Carpenter et al. 1999a). In a more recent study, Blier et al. (2010) reported that fluoxetine plus mirtazapine was significantly more effective than fluoxetine alone in patients with major depression. In contrast, Rush et al. (2011), in the Combining Medications to Enhance Depression Outcomes (CO-MED) study, failed to find differences from the outset among escitalopram plus placebo, bupropion SR plus escitalopram, and venlafaxine plus mirtazapine. Similarly, a randomized trial of adding mirtazapine or switching to mirtazapine monotherapy in a group of MDD patients who did not have an early response to paroxetine found no advantage of adjunctive mirtazapine versus switching to mirtazapine (Xiao et al. 2021). In the STAR*D trial, the combination of mirtazapine (average dosage = 36 mg/day) with venlafaxine (average dosage = 210 mg/day) resulted in remission-level responses in just 13% of patients with three consecutive failed antidepressant trials (McGrath et al. 2006). This result was similar to the remission rate found for tranylcypromine in patients with three failed trials. However, the venlafaxine plus mirtazapine combination was better tolerated than tranylcypromine.

Mirtazapine had been reported to help reverse SSRI-induced sexual side effects (Farah 1999), but a double-blind trial failed to show benefits of mirtazapine in treating sexual side effects (Michelson et al. 2000). In addition, the drug has been reported to help improve negative symptoms in schizophrenia (Berk et al. 2001) and to ameliorate antipsychotic-induced extrapyramidal symptoms.

As reported earlier, mirtazapine has been used as an effective antinausea medication in chemotherapy patients (Kim et al. 2008), in functional vomiting (Bondade et al. 2016), and in the effects of postoperative anesthesia (Chen et al. 2008). In addition, mirtazapine was significantly more effective than placebo in reducing nausea and vomiting in orthopedic patients treated with intrathecal morphine (Chang et al. 2010). Compared with the more commonly used 5-HT$_3$ antagonists such as ondansetron (Zofran), generic mirtazapine is a fraction of the cost and may provide additional benefits, such as sedation and antianxiety effects. Although anecdotal experience suggests mirtazapine might be as useful an antinausea medication as other 5-HT$_3$ antagonists, no comparison study has ever been done.

Side Effects

Mirtazapine has generally been well tolerated in clinical studies. The most common side effects are dry mouth, sedation, somnolence, and weight gain. More than half of all patients treated with mirtazapine, compared with less than 20% of patients treated with placebo, experienced somnolence. Somnolence is more evident at lower doses than at higher doses because antihistaminic effects predominate relative to noradrenergic or serotonergic effects at dosages below 15 mg/day. Thus, vis-à-vis sedation, a starting dosage of 30 mg/day is often better and usually not more poorly tolerated than a dosage of 7.5 mg/day. A trial in Europe did compare mirtazapine at dosages of 15 mg/day and 30 mg/day and found no differences in sedation between the two groups.

Weight gain and increased appetite are clear problems for some patients taking mirtazapine. In short-term trials of 6–12 weeks, about 20% of patients treated with mirtazapine reported increased appetite, and 7.5% of patients had an increase in weight of at least 7%. In our clinical experience, at least 20% of patients gain weight with long-term use of mirtazapine. Weight gain in the elderly appears to be less common. The most reliable strategy for controlling weight when taking mirtazapine is to exercise and to control appetite. The notion that higher doses of mirtazapine may be less problematic for weight gain is less clear than the effects on somnolence. Some clinicians anecdotally report that the use of H$_2$ antagonists, mitigates the weight gain associated with mirtazapine, but this approach is untested. Likewise, some clinicians use stimulants or sibutramine (Orlistat) to help control weight. However, sibutramine is a serotonergic drug and may increase the risk of serotonergic side effects, and stimulants generally require triplicate form prescriptions and have an established abuse potential.

The effects of mirtazapine on cholesterol and triglycerides have become better recognized in recent years. About 15% of patients demonstrate a significant (>20%) increase in cholesterol, and 6% of patients experience a significant increase in triglycerides. It is thus worthwhile to obtain fasting triglyceride and cholesterol levels at baseline and periodically with treatment, especially for patients with known hypercholesterolemia or who have a history of high triglyceride levels. Concurrent use of a 3-hydroxy-3-methyl-glutaryl-coenzyme A reductase inhibitor such as atorvastatin (Lipitor) has been anecdotally reported to reduce the cholesterol and lipid effects of mirtazapine at dosages of 10–80 mg/day. Unless the benefits of mirtazapine are substantial, however, it may be easier to switch to another agent if the patient experiences clinically significant increases in cholesterol or triglyceride levels.

Along with bupropion and nefazodone, mirtazapine is one of the few antidepressants that have limited sexual side effects. Switching from an SSRI to mirtazapine appears to resolve sexual dysfunction associated with the use of an SSRI (Koutouvidis et al. 1999). Case reports indicate that adding mirtazapine at dosages of 15–30 mg/day to an SSRI can mitigate SSRI-induced sexual side effects (Koutouvidis et al. 1999). However, a more recent double-blind trial of mirtazapine in treating SSRI-induced sexual side effects showed no benefit over placebo (Michelson et al. 2002).

Orthostatic hypotension or, conversely, hypertension is occasionally seen in patients treated with mirtazapine. About 7% of patients experience significant dizziness, and some of this may be from postural changes. It is worthwhile to occasionally monitor blood pressure in patients who are being treated with mirtazapine, particularly elderly patients. Other rare but significant side effects associated with mirtazapine include elevations in hepatic transaminases in about 2% of patients—a rate similar to that seen with SSRIs. Worries about agranulocytosis at the time of release of the drug to the market have not been borne out.

Overdose

Mirtazapine appears to be fairly safe in overdose. We are unaware of fatal overdoses with mirtazapine in doses of up to 2 g. The most common effect of overdose with mirtazapine is sedation. Gastric lavage and supportive management have been adequate thus far in dealing with overdoses.

Drug Interactions

As indicated earlier, mirtazapine has a low risk of pharmacokinetic interactions. The most common interaction is synergism with other CNS depressants. Concurrent benzodiazepines, barbiturates, or alcohol increases the risk of significant somnolence and sedation. The combination of mirtazapine and a CNS depressant also has an additive effect on motor impairment.

The proserotonergic effects of mirtazapine impart a potential risk of serotonin syndrome, although this risk is largely obviated via its blocking of 5-HT_2 and 5-HT_3 postsynaptic receptors. The α_2-noradrenergic effects pose a risk of hypertensive crises when the drug is used in combination with an MAOI. As a result, mirtazapine should be discontinued for at least 2 weeks before an MAOI is started and vice versa.

Dosage and Administration

Although the recommended starting dosage of mirtazapine is 15 mg/day, we now advise starting most patients at 30 mg/day. Geriatric patients and those with severe insomnia should be started at 15 mg/day. Mirtazapine is administered once a day, about 1 hour before bedtime. The dose may then be increased by 15 mg every 2 weeks to the maximum recommended dosage of 45 mg/day. In Europe, the maximum dosage is 60 mg/day, and we will sometimes push the dosage to this level in patients with treatment-resistant conditions.

Vilazodone

Vilazodone is a serotonergic agent approved in 2011by the FDA for use in the treatment of major depression. Vilazodone has a multi-ring structure (Figure 3–6) that allows it to bind potently to the serotonin transporter but minimally to the dopamine transporter and norepinephrine transporter. Its mechanism of action is best described as having selective serotonin reuptake inhibition with partial agonist activity at the 5-HT_{1A} receptor (Guay 2012). Thus, vilazodone is, in some respects, like the combination of an SSRI and buspirone.

Vilazodone is well absorbed, and absorption is increased when the drug is given with a fatty meal. It is extensively metabolized via the CYP3A4 isoen-

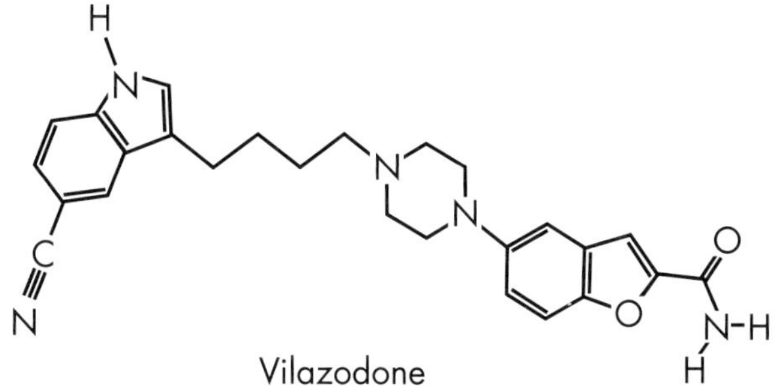

Figure 3–6. Chemical structure of vilazodone.

zyme, with minor contributions by CYP2C19 and CYP2D6. Only 1% of vilazodone is excreted unchanged in the urine. Because vilazodone is primarily a substrate of CYP3A4, strong CYP3A4 inhibitors such as ketoconazole can increase the serum concentration of vilazodone by 50% or more. On the other hand, vilazodone is neither a potent inhibitor nor a potent inducer of any isoenzymes. It may be a mild inducer of CYP2C19.

FDA approval of vilazodone rested primarily on findings from two RCTs. In both trials, a 40-mg dose over an 8-week period was superior to placebo treatment of depression as measured by the MADRS (Khan et al. 2011; Rickels et al. 2009). Patients treated with vilazodone had a 2.5- to 3.2-point greater reduction on the MADRS compared with patients receiving placebo. However, when remission level criteria were used, vilazodone was not much more effective than placebo. From an efficacy standpoint, there is no reason to believe that vilazodone has any efficacy advantages over other antidepressants. As with many other antidepressants, vilazodone also has not demonstrated efficacy in children and adolescents (Findling et al. 2022).

With respect to tolerability, on the other hand, vilazodone might have some relative advantages in some patients. For example, the reported rates of sexual side effects and weight gain are lower than those seen for many other antidepressants. However, vilazodone is associated with high rates of GI side effects such as diarrhea, nausea, and vomiting. As with other serotonergic antidepressants, nausea and vomiting improved over time in most patients, and slow dosing titration, as well as taking the drug with food (but preferably not fatty foods), helps mitigate the nausea. Unfortunately, the diarrhea may persist in some patients.

Vilazodone requires a gradual dose titration to limit the GI side effects. The usual starting dosage is 10 mg/day for the first week, with the dosage increased to 20 mg/day the second week, and a target dosage of 40 mg/day the third week. There is no evidence that speeding up the titration speeds up response, although it is likely to increase the risk of GI side effects. Likewise, there is not much evidence that increasing the dosage above 40 mg/day will increase the response rate, but some individuals may tolerate and respond to 60 or even 80 mg/day.

Vortioxetine

Vortioxetine (Figure 3–7) is a newer agent that is a serotonin reuptake inhibitor like the SSRIs. In addition, vortioxetine appears to directly act on many 5-HT receptors (Stenkrona et al. 2013). In vitro studies indicate that vortioxetine is an antagonist of the 5-HT_3, 5-HT_7, and 5-HT_{1D} receptors, a partial agonist of the 5-HT_{1B} receptor, and an agonist of the 5-HT_{1A} receptor. Vortioxetine is not a potent inhibitor of CYP isoenzymes. However, vortioxetine is extensively metabolized through oxidation via CYP2D6 and other isoenzymes and then undergoes subsequent glucuronidation. It is tightly bound to protein and has linear and dose-proportional pharmacokinetics. Vortioxetine is a substrate of CYP2D6 and CYP2B6, and the dose of vortioxetine may require reduction when it is coadministered with CYP2D6 inhibitors such as paroxetine. Inducers of CYP isoenzymes, such as rifampin, carbamazepine, and phenytoin, will lower serum levels of vortioxetine and may require increasing the dose of vortioxetine.

The registration trials for vortioxetine included six acute controlled trials (e.g., Alvarez et al. 2012; Boulenger et al. 2014), including one in the elderly (Gibb and Deeks 2014). All of these trials were statistically significant compared with placebo on the basis of changes from baseline to the endpoint at 6–8 weeks on the 24-item version of the HDRS and the MADRS. In addition, vortioxetine was also studied as a maintenance treatment for periods up to 64 weeks and appears to have reduced the risk of relapse as we would expect from the continued use of all antidepressants. Also consistent with most other antide-

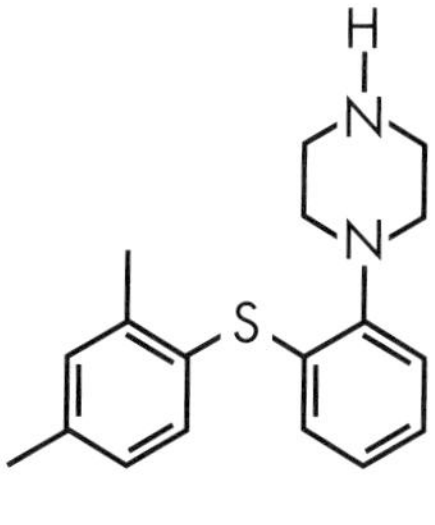

Vortioxetine

Figure 3–7.   Chemical structure of vortioxetine.

pressants, vortioxetine failed to show benefit in the treatment adolescents with MDD (Findling et al. 2022).

Vortioxetine had received an approval by the European Medicines Agency for the treatment of some cognitive symptoms associated with depression. Major depression is well known to be associated with a variety of cognitive deficits, from processing speed to executive functioning. These cognitive deficits can result in large burden for depressed patients that makes it difficult to function. In 2018, the FDA accepted data that showed that vortioxetine was effective in improving the performance of depressed patients on the Digit Symbol Substitution Test (DSST). The DSST is a test of processing speed, and patients treated with vortioxetine showed significant improvement on the DSST. Whether or not vortioxetine is superior to other antidepressants in improving processing speed in major depressive disorder is unclear because the randomized controlled cognitive trials of the type needed to establish efficacy have not been done for any approved antidepressants other than duloxetine.

The most common side effects of vortioxetine were GI side effects, including nausea, vomiting, and constipation (Alam et al. 2014). The nausea effects appear to be dose related, with up to 32% of patients at the 20 mg/day dosage experiencing nausea versus 21% of patients at the 5-mg dose. Likewise, constipation and nausea also appear to be dose related, with twice as many patients experiencing these side effects at 20 mg/day versus 5 mg/day (6% vs. 3%). Nausea was the most common reason that patients discontinued vortioxetine in the clinical trials.

The starting dosage of vortioxetine is usually 10 mg/day for the first week, with a target dosage of 20 mg/day the second week. If a patient cannot tolerate vortioxetine at 10 mg/day, the dosage might be decreased to 5 mg/day and titrated up as tolerated. In the controlled trials, 20 mg/day was superior to either 5 or 10 mg/day in efficacy. However, dosages higher than 20 mg/day have not been well studied, and it is unclear if additional benefits might be seen.

Tricyclic and Tetracyclic Antidepressants

Structures

The chemical structures of TCAs and related compounds are remarkably similar (Figure 3–8). Desipramine and nortriptyline are demethylated metabolites of imipramine and amitriptyline, respectively. Amoxapine is a derivative of the antipsychotic loxapine and has an additional fourth ring off a side chain. Maprotiline is a four-ring compound, with the fourth ring arising perpendicular to the traditional three rings. Its side chain is identical to that of desipramine.

Pharmacological Effects

The pharmacological effects of the tricyclic and tetracyclic antidepressants are highly similar. Initially, particular emphasis was placed on their relative effects in blocking the reuptake of norepinephrine or 5-HT. These differences came to underlie various theories on the biology of depression, particularly the low-norepinephrine hypothesis versus the low-5-HT hypothesis. In recent years, theories have become more complex as the pharmacological effects of these drugs have been shown to go beyond merely their immediate reuptake-blocking effects to include later secondary effects on pre- and postsynaptic receptors, on second-messenger systems, and on other neurotransmitter systems. Such effects may account for differences among the various drugs in both their range of efficacy and their side effects. At one time, the relative effects of norepinephrine reuptake blocking versus 5-HT reuptake blocking were used to explain the relative sedative properties (5-HT) versus activating properties (norepinephrine) of these drugs. Sedation, which early on was ascribed to serotonergic and anticholinergic effects, has in part been ascribed to the antihistamine (H_1 receptor) actions of TCAs. Some investigators have argued that

Tricyclic antidepressants (TCAs): overview

Efficacy	Second- or third-line agents for MDD (FDA approved for all) Panic disorder OCD (FDA approved for clomipramine) Pain syndromes Migraine prophylaxis Enuresis (FDA approved for imipramine)
Side effects	Dry mouth, constipation, urinary retention, blurred vision, confusion Weight gain Sedation Sexual dysfunction Orthostasis Tachycardia Cardiac conduction abnormalities
Dosage and administration	Individualize with low bedtime dosing (25–50 mg) for imipramine and amitriptyline. Increase by 25–50 mg every 3–7 days to target dosage of 150–300 mg/day. (Nortriptyline should be started at 10–25 mg and increased, as needed, to a maximum dosage of 150 mg/day.) Monitor levels and ECGs after dose is stabilized.
Safety in overdose	Lethal in overdose (induces arrhythmias) Lavage and monitor on a cardiac bed for QRS widening
Discontinuation	Flulike and GI symptoms from cholinergic rebound. Reduce by 25–50 mg every 3 days.
Drug interactions	CNS depressants: ↑ sedation, ataxia Anticoagulants: ↑ warfarin levels Antipsychotics: ↑ TCA and antipsychotic levels Cimetidine: ↑ TCA levels Clonidine: hypertensive crisis (**avoid**) L-dopa: TCAs ↓ absorption MAOIs: serotonin syndrome (avoid clomipramine; imipramine and amitriptyline may be used with close monitoring) Stimulants: ↑ TCA levels Oral contraceptives: ↑ TCA levels Quinidine: ↑ arrhythmias (**avoid**) SSRIs: ↑ TCA levels Sympathomimetics: ↑ arrhythmias, hypertension, tachycardia

Note.   ECG = electrocardiogram; GI = gastrointestinal; MAOI = monoamine oxidase inhibitor; MDD = major depressive disorder; SSRI = selective serotonin reuptake inhibitor.

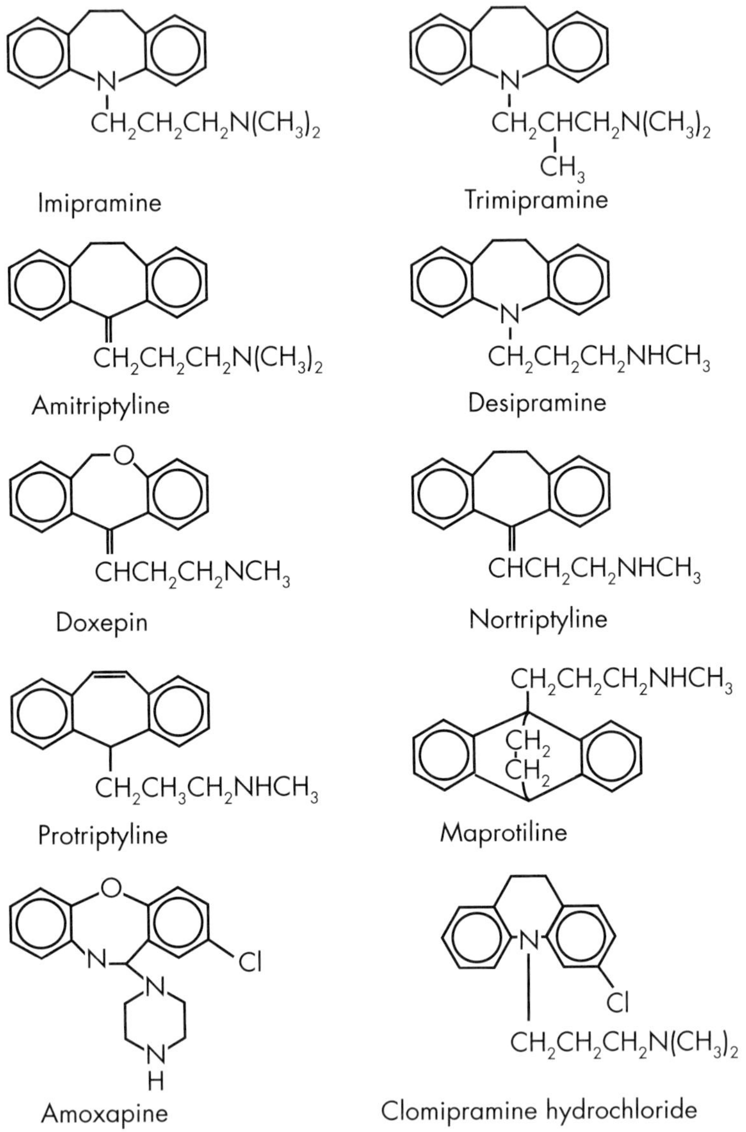

Figure 3–8.   Chemical structures of tricyclic and tetracyclic antidepressants.

weight gain could also be due to H_1 receptor–blocking effects. Anticholinergic effects include dry mouth, constipation, urinary hesitancy, blurred vision, and confusion. The H_2 receptor–blocking effects may play a role in these drugs promoting healing of peptic ulcers.

The relative norepinephrine reuptake–blocking effects, compared with 5-HT reuptake–blocking effects, of the non-MAOI antidepressants are summarized in Table 3–7. The relative effects of these agents on acetylcholine, α_1, H_1, 5-HT$_1$, and 5-HT$_2$ receptors are summarized in Table 3–8. These potencies represent best estimates based on receptor-binding and clinical studies. Note that the TCAs currently available in the United States are relatively weak 5-HT reuptake blockers. Clomipramine is the one exception to this rule. Indeed, in some in vivo models, TCAs—other than clomipramine—are devoid of 5-HT-blocking effects, as is trazodone. Moreover, recent research points to some of the antidepressants as having 5-HT receptor–blocking effects, suggesting that some are 5-HT antagonists. Taken together, laboratory data suggest that the tricyclics—other than clomipramine (see Chapter 6, "Antianxiety Agents")—are weak serotonergic agents. In contrast, the SSRIs are relatively pure 5-HT reuptake blockers, with little in the way of antagonist effects. Thus, these drugs offer an alternative for the clinician. The tricyclic and tetracyclic antidepressants are virtually devoid of dopamine reuptake–blocking effects. Of the available antidepressants, only sertraline and bupropion have such effects, and the effects are somewhat weak. Variations in biological effects help in drug selection, in terms of both clinical efficacy and side effects. The types of side effects that are seen with tricyclic and tetracyclic compounds are summarized in Table 3–9.

Indications

The principal indication for TCAs and related compounds approved by the FDA for marketing is major depression. Other FDA-approved indications include anxiety (for doxepin) and childhood enuresis (for imipramine as an adjunctive treatment). Nonapproved but common uses include insomnia (particularly for amitriptyline and doxepin), headache (most commonly for amitriptyline, imipramine, and doxepin), agoraphobia with panic attacks (for imipramine and clomipramine particularly), chronic pain syndromes (most frequently for doxepin and maprotiline), and bulimia (for imipramine and desipramine). Imipramine has also been reported to be effective in treating

Table 3–7.   Norepinephrine (NE) and serotonin (5-HT) reuptake–blocking effects of the non-MAOI antidepressants

Antidepressant	NE	5-HT
Amitriptyline	+	++
Amoxapine	++	+
Bupropion	+/–	0
Citalopram/escitalopram	0	+++
Clomipramine	++	+++
Desipramine	+++	+
Doxepin	+	+
Fluoxetine	0	+++
Fluvoxamine	0	+++
Imipramine	+	++
Levomilnacipran	++	
Maprotiline	++	0
Mirtazapine	+	–
Nefazodone	0/+	+
Nortriptyline	++	+
Paroxetine	+[a]	+++
Protriptyline	+++	+
Sertraline	0	+++
Trazodone	0	+
Trimipramine	0	0
Venlafaxine	+	++

Note.   Data are approximations of relative activity from in vivo, in vitro, and clinical studies. Data on clomipramine include results on desmethylclomipramine on both active metabolites with pronounced effects on noradrenergic systems. In certain in vivo models, the tricyclic antidepressants (other than clomipramine) and trazodone have been reported not to block 5-HT uptake. MAOI=monoamine oxidase inhibitor. Strength of effect represented on a scale from 0 (no effect) to +++ (marked effect). +/– indicates marginal effect.
[a]Effect at high doses.

GAD, and trimipramine and doxepin were once thought to be effective in treating peptic ulcers. The most recently released TCA, clomipramine, has potent anti-obsessive-compulsive effects, as do the SSRIs, and is FDA approved for that use. Obviously, these drugs exert rather wide pharmacological effects, which account for their potentially broad range of actions. (For further discussion of the use of TCAs in the treatment of anxiety disorders, see the section on antidepressants in Chapter 6.)

Table 3–8. Relative receptor-blocking effects of antidepressants

Antidepressant	ACh	α_1	H_1	5-HT$_1$	5-HT$_2$
Amitriptyline	+++	+++	++	+/–	+/–
Amoxapine	+	++	+	+/–	+++
Bupropion	0	0	0	0	0
Citalopram/escitalopram	0	0	0	0	
Clomipramine	+	++	+	0	+
Desipramine	+	+	+	0	+/–
Doxepin	++	+++	+++	+/–	+/–
Fluoxetine	0	0	0	0	+/–
Fluvoxamine	0	0	0	0	0
Imipramine	++	+	+	0	+/–
Maprotiline	+	+	++	0	+/–
Mirtazapine	0	0	+++	+	+
Nefazodone	0	+	0	+	++
Nortriptyline	+	+	+	+/–	+
Paroxetine	+	0	0	0	0
Protriptyline	+++	+	+	0	+
Sertraline	0	0	0	0	0
Trazodone	0	++	+/–	+	++
Trimipramine	++	++	+++	0	+/–
Venlafaxine	0	0	0	0	0

Note. Data are approximations of relative activity from in vivo, in vitro, and clinical studies. ACh = muscarinic acetylcholine receptor; α_1 = α_1-adrenergic receptor; H_1 = histamine$_1$ receptor; 5-HT$_1$ = serotonin$_1$ receptor; 5-HT$_2$ = serotonin$_2$ receptor. Strength of effect represented on scale from 0 (no effect) to +++ (marked effect). +/– indicates marginal effect.

Table 3–9. Common or troublesome side effects of tricyclic and tetracyclic drugs

Anticholinergic effects
  Dry mouth
  Constipation
  Blurred vision
  Urinary hesitancy
  Esophageal reflux
Cardiovascular effects
  Orthostatic hypotension
  Palpitations
  Conduction slowing
  Hypertension

Central nervous system effects
  Tremor
  Sedation
  Stimulation
  Myoclonic twitches
  Seizure (maprotiline)
  Extrapyramidal symptoms (amoxapine)
Other
  Perspiration
  Weight gain
  Sexual dysfunction
  Impotence

Currently, eight tricyclic and two tetracyclic antidepressants are available in the United States. One tricyclic, clomipramine, is approved for the treatment of OCD but not for depression. It is used worldwide, however, as a major antidepressant, particularly in cases of refractory depression. Generic and brand names, formulations and strengths, and therapeutic dosage ranges of the tricyclic and tetracyclic antidepressants are listed in Table 3–10.

The original patents have expired on all of these drugs, and generic preparations are now available. In the United States, use of generic compounds has not been without controversy. Although generic drugs offered a savings for the consumer, some clinicians questioned their pharmacological equivalence. One difficulty stemmed from the FDA definition of bioequivalence, which relies heavily on the demonstration that an identical dosage of a generic preparation produces blood levels within a specified range (20%–30%) above and below those produced by the original compound. Even with approved generic preparations, some studies had suggested that they were not truly equivalent to standard brands. Moreover, pharmaceutical companies were not required to prove that their generic preparations had equivalence in clinical or biological potency. This area appears to be less of a problem at present because generic drug manufacturers have improved their production methods.

Blood Levels

In past decades, considerable attention has been paid to the use of drug blood levels to monitor treatment with various psychotropic agents. Currently, blood levels are most used in patients treated with TCAs, neuroleptics, clozapine, lithium carbonate, and anticonvulsants. Blood levels have not proved to be useful with the SSRIs and most newer antidepressants. Likewise, blood levels for benzodiazepines are neither widely available nor commonly used. Drug concentrations are determined primarily in serum (e.g., for lithium carbonate and anticonvulsants) or plasma (e.g., for TCAs). In addition to measuring the concentration of neuroleptics in blood, some laboratories measure the relative binding to dopamine receptors (so-called radioreceptor assays). However, this practice has not been widely adopted.

Generally, TCA serum levels are determined in blood drawn 8–12 hours after the patient's last dose to avoid false peaks in blood levels that would occur if blood were drawn immediately after a patient had taken the medication.

Table 3–10. Tricyclic and tetracyclic antidepressants: names, formulations and strengths, and dosages

Generic name	Brand name[a]	Formulations and strengths	Therapeutic dosage range[b] (mg/day)
Tricyclics			
Amitriptyline	Elavil	Tablets: 10, 25, 50, 75, 100, 150 mg	150–300
Clomipramine	Anafranil	Capsules: 25, 50, 75 mg	100–250
Desipramine	Norpramin	Tablets: 10, 25, 50, 75, 100, 150 mg	150–300
Doxepin	Sinequan	Capsules: 10, 25, 50, 75, 100, 150 mg	150–300
		Oral solution: 10 mg/mL (120-mL bottle)	
	Silenor	Tablets: 3, 6 mg	3–6[c]
Imipramine	Tofranil	Tablets: 10, 25, 50 mg	150–300
Imipramine pamoate	Tofranil-PM[d]	Capsules: 75, 100, 125, 150 mg	150–300
Nortriptyline	Aventyl, Pamelor	Capsules: 10, 25, 50, 75 mg	50–150
		Oral solution: 10 mg/5 mL (480-mL bottle)	
Protriptyline	Vivactil	Tablets: 5, 10 mg	15–60
Trimipramine maleate	Surmontil	Capsules: 25, 50, 100 mg	150–300
Tetracyclics			
Amoxapine	Asendin	Tablets: 25, 50, 100, 150 mg	150–400
Maprotiline	Ludiomil	Tablets: 25, 50, 75 mg	150–225

[a]All the tricyclic and tetracyclic antidepressants shown are available generically. Most of the brand-name drugs listed have been discontinued.
[b]Dosage ranges are approximate. Many patients respond at relatively low dosages (even dosages below those in the ranges given in table); others may require higher dosages.
[c]Dosage range for the treatment of insomnia.
[d]Sustained release.

Also, plasma levels are most accurate when the blood is drawn after the patient has achieved steady state—the point at which a specific dose of drug given over a several-day period produces a consistent blood level. For most TCAs, this period is approximately 5–7 days.

Plasma levels can be particularly useful barometers of drug metabolism. There is approximately a 30-fold difference among human subjects in plasma levels of TCAs produced by a single, fixed milligram-per-kilogram dose of a drug, reflecting the degree to which the slowest and fastest metabolizers differ in drug absorption and metabolism. The TCAs are metabolized in part via the CYP2D6 enzyme. Approximately 5%–7% of the white population is deficient in this enzyme. In addition, metabolism of the TCAs is affected by age and by inhibition or activation by other drugs. Obviously, slow metabolizers (such as elderly persons) are at a higher risk for attaining toxic levels of drugs, whereas fast metabolizers may have difficulty building drug levels. Most patients, however, fall in the middle range of the normal bell-shaped curve distribution.

The clearest use of TCAs is for patients with more severe major depression. There is little or no relationship between TCA level and clinical response in patients with nonendogenous depression or in those with dysthymia. Two types of positive relationships between TCA level and clinical response in endogenously depressed patients have been described in the literature. Glassman et al. (1977) reported a sigmoidal relationship between response and imipramine plus desipramine levels; clinical response increases with plasma level up to approximately 250 ng/mL and then levels off thereafter (Figure 3–9). Glassman et al. reported rates of response of 30%, 67%, and 93% for patients with plasma levels in the ranges of less than 150 ng/mL, 150–225 ng/mL, and greater than 225 ng/mL, respectively. For nortriptyline, a curvilinear relationship has been described, as indicated in Figure 3–10. Response increases with plasma level and then plateaus in the range of approximately 50–150 ng/mL, with a decrease in response at plasma levels greater than 150 ng/mL. The critical range of 50–150 ng/mL has been called the *therapeutic window*. Nonresponding patients with plasma levels of approximately 150 ng/mL may respond to a lowering of dosage and plasma level into the window. The decreased response at levels above the window is not due to side effects. Therapeutic windows have at times been described for other drugs, but these windows are not as clear as that seen with nortriptyline. Approximate therapeutic plasma levels for tricyclic and tetracyclic drugs are summarized in Table 3–11.

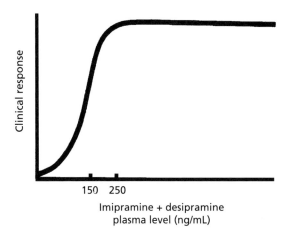

Figure 3–9. Sigmoidal relationship between clinical response and imipramine plus desipramine plasma levels.

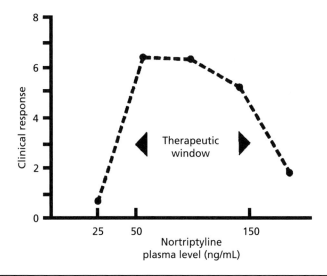

Figure 3–10. Curvilinear relationship between clinical response and nortriptyline plasma levels.

Table 3–11.   Approximate therapeutic serum level ranges for tricyclic and tetracyclic drugs

Drug	Serum level (ng/mL)
Amitriptyline	100–250[a]
Amoxapine	Unknown
Desipramine	150–300
Doxepin	120–250[a]
Imipramine	150–300[a]
Maprotiline	150–250
Nortriptyline[b]	50–150
Protriptyline	75–250
Trimipramine	Unknown

[a]Total concentration of drug and demethylated metabolite.
[b]Has a clear therapeutic window.

A number of medications may increase or decrease plasma levels, generally by interfering with or augmenting liver microsomal enzyme activity. For example, nicotine, barbiturates (including butalbital [Fiorinal]), chloral hydrate, phenytoin, and carbamazepine induce breakdown of TCAs, and clinicians should keep this in mind when prescribing TCAs for patients who are taking these compounds. In contrast, antipsychotics (particularly phenothiazines), the SSRIs, methylphenidate, disulfiram, and fenfluramine increase plasma levels by slowing drug metabolism in the liver. (Fenfluramine [Pondimin] was withdrawn from the market in 1997 when the combination fenfluramine plus phentermine [commonly referred to as *fen-phen*] was found to be associated with heart valve disease.) The SSRIs have become the agents one worries about most because they are potent competitive inhibitors of the CYP2D6 enzyme and thus may substantially increase TCA plasma levels. Conversely, TCAs increase phenothiazine plasma levels. Benzodiazepines and antiparkinsonian medications have little or no effect on TCA levels.

Several issues arise when one considers plasma level data. For one, studies generally use fixed milligram-per-kilogram dosing, and consequently, it is possible that a patient with a given TCA plasma level (e.g., 250 ng/mL) taking the drug at a given dosage (e.g., 300 mg/day of imipramine) might well have responded to a lower dosage and at a lower plasma level. In a sense, then, plasma levels can be viewed as barometers of the adequacy of treatment. Patients who are not responding to a 4- to 6-week trial of imipramine but who have attained a plasma level of 150 ng/mL or less may respond to an increase in dosage and plasma level to greater than 200 ng/mL. On the other hand, other patients who are responding at exactly the same dosage and plasma level do not need to have the dosage or plasma level increased, even if the plasma level is below the therapeutic range. Some investigators have advocated determining the plasma level for any patient who is responding to a TCA in order to record that patient's therapeutic plasma level while taking that drug. This could prove important if the patient has a recurrence and requires retreatment.

Sometimes a routine check of a TCA blood level in a patient who is clinically much improved and has only minor side effects reveals a plasma level of greater than 400 ng/mL, and the patient relapses when the dose is decreased to bring down the plasma level. This result suggests that for that particular patient, a very high plasma level is necessary for improvement. Indeed, there was a prospective report that some patients require very high dosages and blood levels for an adequate response, although there is an inherent risk with this approach. So far, only amitriptyline shows clear toxicity related to plasma levels around 500 ng/mL. Obviously, clinical judgment is necessary. An ECG is useful with patients who do well only at very high plasma levels of the drug to ensure that cardiac conduction is not seriously affected—that is, to ensure that no intracardiac conduction slowing takes place.

Formerly, the variation in TCA assays among laboratories was of major importance because clinicians were unable to interpret a given value in their laboratories. Major national efforts to cross-validate results from laboratories have helped, and this problem appears to have resolved. In summary, plasma levels can provide useful clinical information if the clinician keeps these issues in mind.

Side Effects

A review in the *Physicians' Desk Reference* (PDR) of the package-insert information on each of the TCAs and related agents indicates their myriad side effects. The side effects can be grouped broadly into categories (e.g., anticholinergic, cardiovascular; see Table 3–9). This organization is somewhat artificial because a single side effect (e.g., sedation) may be due to any number of distinct neurochemical effects (e.g., histamine blockade, increased 5-HT availability, 5-HT$_2$ antagonism) or combinations of effects. In addition, some side effects may reflect drug action either in the brain or at the periphery or both (e.g., orthostatic hypotension).

How can clinicians help in the management of side effects? In some patients, particularly those with complicating medical illness, side reactions may not be entirely controllable or manageable. There are, however, some things that can be done, particularly for less severe reactions in medically healthy patients.

One very important issue is *attitude*. Early on, some psychiatrists commonly had rather negative views about medication, which were communicated indirectly or overtly to the patient, particularly if the impetus to try medications had arisen from the patient and not the physician. In our experience, such attitudes can be troubling to the patient, who must rely on the physician's belief in the importance of medication trials and in being able to deal with the side effects. The imperative for clinicians to develop well-reasoned and balanced views about prescribing drugs has obviated this problem somewhat in recent years.

A general principle of drug prescribing is that some side effects can be managed by reducing the dosage or can be avoided by increasing the dosage slowly. In our experience, this is particularly true for the early emergence of "spaciness," depersonalization, confusion, orthostatic hypotension, or marked sedation. If these reactions persist in the presence of more moderate dose escalation, a switch to another TCA or another class of drug may be necessary. In dealing with anticholinergic side effects or sedation, switching to desipramine seems reasonable. For patients who develop orthostatic hypotension, nortriptyline is often a useful alternative because it tends to produce orthostatic changes at plasma levels above the so-called therapeutic window. Thus, nortriptyline is more easily tolerated than imipramine, whose orthostatic effects are often produced at low plasma levels (see previous subsection on TCA blood levels). Nortriptyline has been used successfully in several studies on poststroke and geriatric depression.

Peripheral anticholinergic side effects have also been reported as being ameliorated by administering bethanechol, a procholinergic drug, at dosages of 25–50 mg tid or qid and generally continuing for as long as the patient continues to take TCAs. This drug can be particularly helpful to patients with urinary hesitancy. In cases of anticholinergic delirium, physostigmine (a centrally acting procholinergic agent) may be administered either intravenously or intramuscularly to clarify the diagnosis.

Blurred vision as a result of TCAs can be treated with 4% pilocarpine drops or with oral bethanechol. Patients otherwise doing well with maintenance TCA treatment, and therefore likely to be taking the drug for some time, may require a change in their eyeglasses prescription to correct the blurring of vision. For severe dry mouth, a 1% pilocarpine solution can be created by mixing the 4% solution available as eye drops with three parts water. This solution can be swished around the mouth for a few minutes, 30–60 minutes before an increase in salivation is needed. For example, patients may use this mouthwash before having to give a lecture. Bethanechol in 5-mg or 10-mg tablets may be administered sublingually for a similar effect. Although we know of no studies, anticholinergic effects may be ameliorated with cholinesterase inhibitors.

An important, possibly antihistaminic, side effect of TCAs is weight gain—particularly seen with amitriptyline and doxepin—which can be difficult to control pharmacologically. Often, patients who demonstrate this side effect while taking one TCA will continue to gain weight when switched to another, related drug. In some patients, switching to one of the newer antidepressants may be the only way to maintain an antidepressant effect and promote weight reduction, because MAOIs also cause weight gain. Unfortunately, some patients continue to gain weight while receiving the drug to which they are showing an antidepressant response. In such cases, support and advice about dieting may be the only recourse. Addition of topiramate may facilitate weight loss.

The two tetracyclic agents, maprotiline and amoxapine, have been reported to produce troublesome side effects—seizures and extrapyramidal symptoms—that have been less frequently reported with the standard TCAs. Induced seizures have been reported in several single case reports of patients taking maprotiline. Our group reported on a series of 11 patients with maprotiline-related seizures at one hospital and a study of all U.S. maprotiline-related seizures (Dessain et al. 1986). In our series, prolonged treatment (longer than 6 weeks) at high dosages (225–400 mg/day) appeared to be a major factor. This was confirmed in the U.S. survey. In addition, rapid dose escalation—with the dosage reaching 150 mg/day within 7 days—was a major factor in the general survey. When these two factors were eliminated, the risk of seizures appeared to approximate that associated with classic antidepressants (approximately 0.2%). The manufacturer of maprotiline altered its dosage guidelines, recommending beginning treatment at 75 mg/day for 2 weeks, a maximum dosage of 225 mg/day for up to 6 weeks, and maintenance at 175 mg/day or less. The previous dosage schedule was similar to that of imipramine.

Amoxapine has been reported to produce several side effects associated with dopamine receptor blockade. These side effects are similar to those more commonly found with the neuroleptic loxapine, such as galactorrhea, akathisia, and other extrapyramidal symptoms and even a few cases of dyskinesia. Amoxapine is metabolized to a 7-OH metabolite. In some individuals, alternate hydroxylation at the 8 position results in the accumulation of a neuroleptic metabolite. Generally speaking, we recommend tapering or stopping medications if these symptoms occur (see subsection on blood levels earlier in this section).

Overdose

TCA overdoses can result in death. Tricyclics have narrow safety margins, and intracardiac slowing and arrhythmias may result in death when overdoses are taken. In addition, patients taking overdoses can demonstrate confusion, delirium, and loss of consciousness.

Dosage and Administration

After evaluating a depressed patient, the clinician must determine whether TCAs are an appropriate treatment. In the first edition of this manual, we subscribed to the approach of using a TCA first in the treatment of endogenous or major depression. Because of the superior safety and tolerability of the newer agents, particularly the SSRIs, the TCAs were relegated to second-line status in the second edition. However, some investigators continue to suspect that the TCAs are superior to the newer agents in the treatment of more serious, melancholic depressive episodes. Although it has been difficult to demonstrate greater efficacy for TCAs (see the "Indications" subsection in the section on SSRIs earlier in this chapter), the jury is still out. Because most studies on inpatients and patients with melancholic depression have employed TCAs, these agents still need to be considered early in the treatment of more serious depression.

The choice of which TCA to use is somewhat a matter of personal preference. There is really considerable overlap among these various drugs, although some are a bit more stimulating (desipramine and protriptyline) and others are more sedating (amitriptyline and doxepin). Among the secondary amines, desipramine and nortriptyline have become two of the most popular

TCAs with which to begin treatment. These two drugs have the most favorable side-effect profiles in the TCA group. In addition, these two drugs have reliable plasma level data regarding clinical response. On the other hand, amitriptyline has a very poor side-effect profile secondary to its anticholinergic and antihistaminic side effects and may not be the best first choice for many patients, especially elderly ones. With any of these drugs, the clinician is best advised to start with a relatively low dose, which can then be increased slowly.

For imipramine, the starting doses and regimens vary. One common imipramine regimen is to prescribe 75 mg/day during week 1 and to increase the dosage weekly, as needed, to 150 mg/day during week 2, 225 mg/day during week 3, and 300 mg/day during week 4. Another approach is to start at 50 mg/day, increasing the dosage by 25 mg every few days, as tolerated, to 150 mg/day and then, after about 2 weeks, to increase the dosage from 150 mg/day, at a rate of 50 mg every 3 days, to 300 mg/day. (Similar dosage regimens are recommended for other uses of the drug, such as for panic and pain.)

In prescribing imipramine for some patients, particularly elderly patients (who may be especially intolerant or may be taking other medications), it seems reasonable to begin at 25 mg on day 1 and to increase to 50 mg on day 2, allowing the patient to become acclimated to a single small dose. We also advise a more conservative schedule of increases for elderly patients, keeping the dosage at 50 mg/day for 1 week and thereafter increasing it at a rate of 25 mg every 2 days to 150 mg/day. After 7 days at 150 mg/day, the dosage can be increased further as tolerated. Elderly patients present a somewhat distinctive problem regarding drug-drug interactions (see Chapter 12, "Pharmacotherapy of Specific Populations"). The not uncommon medical problems of elderly persons and their relatively slow drug metabolism usually dictate conservative management. However, clinicians must be careful: some elderly patients are not slow metabolizers but instead require reasonably high dosages and therefore are at risk of being undertreated. The degree of side effects can be a useful barometer of the patient's ability to tolerate a given dosage, and plasma levels may aid in prescribing optimal doses (see subsections on TCA blood levels and side effects earlier in this section).

For doxepin, amitriptyline, and trimipramine, dosage ranges similar to those for imipramine are recommended in both younger and older patients. Trimipramine has a relatively low side-effect profile in elderly patients and has a rapid effect on promoting sleep.

Protriptyline and nortriptyline are prescribed in rather different ways. For younger patients, protriptyline is generally started at 15 mg/day (5 mg tid) in week 1, with an increase each week of 5–10 mg in the daily dose, to a maximum dosage of 60 mg/day. For elderly patients, protriptyline is generally begun at 10 mg/day, aiming for a maximum dosage of 30–40 mg/day. Nortriptyline, which is the only TCA that clearly has a so-called therapeutic window, can be ineffective if plasma levels are either too low or too high. The therapeutic dosage range for nortriptyline in adults is 50–150 mg/day. We recommend starting at 50 mg/day and weekly increasing the daily dosage by 50 mg to 100 mg/day and then to 150 mg/day if needed. (In elderly patients, begin at 25 mg/day and increase the dosage to 50 mg/day after 3–4 days.) After 3 weeks, a decrease in dosage may be helpful—a situation rather different from that of the other TCAs (see subsection on TCA blood levels earlier in this section).

Amoxapine's starting dosage in healthy adults is 150 mg/day, with a maximum dosage of 400 mg/day. A few patients have been treated with up to 600 mg/day. However, this dosage increases the risk of seizures. This drug may be particularly effective in treating psychotic depression (Anton and Sexauer 1983).

Maprotiline's starting and maximum dosages are 75 and 225 mg/day, respectively. To avoid seizures, the starting dose of maprotiline should be maintained for 2 weeks, and after 6 weeks of treatment, the dosage should be reduced to a maximum of 175 mg/day (Dessain et al. 1986).

Discontinuation

When discontinuing or tapering TCAs, it is most prudent to do so at a maximum rate of 25–50 mg every 2–3 days. Many patients will demonstrate symptoms of cholinergic rebound if the TCA is discontinued too abruptly. These symptoms include nausea, queasy stomach, cramping, sweating, headache, neck pain, and vomiting. We have observed several patients who experienced intense GI symptoms during and after TCA withdrawal. For these patients, propantheline bromide (15 mg tid prn) was extremely helpful. Moreover, Nelson et al. (1983) reported that some patients demonstrate "rebound" hypomania or mania with sudden cessation of TCAs, an observation confirmed by others.

When the issue of rebound symptoms versus a medical illness or recurrence of psychiatric symptoms is in doubt, a single dose of the discontinued drug will often relieve the symptoms rapidly, confirming the diagnosis of a withdrawal syndrome. There is one report in which withdrawal mania responded to reinstitution of desipramine therapy (Nelson et al. 1983).

Monoamine Oxidase Inhibitors

Pharmacological Effects

First-generation MAOIs—isocarboxazid, phenelzine, and tranylcypromine—have few direct effects on reuptake or receptor blockade. Instead, they inhibit MAO in various organs, exerting greater effects on monoamine oxidase A (MAO-A)—for which norepinephrine and 5-HT are primary substrates—than on MAO-B, which acts primarily on other amines (e.g., phenylethylamine) and dopamine. Also, MAO-A is found in the gut mucosa and is responsible for degrading various amines that can act as false neurotransmitters and produce hypertensive crises (see later in this section). Isocarboxazid, phenelzine, and tranylcypromine are so-called irreversible inhibitors. When these agents inhibit the enzyme, protein regeneration is required before MAO enzymatic activity is restored. Selegiline (Eldepryl), a selective irreversible MAO inhibitor used in the treatment of Parkinson's disease, exerts its effects on MAO-B and is generally thought to have a very low risk of producing hypertensive crises. However, at the low dosages used in treating parkinsonian patients (5–10 mg/day), this drug is a weak antidepressant, and data from Sunderland et al. (1989) suggested that at higher antidepressant dosages, the drug affects both MAO-A and MAO-B and thus does not protect against hypertensive crises. More information on selegiline is provided in the section "Selective and Reversible Monoamine Oxidase Inhibitors" later in this chapter.

There are two structural classes of MAOIs: the hydrazines (i.e., phenelzine) and the nonhydrazines (tranylcypromine and selegiline) (Figure 3–11 and Table 3–12).

Indications

The primary PDR clinical indication for MAOIs is for treatment of depression refractory to TCA therapy. Phenelzine has an FDA-approved indication for anxious depression. MAOIs are also effective in the treatment of social phobia. With so many other safer antidepressants currently available, MAOIs are now typically indicated when several trials have failed. Still, some patients

Monoamine oxidase inhibitors (MAOIs): overview

Efficacy	Third-line agents for the following: MDD (FDA approved for resistant depression) Social anxiety Panic disorder Second-line agents for Parkinson's disease (selegiline has FDA approval)
Side effects	Weight gain Orthostasis Sexual dysfunction Dry mouth Insomnia/somnolence Headache
Safety in overdose	Can be lethal in overdose. Hypertensive crisis, stroke, and myocardial infarction have been reported. Manage with lavage, emesis induction, and close management of blood pressure and airway.
Dosage and administration	Phenelzine: start at 15 mg bid or tid and increase by 15 mg per week to target dosage of 60–90 mg/day. Tranylcypromine: start at 10 mg bid or tid and increase by 10 mg per week to target dosage of 40–60 mg/day. Isocarboxazid: start at 10 mg bid and increase dosage, if the drug is tolerated, by 10 mg every 2–4 days to 40 mg/day by the end of the first week. Maximum recommended dosage is 60 mg/day, administered in divided doses. Selegiline transdermal system (Emsam): start with 6-mg patch daily for 4 weeks and then increase to 9-mg patch for 2 weeks, and then 12-mg patch as needed. No dietary restrictions at 6 mg/day.
Discontinuation	Flulike symptoms, hallucinations, hypomania, and dysphoria reported with sudden discontinuation. Taper dose by 25% per week.
Drug interactions	Foods containing high levels of tyramine (**contraindicated**) (see Table 3–14): hypertensive crisis β-Blockers: ↑ hypotension, bradycardia Oral hypoglycemics: ↑ hypoglycemic effects Bupropion (**contraindicated**): hypertensive crisis, seizure Carbamazepine (**contraindicated**): hypertensive crisis

Monoamine oxidase inhibitors (MAOIs): overview *(continued)*

Drug interactions *(continued)*	Meperidine (**contraindicated**): serotonin syndrome Nefazodone: possible serotonin syndrome Sympathomimetics: hypertensive crisis SSRIs (**contraindicated**): serotonin syndrome TCAs: clomipramine **contraindicated:** serotonin syndrome Mirtazapine (**contraindicated**): hypertensive crisis SNRIs (**contraindicated**): serotonin syndrome

Note. MDD=major depressive disorder; SNRI=serotonin-norepinephrine reuptake inhibitor; SSRI=selective serotonin reuptake inhibitor; TCA=tricyclic antidepressant.

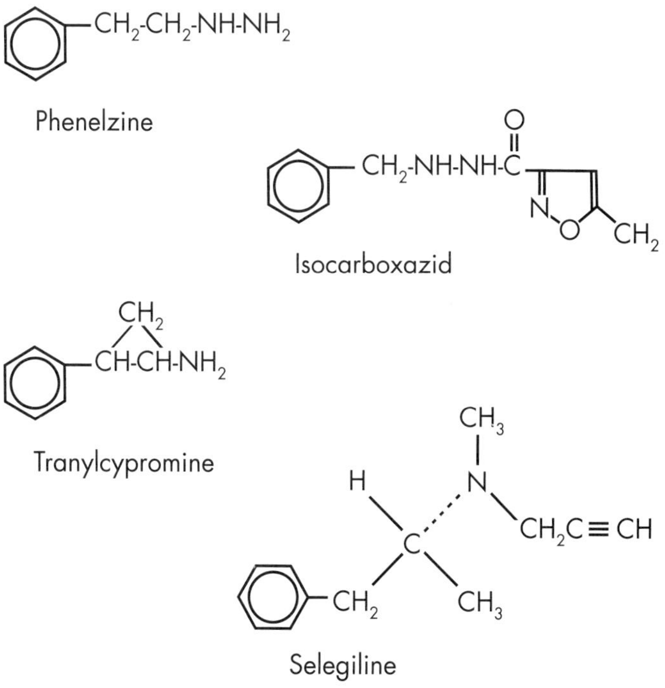

Figure 3–11. Chemical structures of monoamine oxidase inhibitors.

Table 3–12.   Monoamine oxidase inhibitors (MAOIs): names, formulations and strengths, and dosages

Generic name	Brand name	Formulations and strength	Oral concentrate	Therapeutic dosage[a] range (mg/day)
Phenelzine	Nardil	Tablet: 15 mg	None	45–90
Selegiline	Eldepryl	Capsule: 5 mg	None	20–50
	Zelapar	Orally disintegrating tablet: 1.25 mg		
	Emsam	Patch: 6 mg/24 hr, 9 mg/24 hr, 12 mg/24 hr		
Tranylcypromine	Parnate	Tablet: 10 mg	None	30–60
Isocarboxazid	Marplan	Tablet: 10 mg	None	30–60

[a]Dosage ranges are approximate. Many patients respond at relatively low dosages (even dosages below those in the ranges given in table).

respond better to MAOIs than to any other class of agents. Although the British had emphasized frequently that the MAOIs were not particularly helpful in treating the severe forms of major depression referred to in the past as endogenous, the American experience, including our own, was entirely different. These drugs were lifesavers for many severely depressed patients, particularly those whose depression did not respond to TCAs.

Why the discrepancy? For one, there was little doubt that MAOIs were effective in patients with panic attacks or with anxious or atypical depression. However, their effectiveness in patients with melancholic or endogenous depression may require the prescription of considerably higher doses than those used in the early British trials, in which relatively low doses were used. Another difficulty with determining ranges of efficacy revolves around the occurrence of pronounced obsessionality, agitation, and anxiety in many endogenously depressed patients, who, in the early studies, may have been misdiagnosed as only anxiously depressed.

Investigators at Columbia University have attempted to define an atypical depressive syndrome that preferentially responds to phenelzine and other MAOIs such as moclobemide. Their data suggested that patients with atypical depression respond better to MAOIs than to TCAs. The SSRIs are also effective in treating atypical depression. Because the SSRIs are considerably safer than the MAOIs, the use of MAOIs in the treatment of atypical depression has dropped off considerably since the introduction of fluoxetine.

Side Effects

Common side effects of MAOIs are listed in Table 3–13. Because MAOIs do not block acetylcholine receptors, they produce less dry mouth, blurred vision, constipation, and urinary hesitancy than do TCAs. However, we have seen patients who have developed urinary hesitancy, presumably because of an increase in noradrenergic activity. When the problem occurs, a reduction in dosage may help. We have been less impressed with the adjunctive use of bethanechol with MAOIs than with its use with TCAs.

The most common side effect of MAOIs is dizziness, particularly of the orthostatic type. This side effect appears to be somewhat more common with MAOIs than with TCAs. Dose reduction may help, but, again, we have often found reduction in the dose to be problematic because too great a reduction may lead to reemergence of depressive symptoms. Alternative approaches in-

Table 3–13. Common or troublesome side effects of monoamine
oxidase inhibitors (MAOIs)

Orthostatic hypotension
Hypertensive crises (interactions with foodstuffs[a] or medications)
Hyperpyrexic reactions
Anorgasmia or sexual impotence
Insomnia during night
Sedation (particularly in daytime; due to insomnia during night)
Stimulation during day
Muscle cramps and myositis-like reactions
Urinary hesitancy[b]
Constipation[b]
Dry mouth[b]
Weight gain
Myoclonic twitches
Skin irritation at patch site (Emsam)

[a]See Table 3–14.
[b]Less than with tricyclic antidepressants.

clude 1) maintenance of adequate hydration—about eight glasses of fluid a
day—and increased salt intake; 2) use of support stockings, "bellybinders," or
corsets; and 3) addition of a mineralocorticoid (fludrocortisone [Florinef]).
Although this mineralocorticoid has been used in patients with orthostatic
hypotension not induced by medication, we have rarely found it to be helpful
at the usual dosage of 0.3 mg/day. We have been told by colleagues that fludrocortisone can be effective at a total daily dosage of 0.6–0.8 mg. An intriguing
report appeared before our second edition, pointing to the use of small
amounts of cheese to help maintain blood pressure—a counterintuitive but
imaginative solution. However, most clinicians have been wary of the understandable risk of hypertensive crises with cheese, particularly when one does
not really know the tyramine content of the foodstuff. We are not aware of any
more recent reports on this. Similarly, one would intuit that adding a stimulant (D-amphetamine or methylphenidate) to an MAOI would result in
marked surges of blood pressure. In fact, however, Feighner et al. (1985) reported that the addition of stimulants for patients receiving MAOIs or
MAOI-TCA combinations normalized blood pressure in depressed patients
with serious orthostatic hypotension or brought out a clinical response in patients who had previously not had any response. There were no incidents of

hypertensive crises; in fact, several of the patients developed orthostatic hypotension. Daily dosages used were 5–20 mg of D-amphetamine and 10–15 mg of methylphenidate. Feighner et al. recommended beginning at a dosage of 2.5 mg/day of either drug. We have heard of several clinicians in the community who have used these approaches successfully, but we have also heard of occasional hypertensive crises when stimulants were used in combination with MAOIs.

Sedation and activation are also potential problems, the latter being more common. Activation takes two forms: stimulation during the day (particularly with tranylcypromine) and insomnia at night. Tranylcypromine's stimulatory effects have been related to its having a structure similar to that of amphetamines, although this pharmacological link has not been clearly established. Overstimulation can be ameliorated somewhat by dose reduction, although the side effect is not easily eliminated. If a dose reduction does not result in a decrease in stimulation, patients may need to be switched to another medication.

Phenelzine is, overall, far less stimulating and more sedating than tranylcypromine. As such, it offers a major alternative for daytime overstimulation. However, phenelzine may produce both insomnia and secondary daytime sedation. Oddly, one often encounters insomnia in patients who are nevertheless showing a good clinical response to the drug, making it a particularly difficult side effect to manage. Changing the dosage regimen may be helpful. Patients who are not taking phenelzine in the evening may benefit from switching drug taking to the evening hours. Conversely, patients who are taking much of the drug in the evening may respond by taking it earlier in the day. These manipulations can be helpful, although in our experience they are highly variable in their efficacy. Some patients may ultimately require hypnotic agents to overcome persistent insomnia. By the second edition of this manual, we had become very impressed with the addition of low doses of amitriptyline, trimipramine, or trazodone (50–100 mg at bedtime) to counteract MAOI-induced sleep disturbances. Caution should still be exercised in using trazodone or the TCAs with MAOIs because of the slight risk of developing a serotonin syndrome. With trazodone, we recommend trying doses of 50–100 mg per night. An increase to 150 mg hs can be tried if there has been no response at a lower dose and the medication has been well tolerated.

As the dose of an MAOI is increased to high levels to achieve a therapeutic effect, patients occasionally become "intoxicated"—drunk, ataxic, confused, and sometimes euphoric. This is a sign of overdose, and the dose should be reduced. Some patients develop muscle pains or paresthesias, which are probably the result of the MAOIs interfering with pyridoxine (vitamin B_6) metabolism. Pyridoxine administered at a dosage of approximately 100 mg/day can be helpful.

A particularly bothersome side effect is anorgasmia, which in some patients lessens over time. We have not been impressed with any pharmacological attempts to counteract this side effect, although cyproheptadine has been said to be helpful. Agents such as buspirone and bupropion are best avoided in combination with MAOIs.

Overdose

Overdoses are not necessarily lethal. Patients who overdose with an MAOI will show sedation and orthostasis. However, overdoses commonly involve other medications, which can result in serotonin syndromes or hypertensive reactions.

Drug Interactions

The greatest side-effect problems with MAOIs involve untoward interactions with certain foodstuffs or cold remedies, which may produce hypertensive crises with violent cerebrovascular accidents, or serotonin syndromes—consisting of hyperpyrexia, mental status changes, myoclonus, and delirium—that can lead to coma and death. MAO in the intestinal tract degrades tyramine. When MAO is inhibited by MAOIs, the individual is at risk for absorbing large amounts of tyramine and probably other substances (e.g., phenylethylamine), which can act as false neurotransmitters or indirect agonists and elevate blood pressure. Fortunately, dietary restrictions can markedly reduce the risk (Table 3–14). Various prohibited foods are included in lists in the PDR. These lists have been reviewed by several investigators, and relative risks have been attributed to many of the foods. Generally, we have begun to specifically advise patients to avoid eating Chinese food because of the ingredients used (e.g., soy sauce, sherry).

Serotonin syndrome is generally not due to interaction with foodstuffs. It represents increased central 5-HT activity and may be particularly provoked by the addition of certain medications. In some cases of either hypertensive or hyperpyrexic reactions, the exact cause is not clear. Of particular importance regarding medication interactions is warning patients to check with their phy-

Table 3–14.   Foods to be avoided with monoamine oxidase inhibitors

Foods definitely to be avoided:
  Beer, red wine
  Aged cheeses (cottage and cream cheese are allowed)
  Dry sausage
  Fava or Italian green beans
  Brewer's yeast
  Smoked fish
  Liver (beef or chicken)
Foods that may cause problems in large amounts but are otherwise less problematic:
  Alcohol
  Ripe avocado
  Yogurt
  Bananas (ripe)
  Soy sauce
Foods that were thought to be a problem but are probably not problematic in usual quantities:
  Chocolate
  Figs
  Meat tenderizers
  Caffeine-containing beverages
  Raisins

Source.   Based on McCabe and Tsuang 1982.

sician before taking other medications along with the MAOIs. Meperidine (Demerol), epinephrine, local anesthetics (containing sympathomimetic agents), and decongestants can be particularly dangerous.

We are often asked which decongestant or antihistamine can be used with the MAOIs. Unfortunately, there is little in the way of prospective data. Diphenhydramine is used by many practitioners, with apparent success. One problem with this approach, however, is that some over-the-counter diphenhydramine elixirs contain pseudoephedrine, and at least one untoward interaction with the latter agent has been seen by our group. Another option is nasal sprays, but with this form, too, some patients may show increases in blood pressure.

Another issue has to do with general anesthesia—during ECT or surgery—in patients treated with MAOIs. Although at first glance this seems a frightening prospect, many patients have successfully undergone procedures requiring general anesthesia without consequence. Indeed, for the second edition of this manual, Dr. George Murray informed us that Massachusetts General Hospital had collected reports on some 2,000 such cases. Obviously, anesthesiologists need to be apprised of a patient's medications to determine the safest approach. To this end, it is probably wise to have patients taking MAOIs carry a medical alert card. Still, in many settings, surgeons and anesthesiologists advise patients to stop taking MAOIs before undergoing surgery. Further study is needed to determine the most prudent approach to this knotty problem.

If a patient develops a surge in blood pressure with violent headaches, they should be instructed to go to a local emergency department. Phentolamine (Regitine), a central α-blocker, can be administered intravenously to reverse the acute rise in blood pressure. Years ago, some psychopharmacologists recommended that patients take oral chlorpromazine when headache occurred. We have stopped this practice unless patients have not had a documented increase in blood pressure because some patients will display marked headaches secondary to a lowering of blood pressure. Instead, we provide our patients with nifedipine, a calcium channel blocker, in case they experience marked increases in blood pressure; 10 mg per hour until relief occurs (generally one or two doses) appears to be very helpful. To enhance absorption, patients should be instructed to bite into the capsule before swallowing. This approach may prove problematic in elderly patients because acute lowering of blood pressure and myocardial infarction have been reported with this approach for these patients. We advise patients with headaches to have their blood pressure checked. In addition, routine monitoring of blood pressure with an MAOI, particularly during the first 6 weeks of treatment, seems prudent (for both the hypotensive and the hypertensive effects of the drug).

Dosage and Administration

The traditional therapeutic dosage ranges of three MAOIs are as follows: phenelzine, 45–90 mg/day; tranylcypromine, 30–60 mg/day; oral selegiline, 20–50 mg/day. Some patients require treatment at the higher end of the dosage range. For example, 90 mg/day of phenelzine is commonly required in a patient with severe depressive illness.

A patient treated with phenelzine should start taking the medication at 30 mg/day, and the dosage should be increased to 45 mg/day after 3 days. Thereafter, the dosage can be increased at a rate of 15 mg per week to 90 mg/day. We have seen patients who require as much as 120 mg/day; however, many patients cannot tolerate the orthostatic side effects of these drugs. Some investigators have recommended a dosage of 1 mg/kg per day of the drug as a guideline for adequacy of treatment.

For tranylcypromine, a starting dosage of 20 mg/day for 3 days seems reasonable. The dosage can then be increased to 30 mg/day for 1 week, with increases of 10 mg per week to 50–60 mg/day. The manufacturer's current recommended maximum dosage of the drug is 40 mg/day. One investigator, Dr. Jay Amsterdam, reported that extremely high dosages of the drug (110–130 mg/day) may help patients with even the most refractory depression. There is some thought that at such high dosages the drug is exerting alternative, additional effects—possibly acting as a reuptake blocker (Amsterdam and Berwish 1989). Once a patient has responded to the treatment, the medication should be maintained for a length of time similar to that recommended for the TCAs.

Discontinuation

The currently available MAOIs irreversibly bind MAO to such a degree that it takes approximately 2 weeks after the MAOI is stopped for the enzyme to regenerate. During this time, tyramine and drug interactions may occur. Thus, it is important to inform patients that they should maintain their dietary and drug restrictions for 2 weeks after the MAOI is discontinued. In addition, these drugs should be tapered to avoid rebound hypomania. Rarely, the withdrawal of an MAOI elicits a psychiatric excitement or psychosis resembling a delirium more than mania.

If the clinician wants to switch a patient from one MAOI to another, care must be taken to avoid drug-drug interactions. The clinician should taper the first MAOI and allow for a 10- to 14-day drug-free period before beginning another MAOI. Some patients have experienced severe untoward reactions in switching from one MAOI to another, particularly from phenelzine to tranylcypromine—perhaps reflecting the latter's amphetamine-like properties. In general, a good reason to switch from one MAOI to another is intolerance of side effects. If an adequate trial of an MAOI fails, there is little evidence that switching to another MAOI helps.

When a transition between a TCA and an MAOI is being made, the PDR recommends that patients stop taking all medications between trials for 10–14 days. Many clinicians, however, have reported that a briefer drug-free period (i.e., 1–5 days) is sufficient for the transition from a TCA to an MAOI. For the transition from an MAOI to a TCA, the 10- to 14-day period is generally recommended. The difference in these strategies is probably due to the 10- to 14-day period needed to regenerate MAO.

Patients taking MAOIs should wait 2 weeks after discontinuing the MAOI before starting fluoxetine. For the transition from fluoxetine to an MAOI, a 5-week period is recommended by the manufacturer because of the long half-life of the demethylated metabolite norfluoxetine. For the other SSRIs, a 2-week washout is adequate before starting an MAOI. Likewise, a 1- to 2-week washout should ensue before switching to an MAOI from venlafaxine or bupropion. The 5-HT$_2$ antagonists nefazodone and trazodone appear to require very short washouts; 1 week is enough.

Selective and Reversible Monoamine Oxidase Inhibitors

As described earlier, all of the currently available MAOIs at antidepressant doses are nonselective and irreversible inhibitors of MAO; that is, they irreversibly inhibit both MAO-A and MAO-B, and for enzyme activity to commence, new MAO must be generated. Drugs that selectively block MAO-B, such as selegiline, may substantially decrease the risk of hypertensive crises because they do not substantially affect MAO in the gut. Similarly, a reversible inhibitor of MAO-A would have a low affinity for MAO and would be readily displaced by pressor amines, thus reducing the risk of a hypertensive crisis. Two RIMAs, moclobemide and brofaromine, were under investigation, but interest in marketing these drugs in the United States has waned considerably over the years because of limited efficacy in clinical trials.

The FDA approved selegiline in 1991 for use in Parkinson's disease under the trade name Eldepryl. Much of the earlier clinical and scientific literature refers to selegiline by its earlier name, L-deprenyl. Selegiline has proved a useful drug in Parkinson's disease and may be the only antiparkinsonian drug that has neuroprotective qualities and modestly affects the progression of the illness. At the dosages used in Parkinson's disease, 5–10 mg/day, the drug is a selective but irreversible inhibitor of MAO-B. Unfortunately, currently available studies of the use of selegiline in depression suggest that dosages of 20–60 mg/day are required to relieve depression. At these higher dosages, both MAO-A and MAO-B are inhibited and hypertensive crises following ingestion of tyramine in foods are possible. One such case, albeit mild, has been reported in a patient treated with 20 mg/day of selegiline.

A selegiline transdermal system, marketed under the brand name Emsam, was approved by the FDA in February 2006. The transdermal delivery avoids high concentrations of drug in the gut and thus has less MAO-A inhibition in the gut and lower risk of hypertensive crises with the ingestion of specific foodstuffs. The formulation, however, appears to provide reasonably high levels of MAO-A and MAO-B inhibition in the brain.

Numerous clinical studies of the use of selegiline in depression have been published (Agosti et al. 1991; Mann et al. 1989; Sunderland et al. 1994). These studies can be interpreted as confirming the clear therapeutic effect of selegiline in patients with atypical and chronic depression and more serious depression. Furthermore, the Sunderland et al. study suggested that at a dosage of 60 mg/day, selegiline is useful for and well tolerated by geriatric patients with TRD. The drug is of substantial clinical interest because its pattern of side effects at dosages up to 40 mg/day appears quite favorable compared with that of the older MAOIs. Selegiline does not seem to cause clinically significant orthostatic hypotension or sexual dysfunction, and it may cause less insomnia than the older drugs. Several patients who were unable to tolerate the side effects of older MAOIs have tolerated selegiline quite well. It should be noted, however, that most published selegiline trials have lasted only 4–6 weeks, and some patients treated with the older MAOIs develop clinically intolerable side effects only after taking the drug for 2–3 months. Psychiatrists already experienced in the MAOI management of patients may find selegiline worth trying in cases of treatment-resistant conditions. Patients who have a good antidepressant response to MAOIs but who are experiencing intolerable side effects may be the best candidates for selegiline.

Oral selegiline is currently not approved for use in depression; only transdermal selegiline is approved for the treatment of depression. Because selegiline is metabolized to R isomers of amphetamine and methamphetamine in the body and is a dopamine reuptake inhibitor, we strongly urge a 2-week interval between stopping an older MAOI and starting selegiline. Patients treated with transdermal selegiline at dosages higher than 6 mg/day should adhere to the usual restrictions of a low-tyramine diet. That being said, we have done studies of transdermal selegiline at dosages higher than 6 mg/day and have not observed any dietary effects.

Three other comments are worth making here. First, measuring platelet MAOI in patients who are taking selegiline is probably not useful because almost complete inhibition occurs after 1 week at a dosage of 10 mg/day. Second, the drug is very expensive: a local drugstore charges around $5 per 5-mg pill. Finally, selegiline should not be stopped abruptly because sudden cessation is associated with a discontinuation syndrome consisting of nausea, dizziness, and hallucinations.

At least two studies demonstrated efficacy of transdermal selegiline against placebo in major depression (Amsterdam 2003; Bodkin and Amsterdam 2002). Of interest is that in patch delivery, selegiline in brain may be a far more potent MAO-A inhibitor, and this may confer greater efficacy. The drug (in a patch) has earned FDA approval for major depression. As indicated earlier, the transdermal formulation bypasses gut and liver and allows for higher plasma levels with a low risk of foodstuff interactions. The drug is available in patches of 20, 30, and 40 mg/cm^2 (6, 9, and 12 mg/24 hours, respectively) applied daily. In clinical trials, the starting daily dose was typically 20 mg (6 mg/24 hours), and the daily dose was then increased by 10 mg (3 mg/24 hours) every 1–2 weeks to a maximum of 40 mg (12 mg/24 hours). The package insert indicates that dietary modifications are required for patients using Emsam 9 mg/24 hours and 12 mg/24 hours, which pose greater risk of tyramine interaction than does the 6 mg/24 hours patch. This observation is based on a study in healthy control subjects in which a high-tyramine diet was associated with mild increases in blood pressure with the 9- and 12-mg patches. The risk of untoward interactions is largely theoretical. We have carried out studies that used the 9- and 12-mg doses without a restricted diet and have observed no increases in blood pressure.

Rash has been the primary side effect that was observed to be greater with transdermal selegiline than with placebo. Although most patients do not have substantial reactions to the patch, some skin reactions can be quite intense. We have seen a few patients with erythema that extends far beyond the patch site, and pruritis is not uncommon. Oral diphenhydramine seems to help with the itching. After site reactions, insomnia is the next most common side effect and is consistent with the amphetamine-like effects of the drug. Standard sleep medications such as zolpidem or temazepam appear to be helpful and are well tolerated. Although sleep does seem to normalize after the patient has taken the drug for a few weeks, just taking the patch off at night also seems to help. Unfortunately, taking half the dose might also decrease the efficacy of the transdermal selegiline. The patch, designed for 24-hour delivery, needs to be changed daily. Some patients have taken to cutting the 6-mg/24-hour patch in half if they cannot tolerate a full dose. Although cutting the patch should reduce the daily dose in proportion to the amount cut (because surface area of the patch is directly related to total drug dose), the manufacturer recommends against cutting the patch because compromising the integrity of the patch could affect reliability of transdermal drug delivery. The risk of a serotonin syndrome when transdermal selegiline is used in combination with a serotonergic drug appears reduced but not eliminated. Thus, the drug should not be combined with SSRIs, SNRIs, or most TCAs. However, orthostasis, weight gain, and sexual dysfunction appear to be much less of a problem with transdermal selegiline than with oral MAOIs.

Given the ease of use and better tolerability of transdermal selegiline versus oral MAOIs, we are typically using it before considering other MAOIs. The patient profile that may best fit with transdermal selegiline includes patients who have experienced failed trials with one or more classes of antidepressants, depressed patients with prominent fatigue or cognitive deficits, and patients with atypical depression.

Moclobemide is the best-studied RIMA. Its actions on MAO are easily reversed (i.e., do not require regeneration of the enzyme). Moclobemide has a half-life of only 1–3 hours. It is available in Europe, Canada, and other parts of the world, but not in the United States. Several thousand depressed patients have been enrolled in moclobemide studies, and it has been found to be effective in a wide spectrum of depressive illnesses, including melancholic, endogenous, atypical, psychotic (in combination with a neuroleptic), and bipolar subtypes (Fitton et al. 1992).

Moclobemide appears to be effective in elderly as well as younger patients and may be effective in the treatment of social phobia. In unpublished South American trials, moclobemide appeared to be as effective as—if not more effective than—imipramine and superior to placebo. However, one meta-analysis in Europe (Lotufo-Neto et al. 1999) suggested that moclobemide was not a particularly effective antidepressant in comparison with imipramine and placebo. In another South American study, moclobemide was significantly more effective than placebo in the treatment of social phobia.

The primary advantages of moclobemide over standard MAOIs are its tolerability and its safety. Nausea is the only side effect reported more commonly for moclobemide than for placebo. Significant orthostasis and other cardiovascular side effects are usually not seen. Furthermore, moclobemide has proved safe in overdoses to 20 g.

Because moclobemide does not increase tyramine sensitivity (Cusson et al. 1991), the risk of dietary interactions appears low. In Europe, the only significant dietary restriction is avoiding large amounts of aged cheeses after taking a dose of the drug. Moclobemide is usually given after meals or at bedtime to minimize dietary interactions.

The risk of serious drug interactions also appears to be lower with moclobemide. However, serious interactions have been reported with meperidine, clomipramine, and possibly the SSRIs. There is one report that moclobemide has been administered safely with fluvoxamine and fluoxetine (Dingemanse 1993). It is unlikely that moclobemide will be introduced soon in the United States because of a number of failed trials, but it is available through pharmacies in Europe and Canada. Development of another RIMA, brofaromine, was also canceled because of an apparent lack of sufficient efficacy.

Non-monoaminergic Antidepressant Agents

Ketamine and Esketamine

There has been considerable interest in the use of ketamine in the treatment of depression since 2006 when Zarate and colleagues reported rapid onset of response in a group of patients with TRD (Zarate et al. 2006). Ketamine was synthesized by Parke-Davis in the early 1960s as a less toxic analog of phencyclidine, which had been previously produced by the company as a potential anesthetic. The presumed mechanism of ketamine is antagonism of the NMDA receptor. However, ketamine has numerous other effects that could play a role in its antidepressant effects, including opioid and monoamine interactions. Glutamate receptors have long been thought to play a part in the pathophysiology of depression. NMDA antagonists, α-amino-3-hydroxy-5-methyl-4-isoxazolepropionic acid (AMPA), and kainate receptor agonists have antidepressant effects in animal models. Ketamine has been shown in a number of studies to have rapid antidepressant effects in patients with resistant depression when given as a single intravenous dose. Up to 60% of patients unresponsive to other treatments have been reported to have at least short-term benefit from ketamine. The antidepressant effects are often seen within 24 hours and are typically sustained for 3–7 days. Repeated dosing three times per week for 2 or more weeks may allow for better and more sustained improvement (Shiroma et al. 2014). After acute response, some clinicians administer ketamine once every 1–3 weeks to maintain response. In addition, ketamine may be administered intranasally, subcutaneously, or even sublingually. We have combined these approaches in a few patients with refractory depression, starting with one infusion at 0.5 mg/kg per week for 2 weeks and then switching to 56–84 mg intranasally thereafter, with some sustained improvement.

Among the more common short-term risks of ketamine is dissociation. Some patients describe the dissociation as pleasant, but others may experience it as disorienting and even somewhat frightening. We have found it useful to forewarn patients that they may experience dissociation and may feel out of control, but the situation is quite in control and the experience is transient. Other short-term risks include the risks of spikes in blood pressure and heart rate. Thus, it is important to monitor blood pressure and heart rate and to be able to intervene in the rare instance that sympathetic tone increases to dangerous levels. Although it may be possible for ketamine to be administered at 0.5 mg/kg over 40 minutes by potentially any physician with moderate sedation training, our preference to date has been to have ketamine administered by an anesthesiologist who is familiar with ketamine administration.

Although a number of adequately controlled randomized trials of single infusion of ketamine have been conducted, including studies we have participated in, there is a paucity of data on long-term strategies and the risks of chronic ketamine use in patients with major depression. Because depression is potentially a chronic disorder and the effects of ketamine are short-lived, ketamine will require repeated administration. There are a number of known risks with long-term ketamine administration. The most obvious is the risk of abuse. Ketamine is commonly abused in the United States and has the street name Special K. However, in some parts of the world, such as China and

Southeast Asia, ketamine abuse is at epidemic proportions. Because ketamine is a μ opioid receptor agonist, it is unclear whether the effect of intravenous ketamine is simply an analgesic effect akin to getting a shot of heroin. In a report, we demonstrated that the antidepressant effects of ketamine are blocked by pretreatment with the μ opioid receptor antagonist naltrexone (Williams et al. 2018). Although clearly not as addictive as heroin, ketamine is addictive nonetheless. Thus, risks of potential ketamine abuse have to be weighed against the antidepressant benefits.

A second risk is that uropathy may develop. About 30% of ketamine abusers develop what is sometimes referred to as a *K-bladder*, in which they may begin urinating blood. Ketamine is known to inflame the bladder and may result in ulcerations of the bladder wall (Myers et al. 2016). Again, uropathy has not been reported to date in patients using ketamine to treat depression, but it is a defined risk.

A third long-term risk of chronic ketamine use is the development of psychotic symptoms. These risks appear small with short-term intermittent use, but it is not clear whether there are cumulative effects over time, even with low-dose, intermittent use. Because ketamine is a known hallucinogen and is chemically related to phencyclidine, a psychotomimetic effect is possible even with prudent use. Also, it is possible that chronic administration of ketamine may be neurotoxic. Chronic ketamine use is known to be associated with cognitive deficits in executive function, memory, and other cognitive domains (Ke et al. 2018). Beyond these many risks of chronic ketamine use and abuse, many patients seem to lose the antidepressant benefit over time. Thus, although we are increasingly confident that ketamine has short-term benefits in some patients with TRD, we need solid long-term safety and efficacy data in depressed patients before we can routinely recommend its use.

In 2019 the *S*-enantiomer of ketamine, esketamine, was approved for the adjunctive treatment of resistant depression. Esketamine was developed by Janssen to be used in combination with standard oral antidepressants. In the Phase III studies (Popova et al. 2019), researchers reported that patients with depression that was unresponsive in at least two antidepressant trials and who were given two sprays per week of 56 or 84 mg of esketamine in addition to their standard antidepressant were significantly more likely to experience a remission of symptoms by day 28 compared with those who used a placebo nasal spray added to their regimen (52.5% vs. 31%). Likewise, in a proof-of-concept study, Canuso and colleagues (2018) demonstrated that two sprays of intranasal esketamine 84 mg were significantly more likely to reduce or even eliminate suicidal thoughts at 4 hours after the first administration compared with placebo (effect size = 0.61). However, despite dosing twice per week for weeks, the effects were not sustained at 25 days. The Phase III studies generally confirmed the early effectiveness of esketamine in rapidly reducing depressive symptoms. In one trial of 227 MDDs patient with suicidal thoughts, subjects were randomly assigned to adjunctive esketamine 84 mg given two times per week for 4 weeks or adjunctive placebo (Ionescu et al. 2021). Patients in the adjunctive esketamine group showed a more significant drop in suicidal ideation as early as 4 hours after administration and at the 24-hour time point. Thus, the FDA added an indication in 2022 for esketamine in "the treatment of major depressive disorder (MDD) in patients with acute suicidal ideation or behaviors." The most common side effects of esketamine are nausea, dizziness, dissociation, headache, and unpleasant taste in the mouth.

Although it is not clear that esketamine is any more effective or better tolerated than racemic ketamine, there may be a few advantages to esketamine. One advantage is that studies on esketamine will be larger and more comprehensive than any studies done to date with ketamine. As a result, clinicians may have more confidence in the efficacy and limitations of the drug. A second benefit is a readily available and consistent formulation of an intranasal form of the drug. If a clinician wants to prescribe racemic ketamine, it means using a compounding pharmacy, and there may not be as much consistency across individual pharmacies as might be ideal. Clearly, an intranasal formulation is somewhat more convenient to patients than intravenous administration. A meta-analysis of MDD studies suggested that intravenous racemic ketamine is superior to intranasal ketamine in the treatment of MDD, but prospective comparison studies are lacking (Bahji et al. 2021). Furthermore, although racemic ketamine is quite inexpensive and branded intranasal esketamine is costly by comparison, the lack of insurance coverage for intravenous racemic ketamine negates the cost benefit. We typically dose esketamine at 56 mg twice weekly for the first week or two. If there is no substantial response, and the medication is tolerated, we increase the dose to 84 mg for the next 2 weeks. Although there appear to be some late responders to both esketamine and ketamine, we have found that the conditional probability of responding is low if there has been little or no response in the first six treatments. However, it may take more than three inductions to see a response (McInnes et al. 2022). A partial response might prompt a continuation of 2-week treatment for a total of 4–5 weeks. Then treatment is continued once a week for up to 4 weeks and about every 2 weeks subsequently. There are a few patients who can be maintained on 1-month treatment, but they are the exception and not the rule. Except for the esketamine relapse prevention data, we have little long-term safety or efficacy data of ketamine in the treatment of major depression.

We do know much about the long-term risks of ketamine abuse, which can include an increased risk of psychotic symptoms, cystitis and bladder ulceration, and tachyphylaxis. The anesthesia literature includes cases of patients exposed to frequent treatment with ketamine who develop tolerance to it. This may also be the case with some depressed patients who receive long-term treatment with ketamine. Our group hypothesized that ketamine's antidepressant effects are in part mediated via μ opioid receptors (Sanacora and Schatzberg 2015), and because of that, one should be mindful of possible longer-term risks of tolerance and abuse for ketamine and esketamine (Schatzberg 2014, 2019). We demonstrated that naltrexone—a μ opioid antagonist—blocked the antidepressant and antisuicidal effects of intravenous ketamine in depressed patients (Williams et al. 2018), and several groups have demonstrated that behavioral effects of ketamine and esketamine in rodents are blocked by naltrexone or naloxone (Bonaventura et al. 2021; Klein et al. 2020).

So who is the ideal candidate for ketamine treatment of depression? There is not a consensus on this matter, but a possibility is a patient who has not responded to at least two adequate trials of standard antidepressants and probably at least one adequate augmentation strategy. Intravenous and esketamine treatments are logistically challenging in that a patient should not drive to or from treatment and needs to be observed for at least 2 hours. Thus, the patient needs to have someone drive them, although we do have patients who use public transportation or ride-sharing services. Because of the abuse potential of ketamine, we tend to not recommend the treatment for someone with a significant abuse history, even though a family history of alcohol abuse has been associated with better response to ketamine. In addition, psychotomimetic effects of ketamine may suggest that a history of psychosis is a relative contraindication as well. The sympathomimetic effects of ketamine are such that patients with unstable hypertension or a recent myocardial infarction or cerebrovascular accident should be medically cleared for considering treatment.

Patients taking high-dose benzodiazepines are also probably not ideal candidates for ketamine or esketamine because benzodiazepines may attenuate the efficacy of ketamine treatment. These limitations narrow the ideal candidates for ketamine treatment to a small but important subset of patients with resistant MDD. Future studies will help further define the best candidates for long-term treatment with ketamine or its analogs.

Allosteric Modulators of the GABA$_A$ Receptor

Allopregnanolone (Brexanolone)

Allopregnanolone (brexanolone) is a neurosteroid derivative of progesterone approved for the treatment of postpartum depression in 2019. Its primary mechanism of action is thought to be via positive allosteric modulation of the GABA$_A$ receptor. Allopregnanolone is known to have a variety of therapeutic effects on mood, anxiety, and premenstrual dysphoria. At least some of the effects of SSRIs in the treatment of premenstrual dysphoric disorder are thought to be mediated through their effects on allopregnanolone. The allopregnanolone effects of SSRIs are rapid, whereas general antidepressant effects tend to take 4 weeks or longer to be seen. Thus, sertraline may be dosed just 2 weeks out of the month for the treatment of PMDD but not for MDD. Allopregnanolone has a very low oral bioavailability and so is given via intravenous infusion.

In a proof-of-concept study, 21 women with symptoms that met criteria for major depression in the postpartum period were randomly assigned to receive allopregnanolone or placebo over a 60-hour infusion (Kanes et al. 2017). Patients treated with allopregnanolone experienced a 21-point drop in HDRS score at the end of the infusion versus an 8-point drop experienced by the placebo-treated group.

The Phase III program consisted of two RCTs in postpartum depression (Meltzer-Brody et al. 2018). In one trial, 120 women with postpartum depression of greater severity than in the proof-of-concept study were randomly assigned to receive allopregnanolone at either 60 μg/kg/hour or 90 μg/kg/hour or placebo for 60 hours. Both doses of allopregnanolone were significantly more effective than placebo at the 60-hour endpoint, and the effects were sustained at 30 days. The 60 μg/kg/hour dose appeared at least as effective as the 90 μg/kg/hour dose, with a 20-point drop in HDRS score at 60 hours versus 14 points for placebo. In another trial involving 108 moderately depressed patients treated with the 90 μg/kg/hour dose, allopregnanolone-treated patients had a drop in HDRS score of 15 points, versus 12 points in the placebo group, at 60 hours. There were three discontinuations due to adverse events between both studies. The most common side effects reported were headache, nausea, dizziness, and pain at the infusion site. In November 2018, an FDA advisory panel voted 17 to 1 to approve allopregnanolone in the treatment of postpartum depression.

A 60-hour infusion is cumbersome, but given the rapid and apparently sustained response, allopregnanolone appears to be an important option in postpartum depression. However, the expense of the intravenous infusion and its need to take place over 2 nights in a hospital or monitored health care facility limit the accessibility of this treatment.

Zuranolone

A number of follow-up orally active allosteric $GABA_A$ modulators are under development. The oral analog that is farthest along and under current review for possible approval is zuranolone. Like allopregnanolone, zuranolone is a positive allosteric modulator of $GABA_A$, but it has a longer half-life (16–23 hours) and has high bioavailability from an oral tablet, making it suitable for once-daily oral dosing. Zuranolone has been studied extensively for three possible indications: treatment of postpartum depression, monotherapy for major depression, and as an adjunctive treatment for resistant major depression. The data are probably strongest in the treatment of postpartum depression, but there are positive studies for all three indications.

In an RCT Phase III study, 153 patients with postpartum depression of less than 6 months' duration were randomly assigned to 2 weeks of nightly treatment with 30 mg of zuranolone or placebo (Deligiannidis et al. 2021). Patients treated with zuranolone showed significant benefit over those receiving placebo by day 3 ($P=0.03$) that was sustained to day 45 ($P=0.003$) despite only 14 days of active treatment. The remission rate at day 45 (4 weeks after the study drug was discontinued) was 53% in the active group versus 30% in the placebo-treated group ($P=0.009$). Zuranolone was well tolerated, with most side effects, including somnolence, headache, and dizziness, in the mild range.

The Phase II data of zuranolone in nonpostpartum MDD was similarly positive (Gunduz-Bruce et al. 2019). A total of 89 patients between ages 18 and 65 with MDD were treated with zuranolone 30 mg or placebo for 2 weeks. Response rates (50% reduction in HDRS score) were 79% in the zuranolone-treated patients versus 41% in the placebo group; remission rates (HDRS≤7) were 64% in the zuranolone group versus 26% in the placebo-treated patients. However, it is not clear from the study how sustained the benefits were after day 15.

The third possible indication for zuranolone is in the adjunctive treatment of patients with MDD who have not responded adequately to a standard antidepressant. The CORAL Phase III studies evaluated the efficacy of adding 50 mg of zuranolone or placebo to an approved antidepressant in 440 patients with MDD. The primary endpoint was change from baseline on the HDRS to day 15. Two weeks of concurrent treatment with zuranolone was statistically more effective than concurrent treatment with placebo at day 15, with about a 2-point advantage on the HDRS for zuranolone-treated patients. Although this is a modest effect, the finding that adjunctive treatment was well tolerated might represent a relatively benign strategy for rapidly improving antidepressant response.

The hope from early studies with zuranolone was that it could be dosed for just 2 weeks or perhaps might require only intermittent dosing for 2 weeks at a time. However, it is not clear at the time of this writing how effective these dosing strategies might be. Because zuranolone is well tolerated in the 30- to 50-mg dose range, more consistent dosing might yield longer-term benefits. Given zuranolone's purported mechanism of action, there are subsets of patients who might be better candidates for the medication, including MDD patients with anxiety and insomnia. Like brexanolone, zuranolone is likely to be a Schedule IV drug, as are the benzodiazepines. Although the abuse potential appears low, the potential for abuse should be a consideration for prescribers.

Buprenorphine and Other Opioids

One of the factors leading to opioid abuse is that narcotics are mood elevating in some people. Heroin is associated with a transient euphoria and a sense of well-being. Given the mood-elevating properties of some opioids, the analgesic properties of ketamine, and the fact that many antidepressants have analgesic properties, it is reasonable to hypothesize that opioids might also have a role to play in the treatment of depression. Tianeptine—a European antidepressant with a putative odd mechanism of action (i.e., enhanced serotonin reuptake)—has been shown to work as an antidepressant via μ opioid receptor agonism (Samuels et al. 2017).

A study by Bodkin and colleagues suggested that some patients with treatment-refractory depression do well with buprenorphine (Bodkin et al. 1995). Similarly, Nyhuis et al. (2008) found that five of six patients hospitalized with refractory depression achieved remission with 0.6–2 mg/day of buprenorphine. Even smaller doses of buprenorphine (e.g., 0.1 mg bid) have been reported to significantly reduce suicidal ideation in depressed patients, and even patients with borderline personality disorder, over the course of 4 weeks (Yovell et al. 2016). The use of time-limited, ultra-low-dose buprenorphine to manage suicidal ideation would seem a relatively low-risk strategy for getting a patient past a rough period. However, it may not be a practical longer-term intervention. We have occasionally prescribed oral analgesics to patients with refractory depression, with moderate success in patients with a low abuse risk who run out of options. The greatest challenges of using opioids are the significant risk of them being habit-forming and the patient developing tolerance over time. Treatment with buprenorphine generally requires special training and Drug Enforcement Agency (DEA) certification to prescribe as Suboxone (buprenorphine and naloxone) for individuals with opioid addiction, and given the concerns about chronic opioid use expressed by the DEA, psychiatrists should be particularly careful about prescribing opioids for resistant depression outside a sanctioned research protocol.

Another approach to using buprenorphine in depression has been to combine it with a μ opioid receptor antagonist (i.e., samidorphan). The combination of buprenorphine and samidorphan is thought to minimize the risk of abuse through μ opioid receptor antagonism. In a Phase II study, the combination of 2 mg buprenorphine and 2 mg samidorphan was more effective than placebo as an adjunctive treatment to standard antidepressants in patients who had not responded to one or two medication trials. An 8-mg dose each of buprenorphine and samidorphan failed to yield results that achieved statistical significance (Fava et al. 2016). The results of the Phase II study led to a Phase III program of three larger RCTs. In two of the studies, the combination of buprenorphine and samidorphan failed to separate adequately from placebo, but in the third trial, the active drug successfully separated from placebo and met the primary endpoint. In that study of 407 MDD patients, the 2-mg doses of both drugs added to a standard antidepressant was more effective than adjunctive placebo in reducing core symptoms of depression on the MADRS ($P<0.018$) (Thase et al. 2017). The most common side effect was nausea. Nausea, typically in the mild to moderate range of severity, has been probably the most common side effect in clinical trials (27% of patients reported nausea at the 2-mg doses). Dizziness and fatigue were the other two common adverse events. Of note, there was no evidence in any of the trials of abuse potential, tolerance, or withdrawal from the combination. After initially declining to review the new drug application for buprenorphine-samidorphan in the adjunctive treatment of depression, the FDA ultimately agreed to review the application on the basis of one positive Phase III study and pooled data from the two Phase III studies demonstrating greater improvement on the MADRS over placebo with the 2-mg/2-mg dose. As of November 2018, an FDA advisory panel ruled against approval in the adjunctive treatment of major depression, and approval was ultimately denied by the FDA.

Another drug in late Phase III as of this writing is esmethadone. Esmethadone is the D-enantiomer of methadone and appears to have few opioid effects relative to racemic methadone. In fact, dosages up to 7 times the expected standard dosage of 25 mg/day showed much less "likability" or abuse potential than 300 mg of dextromethorphan or ketamine 0.5 mg/kg (Shram et al. 2023). The primary mechanism of action of esmethadone is thought to be antagonism of the NMDA receptor, but it also has some effects on serotonin and norepinephrine transporters. Because no radioligands are currently available for the NMDA receptor, it is not possible to be confident of exactly how esmethadone may work in depression (Nemeroff 2022). Esmethadone has μ opioid agonist effects that may pose issues of abuse and dependence at higher doses.

The Phase II study of esmethadone in the treatment of depression showed promising results (Fava et al. 2022). A total of 62 hospitalized patients with MDD that was resistant to treatment in one to three antidepressant trials were randomly assigned to 25 mg of esmethadone, 50 mg of esmethadone, or placebo for 7 days, with the primary efficacy endpoint being improvement in MADRS scores at days 7 and 14 (7 days after dosing). Both doses of esmethadone were highly efficacious relative to placebo, with separation from placebo by day 4 sustained to day 14. Remission rates (MADRS ≤ 10) at day 14 were 5% in the placebo-treated group and 31% and 39% in the 25- and 50-mg groups, respectively. This represented a very large effect size of 0.7–1.1 for esmethadone treatment. Esmethadone side effects included headache, constipation, and nausea. There was no evidence of opioid withdrawal in any subject.

On the basis of the exceptional Phase II data, a Phase III program was initiated for both monotherapy with esmethadone in MDD and esmethadone as adjunctive treatment with standard antidepressants in TRD. The Phase III monotherapy study did not go as well as hoped. In the study, 232 outpatients with MDD were randomly assigned to 25 mg of esmethadone or placebo for 28 days (after a loading dose of 75 mg the first day), with the primary endpoint being change from baseline in MADRS score on day 28. The topline results showed that the esmethadone group did not separate from placebo, and in many sites, placebo beat the active drug. One possible explanation is that the drug is underdosed in the studies. Increasing the dose may provide greater efficacy but also greater risk due to inherent μ opioid agonism. If sites with a paradoxically high placebo response were excluded, there were significant differences favoring esmethadone. However, this is cherry-picking the results, and no clear benefit of esmethadone could be determined. On a more positive note, esmethadone appeared to be very well tolerated. Early data from the Phase III adjunctive studies with esmethadone in TRD also did not show a significant improvement over placebo but at least were trending in the right direction. Additional studies with adjunctive esmethadone are under way, and if positive, they might represent a relatively benign alternative to currently approved adjunctive agents for depression such as the antipsychotics.

Tianeptine is a serotonin reuptake enhancer and μ opioid agonist currently approved in France and several other countries. One of its purported mechanisms of action is opposite that of the SSRIs in that it increases the uptake of serotonin in the synaptic cleft rather than blocking the reuptake as do SSRIs. In addition, tianeptine has a variety of other actions, including enhancing dopamine release and actions on the AMPA and NMDA glutamate receptors. Despite a number of pharmacodynamic effects, much of tianeptine antidepressant actions might be related to its opioid agonism. Tianeptine is banned from a number of countries because of its abuse potential, and the FDA issued a warning in 2022 about the risk of abuse, overdose, and other harmful effects of tianeptine. Tianeptine is not likely to ever be approved in the United States because of its liabilities, but it may have a limited role in TRD and is currently being studied at Stanford University and Mount Sinai Medical School for this indication.

κ Opioid antagonists (KOAs) are also in development for the treatment of major depression and anxiety. Agonists of the κ opioid receptor have been shown to increase anxiety-like, dysphoric, and drug-seeking behavior in animal models. Antagonists of the κ opioid receptor thus have potential as anxiolytic and antidepressant drugs. In a proof-of-concept study, Fava and colleagues (2020) examined the adjunctive use of a κ opioid antagonist (CERC-501) in eight patients with inadequate response to an antidepressant. The adjunctive κ opioid antagonist was numerically but not statistically superior to adjunctive placebo in this small study. Aticaprant is a KOA with high affinity for the κ opioid receptor and very low affinity for the μ and δ opioid receptors. It has apparent antidepressant effects in some animal models of depression, such as the forced swim test, and appears to have synergistic properties when combined with antidepressants in these models. Aticaprant is being studied as an adjunctive treatment with SSRIs and SNRIs for targeting anhedonia in depression in both younger and elderly patients.

Psychedelics

When famed medicinal chemist Albert Hoffman at Sandoz Laboratories in Basel, Switzerland, first synthesized LSD in 1938 as a potential circulatory and respiratory stimulant, it did not have the desired effect and was shelved. Approximately 5 years later, he accidentally dropped a small amount of LSD on his hand and subsequently experienced some dizziness and restlessness. He then decided to self-administer a much larger dose and experienced profound changes in perception that were frightening to him. He decided to ride his bike back home (now celebrated as "bicycle day") and was convinced that he had poisoned himself. He was experiencing psychotic symptoms, including visual hallucinations and paranoid ideas. However, by the next day, he felt a significant sense of well-being and a zest for life. Hoffman and, eventually, Sandoz, saw a potential for LSD as a psychotherapeutic agent, and it was released in the United States in 1947 under the tradename Delsid. Over the next 15 years, LSD was studied in the treatment of alcohol use disorders, depression, anxiety, and other mental health conditions.

Although Hoffman could not conceive of the possibility that a drug with such profound perceptual effects could be abused, LSD found evangelical endorsement in prominent representatives of the counterculture movement of the 1960s, including Timothy Leary and Ken Kesey. As abuse of psychedelics expanded throughout the 1960s, LSD and psilocybin, which had also been isolated by Hoffman from psilocybin mushrooms in 1955, were eventually banned under the Comprehensive Drug Abuse Prevention and Control Act of 1970. Notably, however, Oregon has debuted a first-of-its-kind legal market for psilocybin mushrooms. Research on psychedelics otherwise dried up. However, a resurgence of interest in the potential of psychedelics began in the late 1990s with studies from the University of Zurich and Johns Hopkins University suggesting an important therapeutic benefit of psilocybin in some populations. As of this writing, psilocybin is in late-stage development for the treatment of resistant depression, and MDMA is in Phase III for the treatment of PTSD. Numerous other psychedelics are currently being studied for a variety of other indications, including anxiety disorders and substance use disorders.

The mechanisms by which psychedelics work have not been established. The most studied psychedelics are the 5-HT$_{2A}$ agonists, which include psilocybin, LSD, and dimethyltryptamine. The serotonergic agonist effects of these drugs habituate and saturate serotonergic receptors throughout the cortex. A 25-mg dose of psilocybin will saturate 70% or more of all 5-HT$_2$ receptors in the cortex, and the psychedelic experience appears to be correlated with the degree of serotonin receptor saturation. This saturation is known to inhibit some of the regulatory processes of the serotonergic system, including the suppression of dopamine. Thus, dopaminergic neurotransmission is enhanced with 5-HT$_{2A}$ agonism. Downstream effects result in a rapid change in plasticity across cortico-striatal-thalamic tracts. The psychedelics appear to result in more connections between discrete tracts but less connectivity within a given tract. This psychedelic disruption in cortical connectivity might allow for disintegration of persistent maladaptive patterns of thought or behavior and reintegration into something more adaptive and less destructive. Among the most consistent effects of the psychedelics is the temporary suppression of the default mode network (DMN). The DMN is a set of brain regions that are active during passive tasks such as daydreaming, rest, and sleep and inactive in tasks that require active attention. In depression and anxiety states, there appears to be an abnormality in the functional connectivity of the DMN. Psychedelics may alter the functional connectivity of the DMN in ways that benefit depression and anxiety states.

Evidence of a therapeutic effect of psilocybin in the treatment of anxiety and depression associated with terminal illness began to emerge with the work of Roland Griffiths at Johns Hopkins and other investigators. A single dose of psilocybin combined with a nondirective, supportive form of psychedelic psychotherapy that was used in the LSD studies in the 1960s resulted in the rapid reduction of depressive symptoms and anxiety in terminal cancer patients (Griffiths et al. 2016; Ross et al. 2016). Notably, the effects of a single dose of psilocybin were often sustained for 6 months or longer.

The potential of psilocybin in patients with TRD resulted in the FDA granting psilocybin a "breakthrough" designation for the treatment of TRD in 2019. Thus, if a series of RCTs confirm the efficacy and safety of psilocybin in the treatment of TRD, the drug could receive rapid review, leading to FDA approval. The first carefully controlled Phase II study of psilocybin in the treatment of resistant depression was completed in 2022 (Goodwin et al. 2022). In this study, 233 patients with MDD unresponsive to two to four adequate antidepressant trials for the current episode were randomly assigned to either 1 mg, 10 mg, or 25 mg of psilocybin. Although there is no ideal placebo for a psychedelic, a 1-mg dose of psilocybin is not associated with perceptual changes and thus was the placebo dose. Patients were tapered off existing antidepressants and had three pretreatment sessions with a therapist. A single induction with one of the psilocybin doses was then completed with two therapists in the room for 6–8 hours. Subsequently, subjects were seen for integration therapy sessions and were followed for a total of 12 weeks. The results showed a significant improvement in the 25-mg group compared with both the 10-mg and 1-mg groups at the week 3 endpoint. Significant benefits in the 25-mg group were seen by day 2. There was a 29% remission rate in the 25-mg group, versus 9% and 8%, respectively, in the 10-mg and 1-mg groups. The most common side effects were headache, nausea, and dizziness. The conclusion of this study was that a single 25-mg dose could provide significant rapid, sustained benefit in a subset of patients with TRD. The Phase III studies, which are under way as of this writing, will attempt to replicate these results and address a number of issues, including the utility of repeated doses, determination of appropriate candidates for psilocybin treatment, and the long-term efficacy and safety of psilocybin. One caveat for psilocybin and ketamine trials is that it is almost impossible to maintain a blind, leading to skepticism on the part of many investigators.

Other Novel/Future Antidepressants

Although is unlikely that another SSRI or SNRI is in the offing, a number of *triple reuptake inhibitors* are under investigation. These drugs block the reuptake of dopamine in addition to 5-HT and norepinephrine. It is speculated that the dopamine-enhancing effects of these drugs might lead to earlier response and greater efficacy in some patients. Two triple reuptake inhibitor drugs that are in early development are DOV-216,303 and tesofensine. Tesofensine has shown consistent benefits as an anorexiant in early trials. Patients have lost an average of 14 kg after 24 weeks of taking 0.5 mg of tesofensine. This drug also might help with glucose control in type 2 diabetes and might help manage the motor symptoms of Parkinson's disease. However, few data exist on its utility as an antidepressant other than from animal studies, in which the results are promising. Like tesofensine, DOV-216,303 has shown antidepressant effects in animal models and appears well tolerated in Phase I trials. A concern about the dopamine reuptake inhibitors is abuse potential. Studies with tesofensine thus far have not indicated tolerance or withdrawal.

Another novel approach to the treatment of depression has been the use of cortisol-specific agents. Depression—particularly more serious forms, such as psychotic depression—is known to be associated with abnormalities in the hypothalamic-pituitary-adrenal axis, including changes in cortisol levels and secretion and increases in levels of corticotropin-releasing factor (CRF). Cortisol and its analogs, the glucocorticoids, are known to produce mood, cognitive, and psychotic symptoms that mimic, to some degree, what is observed in serious forms of depression. Cortisol synthesis inhibitors such as ketoconazole have shown some benefits in a subset of patients with hypercortisolemia. However, ketoconazole can be quite toxic at the doses required to inhibit cortisol synthesis. A CRF receptor-1 (CRFR1) antagonist had shown efficacy in early open-label studies, but a large controlled trial completed with a CRF antagonist failed to show benefit in the treatment of depression (Binneman et al. 2008.) In addition, other reports on CRFR1 antagonists in the treatment of GAD and alcohol abuse have also been negative. We have studied the glucocorticoid receptor antagonist mifepristone, which showed benefits in the treatment of psychotic symptoms of psychotic depression in early pilot trials and a multicenter Phase II trial. (A.F.S. and C.D. have a conflict of interest in owning equity in the company pursuing this indication.) However, three subsequent trials have failed to replicate the earlier findings. The roll-up data were recently published and pointed to mifepristone being rapidly effective for reducing psychotic symptoms when so-called therapeutic blood levels were attained (Block et al. 2018). The clinical efficacy of cortisol-specific treatments of depression awaits potential further study.

Inflammatory cytokines are thought to play a role in the pathophysiology of depression. Levels of cytokines such as interleukin-6 and tumor necrosis factor-α are known to be increased in depression. These elevations appear to play a role in increasing CRF and cortisol levels in depression. In animal models, acute administration of these cytokines induces anhedonia, decreased libido, and decreased social interaction. It makes sense, therefore, that an anti-inflammatory drug might have antidepressant properties. In a study of etanercept, a tumor necrosis factor–specific agent being investigated for the treatment of psoriasis, patients treated with the drug had significantly greater improvement in mood on the Beck Depression Inventory than did the patients receiving placebo (Krishnan et al. 2007). This benefit was independent of the magnitude of response obtained for the psoriasis. As we wrote previously, a variety of other drugs, including the tumor necrosis factor antibody infliximab, were thought to be candidates for investigation in the treatment of depression. Raison et al. (2013) reported that infliximab was ineffective in patients with refractory depression, although it did have efficacy in patients with elevated C-reactive protein levels indicative of inflammatory processes. Thus far, anti-inflammatory agents have not proven consistently helpful in the treatment of MDD, but there may be a subgroup of patients with elevated inflammatory biomarkers who may benefit from anti-inflammatory drugs (Raison 2017).

Many new targets for the treatment of depression exist. Because many patients do not respond adequately to monoamine drugs, it is the hope of clinicians and patients everywhere that new advantageous agents will become available in the coming years.

Suggested Readings

Aguglia E, Casacchia M, Cassano GB, et al: Double-blind study of the efficacy and safety of sertraline versus fluoxetine in major depression. Int Clin Psychopharmacol 8(3):197–202, 1993 8263318

Alphs LD, Cooper K, Popova V, et al: Clinical efficacy and safety of flexibly dosed intranasal esketamine in a U.S. population of patients with treatment-resistant depression. Paper presented at the Annual Meeting of the American Psychiatric Association, New York, May 5–9, 2018

Amsterdam JD, Hornig-Rohan M, Maislin G: Efficacy of alprazolam in reducing fluoxetine-induced jitteriness in patients with major depression. J Clin Psychiatry 55(9):394–400, 1994 7929020

Amsterdam JD, Maislin G, Potter L: Fluoxetine efficacy in treatment resistant depression. Prog Neuropsychopharmacol Biol Psychiatry 18(2):243–261, 1994 8208976

Aranow AB, Hudson JI, Pope HG Jr, et al: Elevated antidepressant plasma levels after addition of fluoxetine. Am J Psychiatry 146(7):911–913, 1989 2787124

Arminen SL, Ikonen U, Pulkkinen P, et al: A 12-week double-blind multi-centre study of paroxetine and imipramine in hospitalized depressed patients. Acta Psychiatr Scand 89(6):382–389, 1994 8085467

Asakura S, Tajima O, Koyama T: Fluvoxamine treatment of generalized social anxiety disorder in Japan: a randomized double-blind, placebo-controlled study. Int J Neuropsychopharmacol 10(2):263–274, 2007 16573847

Åsberg M, Crönholm B, Sjöqvist F, et al: Relationship between plasma level and therapeutic effect of nortriptyline. BMJ 3(5770):331–334, 1971 5558186

Asnis GM, Bose A, Gommoll CP, et al: Efficacy and safety of levomilnacipran sustained release 40 mg, 80 mg, or 120 mg in major depressive disorder: a phase 3, randomized, double-blind, placebo-controlled study. J Clin Psychiatry 74(3):242–248, 2013 23561229

Bakish D, Bose A, Gommoll C, et al: Levomilnacipran ER 40 mg and 80 mg in patients with major depressive disorder: a Phase III, randomized, double-blind, fixed-dose, placebo-controlled study. J Psychiatry Neurosci 39(1):40–49, 2014 24144196

Banasr M, Soumier A, Hery M, et al: Agomelatine, a new antidepressant, induces regional changes in hippocampal neurogenesis. Biol Psychiatry 59(11):1087–1096, 2006 16499883

Banham ND: Fatal venlafaxine overdose. Med J Aust 169(8):445, 448, 1998 9830400

Belanoff JK, Flores BH, Kalezhan M, et al: Rapid reversal of psychotic depression using mifepristone. J Clin Psychopharmacol 21(5):516–521, 2001 11593077

Belanoff JK, Rothschild AJ, Cassidy F, et al: An open label trial of C-1073 (mifepristone) for psychotic major depression. Biol Psychiatry 52(5):386–392, 2002 12242054

Bell IR, Cole JO: Fluoxetine induces elevation of desipramine level and exacerbation of geriatric nonpsychotic depression. J Clin Psychopharmacol 8(6):447–448, 1988 3266222

Bellino S, Paradiso E, Bogetto F: Efficacy and tolerability of pharmacotherapies for borderline personality disorder. CNS Drugs 22(8):671–692, 2008 18601305

Bhagwagar Z, Cowen PJ: "It's not over when it's over": persistent neurobiological abnormalities in recovered depressed patients. Psychol Med 38(3):307–313, 2008 18444278

Bhatara VS, Bandettini FC: Possible interaction between sertraline and tranylcypromine. Clin Pharm 12(3):222–225, 1993 8491079

Bielski RJ, Cunningham L, Horrigan JP, et al: Gepirone extended-release in the treatment of adult outpatients with major depressive disorder: a double-blind, randomized, placebo-controlled, parallel-group study. J Clin Psychiatry 69(4):571–577, 2008 18373383

Black DW, Wesner R, Gabel J: The abrupt discontinuation of fluvoxamine in patients with panic disorder. J Clin Psychiatry 54(4):146–149, 1993 8486592

Boyd IW: Venlafaxine withdrawal reactions. Med J Aust 169(2):91–92, 1998 9700345

Cankurtaran ES, Ozalp E, Soygur H, et al: Mirtazapine improves sleep and lowers anxiety and depression in cancer patients: superiority over imipramine. Support Care Cancer 16(11):1291–1298, 2008 18299900

Carhart-Harris RL, Bolstridge M, Day CMJ, et al: Psilocybin with psychological support for treatment-resistant depression: six-month follow-up. Psychopharmacology (Berl) 235(2):399–408, 2018 29119217

Carhart-Harris R, Giribaldi B, Watts R, et al: Trial of psilocybin versus escitalopram for depression. N Engl J Med 384(15):1402–1411, 2021 33852780

Citrome L: Vilazodone for major depressive disorder: a systematic review of the efficacy and safety profile for this newly approved antidepressant—what is the number needed to treat, number needed to harm and likelihood to be helped or harmed? Int J Clin Pract 66(4):356–368, 2012 22284853

Citrome L: Levomilnacipran for major depressive disorder: a systematic review of the efficacy and safety profile for this newly approved antidepressant—what is the number needed to treat, number needed to harm and likelihood to be helped or harmed? Int J Clin Pract 67(11):1089–1104, 2013 24016209

Citrome L: Vortioxetine for major depressive disorder: a systematic review of the efficacy and safety profile for this newly approved antidepressant—what is the number needed to treat, number needed to harm and likelihood to be helped or harmed? Int J Clin Pract 68(1):60–82, 2014 24165478

Claghorn J: A double-blind comparison of paroxetine and placebo in the treatment of depressed outpatients. Int Clin Psychopharmacol 6(Suppl 4):25–30, 1992 1431007

Claghorn JL, Feighner JP: A double-blind comparison of paroxetine with imipramine in the long-term treatment of depression. J Clin Psychopharmacol 13(6)(Suppl 2):23S–27S, 1993 8106652

Cohn CK, Shrivastava R, Mendels J, et al: Double-blind, multicenter comparison of sertraline and amitriptyline in elderly depressed patients. J Clin Psychiatry 51(12)(Suppl B):28–33, 1990 2258379

Cole JO, Bodkin JA: Antidepressant drug side effects. J Clin Psychiatry 51(1 Suppl):21–26, 1990 2404000

Cooper GL: The safety of fluoxetine—an update. Br J Psychiatry Suppl 153(3):77–86, 1988 3074869

Dallal A, Chouinard G: Withdrawal and rebound symptoms associated with abrupt discontinuation of venlafaxine. J Clin Psychopharmacol 18(4):343–344, 1998 9690703

Daniels RJ: Serotonin syndrome due to venlafaxine overdose. J Accid Emerg Med 15(5):333–334, 1998 9785164

Davidson JR, Weisler RH, Butterfield MI, et al: Mirtazapine vs. placebo in posttraumatic stress disorder: a pilot trial. Biol Psychiatry 53(2):188–191, 2003 12547477

Daly EJ, Singh JB, Fedgchin M, et al: Efficacy and safety of intranasal esketamine adjunctive to oral antidepressant therapy in treatment-resistant depression: a randomized clinical trial. JAMA Psychiatry 75(2):139–148, 2018 29282469

Daly EJ, Trivedi MH, Janik A, et al: Efficacy of esketamine nasal spray plus oral antidepressant treatment for relapse prevention in patients with treatment-resistant depression: a randomized clinical trial. JAMA Psychiatry 76(9):893–903, 2019 31166571

DeBattista C, Lembke A, Solvason HB, et al: A prospective trial of modafinil as an adjunctive treatment of major depression. J Clin Psychopharmacol 24(1):87–90, 2004 14709953

DeBattista C, Belanoff J, Glass S, et al: Mifepristone versus placebo in the treatment of psychosis in patients with psychotic major depression. Biol Psychiatry 60(12):1343–1349, 2006 16889757

den Boer JA, Bosker FJ, Meesters Y: Clinical efficacy of agomelatine in depression: the evidence. Int Clin Psychopharmacol 21(Suppl 1):S21–S24, 2006 16436936

Dolder CR, Nelson M, Snider M: Agomelatine treatment of major depressive disorder. Ann Pharmacother 42(12):1822–1831, 2008 19033480

Doogan DP, Langdon CJ: A double-blind, placebo-controlled comparison of sertraline and dothiepin in the treatment of major depression in general practice. Int Clin Psychopharmacol 9(2):95–100, 1994 8057000

Dubocovich ML: Agomelatine targets a range of major depressive disorder symptoms. Curr Opin Investig Drugs 7(7):670–680, 2006 16869122

Dunner DL: An overview of paroxetine in the elderly. Gerontology 40(Suppl 1):21–27, 1994 8020767

Einarson TR, Arikian SR, Casciano J, et al: Comparison of extended-release venlafaxine, selective serotonin reuptake inhibitors, and tricyclic antidepressants in the treatment of depression: a meta-analysis of randomized controlled trials. Clin Ther 21(2):296–308, 1999 10211533

Ellingrod VL, Perry PJ: Venlafaxine: a heterocyclic antidepressant. Am J Hosp Pharm 51(24):3033–3046, 1994 7856622

Feiger AD: A double-blind comparison of gepirone extended release, imipramine, and placebo in the treatment of outpatient major depression. Psychopharmacol Bull 32(4):659–665, 1996 8993088

Feiger AD, Tourian KA, Rosas GR, et al: A placebo-controlled study evaluating the efficacy and safety of flexible-dose desvenlafaxine treatment in outpatients with major depressive disorder. CNS Spectr 14(1):41–50, 2009 19169187

Feighner JP, Aden GC, Fabre LF, et al: Comparison of alprazolam, imipramine, and placebo in the treatment of depression. JAMA 249(22):3057–3064, 1983 6133970

Friel PN, Logan BK, Fligner CL: Three fatal drug overdoses involving bupropion. J Anal Toxicol 17(7):436–438, 1993 8309220

Gambi F, De Berardis D, Campanella D, et al: Mirtazapine treatment of generalized anxiety disorder: a fixed dose, open label study. J Psychopharmacol 19(5):483–487, 2005 16166185

Goodnick PJ: Pharmacokinetics of second generation antidepressants: bupropion. Psychopharmacol Bull 27(4):513–519, 1991 1813898

Grimsley SR, Jann MW: Paroxetine, sertraline, and fluvoxamine: new selective serotonin reuptake inhibitors. Clin Pharm 11(11):930–957, 1992 1464219

Gupta S, Ghaly N, Dewan M: Augmenting fluoxetine with dextroamphetamine to treat refractory depression. Hosp Community Psychiatry 43(3):281–283, 1992 1555827

Hamilton MS, Opler LA: Akathisia, suicidality, and fluoxetine. J Clin Psychiatry 53(11):401–406, 1992 1364815

Haria M, Fitton A, McTavish D: Trazodone: a review of its pharmacology, therapeutic use in depression and therapeutic potential in other disorders. Drugs Aging 4(4):331–355, 1994 8019056

Harris MG, Benfield P: Fluoxetine: a review of its pharmacodynamic and pharmacokinetic properties, and therapeutic use in older patients with depressive illness. Drugs Aging 6(1):64–84, 1995 7696780

Henry JA: Overdose and safety with fluvoxamine. Int Clin Psychopharmacol 6(Suppl 3):41–45, 1991 1806634

Holliday SM, Benfield P: Venlafaxine: a review of its pharmacology and therapeutic potential in depression. Drugs 49(2):280–294, 1995 7729333

Holliday SM, Plosker GL: Paroxetine: a review of its pharmacology, therapeutic use in depression and therapeutic potential in diabetic neuropathy. Drugs Aging 3(3):278–299, 1993 8324301

Howland RH: Pharmacotherapy of dysthymia: a review. J Clin Psychopharmacol 11(2):83–92, 1991 2056146

Jaffe PD, Batziris HP, van der Hoeven P, et al: A study involving venlafaxine overdoses: comparison of fatal and therapeutic concentrations in postmortem specimens. J Forensic Sci 44(1):193–196, 1999 9987886

Jain R, Chen D, Edwards J, et al: Early and sustained improvement with vilazodone in adult patients with major depressive disorder: post hoc analyses of two Phase III trials. Curr Med Res Opin 30(2):263–270, 2014 24127687

Johnson H, Bouman WP, Lawton J: Withdrawal reaction associated with venlafaxine. BMJ 317(7161):787, 1998 9740568

Kamath J, Handratta V: Desvenlafaxine succinate for major depressive disorder: a critical review of the evidence. Expert Rev Neurother 8(12):1787–1797, 2008 19086875

Katona CL, Abou-Saleh MT, Harrison DA, et al: Placebo-controlled trial of lithium augmentation of fluoxetine and lofepramine. Br J Psychiatry 166(1):80–86, 1995 7894881

Keller M, Montgomery S, Ball W, et al: Lack of efficacy of the substance P (neurokinin 1 receptor) antagonist aprepitant in the treatment of major depressive disorder. Biol Psychiatry 59(3):216–223, 2006 16248986

Keller MB, Trivedi MH, Thase ME, et al: The Prevention of Recurrent Episodes of Depression with Venlafaxine for Two Years (PREVENT) study: outcomes from the 2-year and combined maintenance phases. J Clin Psychiatry 68(8):1246–1256, 2007 17854250

Kennedy SH, Emsley R: Placebo-controlled trial of agomelatine in the treatment of major depressive disorder. Eur Neuropsychopharmacol 16(2):93–100, 2006 16249073

Keppel Hesselink JM, de Jongh PM: Sertraline in the prevention of depression (comment). Br J Psychiatry 161:270–271, 1992 1521116

Khan A, Khan S: Placebo response in depression: a perspective for clinical practice. Psychopharmacol Bull 41(3):91–98, 2008 18779778

Kline NS: Clinical experience with iproniazid (Marsilid). J Clin Exp Psychopathol 19(2) (Suppl 1):72–78, 1958 18289144

Kramer MS, Cutler N, Feighner J, et al: Distinct mechanism for antidepressant activity by blockade of central substance P receptors. Science 281(5383):1640–1645, 1998 9733503

Kramer MS, Winokur A, Kelsey J, et al: Demonstration of the efficacy and safety of a novel substance P (NK1) receptor antagonist in major depression. Neuropsychopharmacology 29(2):385–392, 2004 14666114

Kuhn R: Treatment of depressive states with an iminodibenzyl derivative (G 22355) [in German]. Schweiz Med Wochenschr 87(35–36):1135–1140, 1957 13467194

Kupfer DJ, Frank E, Perel JM, et al: Five-year outcome for maintenance therapies in recurrent depression. Arch Gen Psychiatry 49(10):769–773, 1992 1417428

Leaf EV: Comment: venlafaxine overdose and seizure. Ann Pharmacother 32(1):135–136, 1998 9475842

Liappas J, Paparrigopoulos T, Tzavellas E, et al: Mirtazapine and venlafaxine in the management of collateral psychopathology during alcohol detoxification. Prog Neuropsychopharmacol Biol Psychiatry 29(1):55–60, 2005 15610945

Liebowitz MR, Quitkin FM, Stewart JW, et al: Antidepressant specificity in atypical depression. Arch Gen Psychiatry 45(2):129–137, 1988 3276282

Lonnqvist J, Sihvo S, Syvälahti E, et al: Moclobemide and fluoxetine in atypical depression: a double-blind trial. J Affect Disord 32(3):169–177, 1994 7852659

Lôo H, Daléry J, Macher JP, et al: Pilot study comparing in blind the therapeutic effect of two doses of agomelatine, melatoninergic agonist and selective 5HT2C receptors antagonist, in the treatment of major depressive disorders [in French]. Encephale 28(4):356–362, 2002 12232545

Lôo H, Hale A, D'haenen H: Determination of the dose of agomelatine, a melatoninergic agonist and selective 5-HT(2C) antagonist, in the treatment of major depressive disorder: a placebo-controlled dose range study. Int Clin Psychopharmacol 17(5):239–247, 2002 12177586

Louie AK, Lewis TB, Lannon RA: Use of low-dose fluoxetine in major depression and panic disorder. J Clin Psychiatry 54(11):435–438, 1993 8270588

Mago R, Forero G, Greenberg WM, et al: Safety and tolerability of levomilnacipran ER in major depressive disorder: results from an open-label, 48-week extension study. Clin Drug Investig 33(10):761–771, 2013 23999912

Mahableshwarkar AR, Jacobsen PL, Chen Y: A randomized, double-blind trial of 2.5 mg and 5 mg vortioxetine (Lu AA21004) versus placebo for 8 weeks in adults with major depressive disorder. Curr Med Res Opin 29(3):217–226, 2013 23252878

Mahableshwarkar AR, Jacobsen PL, Chen Y, et al: A randomised, double-blind, placebo-controlled, duloxetine-referenced study of the efficacy and tolerability of vortioxetine in the acute treatment of adults with generalised anxiety disorder. Int J Clin Pract 68(1):49–59, 2014 24341301

McGrath PJ, Quitkin FM, Harrison W, et al: Treatment of melancholia with tranylcypromine. Am J Psychiatry 141(2):288–289, 1984 6691499

McGrath PJ, Stewart JW, Quitkin FM, et al: Gepirone treatment of atypical depression: preliminary evidence of serotonergic involvement. J Clin Psychopharmacol 14(5):347–352, 1994 7806692

Mendlewicz J: Efficacy of fluvoxamine in severe depression. Drugs 43(Suppl 2):32–37, 1992 1378372

Mertens LJ, Wall MB, Roseman L, et al: Therapeutic mechanisms of psilocybin: changes in amygdala and prefrontal functional connectivity during emotional processing after psilocybin for treatment-resistant depression. J Psychopharmacol 34(2):167–180, 2020 31941394

Mitchell AJ: The role of corticotropin releasing factor in depressive illness: a critical review. Neurosci Biobehav Rev 22(5):635–651, 1998 9662725

Monoamine oxidase inhibitors and anesthesia: update. Int Drug Ther Newsl 24:13–14, 1989

Montgomery SA, Mansuy L, Ruth AC, et al: The efficacy of extended-release levomilnacipran in moderate to severe major depressive disorder: secondary and post-hoc analyses from a randomized, double-blind, placebo-controlled study. Int Clin Psychopharmacol 29(1):26–35, 2014 24172160

Mooney JJ, Schatzberg AF, Cole JO, et al: Enhanced signal transduction by adenylate cyclase in platelet membranes of patients showing antidepressant responses to alprazolam: preliminary data. J Psychiatr Res 19(1):65–75, 1985 2985777

Muehlbacher M, Nickel MK, Nickel C, et al: Mirtazapine treatment of social phobia in women: a randomized, double-blind, placebo-controlled study. J Clin Psychopharmacol 25(6):580–583, 2005 16282842

Murdoch D, McTavish D: Sertraline: a review of its pharmacodynamic and pharmacokinetic properties, and therapeutic potential in depression and obsessive-compulsive disorder. Drugs 44(4):604–624, 1992 1281075

National Center for Health Statistics: Health, United States, 2007, With Chartbook on Trends in the Health of Americans. Hyattsville, MD, Centers for Disease Control and Prevention, U.S. Department of Health and Human Services, 2007. Available at: www.cdc.gov/nchs/data/hus/hus07.pdf. Accessed August 5, 2009.

Nefazodone for depression. Med Lett Drugs Ther 37(946):33–35, 1995 7707998

Nemeroff CB: The clinical pharmacology and use of paroxetine, a new selective serotonin reuptake inhibitor. Pharmacotherapy 14(2):127–138, 1994 8197030

Nierenberg AA: The treatment of severe depression: is there an efficacy gap between the SSRIs and TCA antidepressant generations? J Clin Psychiatry 55(9 Suppl):55–61 [discussion 60–61, 98–100], 1994 7961543

Nierenberg AA, Keck PE Jr: Management of monoamine oxidase inhibitor-associated insomnia with trazodone. J Clin Psychopharmacol 9(1):42–45, 1989 2708555

Nierenberg AA, Cole JO, Glass L: Possible trazodone potentiation of fluoxetine: a case series. J Clin Psychiatry 53(3):83–85, 1992 1548249

Nierenberg AA, Feighner JP, Rudolph R, et al: Venlafaxine for treatment-resistant unipolar depression. J Clin Psychopharmacol 14(6):419–423, 1994 7884023

Norden MJ: Fluoxetine in borderline personality disorder. Prog Neuropsychopharmacol Biol Psychiatry 13(6):885–893, 1989 2813806

Olfson M, Marcus SC, Shaffer D: Antidepressant drug therapy and suicide in severely depressed children and adults: a case-control study. Arch Gen Psychiatry 63(8):865–872, 2006 16894062

Pande AC, Sayler ME: Severity of depression and response to fluoxetine. Int Clin Psychopharmacol 8(4):243–245, 1993 8277142

Papakostas GI, Thase ME, Fava M, et al: Are antidepressant drugs that combine serotonergic and noradrenergic mechanisms of action more effective than the selective serotonin reuptake inhibitors in treating major depressive disorder? A meta-analysis of studies of newer agents. Biol Psychiatry 62(11):1217–1227, 2007 17588546

Papp M, Litwa E, Gruca P, et al: Anxiolytic-like activity of agomelatine and melatonin in three animal models of anxiety. Behav Pharmacol 17(1):9–18, 2006 16377959

Paris PA, Saucier JR: ECG conduction delays associated with massive bupropion overdose. J Toxicol Clin Toxicol 36(6):595–598, 1998 9776964

Patten SB: The comparative efficacy of trazodone and imipramine in the treatment of depression. CMAJ 146(7):1177–1182, 1992 1532532

Pearlstein TB, Stone AB: Long-term fluoxetine treatment of late luteal phase dysphoric disorder. J Clin Psychiatry 55(8):332–335, 1994 8071300

Phanjoo A: The elderly depressed and treatment with fluvoxamine. Int Clin Psychopharmacol 6(Suppl 3):33–37 [discussion 37–39], 1991 1806633

Pinzani V, Giniès E, Robert L, et al: Venlafaxine withdrawal syndrome: report of six cases and review of the literature [in French]. Rev Med Interne 21(3):282–284, 2000 10763190

Pope HG Jr, Hudson JI, Jonas JM, et al: Bulimia treated with imipramine: a placebo-controlled, double-blind study. Am J Psychiatry 140(5):554–558, 1983 6342421

Preskorn S, Macaluso M, Mehra DO, et al: Randomized proof of concept trial of GLYX-13, an N-methyl-D-aspartate receptor glycine site partial agonist, in major depressive disorder nonresponsive to a previous antidepressant agent. J Psychiatr Pract 21(2):140–149, 2015 25782764

Quitkin F, Gibertine M: Patients with probable atypical depression are responsive to the 5-HT1A partial agonist, gepirone-ER. Presentation at the annual meeting of the American College of Neuropsychopharmacology, San Juan, Puerto Rico, 2001

Quitkin F, Rifkin A, Klein DF: Monoamine oxidase inhibitors: a review of antidepressant effectiveness. Arch Gen Psychiatry 36(7):749–760, 1979 454092

Reimherr FW, Chouinard G, Cohn CK, et al: Antidepressant efficacy of sertraline: a double-blind, placebo- and amitriptyline-controlled, multicenter comparison study in outpatients with major depression. J Clin Psychiatry 51(12)(Suppl B):18–27, 1990 2258378

Richelson E: Synaptic pharmacology of antidepressants: an update. McLean Hospital Journal 13:67–88, 1988

Richelson E, Nelson A: Antagonism by antidepressants of neurotransmitter receptors of normal human brain in vitro. J Pharmacol Exp Ther 230(1):94–102, 1984 6086881

Rickels K, Chung HR, Csanalosi IB, et al: Alprazolam, diazepam, imipramine, and placebo in outpatients with major depression. Arch Gen Psychiatry 44(10):862–866, 1987 3310952

Rickels K, Schweizer E, Clary C, et al: Nefazodone and imipramine in major depression: a placebo-controlled trial. Br J Psychiatry 164(6):802–805, 1994 7952987

Roose SP, Glassman AH: Cardiovascular effects of tricyclic antidepressants in depressed patients with and without heart disease. J Clin Psychiatry 50(suppl):1–18, 1989

Rothschild AJ, Samson JA, Bessette MP, et al: Efficacy of the combination of fluoxetine and perphenazine in the treatment of psychotic depression. J Clin Psychiatry 54(9):338–342, 1993 8104930

Rothschild BS: Fluoxetine-nortriptyline therapy of treatment-resistant major depression in a geriatric patient. J Geriatr Psychiatry Neurol 7(3):137–138, 1994 7916935

Sambunaris A, Bose A, Gommoll CP, et al: A phase III, double-blind, placebo-controlled, flexible-dose study of levomilnacipran extended-release in patients with major depressive disorder. J Clin Psychopharmacol 34(1):47–56, 2014 24172209

Saraceni MM, Venci JV, Gandhi MA: Levomilnacipran (Fetzima): a new serotonin-norepinephrine reuptake inhibitor for the treatment of major depressive disorder. J Pharm Pract 27(4):389–395, 2014 24381243

Sarchiapone M, Amore M, De Risio S, et al: Mirtazapine in the treatment of panic disorder: an open-label trial. Int Clin Psychopharmacol 18(1):35–38, 2003 12490773

Sargant W: The treatment of anxiety states and atypical depressions by the monoamine oxidase inhibitor drugs. J Neuropsychiatry 3(Suppl 1):96–103, 1962 13991481

Schatzberg AF, Cole JO: Benzodiazepines in depressive disorders. Arch Gen Psychiatry 35(11):1359–1365, 1978 30428

Shrivastava RK, Cohn C, Crowder J, et al: Long-term safety and clinical acceptability of venlafaxine and imipramine in outpatients with major depression. J Clin Psychopharmacol 14(5):322–329, 1994 7806687

Simon GE, VonKorff M, Heiligenstein JH, et al: Initial antidepressant choice in primary care: effectiveness and cost of fluoxetine vs tricyclic antidepressants. JAMA 275(24):1897–1902, 1996 8648870

Spiegel K, Kalb R, Pasternak GW: Analgesic activity of tricyclic antidepressants. Ann Neurol 13(4):462–465, 1983 6838179

Stark P, Fuller RW, Wong DT: The pharmacologic profile of fluoxetine. J Clin Psychiatry 46(3 Pt 2):7–13, 1985 3871767

Stokes PE: Fluoxetine: a five-year review. Clin Ther 15(2):216–243 [discussion 215], 1993 8519034

Stuppaeck CH, Geretsegger C, Whitworth AB, et al: A multicenter double-blind trial of paroxetine versus amitriptyline in depressed inpatients. J Clin Psychopharmacol 14(4):241–246, 1994 7962679

Taylor MJ, Rudkin L, Hawton K: Strategies for managing antidepressant-induced sexual dysfunction: systematic review of randomised controlled trials. J Affect Disord 88(3):241–254, 2005 16162361

Teicher MH, Cohen BM, Baldessarini RJ, et al: Severe daytime somnolence in patients treated with an MAOI. Am J Psychiatry 145(12):1552–1556, 1988 3273886

Teicher MH, Glod CA, Cole JO: Antidepressant drugs and the emergence of suicidal tendencies. Drug Saf 8(3):186–212, 1993 8452661

Thase ME: Are SNRIs more effective than SSRIs? A review of the current state of the controversy. Psychopharmacol Bull 41(2):58–85, 2008 18668017

Tignol J, Stoker MJ, Dunbar GC: Paroxetine in the treatment of melancholia and severe depression. Int Clin Psychopharmacol 7(2):91–94, 1992 1487627

van Bemmel AL, Havermans RG, van Diest R: Effects of trazodone on EEG sleep and clinical state in major depression. Psychopharmacology (Berl) 107(4):569–574, 1992 1603901

van Laar MW, van Willigenburg AP, Volkerts ER: Acute and subchronic effects of nefazodone and imipramine on highway driving, cognitive functions, and daytime sleepiness in healthy adult and elderly subjects. J Clin Psychopharmacol 15(1):30–40, 1995 7714226

Vartiainen H, Leinonen E: Double-blind study of mirtazapine and placebo in hospitalized patients with major depression. Eur Neuropsychopharmacol 4(2):145–150, 1994 7919944

Volicer L, Rheaume Y, Cyr D: Treatment of depression in advanced Alzheimer's disease using sertraline. J Geriatr Psychiatry Neurol 7(4):227–229, 1994 7826491

Wajs E, Aluisio L, Holder R, et al: Esketamine nasal spray plus oral antidepressant in patients with treatment-resistant depression: assessment of long-term safety in a phase 3, open-label study (SUSTAIN-2). J Clin Psychiatry 81(3):19m12891, 2020 32316080

Wang SM, Han C, Lee SJ, et al: A review of current evidence for vilazodone in major depressive disorder. Int J Psychiatry Clin Pract 17(3):160–169, 2013 23578403

Weilburg JB, Rosenbaum JF, Biederman J, et al: Fluoxetine added to non-MAOI antidepressants converts nonresponders to responders: a preliminary report. J Clin Psychiatry 50(12):447–449, 1989 2600061

Weisler RH, Johnston JA, Lineberry CG, et al: Comparison of bupropion and trazodone for the treatment of major depression. J Clin Psychopharmacol 14(3):170–179, 1994 8027413

Wilcox CS, Ferguson JM, Dale JL, et al: A double-blind trial of low- and high-dose ranges of gepirone-ER compared with placebo in the treatment of depressed outpatients. Psychopharmacol Bull 32(3):335–342, 1996 8961776

Wolfersdorf M, Barg T, König F, et al: Paroxetine in the treatment of inpatients with non-delusional endogenous or neurotic depression. Schweiz Arch Neurol Psychiatr 145(6):15–18, 1994 7533940

Yoon SJ, Pae CU, Kim DJ, et al: Mirtazapine for patients with alcohol dependence and comorbid depressive disorders: a multicentre, open label study. Prog Neuropsychopharmacol Biol Psychiatry 30(7):1196–1201, 2006 16624467

Young AH, Gallagher P, Watson S, et al: Improvements in neurocognitive function and mood following adjunctive treatment with mifepristone (RU-486) in bipolar disorder. Neuropsychopharmacology 29(8):1538–1545, 2004 15127079

Zisook S, Rush AJ, Haight BR, et al: Use of bupropion in combination with serotonin reuptake inhibitors. Biol Psychiatry 59(3):203–210, 2006 16165100

Zobel AW, Nickel T, Künzel HE, et al: Effects of the high-affinity corticotropin-releasing hormone receptor 1 antagonist R121919 in major depression: the first 20 patients treated. J Psychiatr Res 34(3):171–181, 2000 10867111

References

Agosti V, Stewart JW, Quitkin FM: Life satisfaction and psychosocial functioning in chronic depression: effect of acute treatment with antidepressants. J Affect Disord 23(1):35–41, 1991 1774421

Aizenberg D, Zemishlany Z, Weizman A: Cyproheptadine treatment of sexual dysfunction induced by serotonin reuptake inhibitors. Clin Neuropharmacol 18(4):320–324, 1995 8665544

Alam MY, Jacobsen PL, Chen Y, et al: Safety, tolerability, and efficacy of vortioxetine (Lu AA21004) in major depressive disorder: results of an open-label, flexible-dose, 52-week extension study. Int Clin Psychopharmacol 29(1):36–44, 2014 24169027

Altamura AC, Pioli R, Vitto M, et al: Venlafaxine in social phobia: a study in selective serotonin reuptake inhibitor non-responders. Int Clin Psychopharmacol 14(4):239–245, 1999 10468317

Alvarez E, Perez V, Dragheim M, et al: A double-blind, randomized, placebo-controlled, active reference study of Lu AA21004 in patients with major depressive disorder. Int J Neuropsychopharmacol 15(5):589–600, 2012 21767441

American Psychiatric Association: Diagnostic and Statistical Manual of Mental Disorders, 4th Edition. Washington, DC, American Psychiatric Association, 1994

Amsterdam JD: A double-blind, placebo-controlled trial of the safety and efficacy of selegiline transdermal system without dietary restrictions in patients with major depressive disorder. J Clin Psychiatry 64(2):208–214, 2003 12633131

Amsterdam JD, Berwish NJ: High dose tranylcypromine therapy for refractory depression. Pharmacopsychiatry 22(1):21–25, 1989 2710808

Ansseau M, Darimont P, Lecoq A, et al: Controlled comparison of nefazodone and amitriptyline in major depressive inpatients. Psychopharmacology (Berl) 115(1–2):254–260, 1994 7862904

Anton RF, Sexauer JD: Efficacy of amoxapine in psychotic depression. Am J Psychiatry 140(10):1344–1347, 1983 6624968

Aranda-Michel J, Koehler A, Bejarano PA, et al: Nefazodone-induced liver failure: report of three cases. Ann Intern Med 130(4 Pt 1):285–288, 1999 10068386

Archer DF, Dupont CM, Constantine GD, et al: Desvenlafaxine for the treatment of vasomotor symptoms associated with menopause: a double-blind, randomized, placebo-controlled trial of efficacy and safety. Am J Obstet Gynecol 200(3):238.e1–238.e10, 2009 19167693

Armitage R, Rush AJ, Trivedi M, et al: The effects of nefazodone on sleep architecture in depression. Neuropsychopharmacology 10(2):123–127, 1994 8024673

Arnow BA, Blasey C, Williams LM, et al: Depression subtypes in predicting antidepressant response: a report from the iSPOT-D trial. Am J Psychiatry 172(8):743–750, 2015 25815419

Ashton AK, Bennett RG: Sildenafil treatment of serotonin reuptake inhibitor-induced sexual dysfunction. J Clin Psychiatry 60(3):194–195, 1999 10192597

Ashton AK, Rosen RC: Bupropion as an antidote for serotonin reuptake inhibitor-induced sexual dysfunction. J Clin Psychiatry 59(3):112–115, 1998 9541153

Bahji A, Vazquez GH, Zarate CA: Comparative efficacy of racemic ketamine and esketamine for depression: a systematic review and meta-analysis. J Affect Disord 278:542–555, 2021 33022440

Balon R: Intermittent amantadine for fluoxetine-induced anorgasmia. J Sex Marital Ther 22(4):290–292, 1996 9018655

Barbey JT, Roose SP: SSRI safety in overdose. J Clin Psychiatry 59(Suppl 15):42–48, 1998 9786310

Beasley CM Jr, Dornseif BE, Bosomworth JC, et al: Fluoxetine and suicide: a meta-analysis of controlled trials of treatment for depression. BMJ 303(6804):685–692, 1991 1833012 (also see comments) (erratum: BMJ 23:968, 1991)

Beasley CM Jr, Potvin JH, Masica DN, et al: Fluoxetine: no association with suicidality in obsessive-compulsive disorder. J Affect Disord 24(1):1–10, 1992 1545040

Benazzi F: Nefazodone withdrawal symptoms. Can J Psychiatry 43(2):194–195, 1998 9533975

Berk M, Ichim C, Brook S: Efficacy of mirtazapine add on therapy to haloperidol in the treatment of the negative symptoms of schizophrenia: a double-blind randomized placebo-controlled study. Int Clin Psychopharmacol 16(2):87–92, 2001 11236073

Bertschy G, Vandel S, Vandel B, et al: Fluvoxamine-tricyclic antidepressant interaction: an accidental finding. Eur J Clin Pharmacol 40(1):119–120, 1991 1905641

Bhattacharjee C, Smith M, Todd F, et al: Bupropion overdose: a potential problem with the new "miracle" anti-smoking drug. Int J Clin Pract 55(3):221–222, 2001 11351778

Bielski RJ, Ventura D, Chang CC: A double-blind comparison of escitalopram and venlafaxine extended release in the treatment of major depressive disorder. J Clin Psychiatry 65(9):1190–1196, 2004 15367045

Binneman B, Feltner D, Kolluri S, et al: A 6-week randomized, placebo-controlled trial of CP-316,311 (a selective CRH1 antagonist) in the treatment of major depression. Am J Psychiatry 165(5):617–620, 2008 18413705

Blier P, Ward HE, Tremblay P, et al: Combination of antidepressant medications from treatment initiation for major depressive disorder: a double-blind randomized study. Am J Psychiatry 167(3):281–288, 2010 20008946

Block TS, Kushner H, Kalin N, et al: Combined analysis of mifepristone for psychotic depression: plasma levels associated with clinical response. Biol Psychiatry 84(1):46–54, 2018 29523415

Bodkin JA, Amsterdam JD: Transdermal selegiline in major depression: a double-blind, placebo-controlled, parallel-group study in outpatients. Am J Psychiatry 159(11):1869–1875, 2002 12411221

Bodkin JA, Zornberg GL, Lukas SE, et al: Buprenorphine treatment of refractory depression. J Clin Psychopharmacol 15(1):49–57, 1995 7714228

Bonaventura J, Lam S, Carlton M, et al: Pharmacological and behavioral divergence of ketamine enantiomers: implications for abuse liability. Mol Psychiatry 26(11):6704–6722, 2021 33859356

Bondade S, Basavaraju V, Singh N: Use of mirtazapine in functional vomiting. Aust N Z J Psychiatry 50(1):102–103, 2016 26320233

Borys DJ, Setzer SC, Ling LJ, et al: Acute fluoxetine overdose: a report of 234 cases. Am J Emerg Med 10(2):115–120, 1992 1586402

Boulenger JP, Loft H, Olsen CK: Efficacy and safety of vortioxetine (Lu AA21004), 15 and 20 mg/day: a randomized, double-blind, placebo-controlled, duloxetine-referenced study in the acute treatment of adult patients with major depressive disorder. Int Clin Psychopharmacol 29(3):138–149, 2014 24257717

Brown WA, Harrison W: Are patients who are intolerant to one serotonin selective reuptake inhibitor intolerant to another? J Clin Psychiatry 56(1):30–34, 1995 7836337

Buckley NA, McManus PR: Fatal toxicity of serotoninergic and other antidepressant drugs: analysis of United Kingdom mortality data. BMJ 325(7376):1332–1333, 2002 12468481

Cantwell DP: ADHD through the life span: the role of bupropion in treatment. J Clin Psychiatry 59(4)(Suppl 4):92–94, 1998 9554326

Canuso CM, Singh JB, Fedgchin M, et al: Efficacy and safety of intranasal esketamine for the rapid reduction of symptoms of depression and suicidality in patients at imminent risk for suicide: results of a double-blind, randomized, placebo-controlled study. Am J Psychiatry 175(7):620–630, 2018 29656663

Carpenter LL, Jocic Z, Hall JM, et al: Mirtazapine augmentation in the treatment of refractory depression. J Clin Psychiatry 60(1):45–49, 1999a 10074878

Carpenter LL, Leon Z, Yasmin S, et al: Clinical experience with mirtazapine in the treatment of panic disorder. Ann Clin Psychiatry 11(2):81–86, 1999b 10440525

Chang FL, Ho ST, Sheen MJ: Efficacy of mirtazapine in preventing intrathecal morphine-induced nausea and vomiting after orthopaedic surgery. Anaesthesia 65(12):1206–1211, 2010 21182602

Chen CC, Lin CS, Ko YP, et al: Premedication with mirtazapine reduces preoperative anxiety and postoperative nausea and vomiting. Anesth Analg 106(1):109–113, 2008 18165563

Chouinard G, Goodman W, Greist J, et al: Results of a double-blind placebo controlled trial of a new serotonin uptake inhibitor, sertraline, in the treatment of obsessive-compulsive disorder. Psychopharmacol Bull 26(3):279–284, 1990 2274626

Clayton AH, Warnock JK, Kornstein SG, et al: A placebo-controlled trial of bupropion SR as an antidote for selective serotonin reuptake inhibitor-induced sexual dysfunction. J Clin Psychiatry 65(1):62–67, 2004 14744170

Clerc GE, Ruimy P, Verdeau-Pallès J, et al: A double-blind comparison of venlafaxine and fluoxetine in patients hospitalized for major depression and melancholia. Int Clin Psychopharmacol 9(3):139–143, 1994 7814822

Connor KM, Davidson JR, Weisler RH, et al: A pilot study of mirtazapine in post-traumatic stress disorder. Int Clin Psychopharmacol 14(1):29–31, 1999 10221639

Cooper JM, Brown JA, Cairns R, et al: Desvenlafaxine overdose and the occurrence of serotonin toxicity, seizures and cardiovascular effects. Clin Toxicol (Phila) 55(1):18–24, 2017 27622824

Cougnard A, Verdoux H, Grolleau A, et al: Impact of antidepressants on the risk of suicide in patients with depression in real-life conditions: a decision analysis model. Psychol Med 39(8):1307–1315, 2009 19063772

Cusson JR, Goldenberg E, Larochelle P: Effect of a novel monoamine-oxidase inhibitor, moclobemide on the sensitivity to intravenous tyramine and norepinephrine in humans. J Clin Pharmacol 31(5):462–467, 1991 2050833

Dalfen AK, Stewart DE: Who develops severe or fatal adverse drug reactions to selective serotonin reuptake inhibitors? Can J Psychiatry 46(3):258–263, 2001 11320680

Danish University Antidepressant Group: Paroxetine: a selective serotonin reuptake inhibitor showing better tolerance, but weaker antidepressant effect than clomipramine in a controlled multicenter study. J Affect Disord 18(4):289–299, 1990 2140382

Davidson JR, DuPont RL, Hedges D, et al: Efficacy, safety, and tolerability of venlafaxine extended release and buspirone in outpatients with generalized anxiety disorder. J Clin Psychiatry 60(8):528–535, 1999 10485635

Davis JL, Smith RL: Painful peripheral diabetic neuropathy treated with venlafaxine HCl extended release capsules. Diabetes Care 22(11):1909–1910, 1999 10546032

DeBattista C, Doghramji K, Menza MA, et al: Adjunct modafinil for the short-term treatment of fatigue and sleepiness in patients with major depressive disorder: a preliminary double-blind, placebo-controlled study. J Clin Psychiatry 64(9):1057–1064, 2003 14628981

DeBattista C, Solvason B, Poirier J, et al: A placebo-controlled, randomized, double-blind study of adjunctive bupropion sustained release in the treatment of SSRI-induced sexual dysfunction. J Clin Psychiatry 66(7):844–848, 2005 16013899

Deligiannidis KM, Meltzer-Brody S, Gunduz-Bruce H, et al: Effect of zuranolone vs placebo in postpartum depression: a randomized clinical trial. JAMA Psychiatry 78(9):951–959, 2021 34190962

Dessain EC, Schatzberg AF, Woods BT, et al: Maprotiline treatment in depression: a perspective on seizures. Arch Gen Psychiatry 43(1):86–90, 1986 3942475

Detke MJ, Lu Y, Goldstein DJ, et al: Duloxetine, 60 mg once daily, for major depressive disorder: a randomized double-blind placebo-controlled trial. J Clin Psychiatry 63(4):308–315, 2002 12000204

Diaz-Martinez A, Benassinni O, Ontiveros A, et al: A randomized, open-label comparison of venlafaxine and fluoxetine in depressed outpatients. Clin Ther 20(3):467–476, 1998 9663362

Dingemanse J: An update of recent moclobemide interaction data. Int Clin Psycho-pharmacol 7(3–4):167–180, 1993 8468439

Falkai P: Mirtazapine: other indications. J Clin Psychiatry 60 (Suppl 17):36–40 [discussion 46–48], 1999 10446741

Farah A: Relief of SSRI-induced sexual dysfunction with mirtazapine treatment. J Clin Psychiatry 60(4):260–261, 1999 10221289

Fava M, Rosenbaum JF, McGrath PJ, et al: Lithium and tricyclic augmentation of fluoxetine treatment for resistant major depression: a double-blind, controlled study. Am J Psychiatry 151(9):1372–1374, 1994 8067495

Fava M, Dunner DL, Greist JH, et al: Efficacy and safety of mirtazapine in major depressive disorder patients after SSRI treatment failure: an open-label trial. J Clin Psychiatry 62(6):413–420, 2001 11465517

Fava M, Nurnberg HG, Seidman SN, et al: Efficacy and safety of sildenafil in men with serotonergic antidepressant-associated erectile dysfunction: results from a randomized, double-blind, placebo-controlled trial. J Clin Psychiatry 67(2):240–246, 2006a 16566619

Fava M, Rush AJ, Wisniewski SR, et al: A comparison of mirtazapine and nortriptyline following two consecutive failed medication treatments for depressed outpatients: a STAR*D report. Am J Psychiatry 163(7):1161–1172, 2006b 16816220

Fava M, Rush AJ, Alpert JE, et al: Difference in treatment outcome in outpatients with anxious versus nonanxious depression: a STAR*D report. Am J Psychiatry 165(3):342–351, 2008 1817 2020

Fava M, Memisoglu A, Thase ME, et al: Opioid modulation with buprenorphine/samidorphan as adjunctive treatment for inadequate response to antidepressants: a randomized double-blind placebo-controlled trial. Am J Psychiatry 173(5):499–508, 2016 26869247

Fava M, Mazzone E, Freeman M, et al. Double-blind, placebo-controlled, proof-of-concept trial of a kappa-selective opioid receptor antagonist augmentation in treatment-resistant depression. Ann Clin Psychiatry 32(4):18-26, 2020 33125454

Fava M, Stahl S, Pani L, et al: REL-1017 (esmethadone) as adjunctive treatment in patients with major depressive disorder: a phase 2a randomized double-blind trial. Am J Psychiatry 179(2):122–131, 2022 34933568

Fawcett J, Barkin RL: Review of the results from clinical studies on the efficacy, safety and tolerability of mirtazapine for the treatment of patients with major depression. J Affect Disord 51(3):267–285, 1998 10333982

Feiger A, Kiev A, Shrivastava RK, et al: Nefazodone versus sertraline in outpatients with major depression: focus on efficacy, tolerability, and effects on sexual function and satisfaction. J Clin Psychiatry 57(2)(Suppl 2):53–62, 1996 8626364

Feighner JP, Herbstein J, Damlouji N: Combined MAOI, TCA, and direct stimulant therapy of treatment-resistant depression. J Clin Psychiatry 46(6):206–209, 1985 3997787

Findling RL, DelBello MP, Zuddas A, et al: Vortioxetine for major depressive disorder in adolescents: 12-week randomized, placebo-controlled, fluoxetine-referenced, fixed-dose study. J Am Acad Child Adolesc Psychiatry 61(9):1106–1118.e2, 2022 35033635

Fisher S, Bryant SG, Kent TA: Postmarketing surveillance by patient self-monitoring: trazodone versus fluoxetine. J Clin Psychopharmacol 13(4):235–242, 1993 8376610

Fitton A, Faulds D, Goa KL: Moclobemide: a review of its pharmacological properties and therapeutic use in depressive illness. Drugs 43(4):561–596, 1992 1377119

Fluoxetine Bulimia Nervosa Collaborative Study Group: Fluoxetine in the treatment of bulimia nervosa: a multicenter, placebo-controlled, double-blind trial. Arch Gen Psychiatry 49(2):139–147, 1992 1550466

Fontaine R, Ontiveros A, Elie R, et al: A double-blind comparison of nefazodone, imipramine, and placebo in major depression. J Clin Psychiatry 55(6):234–241, 1994 8071277

Frank E, Kupfer DJ, Perel JM, et al: Three-year outcomes for maintenance therapies in recurrent depression. Arch Gen Psychiatry 47(12):1093–1099, 1990 2244793

Furukawa TA, Cipriani A, Atkinson LZ et al: Placebo response rates in antidepressant trials: a systematic review of published and unpublished double-blind randomized controlled studies. Lancet Psychiatry 3(11):1059–1066, 2016 27726982

Gelenberg AJ, Lydiard RB, Rudolph RL, et al: Efficacy of venlafaxine extended-release capsules in nondepressed outpatients with generalized anxiety disorder: a 6-month randomized controlled trial. JAMA 283(23):3082–3088, 2000 10865302

Gibb A, Deeks ED: Vortioxetine: first global approval. Drugs 74(1):135–145, 2014 24311349

Gittelman DK, Kirby MG: A seizure following bupropion overdose. J Clin Psychiatry 54(4):162, 1993 8486598

Glassman AH, Perel JM, Shostak M, et al: Clinical implications of imipramine plasma levels for depressive illness. Arch Gen Psychiatry 34(2):197–204, 1977 843179

Golden RN, Rudorfer MV, Sherer MA, et al: Bupropion in depression I: biochemical effects and clinical response. Arch Gen Psychiatry 45(2):139–143, 1988 3122698

Goldstein D, Bitter I, Lu Y, et al: Duloxetine in the treatment of depression: a double-blind, placebo-controlled comparison with paroxetine. Eur Psychiatry 17(Suppl 1):98, 2002

Goldstein MG: Bupropion sustained release and smoking cessation. J Clin Psychiatry 59(4)(Suppl 4):66–72, 1998 9554323

Goodnick PJ, Puig A, DeVane CL, et al: Mirtazapine in major depression with comorbid generalized anxiety disorder. J Clin Psychiatry 60(7):446–448, 1999 10453798

Goodwin GM, Aaronson ST, Alvarez O, et al: Single-dose psilocybin for a treatment-resistant episode of major depression. N Engl J Med 387(18):1637–1648, 2022 36322843

Gorwood P, Corruble E, Falissard B, et al: Toxic effects of depression on brain function: impairment of delayed recall and the cumulative length of depressive disorder in a large sample of depressed outpatients. Am J Psychiatry 165(6):731–739, 2008 18381906

Griffiths RR, Johnson MW, Carducci MA, et al: Psilocybin produces substantial and sustained decreases in depression and anxiety in patients with life-threatening cancer: a randomized double-blind trial. J Psychopharmacol 30(12):1181–1197, 2016 27909165

Guay DR: Vilazodone hydrochloride, a combined SSRI and 5-HT1A receptor agonist for major depressive disorder. Consult Pharm 27(12):857–867, 2012 23229074

Gunduz-Bruce H, Kanes SJ, Zorumski CF: Trial of SAGE-217 in patients with major depressive disorder. N Engl J Med 381(10):903–911, 2019 31483961

Gupta S, Droney T, Masand P, et al: SSRI-induced sexual dysfunction treated with sildenafil. Depress Anxiety 9(4):180–182, 1999 10431684

Hammad TA, Laughren T, Racoosin J: Suicidality in pediatric patients treated with antidepressant drugs. Arch Gen Psychiatry 63(3):332–339, 2006a 16520440

Hammad TA, Laughren TP, Racoosin JA: Suicide rates in short-term randomized controlled trials of newer antidepressants. J Clin Psychopharmacol 26(2):203–207, 2006b 16633153

Hamner MB, Frueh BC: Response to venlafaxine in a previously antidepressant treatment-resistant combat veteran with post-traumatic stress disorder. Int Clin Psychopharmacol 13(5):233–234, 1998 9817630

Hidalgo R, Hertzberg MA, Mellman T, et al: Nefazodone in post-traumatic stress disorder: results from six open-label trials. Int Clin Psychopharmacol 14(2):61–68, 1999 10220119

Hirschfeld RM: Efficacy of SSRIs and newer antidepressants in severe depression: comparison with TCAs. J Clin Psychiatry 60(5):326–335, 1999 10362442

Ionescu DF, Fu DJ, Qiu X, et al: Esketamine nasal spray for rapid reduction of depressive symptoms in patients with major depressive disorder who have active suicide ideation with intent: results of a phase 3, double-blind, randomized study (ASPIRE II). Int J Neuropsychopharmacol 24(1):22–31, 2021 32861217

Iosifescu DV, Jones A, O'Gorman C, et al: Efficacy and safety of AXS-05 (dextromethorphan-bupropion) in patients with major depressive disorder: a phase 3 randomized clinical trial (GEMINI). J Clin Psychiatry 30(4):21m14345, 2022 35649167

Jacobsen FM: Fluoxetine-induced sexual dysfunction and an open trial of yohimbine. J Clin Psychiatry 53(4):119–122, 1992 1564046

Jermain DM, Preece CK, Sykes RL, et al: Luteal phase sertraline treatment for premenstrual dysphoric disorder: results of a double-blind, placebo-controlled, crossover study. Arch Fam Med 8(4):328–332, 1999 10418540

Kaizar EE, Greenhouse JB, Seltman H, et al: Do antidepressants cause suicidality in children? A Bayesian meta-analysis. Clin Trials 3(2):73–90 [discussion 91–98], 2006 16773951

Kanes S, Colquhoun H, Gunduz-Bruce H, et al: Brexanolone (SAGE-547 injection) in post-partum depression: a randomised controlled trial. Lancet 390(10093):480–489, 2017 28619476

Kast RE, Foley KF: Cancer chemotherapy and cachexia: mirtazapine and olanzapine are 5-HT3 antagonists with good antinausea effects. Eur J Cancer Care (Engl) 16(4):351–354, 2007 17587360

Kavoussi RJ, Liu J, Coccaro EF: An open trial of sertraline in personality disordered patients with impulsive aggression. J Clin Psychiatry 55(4):137–141, 1994 8071257

Kaye WH, Weltzin TE, Hsu LK, et al: An open trial of fluoxetine in patients with anorexia nervosa. J Clin Psychiatry 52(11):464–471, 1991 1744064

Ke X, Ding Y, Xu K, et al: The profile of cognitive impairments in chronic ketamine users. Psychiatry Res 266:124–131, 2018 29864611

Keller Ashton A, Hamer R, Rosen RC: Serotonin reuptake inhibitor-induced sexual dysfunction and its treatment: a large-scale retrospective study of 596 psychiatric outpatients. J Sex Marital Ther 23(3):165–175, 1997 9292832

Khan A, Cutler AJ, Kajdasz DK, et al: A randomized, double-blind, placebo-controlled, 8-week study of vilazodone, a serotonergic agent for the treatment of major depressive disorder. J Clin Psychiatry 72(4):441–447, 2011 21527122

Kiayias JA, Vlachou ED, Lakka-Papadodima E: Venlafaxine HCl in the treatment of painful peripheral diabetic neuropathy. Diabetes Care 23(5):699, 2000 10834432

Killen JD, Robinson TN, Ammerman S, et al: Randomized clinical trial of the efficacy of bupropion combined with nicotine patch in the treatment of adolescent smokers. J Consult Clin Psychol 72(4):729–735, 2004 15301658

Kim SW, Shin IS, Kim JM, et al: Effectiveness of mirtazapine for nausea and insomnia in cancer patients with depression. Psychiatry Clin Neurosci 62(1):75–83, 2008 18289144

Klein ME, Chandra J, Sheriff S, et al: Opioid system is necessary but not sufficient for antidepressive actions of ketamine in rodents. Proc Natl Acad Sci USA 117(5):2656–2662, 2020 31941713

Kornstein SG: Maintenance therapy to prevent recurrence of depression: summary and implications of the PREVENT study. Expert Rev Neurother 8(5):737–742, 2008 18457530

Kotlyar M, Golding M, Brewer ER, et al: Possible nefazodone withdrawal syndrome (letter). Am J Psychiatry 156(7):1117, 1999 10401469

Koutouvidis N, Pratikakis M, Fotiadou A: The use of mirtazapine in a group of 11 patients following poor compliance to selective serotonin reuptake inhibitor treatment due to sexual dysfunction. Int Clin Psychopharmacol 14(4):253–255, 1999 10468319

Krishnan R, Cella D, Leonardi C, et al: Effects of etanercept therapy on fatigue and symptoms of depression in subjects treated for moderate to severe plaque psoriasis for up to 96 weeks. Br J Dermatol 157(6):1275–1277, 2007 17916204

Kuhn R: The treatment of depressive states with G 22355 (imipramine hydrochloride). Am J Psychiatry 115(5):459–464, 1958 13583250

Labbate LA, Pollack MH: Treatment of fluoxetine-induced sexual dysfunction with bupropion: a case report. Ann Clin Psychiatry 6(1):13–15, 1994 7951639

Landén M, Eriksson E, Agren H, et al: Effect of buspirone on sexual dysfunction in depressed patients treated with selective serotonin reuptake inhibitors. J Clin Psychopharmacol 19(3):268–271, 1999 10350034

Lauber C: Nefazodone withdrawal syndrome. Can J Psychiatry 44(3):285–286, 1999 10225135

Leinonen E, Skarstein J, Behnke K, et al: Efficacy and tolerability of mirtazapine versus citalopram: a double-blind, randomized study in patients with major depressive disorder. Int Clin Psychopharmacol 14(6):329–337, 1999 10565799

Lenderking WR, Tennen H, Nackley JF, et al: The effects of venlafaxine on social activity level in depressed outpatients. J Clin Psychiatry 60(3):157–163, 1999 10192590

Lohoff FW, Rickels K: Desvenlafaxine succinate for the treatment of major depressive disorder. Expert Opin Pharmacother 9(12):2129–2136, 2008 18671467

Lotufo-Neto F, Trivedi M, Thase ME: Meta-analysis of the reversible inhibitors of monoamine oxidase type A moclobemide and brofaromine for the treatment of depression. Neuropsychopharmacology 20(3):226–247, 1999 10063483

Luckhaus C, Jacob C: Venlafaxine withdrawal syndrome not prevented by maprotiline, but resolved by sertraline (letter). Int J Neuropsychopharmacol 4(1):43–44, 2001 11343628

Mainie I, McGurk C, McClintock G, et al: Seizures after bupropion overdose. Lancet 357(9268):1624, 2001 11386326

Maletic V, Robinson M, Oakes T, et al: Neurobiology of depression: an integrated view of key findings. Int J Clin Pract 61(12):2030–2040, 2007 17944926

Mann JJ, Aarons SF, Wilner PJ, et al: A controlled study of the antidepressant efficacy and side effects of (-)-deprenyl: a selective monoamine oxidase inhibitor. Arch Gen Psychiatry 46(1):45–50, 1989 2491941

Markowitz JS: Re: Nefazodone withdrawal. Can J Psychiatry 44(3):286–287, 1999 10225136

McCabe B, Tsuang MT: Dietary consideration in MAO inhibitor regimens. J Clin Psychiatry 43(5):178–181, 1982 7076627

McGrath PJ, Quitkin FM, Klein DF: Bromocriptine treatment of relapses seen during selective serotonin re-uptake inhibitor treatment of depression. J Clin Psychopharmacol 15(4):289–291, 1995 7593717

McGrath PJ, Stewart JW, Fava M, et al: Tranylcypromine versus venlafaxine plus mirtazapine following three failed antidepressant medication trials for depression: a STAR*D report. Am J Psychiatry 163(9):1531–1541, quiz 1666, 2006 16946177

McInnes LA, Qian JJ, Gargeya RS, et al: A retrospective analysis of ketamine intravenous therapy for depression in real-world care settings. J Affect Disord 301:486–495, 2022 35027209

McIntyre RS, Lophaven S, Olsen CK: A randomized, double-blind, placebo-controlled study of vortioxetine on cognitive function in depressed adults. Int J Neuropsychopharmacol 17(10):1557–1567, 2014 24787143

McKenzie MS, McFarland BH: Trends in antidepressant overdoses. Pharmacoepidemiol Drug Saf 16(5):513–523, 2007 17200994

Meltzer-Brody S, Colquhoun H, Riesenberg R, et al: Brexanolone injection in postpartum depression: two multicentre, double-blind, randomised, placebo-controlled, phase 3 trials. Lancet 392(10152):1058–1070, 2018 17200994

Michelson D, Bancroft J, Targum S, et al: Female sexual dysfunction associated with antidepressant administration: a randomized, placebo-controlled study of pharmacologic intervention. Am J Psychiatry 157(2):239–243, 2000 10671393

Michelson D, Kociban K, Tamura R, et al: Mirtazapine, yohimbine or olanzapine augmentation therapy for serotonin reuptake-associated female sexual dysfunction: a randomized, placebo controlled trial. J Psychiatr Res 36(3):147–152, 2002 11886692

Mitchell JM, Ot'alora GM, Van der Kolk B, et al: MDMA-assisted therapy for moderate to severe PTSD: a randomized, placebo-controlled phase 3 trial. Nat Med 29(10):2473–2480, 2023 37709999

Modell JG, Rosenthal NE, Harriett AE, et al: Seasonal affective disorder and its prevention by anticipatory treatment with bupropion XL. Biol Psychiatry 58(8):658–667, 2005 16271314

Monteleone P, Gnocchi G: Evidence for a linear relationship between plasma trazodone levels and clinical response in depression in the elderly. Clin Neuropharmacol 13(Suppl 1):S84–S89, 1990 2379183

Montgomery SA, Baldwin DS, Blier P, et al: Which antidepressants have demonstrated superior efficacy? A review of the evidence. Int Clin Psychopharmacol 22(6):323–329, 2007 17917550

Murphy GM Jr, Kremer C, Rodrigues HE, et al: Pharmacogenetics of antidepressant medication intolerance. Am J Psychiatry 160(10):1830–1835, 2003 14514498

Murrough JW, Wade E, Sayed S, et al: Dextromethorphan/quinidine pharmacotherapy in pa-tients with treatment resistant depression: a proof of concept clinical trial. J Affect Disord 218:277–283, 2017 28478356

Myers FA Jr, Bluth MH, Cheung WW: Ketamine: a cause of urinary tract dysfunction. Clin Lab Med 36(4):721–744, 2016 27842789

Nelson JC, Schottenfeld RS, Conrad CD: Hypomania after desipramine withdrawal. Am J Psychiatry 140(5):624–625, 1983 6846597

Nemeroff CB: Back to the future: esmethadone, the (maybe) nonopiate opiate, and depression. Am J Psychiatry 179(2):83–84, 2022 35105159

Nemeroff CB, Entsuah RA, Willard B, et al: Venlafaxine and SSRIs pooled remission analysis (NR263), in 2003 New Research Program and Abstracts, American Psychiatric Association 156th Annual Meeting, San Francisco, CA, May 17–22, 2003. Washington, DC, American Psychiatric Association, 2003

Nierenberg AA, McLean NE, Alpert JE, et al: Early nonresponse to fluoxetine as a predictor of poor 8-week outcome. Am J Psychiatry 152(10):1500–1503, 1995 7573590

Nierenberg AA, Farabaugh AH, Alpert JE, et al: Timing of onset of antidepressant response with fluoxetine treatment. Am J Psychiatry 157(9):1423–1428, 2000 10964858

Norden MJ: Buspirone treatment of sexual dysfunction associated with selective serotonin reuptake inhibitors. Depression 2:109–112, 1994

Norton PA, Zinner NR, Yalcin I, et al: Duloxetine versus placebo in the treatment of stress urinary incontinence. Am J Obstet Gynecol 187(1):40–48, 2002 12114886

Nurnberg HG, Hensley PL, Lauriello J, et al: Sildenafil for women patients with antidepressant-induced sexual dysfunction. Psychiatr Serv 50(8):1076–1078, 1999a 10445658

Nurnberg HG, Lauriello J, Hensley PL, et al: Sildenafil for iatrogenic serotonergic antidepressant medication-induced sexual dysfunction in 4 patients. J Clin Psychiatry 60(1):33–35, 1999b 10074875

Nurnberg HG, Thompson PM, Hensley PL: Antidepressant medication change in a clinical treatment setting: a comparison of the effectiveness of selective serotonin reuptake inhibitors. J Clin Psychiatry 60(9):574–579, 1999c 10520974

Nurnberg HG, Gelenberg A, Hargreave TB, et al: Efficacy of sildenafil citrate for the treatment of erectile dysfunction in men taking serotonin reuptake inhibitors. Am J Psychiatry 158(11):1926–1928, 2001 11691705

Nurnberg HG, Hensley PL, Heiman JR, et al: Sildenafil treatment of women with antidepressant-associated sexual dysfunction: a randomized controlled trial. JAMA 300(4):395–404, 2008 18647982

Nyhuis PW, Gastpar M, Scherbaum N: Opiate treatment in depression refractory to antidepressants and electroconvulsive therapy. J Clin Psychopharmacol 28(5):593–595, 2008 18794671

Oslin DW, Ten Have TR, Streim JE, et al: Probing the safety of medications in the frail elderly: evidence from a randomized clinical trial of sertraline and venlafaxine in depressed nursing home residents. J Clin Psychiatry 64(8):875–882, 2003 12927001

Otani K, Tanaka O, Kaneko S, et al: Mechanisms of the development of trazodone withdrawal symptoms. Int Clin Psychopharmacol 9(2):131–133, 1994 8056996

Papakostas GI, Homberger CH, Fava M: A meta-analysis of clinical trials comparing mirtazapine with selective serotonin reuptake inhibitors for the treatment of major depressive disorder. J Psychopharmacol 22(8):843–848, 2008 18308801

Parikh SV, Aaronson ST, Mathew SJ, et al: Efficacy and safety of zuranolone co-initiated with an antidepressant in adults with major depressive disorder: results from the phase 3 CORAL study. Neuropsychopharmacology Oct 24, 2023 37875578 Epub ahead of print

Pernia A, Micó JA, Calderón E, et al: Venlafaxine for the treatment of neuropathic pain. J Pain Symptom Manage 19(6):408–410, 2000 10991644

Pescatori ES, Engelman JC, Davis G, et al: Priapism of the clitoris: a case report following trazodone use. J Urol 149(6):1557–1559, 1993 8501813

Popova V, Daly EJ, Trivedi M, et al: Efficacy and safety of flexibly dosed esketamine nasal spray combined with a newly initiated oral antidepressant in treatment-resistant depression: a randomized double-blind active-controlled study. Am J Psychiatry 176(6):428–438, 2019 31109201

Pratt LA, Brody DJ, Gu Q: Antidepressant Use Among Persons Aged 12 and Over: United States, 2011–2014. NCHS Data Brief No 283. Hyattsville, MD, National Center for Health Statistics, August 2017. Available at: www.cdc.gov/nchs/data/databriefs/db283.pdf. Accessed September 2017.

Preskorn SH: Recent pharmacologic advances in antidepressant therapy for the elderly. Am J Med 94(5A):2S–12S, 1993 8503477

Price J, Grunhaus LJ: Treatment of clomipramine-induced anorgasmia with yohimbine: a case report. J Clin Psychiatry 51(1):32–33, 1990 2295589

Prien RF, Kupfer DJ, Mansky PA, et al: Drug therapy in the prevention of recurrences in unipolar and bipolar affective disorders: report of the NIMH Collaborative Study Group comparing lithium carbonate, imipramine, and a lithium carbonate-imipramine combination. Arch Gen Psychiatry 41(11):1096–1104, 1984 6437366

Quitkin FM, Rabkin JG, Ross D, et al: Duration of antidepressant drug treatment: what is an adequate trial? Arch Gen Psychiatry 41(3):238–245, 1984 6367689

Quitkin FM, McGrath PJ, Stewart JW, et al: Chronological milestones to guide drug change: when should clinicians switch antidepressants? Arch Gen Psychiatry 53(9):785–792, 1996 8792755

Quitkin FM, Taylor BP, Kremer C: Does mirtazapine have a more rapid onset than SSRIs? J Clin Psychiatry 62(5):358–361, 2001 11411818

Raby WN: Treatment of venlafaxine discontinuation symptoms with ondansetron. J Clin Psychiatry 59(11):621–622, 1998 9862610

Raison CL: The promise and limitations of anti-inflammatory agents for the treatment of major depressive disorder. Curr Top Behav Neurosci 31:287–302, 2017 27278642

Raison CL, Rutherford RE, Woolwine BJ, et al: A randomized controlled trial of the tumor necrosis factor antagonist infliximab for treatment-resistant depression: the role of baseline inflammatory biomarkers. JAMA Psychiatry 70(1):31–41, 2013 22945416

Raison CL, Sanacora G, Woolley J, et al: Single-dose psilocybin treatment for major depressive disorder: a randomized clinical trial. JAMA 330 (9):843–853, 2023 37709999

Raskin J, Wiltse CG, Siegal A, et al: Efficacy of duloxetine on cognition, depression, and pain in elderly patients with major depressive disorder: an 8-week, double-blind, placebo-controlled trial. Am J Psychiatry 164(6):900–909, 2007 17541049

Rickels K, Schweizer E: Clinical overview of serotonin reuptake inhibitors. J Clin Psychiatry 51(12)(Suppl B):9–12, 1990 2147922

Rickels K, Downing R, Schweizer E, et al: Antidepressants for the treatment of generalized anxiety disorder: a placebo-controlled comparison of imipramine, trazodone, and diazepam. Arch Gen Psychiatry 50(11):884–895, 1993 8215814

Rickels K, Athanasiou M, Robinson DS, et al: Evidence for efficacy and tolerability of vilazodone in the treatment of major depressive disorder: a randomized, double-blind, placebo-controlled trial. J Clin Psychiatry 70(3):326–333, 2009 19284933

Riggs PD, Leon SL, Mikulich SK, et al: An open trial of bupropion for ADHD in adolescents with substance use disorders and conduct disorder. J Am Acad Child Adolesc Psychiatry 37(12):1271–1278, 1998 9847499

Rinne T, van den Brink W, Wouters L, et al: SSRI treatment of borderline personality disorder: a randomized, placebo-controlled clinical trial for female patients with borderline personality disorder. Am J Psychiatry 159(12):2048–2054, 2002 12450955

Rohrig TP, Ray NG: Tissue distribution of bupropion in a fatal overdose. J Anal Toxicol 16(5):343–345, 1992 1294844

Roose SP, Glassman AH, Attia E, et al: Selective serotonin reuptake inhibitor efficacy in melancholia and atypical depression. Paper presented at the 147th Annual Meeting of the American Psychiatric Association, Philadelphia, PA, May 21–26, 1994

Rosen R, Shabsigh R, Berber M, et al: Efficacy and tolerability of vardenafil in men with mild depression and erectile dysfunction: the depression-related improvement with vardenafil for erectile response study. Am J Psychiatry 163(1):79–87, 2006 16390893

Ross S, Bossis A, Guss J, et al: Rapid and sustained symptom reduction following psilocybin treatment for anxiety and depression in patients with life-threatening cancer: a randomized controlled trial. J Psychopharmacol 30(12):1165–1180, 2016 27909164

Rothschild AJ, Locke CA: Reexposure to fluoxetine after serious suicide attempts by three patients: the role of akathisia. J Clin Psychiatry 52(12):491–493, 1991 1752848

Rush AJ, Trivedi MH, Wisniewski SR, et al: Bupropion-SR, sertraline, or venlafaxine-XR after failure of SSRIs for depression. N Engl J Med 354(12):1231–1242, 2006 16554525

Rush AJ, Trivedi MH, Stewart JW, et al: Combining Medications to Enhance Depression Outcomes (CO-MED): acute and long-term outcomes of a single-blind randomized study. Am J Psychiatry 168(7):689–701, 2011 21536692

Russell JI, Mease PJ, Smith TR, et al: Efficacy and safety of duloxetine for treatment of fibromyalgia in patients with or without major depressive disorder: results from a 6-month, randomized, double-blind, placebo-controlled, fixed-dose trial. Pain 136(3):432–444, 2008 18395345

Rynn M, Russell J, Erickson J, et al: Efficacy and safety of duloxetine in the treatment of generalized anxiety disorder: a flexible-dose, progressive-titration, placebo-controlled trial. Depress Anxiety 25(3):182–189, 2008 17311303

Sacchetti E, Conte G, Guarneri L: Are SSRI antidepressants a clinically homogeneous class of compounds? Lancet 344(8915):126–127, 1994 7912358

Sackeim HA, Roose SP, Burt T: Optimal length of antidepressant trials in late-life depression. J Clin Psychopharmacol 25(4)(Suppl 1):S34–S37, 2005 16027559

Samuels BA, Nautiyal KM, Kruegel AC, et al: The behavioral effects of the antidepressant tianeptine require the mu-opioid receptor. Neuropsychopharmacology 42(10):2052–2063, 2017 28303899

Sanacora G, Schatzberg AF: Ketamine: promising path or false prophecy in the development of novel therapeutics for mood disorders? Neuropsychopharmacology 40(2):259–267, 2015 25257213

Saveanu R, Etkin A, Duchemin AM, et al: The international Study to Predict Optimized Treatment in Depression (iSPOT-D): outcomes from the acute phase of antidepressant treatment. J Psychiatr Res 61:1–12, 2015 25586212

Schatzberg AF: Trazodone: a 5-year review of antidepressant efficacy. Psychopathology 20(Suppl 1):48–56, 1987 3321130

Schatzberg AF: A word to the wise about ketamine. Am J Psychiatry 171(3):262–264, 2014 24585328

Schatzberg AF: A word to the wise about intranasal esketamine. Am J Psychiatry 176(6):422–424, 2019 31109197

Schatzberg AF: Understanding the efficacy and mechanism of action of a dextromethorphan-bupropion combination: where does it fit in the NMDA versus mu-opioid story? Am J Psychiatry 179(7):448–450, 2022 35775155

Schatzberg AF, Rosenbaum AH, Orsulak PJ, et al: Toward a biochemical classification of depressive disorders III: pretreatment urinary MHPG levels as predictors of response to treatment with maprotiline. Psychopharmacology (Berl) 75(1):34–38, 1981 6795656

Schatzberg AF, Kremer C, Rodrigues HE, et al: Double-blind, randomized comparison of mirtazapine and paroxetine in elderly depressed patients. Am J Geriatr Psychiatry 10(5):541–550, 2002 12213688

Schmit G, De Boosere E, Vanhaebost J, et al: Bupropion overdose resulted in a pharmacobezoar in a fatal bupropion (Wellbutrin) sustained-release overdose: postmortem distribution of bupropion and its major metabolites. J Forensic Sci 62(6):1674–1676, 2017 28631318

Schneier FR, Liebowitz MR, Davies SO, et al: Fluoxetine in panic disorder. J Clin Psychopharmacol 10(2):119–121, 1990 2341585

Schwartz D, Blendl M: Sedation and anxiety reducing properties of trazodone, in Trazodone (Modern Problems in Pharmacopsychiatry, Vol 9). Edited by Ban TA, Silvestrini B. Basel, Switzerland, S Karger, 1974, pp 29–46

Segraves RT, Lee J, Stevenson R, et al: Tadalafil for treatment of erectile dysfunction in men on antidepressants. J Clin Psychopharmacol 27(1):62–66, 2007 17224715

Sheehan DV, Davidson J, Manschreck T, et al: Lack of efficacy of a new antidepressant (bupropion) in the treatment of panic disorder with phobias. J Clin Psychopharmacol 3(1):28–31, 1983 6403599

Shiroma PR, Johns B, Kuskowski M, et al: Augmentation of response and remission to serial intravenous subanesthetic ketamine in treatment resistant depression. J Affect Disord 155:123–129, 2014 24268616

Shram MJ, Henningfield JE, Apseloff G, et al: The novel uncompetitive NMDA receptor antagonist esmethadone (REL-1017) has no meaningful abuse potential in recreational drug users. Transl Psychiatry 13(1):192 2023 37286536

Shrivastava RK, Shrivastava S, Overweg N, et al: Amantadine in the treatment of sexual dysfunction associated with selective serotonin reuptake inhibitors. J Clin Psychopharmacol 15(1):83–84, 1995 7714234

Simon GE, Savarino J, Operskalski B, et al: Suicide risk during antidepressant treatment. Am J Psychiatry 163(1):41–47, 2006 16390887

Søndergård L, Kvist K, Andersen PK, et al: Do antidepressants precipitate youth suicide? A nationwide pharmacoepidemiological study. Eur Child Adolesc Psychiatry 15(4):232–240, 2006a 16502208

Søndergård L, Kvist K, Andersen PK, et al: Do antidepressants prevent suicide? Int Clin Psychopharmacol 21(4):211–218, 2006b 16687992

Spar JE: Plasma trazodone concentrations in elderly depressed inpatients: cardiac effects and short-term efficacy. J Clin Psychopharmacol 7(6):406–409, 1987 3429702

Spiller HA, Ramoska EA, Krenzelok EP, et al: Bupropion overdose: a 3-year multicenter retrospective analysis. Am J Emerg Med 12(1):43–45, 1994 8285970

Stamenkovic M, Pezawas L, de Zwaan M, et al: Mirtazapine in recurrent brief depression. Int Clin Psychopharmacol 13(1):39–40, 1998 9988366

Stein MB, Liebowitz MR, Lydiard RB, et al: Paroxetine treatment of generalized social phobia (social anxiety disorder): a randomized controlled trial. JAMA 280(8):708–713, 1998 9728642

Steiner M, Steinberg S, Stewart D, et al: Fluoxetine in the treatment of premenstrual dysphoria. N Engl J Med 332(23):1529–1534, 1995 7739706

Stenkrona P, Halldin C, Lundberg J: 5-HTT and 5-HT(1A) receptor occupancy of the novel substance vortioxetine (Lu AA21004): a PET study in control subjects. Eur Neuropsychopharmacol 23(10):1190–1198, 2013 23428337

Storrow AB: Bupropion overdose and seizure. Am J Emerg Med 12(2):183–184, 1994 8161393

Sunderland T, Cohen RM, Thompson KE, et al: L-deprenyl treatment of older depressives (NR159), in 1989 New Research Program and Abstracts, American Psychiatric Association 142nd Annual Meeting, San Francisco, May 6–11, 1989. Washington, DC, American Psychiatric Association, 1989, p 101

Sunderland T, Cohen RM, Molchan S, et al: High-dose selegiline in treatment-resistant older depressive patients. Arch Gen Psychiatry 51(8):607–615, 1994 7519005

Tabuteau H, Jones A, Anderson A, et al: Effect of AXS-05 (dextromethorphan-bupropion) in major depressive disorder: a randomized double-blind controlled trial. Am J Psychiatry 179(7):490–499, 2022 35582785

Taylor D, Lenox-Smith A, Bradley A: A review of the suitability of duloxetine and venlafaxine for use in patients with depression in primary care with a focus on cardiovascular safety, suicide and mortality due to antidepressant overdose. Ther Adv Psychopharmacol 3(3):151–161, 2013 24167687

Teicher MH, Glod C, Cole JO: Emergence of intense suicidal preoccupation during fluoxetine treatment. Am J Psychiatry 147(2):207–210, 1990 2301661

Thase ME: Effectiveness of antidepressants: comparative remission rates. J Clin Psychiatry 64(Suppl 2):3–7, 2003 12625792

Thase ME, Blomgren SL, Birkett MA, et al: Fluoxetine treatment of patients with major depressive disorder who failed initial treatment with sertraline. J Clin Psychiatry 58(1):16–21, 1997 9055832

Thase ME, Entsuah AR, Rudolph RL: Remission rates during treatment with venlafaxine or selective serotonin reuptake inhibitors. Br J Psychiatry 178:234–241, 2001 11230034

Thase M, Martin W, Memisoglu A, et al: ALKS 5461: a buprenorphine-samidorphan combination for major depression. Poster presented at the 30th Annual Psychiatric Congress, New Orleans, LA, September 17, 2017. Available at: www.psychcongress.com/posters/alks-5461-buprenorphine-samidorphan-combination-major-depression. Accessed October 1, 2018.

Thompson C: Mirtazapine versus selective serotonin reuptake inhibitors. J Clin Psychiatry 60(Suppl 17):18–22, 1999 10446737

Tollefson GD, Rampey AH Jr, Potvin JH, et al: A multicenter investigation of fixed-dose fluoxetine in the treatment of obsessive-compulsive disorder. Arch Gen Psychiatry 51(7):559–567, 1994 8031229

Trivedi MH, Fava M, Wisniewski SR, et al: Medication augmentation after the failure of SSRIs for depression. N Engl J Med 354(12):1243–1252, 2006 16554526 van Moffaert M, de Wilde J, Vereecken A, et al: Mirtazapine is more effective than trazodone: a double-blind controlled study in hospitalized patients with major depression. Int Clin Psychopharmacol 10(1):3–9, 1995 7622801

van Rooij K, Poels S, Worst P, et al: Efficacy of testosterone combined with a PDE5 inhibitor and testosterone combined with a serotonin (1A) receptor agonist in women with SSRI-induced sexual dysfunction: a preliminary study. Eur J Pharmacol 753:246–251, 2015 25460030

Verbeeck W, Bekkering GE, Van den Noortgate W, et al: Bupropion for attention deficit hyperactivity disorder (ADHD) in adults. Cochrane Database Syst Rev 10(10):CD009504, 2017 28965364

Walker PW, Cole JO, Gardner EA, et al: Improvement in fluoxetine-associated sexual dysfunction in patients switched to bupropion. J Clin Psychiatry 54(12):459–465, 1993 8276736

Walsh BT, Kaplan AS, Attia E, et al: Fluoxetine after weight restoration in anorexia nervosa: a randomized controlled trial. JAMA 295(22):2605–2612, 2006 16772623

Weinmann S, Becker T, Koesters M: Re-evaluation of the efficacy and tolerability of venlafaxine vs SSRI: meta-analysis. Psychopharmacology (Berl) 196(4):511–520, 521–522, 2008 17955213

Wheadon DE, Rampey AH Jr, Thompson VL, et al: Lack of association between fluoxetine and suicidality in bulimia nervosa. J Clin Psychiatry 53(7):235–241, 1992 1639742

Wheatley D: Triple-blind, placebo-controlled trial of Ginkgo biloba in sexual dysfunction due to antidepressant drugs. Hum Psychopharmacol 19(8):545–548, 2004 15378664

Wheatley DP, van Moffaert M, Timmerman L et al: Mirtazapine: efficacy and tolerability in comparison with fluoxetine in patients with moderate to severe major depressive disorder. J Clin Psychiatry 59(6):306–312, 1998 9671343

Williams NR, Heifets BD, Blasey C, et al: Attenuation of antidepressant effects of ketamine by opioid receptor antagonism. Am J Psychiatry 175(12):1205–1215, 2018 30153752

Williams T, Phillips NJ, Stein DJ, et al: Pharmacotherapy for post traumatic stress disorder (PTSD). Cochrane Database Syst Rev Mar 2 3(3):CD002795, 2022 35234292

Wolfe F, Cathey MA, Hawley DJ: A double-blind placebo controlled trial of fluoxetine in fibromyalgia. Scand J Rheumatol 23(5):255–259, 1994 7973479

Xiao L, Zhu X, Gillespie A, et al: Effectiveness of mirtazapine as add-on to paroxetine v. paroxetine or mirtazapine monotherapy in patients with major depressive disorder with early non-response to paroxetine: a two-phase, multicentre, randomized, double-blind clinical trial. Psychol Med 51(7):1166–1174, 2021 31931894

Yovell Y, Bar G, Mashiah M, et al: Ultra-low-dose buprenorphine as a time-limited treatment for severe suicidal ideation: a randomized controlled trial. Am J Psychiatry 173(5):491–498, 2016 26684923

Zarate CA Jr, Singh JB, Carlson PJ, et al: A randomized trial of an N-methyl-D-aspartate antagonist in treatment-resistant major depression. Arch Gen Psychiatry 63(8):856–864, 2006 16894061

4

Antipsychotic Drugs

O bservations in the late nineteenth century that aniline dyes had calming and sedating effects ultimately led to the development of the first phenothiazine, promethazine. In 1952, a related phenothiazine, chlorpromazine, was investigated as an antiautonomic drug to protect the body against its own excessive compensatory reactions during major surgery. It spread into psychiatry from the field of anesthesia after an initial clinical report by Delay et al. (1952) demonstrated the drug's favorable side-effect profile and its efficacy in treating acute psychosis. Endless subsequent double-blind studies have served chiefly to confirm the effects already obvious to the original French clinicians.

We now know substantially more about the side effects and limitations of the currently available antipsychotic drugs and more about their mechanisms of action. We are beginning to understand dose-response relationships and have second-generation antipsychotics (SGAs) that now represent the most commonly prescribed antipsychotics. There is considerable debate as to whether the benefits of the second-generation agents over their first-generation counterparts are outweighed by their cost and side effects. However, as an increasing number of the second-generation drugs have become generically available, the debate has shifted primarily to the trade-off of more metabolic side effects for many of the newer agents versus more extrapyramidal symptoms (EPS) for the first-generation drugs.

The second-generation, or atypical, antipsychotics, which include clozapine, olanzapine, risperidone, quetiapine, ziprasidone, aripiprazole, paliperidone, iloperidone, lurasidone, asenapine, and, most recently, brexpiprazole and cariprazine, have now largely supplanted the first-generation, "typical" antipsychotics such as perphenazine and haloperidol. The concept of atypicality arose from the finding that the SGAs had a greater serotonin (5-HT)/dopamine ratio than did earlier drugs and might be associated with improved efficacy (particularly for so-called negative symptoms) and reduced EPS. For example, the greater serotonergic effects of SGAs were thought to be associated with fewer EPS and greater efficacy in reducing cognitive and negative symptoms. However, recent data have not always found that the second-generation, atypical agents are that different from the first-generation, typical agents. Thus, the atypicals may not be that "atypical" after all (Gründer et al. 2009).

The SGAs, like the first-generation antipsychotics (FGAs), are a heterogeneous group of agents, each with potential advantages and disadvantages over individual first-generation drugs. For example, the rate of EPS does appear to be lower in most SGAs compared with the first-generation drugs. The Clinical Antipsychotic Trials of Intervention Effectiveness (CATIE; Lieberman et al. 2005) did not show clear advantages of the SGAs over perphenazine, including in rates of EPS. However, the relatively short duration of CATIE might prevent a clear determination of EPS, such as parkinsonism and tardive dyskinesia, that may take years to develop. Also, in CATIE, patients with a history of EPS while taking neuroleptics were not randomly assigned to the typical agent, potentially affecting incidence of EPS in the perphenazine cell.

On the other hand, the rates of tardive dyskinesia associated with typical antipsychotics might have been inflated historically by the high doses of these agents that were used. For example, haloperidol in early trials and in clinical use was commonly given at a dosage of 20 mg/day or higher. We now know that 2–5 mg/day of haloperidol results in the 80% binding to dopamine$_2$ (D$_2$) receptors needed for efficacy. Because doses resulting in >80% binding increase EPS without necessarily increasing efficacy, the real rates of tardive dyskinesia in the first-generation drugs are probably less than the 4% per year rate that is frequently quoted. Some clinicians, particularly in primary care settings, have mistakenly assumed that there is no risk for akathisia, dystonias, and tardive dyskinesia with the SGAs. Although the risk of EPS with SGAs is somewhat smaller than the risk with typical antipsychotics, the risk is not negligible, particularly with risperidone at higher doses.

The SGAs are thought to have a number of other advantages over the typical antipsychotic agents. As indicated above, the SGAs may be somewhat more helpful than typical agents in treating the negative symptoms of schizophrenia. The negative symptoms result in considerably more disability for patients with schizophrenia than do positive symptoms such as hallucinations and delusions. Results from CATIE and the European Cost Utility of the Latest Antipsychotic Drugs in Schizophrenia Study (CUtLASS) trial do not necessarily support the benefit of SGAs over first-generation agents in treating negative symptoms. Likewise, a meta-analysis of randomized controlled trials to date did not find that the SGAs had any greater efficacy than the first-generation agents in reducing negative symptoms (Leucht et al. 2009b). In addition, the SGAs may have benefit in treating the cognitive disturbance and executive dysfunction that can be so disabling in schizophrenia patients. Some, but not all, studies suggest a modest advantage of the SGAs versus the FGAs. However, these apparent benefits have not translated into evidence that the SGAs are superior to the typical agents on measures of quality of life (Jones et al. 2006). Clozapine has shown clear utility in the treatment of schizophrenia that has not responded to typical agents. Both the CATIE and CUtLASS trials appear to confirm this finding. It was this utility in patients with treatment-refractory schizophrenia that ultimately led to the approval of clozapine in the United States. Finally, the SGAs appear to have more mood-stabilizing and perhaps mood-elevating properties than do typical antipsychotics. Although the typical agents such as chlorpromazine are clearly effective antimanic agents, evidence that the typical agents are effective in the maintenance treatment of bipolar disorder or are effective in treating bipolar depression is lacking. Depressive symptoms in schizophrenia are often improved by SGAs more than by the older drugs. In fact, clozapine became the first drug with a specific indication for reducing suicidality in patients with schizophrenia.

Although there may be some benefits of the SGAs in schizophrenia, the effect size of the SGAs in treating this disorder is probably no greater than that seen with the first-generation agents. In a meta-analysis of 127 comparison trials, Davis and colleagues (2003) found that only clozapine had a robustly larger effect size than haloperidol in the treatment of schizophrenia. More recent studies have confirmed these earlier findings (Leucht et al. 2009a, 2009c). The rest of the SGAs had impacts on somewhat different aspects of the illness, but their overall effect was about equal to that of haloperidol. However, the utility of second-generation (atypical) versus first-generation (typical) agents in the treatment of mood disorders may be a different matter.

It is now clear that virtually all of the SGAs are effective antimanic drugs and probably work faster than and at least as well as mood-stabilizing agents such as lithium in this regard (see Chapter 5, "Mood Stabilizers"). The use of second-generation agents in mood disorders appears to have eclipsed their use in schizophrenia some time ago. Olanzapine, already approved by the FDA for the treatment of acute mania, has also received FDA approval for the maintenance monotherapy of bipolar disorder. In addition, olanzapine was approved in a combination formulation with fluoxetine (Symbyax) first for the treatment of bipolar depression and recently for refractory depression. Olanzapine and other SGAs such as quetiapine are also increasingly being used as adjunctive and augmentation agents in the treatment of unipolar depression. Cariprazine was recently given FDA approval for augmentation in refractory major depression. Quetiapine has been approved as a monotherapy for bipolar depression. In addition, lurasidone, cariprazine, and lumateperone are now also approved for the treatment of bipolar depression. The role of the SGAs in the treatment of mood disorders continues to be defined (see Chapter 5).

Although the D_2/5-HT_2 antagonists offer many advantages over the typical antipsychotics, they have some distinct disadvantages as well. Among them is cost. The branded SGAs cost many times what older drugs do, and some formularies and third-party payers have limited the use of more expensive SGAs that are still on patent. Of course, many of the SGAs, including olanzapine, risperidone, quetiapine, and ziprasidone, are now available in generic forms. Thus, cost is not as much an issue as it once was. As reported earlier, it is difficult to demonstrate a clear advantage of the SGAs in efficacy (for the treatment of schizophrenia, at least) to justify the enormously greater costs of branded SGAs. Another important disadvantage of the D_2/5-HT_2 antagonists is their metabolic effect. In 2003, the FDA advised all manufacturers of SGAs that their labels should be changed to reflect that these drugs are associated with an enhanced risk of hyperglycemia and diabetes. Although the extent of the metabolic risks associated with the SGAs continues to be debated, there is little doubt that some enhanced risk of weight gain and metabolic effects occurs with most, although probably not all, of the second-generation agents.

General Principles of Antipsychotic Use

Available Drugs

At the time of this writing, 22 antipsychotic drugs are available for prescription use in the United States: 10 FGA agents and 12 SGA agents (Table 4–1 and Figure 4–1). One of the first-generation agents, pimozide, is FDA approved for use only in Tourette's disorder and is now rarely used because of the known risk of QTc prolongation. Likewise, droperidol, another agent with a black box warning of QTc prolongation, is approved only for parenteral use in anesthesia. However, studies done on the rate of arrhythmias in droperidol-treated patients since the black box warning in 2001 have not necessarily supported an enhanced risk (Nuttall et al. 2007). All the antipsychotic agents, except clozapine and pimavanserin, are reasonably potent postsynaptic dopamine receptor blockers (dopamine antagonists). Some, such as aripiprazole and brexpiprazole, are partial agonists that at typical therapeutic doses act as dopamine antagonists. Although it is conceivable that the antipsychotic effects of these drugs might be attributable to some other mechanism, it seems unlikely. Although some of the efficacy of the SGAs is due to $5\text{-}HT_2$ antagonism or the blockade of other dopamine receptors, for most antipsychotics, it is the D_2 blockade that likely drives much of the antipsychotic effect.

All the effective antipsychotic drugs, except clozapine and pimavanserin, act on the nigrostriatal system in the predicted manner and can potentially produce EPS. For an antipsychotic to be effective, it generally requires a dopamine antagonism of 60%–80% of dopamine D_2 receptors. Lower levels of dopamine antagonism tend not to be associated with antipsychotic properties, whereas higher levels tend to produce more extensive EPS. PET studies indicate that a dosage of about 2.5–6.0 mg/day of haloperidol results in occupation of about 60%–80% of D_2 receptors (Remington and Kapur 1999). These studies also indicated that the standard therapeutic dosages of olanzapine (10–20 mg/day) and risperidone (2–6 mg/day) result in a 60%–80% binding of D_2 receptors. Only clozapine showed a D_2 binding affinity of less than 60% at therapeutic dosages. In typical antipsychotics, dosages higher than these are not clearly as-

Table 4–1.　Antipsychotic drugs: names, formulations, and strengths

Generic name	Brand name[a]	Formulations and strengths
Aripiprazole	Abilify	Tablets: 2, 5, 10, 15, 20, 30 mg
	Abilify Asimtufii	Suspension (extended release): 720 mg/2.4 mL (300 mg/mL)
		Suspension (extended release): 960 mg/3.2 mL (300 mg/mL)
	Abilify Maintena kit	For suspension (extended release): 300 mg/vial
		For suspension (extended release): 400 mg/vial
	Aripiprazole	Solution: 1 mg/mL
		Orally disintegrating tablets: 10, 15, 20, 30 mg
Aripiprazole lauroxil	Aristada	Suspension (extended release): 441 mg/1.6 mL (275.63 mg/mL)
		Suspension (extended release): 662 mg/2.4 mL (275.83 mg/mL)
		Suspension (extended release): 882 mg/3.2 mL (275.63 mg/mL)
		Suspension (extended release): 1,064 mg/3.9 mL (272.82 mg/mL)
	Aristada Initio kit	Suspension (extended release): 675 mg/2.4 mL
Asenapine	Secuado	System: 3.8, 5.7, 7.6 mg/24 hr
Asenapine maleate	Saphris	Tablets (sublingual): 2.5, 5, 10 mg
Brexpiprazole	Rexulti	Tablets: 0.25, 0.5, 1, 2, 3, 4 mg
Cariprazine hydrochloride	Vraylar	Capsules: 1.5, 3, 4.5, 6 mg
Chlorpromazine hydrochloride	Chlorpromazine hydrochloride	Concentrate: 30, 100 mg/mL
		Injection: 25 mg/mL
		Tablets: 10, 25, 50, 100, 200 mg
Clozapine	Clozapine	Orally disintegrating tablets: 12.5, 25, 100, 150, 200 mg
		Tablets: 12.5, 25, 50, 100, 200 mg
	Clozaril	Tablets: 25, 50, 100, 200 mg
	Versacloz	Suspension: 50 mg/mL

Table 4–1.   Antipsychotic drugs: names, formulations, and strengths *(continued)*

Generic name	Brand name[a]	Formulations and strengths
Droperidol	Inapsine	Injection: 2.5 mg/mL
Fluphenazine decanoate	Fluphenazine decanoate	Injection: 25 mg/mL
Fluphenazine hydrochloride	Fluphenazine hydrochloride	Concentrate: 5 mg/mL
		Elixir: 2.5 mg
		Injection: 2.5 mg/mL
		Tablets: 1, 2.5, 5, 10 mg
Haloperidol	Haloperidol	Tablets: 0.5, 1, 2, 5, 10, 20 mg
Haloperidol decanoate	Haldol	Injection: 50, 100 mg/mL
Haloperidol lactate	Haloperidol	Concentrate: 2 mg/mL
		Injection: 5 mg/mL
Iloperidone	Fanapt	Tablets: 1, 2, 4, 6, 8, 10, 12 mg
Loxapine	Adasuve	Inhalation powder: 10 mg
Loxapine succinate	Loxitane	Capsules: 5, 10, 25, 50 mg
Lurasidone hydrochloride	Latuda	Tablets: 20, 40, 60, 80, 120 mg
Molindone hydrochloride	Molindone hydrochloride	Tablets: 5, 10, 25 mg
Olanzapine	Zyprexa	Injection: 10 mg/vial
		Tablets: 2.5, 5, 7.5, 10, 15, 20 mg
		Orally disintegrating tablets: 5, 10, 15, 20 mg
Olanzapine pamoate	Zyprexa Zydis	Suspension (extended release): 210 mg/vial
	Zyprexa Relprevv	Suspension (extended release): 300 mg/vial
		Suspension (extended release): 405 mg/vial

Table 4–1.   Antipsychotic drugs: names, formulations, and strengths *(continued)*

Generic name	Brand name[a]	Formulations and strengths
Olanzapine+samidorphan L-malate	Lybalvi	Tablets: 5 mg/10 mg Tablets: 10 mg/10 mg Tablets: 15 mg/10 mg Tablets: 20 mg/10 mg
Paliperidone	Invega	Tablets (extended release): 1.5, 3, 6, 9 mg
Paliperidone palmitate	Invega Hafyera	Suspension (extended release): 1.092 mg/3.5 mL (312 mg/mL) Suspension (extended release): 1.560 mg/5 mL (312 mg/mL)
	Invega Sustenna	Suspension (extended release): 39 mg/0.25 mL (39 mg/0.25 mL) Suspension (extended release): 78 mg/0.5 mL (78 mg/0.2 mL) Suspension (extended release): 117 mg/0.75 mL (117 mg/0.75 mL) Suspension (extended release): 156 mg/mL (156 mg/mL) Suspension (extended release): 234 mg/1.5 mL (156 mg/mL)
	Invega Trinza	Suspension (extended release): 273 mg/0.875 mL (273 mg/0.875 mL) Suspension (extended release): 410 mg/1.315 mL (311.79 mg/mL) Suspension (extended release): 546 mg/1.75 mL (312 mg/mL) Suspension (extended release): 819 mg/2.625 mL (312 mg/mL)
Perphenazine	Perphenazine	Tablets: 2, 4, 8, 16 mg
Pimavanserin tartrate	Nuplazid	Capsules: 34 mg
Pimozide	Pimozide	Tablets: 10 mg
Quetiapine fumarate	Quetiapine fumarate	Tablets: 1, 2 mg
	Seroquel	Tablets: 25, 50, 100, 150, 200, 300, 400 mg
	Seroquel XR	Tablets: 25, 50, 100, 200, 300, 400 mg Tablets (extended release): 50, 150, 200, 300, 400 mg

Table 4–1. Antipsychotic drugs: names, formulations, and strengths *(continued)*

Generic name	Brand name[a]	Formulations and strengths
Risperidone	Perseris kit	For suspension (extended release): 90, 120 mg
	Risperdal	Solution: 1 mg/mL
		Tablets: 0.25, 0.5, 1, 2, 3, 4 mg
	Risperdal Consta	Injection: 12.5 mg/vial
		Injection: 25 mg/vial
		Injection: 37.5 mg/vial
		Injection: 50 mg/vial
	Risperidone	Orally disintegrating tablets: 0.25, 0.5, 1, 2, 3, 4 mg
	Rykindo	For suspension (extended release): 12.5 mg
		For suspension (extended release): 25 mg
		For suspension (extended release): 37.5 mg
		For suspension (extended release): 50 mg
	Uzedy	Suspension (extended release, subcutaneous): 50, 75, 100, 125, 150, 200, 250 mg
Thioridazine hydrochloride	Thioridazine hydrochloride	Tablets: 10, 25, 50, 100 mg
Thiothixene	Thiothixene	Capsules: 1, 2, 5, 10 mg
Trifluoperazine hydrochloride	Trifluoperazine hydrochloride	Tablets: 1, 2, 5, 10 mg
Ziprasidone hydrochloride	Geodon	Capsules: 20, 40, 60, 80 mg
Ziprasidone mesylate	Geodon	Powder: 20 mg/vial

[a]Where the brand name is the same as the generic name, the brand-name products may be no longer available.

A. Phenothiazines

1. Aliphatic

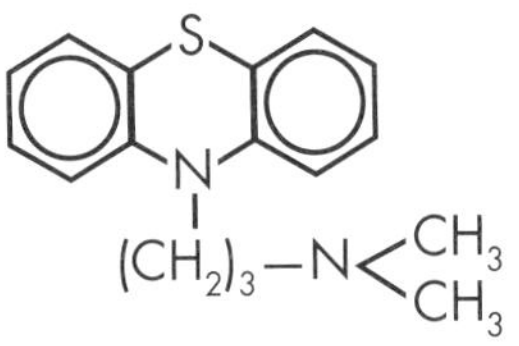

$(CH_2)_3-N\begin{subarray}{l}CH_3\\CH_3\end{subarray}$

Promazine*

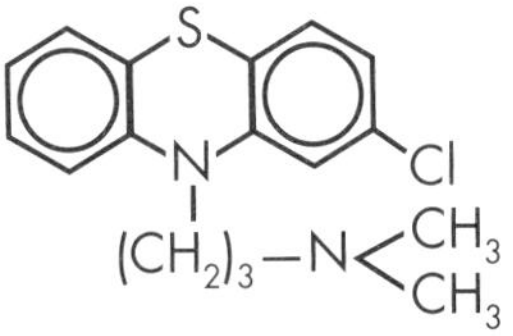

$(CH_2)_3-N\begin{subarray}{l}CH_3\\CH_3\end{subarray}$

Chlorpromazine

$(CH_2)_3-N\begin{subarray}{l}CH_3\\CH_3\end{subarray}$

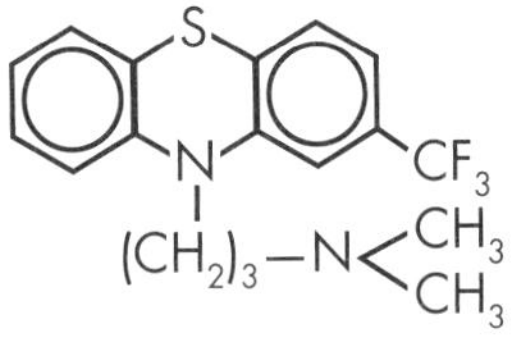

Triflupromazine

2. Piperidine

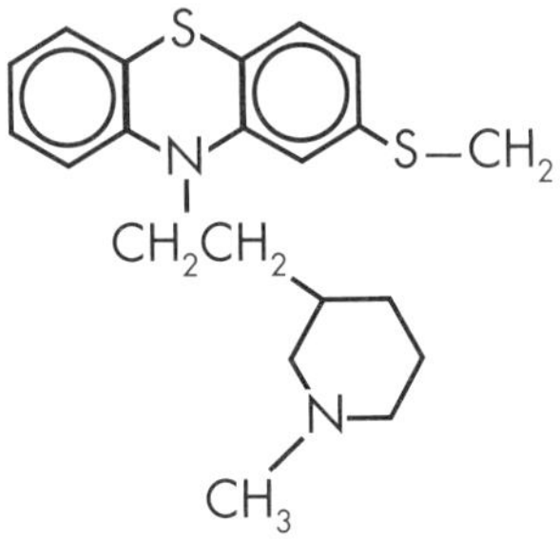

$S-CH_2$

CH_2CH_2

CH_3

Thioridazine

$S-CH_3$

CH_2CH_2

CH_3

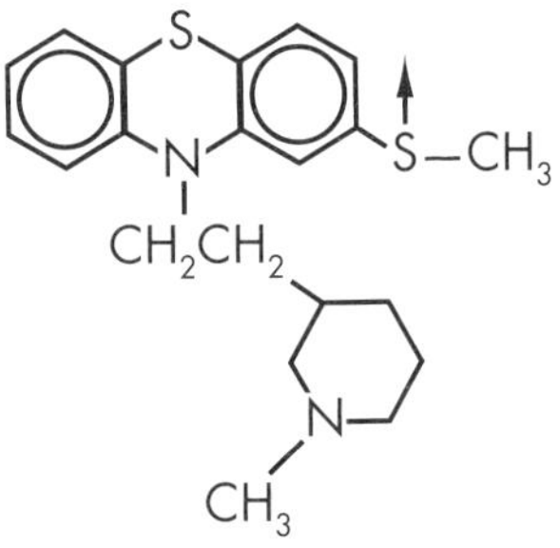

Mesoridazine*

Figure 4–1.   Chemical structures of antipsychotic drugs.
*No longer available in the United States.

3. Piperazine

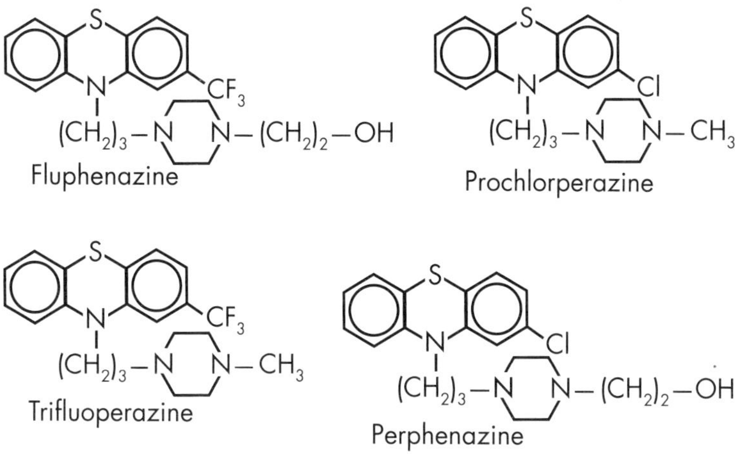

Fluphenazine

Prochlorperazine

Trifluoperazine

Perphenazine

B. Butyrophenone-like

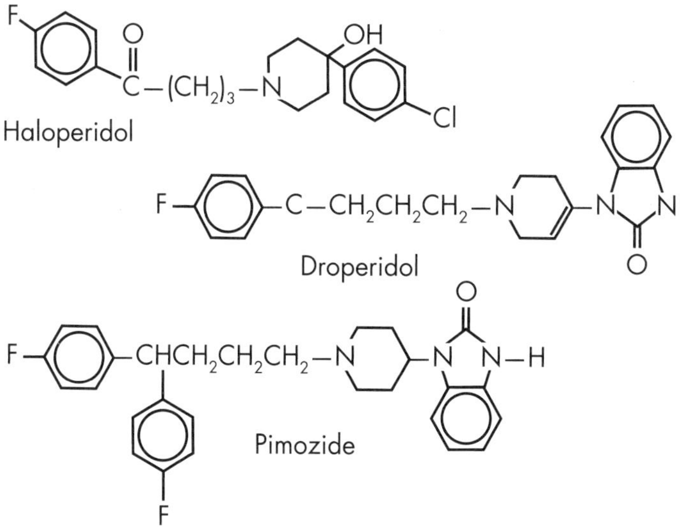

Haloperidol

Droperidol

Pimozide

Figure 4–1. Chemical structures of antipsychotic drugs *(continued)*.

C. Thioxanthenes

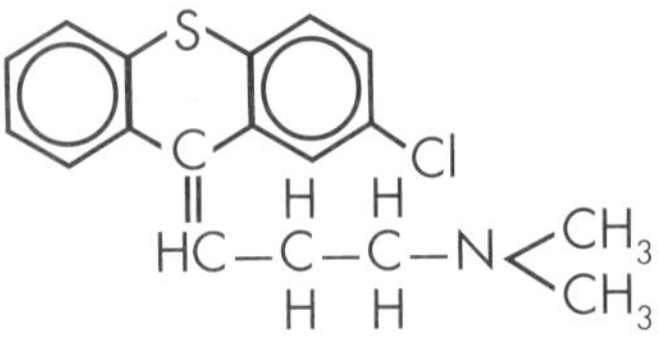

Chlorprothixene*

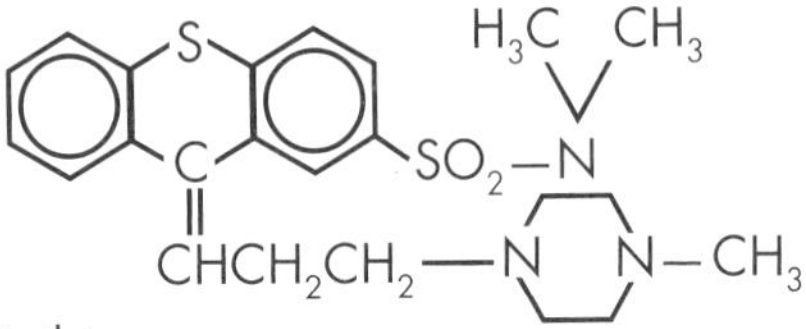

Thiothixene

D. Indole

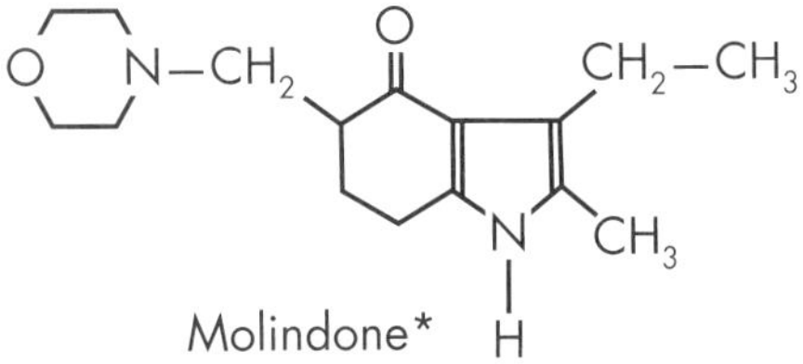

Molindone*

E. Dibenzazepines

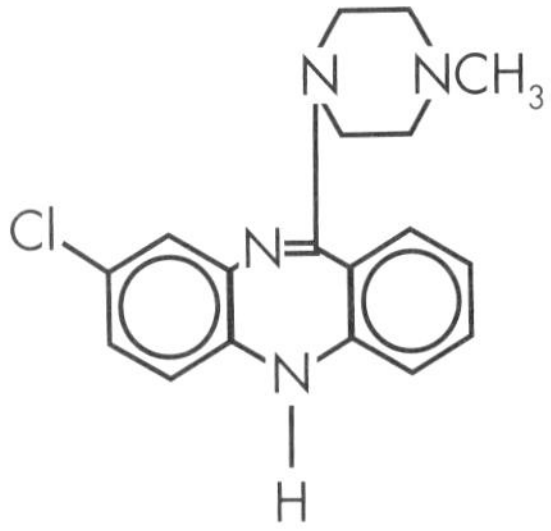

Clozapine

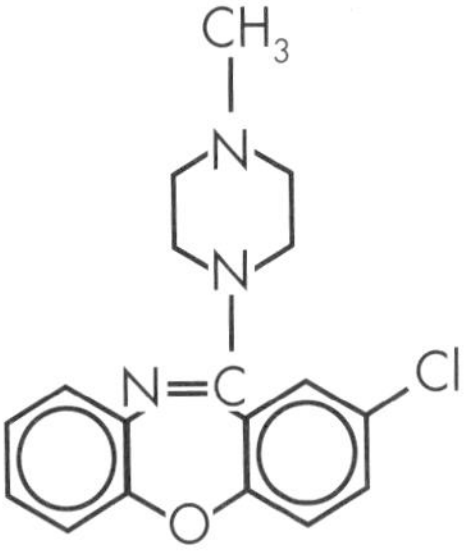

Loxapine

Figure 4–1. Chemical structures of antipsychotic drugs *(continued).*
*No longer available in the United States.

F. Benzisoxazole

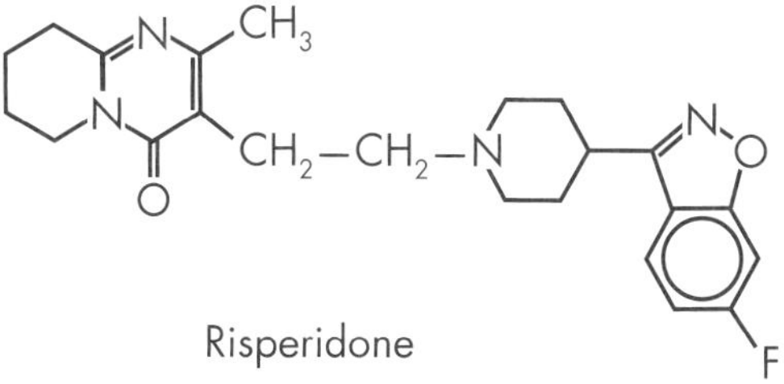

Risperidone

G. Thienobenzodiazepine

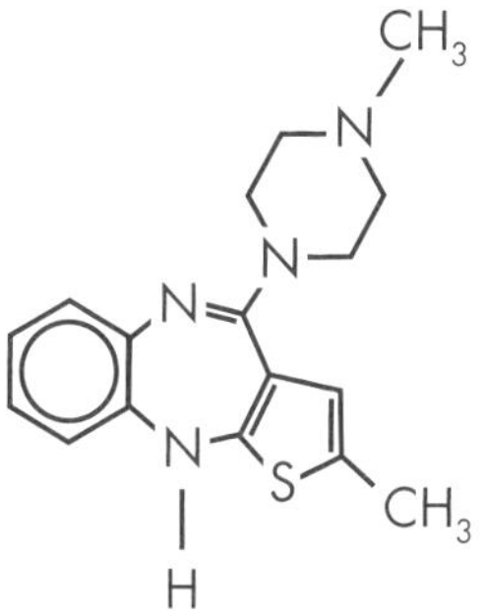

Olanzapine

Figure 4–1. Chemical structures of antipsychotic drugs *(continued)*.

H. Other

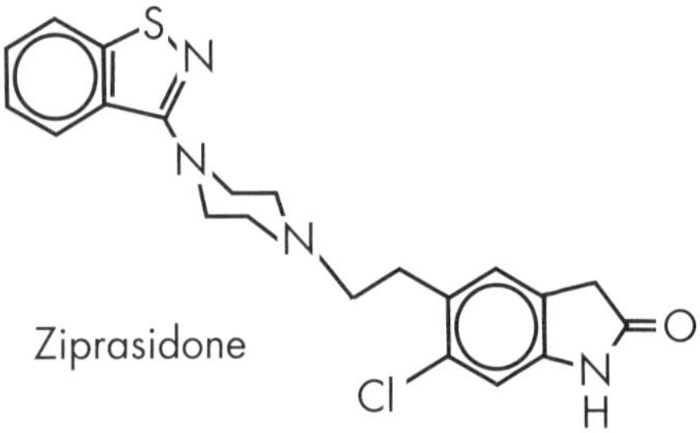

Ziprasidone

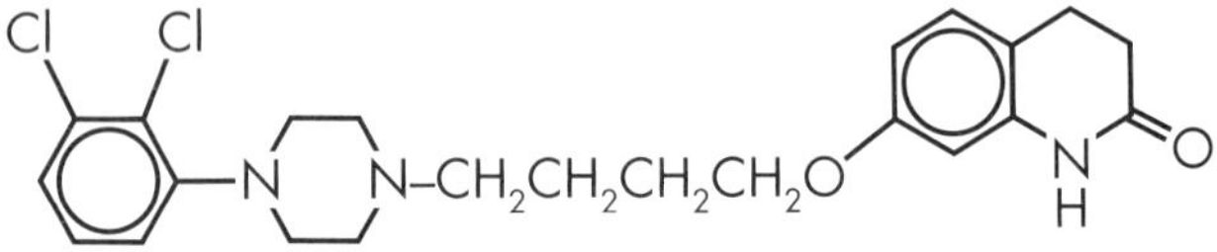

Aripiprazole

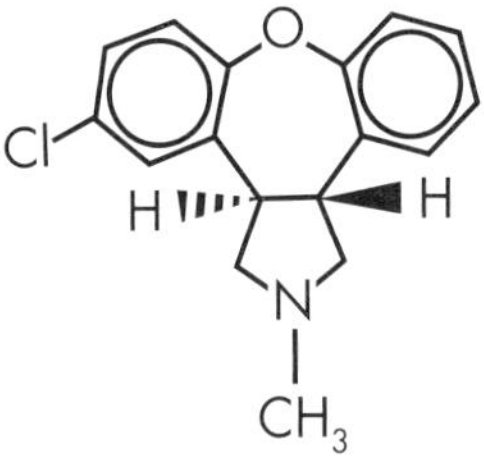

Asenapine

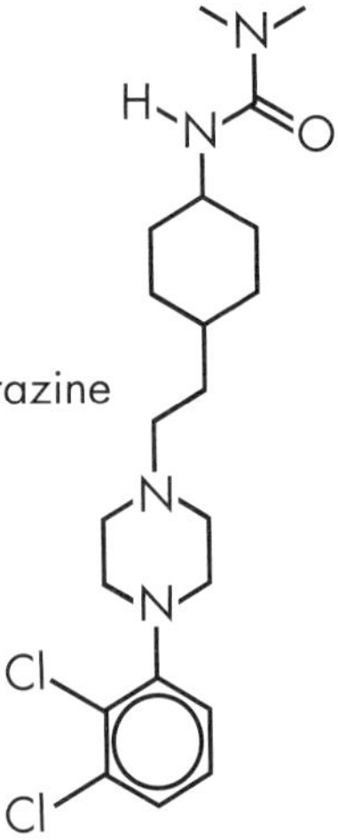

Cariprazine

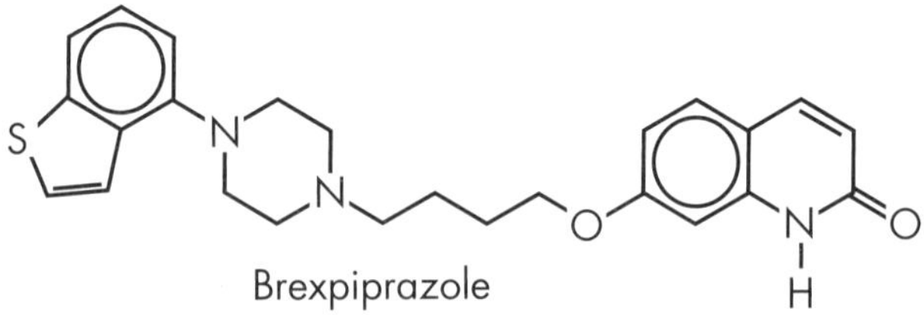

Brexpiprazole

Figure 4–1. Chemical structures of antipsychotic drugs *(continued)*.

H. Other (*continued*)

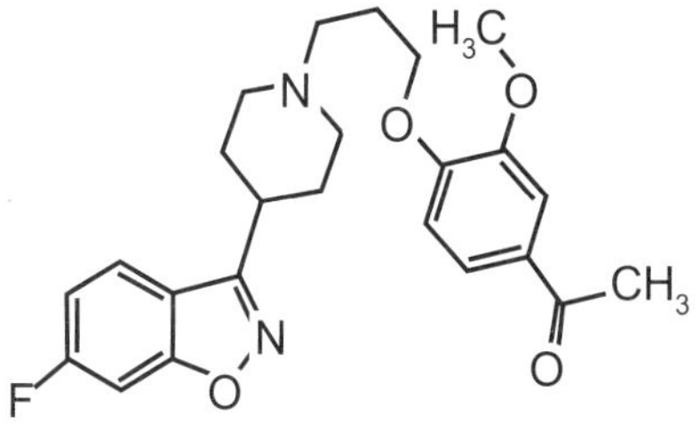

Iloperidone

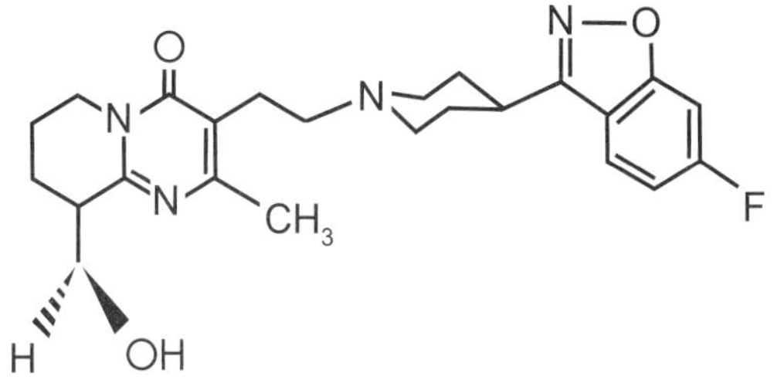

Paliperidone

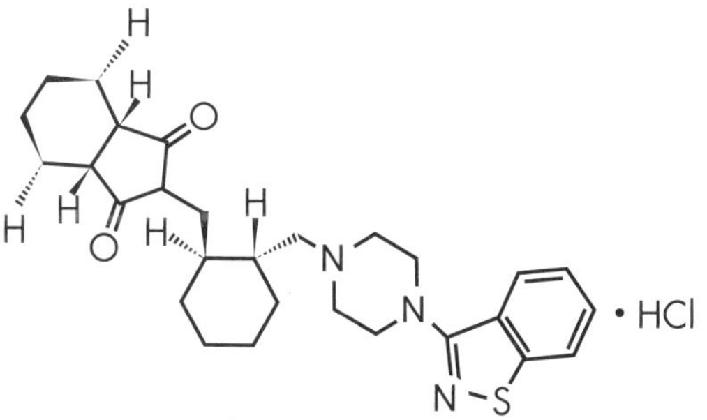

Lurasidone

Figure 4–1. Chemical structures of antipsychotic drugs (*continued*).

sociated with improvement in psychosis but do increase the risk of EPS (Kapur et al. 1999). The lack of parkinsonian side effects may also reflect the limited time these agents occupy dopamine receptors. More recently, SGAs have been thought to bind less tightly—or for briefer periods—to D_2 receptors than do typical agents, resulting in fewer EPS.

Clozapine, with its risk of agranulocytosis, has been known to be unique in its action on psychosis for more than 30 years and to be relatively free of EPS other than akathisia. Until recently, however, no really comparable drug had been discovered to replace it, despite the efforts of many major pharmaceutical firms. Olanzapine appears quite similar to clozapine in its pharmacological effects but superior in side-effect profile. In the CATIE and CUtLASS trials, olanzapine did seem to do better on measures of efficacy in schizophrenia relative to other SGAs and some first-generation agents. However, clozapine tends to be even more consistently effective in patients who have not responded to other antipsychotic agents.

Efficacy

All the available antipsychotic drugs have been clearly shown to be more effective than placebo in treating schizophrenia, both acutely and chronically. Most major studies on FGAs were done many years ago and used some variant of DSM-II criteria (American Psychiatric Association 1968). They involved an unknown but possibly large proportion of acute patients who might be judged, by DSM-5 (American Psychiatric Association 2013) standards, to have schizophreniform, bipolar, or schizoaffective disorder. It is therefore clinically sensible to assume that all the drugs are effective in all these DSM-5 conditions and to include mania as a proven indication as well. The SGAs have all been studied with DSM-III-R, DSM-IV, and DSM-5 criteria for schizophrenia and bipolar disorder.

In many respects, the nature and timing of clinical response to antipsychotics are unsatisfactory. In large-scale 6-week placebo-controlled trials involving hospitalized patients, 75% of drug-treated patients showed at least moderate improvement, whereas only 25% of placebo-treated patients did as well, and some got worse. However, most patients never achieve complete remission, and few are able to function at a fully effective level on return to the community. Some SGAs may be better than first-generation agents in improving social functioning. Studies of quality of life of patients who are administered clozapine for treatment-refractory schizophrenia have sometimes shown a dramatic improvement in work-related activity and a substantial decrease in the rate of rehospitalization. About 30% of patients who do not respond to FGAs will respond to clozapine in a 12-week trial. In addition, another 15%–30% of patients who do not respond in the first few months will respond in 6–12 months (Meltzer 1997; Meltzer et al. 1989).

Antipsychotics tend to act in a slow, approximate manner in the treatment of psychotic symptoms. Symptoms such as agitation may respond quite rapidly. A few patients show rapid, excellent antipsychotic response, but most get better more slowly, and some do not respond at all or do so only very slowly. Sometimes the response is so slow and variable that clinicians, in an understandable but probably misguided effort to speed clinical response, may prescribe very high drug dosages early in treatment. In recent studies, as well as in studies done more than five decades ago, improvement increased relatively rapidly between the first and sixth week of taking the drug. Thereafter, modest further improvement occurred between the sixth and thirteenth week, with little additional improvement by the twenty-sixth week. These changes are, of course, *average* improvement—individual patients may improve more or less, earlier or later. Similarly, once a patient's condition has improved, it is difficult to find the minimal effective maintenance dose in any reliable way. One might imagine that the physician could gradually reduce the dosage from that at which the patient had recovered. Unfortunately, when patients whose condition is stable are shifted abruptly from an antipsychotic drug to placebo, some experience relapse relatively soon, but others experience relapse at a leisurely and completely unpredictable rate over months and even years. In only a few cases is the relapse so rapid that a minimum maintenance dosage can be easily determined.

Reviews of the antipsychotic discontinuation literature (Baldessarini and Viguera 1995; Emsley et al. 2018) show that relapse rates are higher in the first 3 months after abrupt discontinuation of antipsychotics. Nonadherence with prescribed SGAs, quite common in schizophrenia, also consistently results in higher relapse rates and greater likelihood of hospitalization (Sun et al. 2007). The reviews also show that slowly tapering antipsychotics (or stopping depot antipsychotics, with their long half-lives) not only substantially decreases the early relapse rate but also leaves more patients with stable functioning in the community 2 years later than does rapid termination of neuroleptic therapy. It appears that abrupt discontinuation of antipsychotic medication by treaters or unilaterally by patients is almost as bad for patients with chronic schizophrenia as abrupt discontinuation of lithium carbonate is for patients with bipolar disorder (Suppes et al. 1993).

This updated look at old data, supported by a study by Green et al. (1990), throws into question many old reports about the differences between drug and placebo observed in follow-up studies designed to assess the relative values of active and inert therapies for chronic psychosis. If abrupt termination of drug therapy artificially increases relapse rates, much work needs to be reassessed or redone.

The value of depot or long-acting injectable drugs in the long-term management of schizophrenia also needs more positive consideration (Glazer and Kane 1992; Kishimoto et al. 2018; Titus-Lay et al. 2018). There is ample evidence that long-acting injectables are superior to oral antipsychotics in maintaining adherence, reducing relapse rates, and limiting hospitalizations. In past years, clinicians working with intermittent antipsychotic medication strategies for patients with schizophrenia claimed that identifying the individual patient's unique signs of impending relapse (e.g., poor sleep, pacing, special fears or worries) could enable the treating psychiatrist to reinstitute antipsychotic medication rapidly and thus avert a full psychotic episode (Carpenter and Heinrichs 1983; Herz et al. 1982). Enlisting both patient and family to identify such early warning signs and symptoms and to watch for their reemergence may be beneficial. This technique can be applied as well to gradual dose-tapering strategies. For this strategy to work well, careful patient monitoring by both family or caretakers and mental health professionals is necessary. Unfortunately, studies attempting to demonstrate the efficacy of this approach have not been successful. Intermittent medication strategies have been repeatedly shown to be less effective than low, fixed, steady dosage regimens (Carpenter et al. 1990; Herz et al. 1991). Moreover, one trial indicated that higher doses of maintenance depot haloperidol were more effective in preventing relapse than were lower doses (Kane et al. 2002). Still, lower doses are clearly better tolerated than higher doses and are more effective than placebo in preventing relapse. The availability of a long-acting form of a number of SGAs (Risperdal Consta, Abilify Maintena, Zyprexa Relprevv, Invega Sustenna, Invega Trinza) now provides clinicians with an SGA that can be given as infrequently as once every 3 months.

Acute Antipsychotic Treatment

The decision of which antipsychotic agent to administer for a first break of psychosis or in the emergency department setting has become more complex with the availability of the SGAs. In general, second-generation agents are now the first-line antipsychotics in the treatment of most psychotic episodes. Although studies such as CATIE and CUtLASS 1 have failed to show any efficacy benefit of the SGAs over FGAs in the treatment of schizophrenia, clinicians have not generally embraced the first-generation agents again. A number of factors might explain why clinicians have been hesitant to return to the older agents despite potentially enormous cost savings over nongeneric SGAs. One is concern about the risk of EPS, particularly tardive dyskinesia. Although CATIE did not show great differences between perphenazine and second-generation drugs, perphenazine and risperidone were somewhat more likely to be associated with akathisia (Miller et al. 2005). The rates of tardive dyskinesia and dystonia in CATIE were equivalent with the SGAs and perphenazine. However, as alluded to earlier, CATIE may not have been long enough to show differences in rates of tardive dyskinesia. The known rates of tardive dyskinesia with the SGAs in long-term schizophrenia trials do appear to be lower than those reported in trials of first-generation agents in schizophrenia, even after the more aggressive dosing is taken into account. The overall rate of tardive dyskinesia with the SGAs seems to be around 1%–3% per year or less, whereas the reported rates of tardive dyskinesia for even midpotency first-generation drugs appear to be about twice as high. However, some studies have suggested that the tardive dyskinesia prevalence may be more similar with FGAs versus SGAs than previously believed. Carbon and colleagues (2017) found the prevalence of tardive dyskinesia with the second-generation agents to be about 20%, versus 30% with the FGAs. These data may be difficult to interpret because many patients taking SGAs long-term may have also been treated with FGAs first. Even if the overall rate of tardive dyskinesia with the SGAs turns out to be two-thirds of the rate with the FGAs, that would still probably be enough to favor the SGAs, given the persistent and sometimes disabling nature of tardive dyskinesia. Since the standard of care is currently to use SGAs, the application of first-generation drugs for cost savings presents a legal dilemma should a patient develop an irreversible tardive dyskinesia while taking an FGA.

Oral FGAs have largely been supplanted by the SGAs, but the same is not true for short-acting intramuscular FGAs. Whereas many SGAs, including olanzapine, ziprasidone, and aripiprazole, have short-acting intramuscular formulations, haloperidol remains the most popular medication for managing

224 Schatzberg's Manual of Clinical Psychopharmacology

acute psychosis and agitation in the emergency department (Campillo et al. 2015). Despite being more likely to cause EPS than the intramuscular forms of the SGAs (Bosanac et al. 2013), intramuscular haloperidol is inexpensive and has a track record of decades of use in the emergency department.

There are new formulations of first-generation drugs, such as an inhaled form of loxapine, that would be useful in some acute situations as an alternative to intramuscular haloperidol. The inhaled form of loxapine (Adasuve) has been available since 2012 for the management of acute agitation in patients with schizophrenia or bipolar disorder. An inhaled antipsychotic would appear to be a more benign, fast-acting alternative to an injection. Unfortunately, an agitated patient may be unable to cooperate with the instructions necessary to use the inhaler properly. This includes having the patient take a deep breath and then hold their breath as long as possible (ideally at least 10 seconds). Inhaled loxapine is also quite expensive and has not gained much popularity. The typical inhaled dose is 10 mg and should not be repeated for a 24-hour period. Cost and practicality of administering inhaled antipsychotics have limited the use of this formulation.

Choosing among the oral SGAs to use acutely is a matter of best matching patient characteristics to the side-effect profiles of the available agents. For rapid oral titration in the treatment of an acutely psychotic patient, the best choices currently are sublingual risperidone (Risperdal M-TAB), aripiprazole (Abilify Disc Melt), and olanzapine (Zyprexa Zydis) in orally disintegrating tablets.

Quetiapine and clozapine require more time to achieve a therapeutic dose than do other SGAs and therefore may be less advantageous in the acute setting. As in the emergency setting, we sometimes employ a high-potency antipsychotic such as orally administered haloperidol concurrently with upward titration of quetiapine. Then, at about 2–4 weeks, we taper the haloperidol and continue the titration of the SGA.

Choosing among the FGAs follows the same principle of matching patient characteristics to the side-effect profiles of agents. We tend to favor mid-potency first-generation drugs such as perphenazine as the best balance of side effects, including EPS and weight gain. The clinician might guess that a sedating drug such as chlorpromazine may elicit a better response in an anxious, excited, acutely psychotic patient, or the clinician might judge that a less sedating drug such as haloperidol is a better choice because relatively larger doses are likely to be better tolerated. Either choice is acceptable. A small series of studies by Van Putten (1974) showed that if the first dose of an antipsychotic was judged even slightly helpful by a patient, that patient had a good response to the drug over a 4-week trial. On the other hand, if the first dose was unpleasant because of oversedation or early signs of akathisia, the patient did badly during a 4-week trial, even if antiparkinsonian drugs and dosage adjustment were used to their best advantage. It may be—although no one has tried such an irregular approach—that one should give acutely ill patients a different drug every day until finding one that the patient does not dislike. The inverse of this approach is to take good drug histories whenever possible and to avoid using drugs that the patient remembers to have been unpleasant.

Antipsychotic drugs differ in the dosages and formulations in which they are available. Thioridazine and pimozide, and some SGAs, are not available in parenteral forms. Generic, and therefore less expensive, forms are available for chlorpromazine, haloperidol, fluphenazine, and pimozide. Among the second-generation agents, aripiprazole, clozapine, olanzapine, paliperidone, quetiapine, risperidone, and ziprasidone are available generically. So far there is no evidence that generic forms of antipsychotic drugs are significantly different from the original product, but some patients strongly prefer the brand version. Haloperidol may have a special tactical advantage in being available as a tasteless, colorless concentrate. For a list of available formulations and strengths of antipsychotic agents, see Table 4–1.

Several experts have tried to compare the potencies of the various available antipsychotic agents. Our version of the comparative potencies of the various available antipsychotics, based on D_2 binding data, is presented in Table 4–2.

Early Intervention in First-Episode Psychosis

There is some evidence that the earlier the treatment of a first-episode psychosis, the more favorable the long-term outcome. As with depression, some loss of gray matter has been noted to commence with the beginning of psychosis in schizophrenia (Pantelis et al. 2003). Gray matter loss that progresses over time has been noted in early schizophrenia in the cingulate gyrus, orbital frontal cortex, and cerebellar cortex, among other areas. In addition, there is often a loss of function that precedes the emergence of psychotic symptoms in patients with schizophrenia. Thus, there is hope that early intervention might improve long-term outcome or even prevent the full-blown development of schizophrenia in patients with prodromal symptoms.

Table 4–2.　Antipsychotic drug potency

Generic name	Brand name	Chlorpromazine equivalence
Aripiprazole	Abilify	10 mg
Chlorpromazine	Thorazine	100 mg
Clozapine	Clozaril	50 mg
Fluphenazine hydrochloride	Prolixin	2 mg
Fluphenazine decanoate	Prolixin Decanoate	0.25 cc/month
Haloperidol	Haldol	2 mg
Loxapine	Loxitane	10 mg
	Adusave (inhaler)	10 mg
Molindone	Moban	10 mg
Olanzapine	Zyprexa	~5 mg
Perphenazine	Trilafon	10 mg
Prochlorperazine	Compazine	15 mg
Quetiapine	Seroquel	63 mg
Risperidone	Risperdal	0.5 mg
Thioridazine	Mellaril	100 mg
Thiothixene	Navane	4 mg
Trifluoperazine	Stelazine	5 mg

In general, there appears to be a negative relationship between time to treatment of a first-episode psychosis and outcome across a number of measures. For example, the shorter the duration of untreated psychotic symptoms, the greater the response to antipsychotics (Perkins et al. 2005). The longer the patient stays psychotic, the less likely medications will be successful in alleviating symptoms. This appears to be true for response to both positive and negative symptoms, but the effects are most notable in the treatment of positive symptoms. Shorter duration of illness to first treatment may also be associated with an improvement in functional outcome and cognition and a reduced risk of relapse.

Does early treatment in first-episode psychotic patients affect the progressive morphological changes that have been observed in schizophrenia? There is some suggestion that early treatment might have a neuroprotective effect that presumably could be associated with improved prognosis. Lieberman and colleagues (2003) randomly assigned a group of 300 patients with first-episode psychosis to treatment with either haloperidol or olanzapine. The patients treated with olanzapine did not appear to show morphological changes, whereas the patients treated with haloperidol did. Over the course of 2 years, the olanzapine-treated patients did not have loss in frontal gray matter as did the haloperidol-treated patients. In addition, there was a modest increase in volume in the temporal areas in the patients treated with olanzapine but not in the patients treated with haloperidol. The implications of this study are unclear, but the findings suggest that early intervention may have impacts on cortical areas in important ways and that different antipsychotics might act differently. More generally, intervening early and attempting to prevent relapse in schizophrenia may substantially improve long-term outcome. The possibility that we might prevent the syndrome of schizophrenia altogether through early identification of at-risk children and adolescents is intriguing. However, the tools for identifying at-risk patients and the interventions that might prevent schizophrenia from emerging are not yet fully developed. Few, if any, data exist to indicate that the transition of prodromal schizophrenia to full schizophrenia can be prevented with SGAs (McGlashan et al. 2006); however, there is some suggestion that omega-3 fatty acids and cognitive training may actually prevent full expression of the disorder (see, e.g., Amminger et al. 2010). Longer-term studies of early medication intervention alone for first-break schizophrenia have not shown consistent benefits in preventing relapse or decreasing the number of hospital days over the subsequent 3–5 years (Chang et al. 2017). However, a comprehensive approach to first-onset psychosis that includes family education, assertive community treatment, and social skills training, such as in the Dutch OPUS trials, does appear to have long-term benefits in some outcome measures such as reduced need for supportive housing, lower mortality, and fewer hospitalizations (Posselt et al. 2021).

Inpatient Treatment

In the age of managed care, with dwindling length of hospital stays, there is considerable pressure to move acutely psychotic patients out of the hospital rapidly. Unfortunately, as previously described, all antipsychotics work in a slow, approximate manner. There is no evidence that pushing doses higher than that which is known to produce a 60%–80% D_2 receptor blockade speeds response. Controlled acute-treatment drug studies generally fail to find an antipsychotic dosage so low that improvement does not occur, and such studies also find that very high dosages are often less effective than lower dosages. So far, we know of no study of acutely psychotic inpatients that has found a dosage too low to be effective. The psychiatrist faced with a disturbed patient and a concerned or even frightened ward staff who ordinarily use high antipsychotic dosages and frequent as-needed medication may be hard put to keep to a low- and steady-dosage regimen, however sensible, but we strongly believe that the latter alternative is best. Again, using oral and parenteral benzodiazepines such as lorazepam may be more useful than administering higher dosages of an antipsychotic, and the former may provide more benefit to both patient and staff.

Choosing the "right" drug for the patient may not be possible, and the actual drug used may often be irrelevant because all available FGAs and SGAs are essentially equivalent in average efficacy. Nevertheless, for patients who previously received antipsychotic therapy, it is well worth getting a detailed drug history from them and from their family and past physicians. The point is to know the drugs that the patient has received and responded to—or those that the patient has had bad reactions to or disliked actively—and to try to choose a drug that the patient will both accept and respond to.

If a patient's condition does not improve with an adequate dosage of an antipsychotic, several approaches are available, although the reasons for selecting a specific one remain obscure. A different antipsychotic drug can be tried, of course. However, in the absence of undesirable side effects, it is always difficult to be sure whether a shift to a different drug at a more or less equivalent dosage will be better than continuing the original drug for a longer period. Pragmatically, 2 weeks without response in markedly psychotic patients and 5–6 weeks in patients with milder symptoms or with detectable but quite inadequate improvement generally forces the clinician to make a change. Again, the choice of the second drug is determined more clearly by the patient's past untoward reactions to specific antipsychotics than by any rational strategy based on the patient's specific pattern of psychopathology. Some clinicians end up selecting the last drug that worked for them for a patient with a similar treatment-resistant condition. For patients who are not experiencing a response, higher dosages of the original antipsychotic have usually already been tried without benefit, so it is better to use the time of change to see whether a substantially lower equivalent dosage of the new drug is any better. Again, if the second drug is well tolerated, it should be continued for several weeks. The only situation in which changing drugs can be dramatic is a shift to parenteral or depot medication in a patient who has not actually been taking their oral medication. As Donald Klein once said, "The first thing to do when a drug isn't working is to make sure the patient is actually taking it!" When the patient is taking a substantial dose of an antipsychotic and their condition is not improving, it is possible that akinesia, akathisia, or confusion due to the anticholinergic effects of antiparkinsonian drugs may be responsible. The clinician can decrease the dosage rapidly and expect some rebound agitation, followed, sometimes, by significant improvement.

It is still unclear whether antipsychotic plasma levels are of major value in titrating dose, but there are enough suggestions of the existence of a therapeutic window with some antipsychotics that the clinician can try, with caution, using plasma levels as a gauge of clinical response in patients who are not experiencing improvement. Therapeutic ranges of antipsychotics, except for haloperidol and perhaps clozapine, really do not exist, but laboratories can provide commonly observed blood level ranges. If a patient's blood level (12 hours after an oral dose or 1 week after a depot injection) is either very high or almost undetectable, appropriate changes can be tried. If the patient is already on a very high dosage of a neuroleptic and the laboratory finds almost none of the agent in the blood, the clinician should change drugs (or laboratories) or double-check that compliance is not a factor. We worry about escalating antipsychotics to huge dosages on the basis of laboratory data alone unless the clincian has access to an outstandingly competent laboratory.

At this time, the best evidence for a rational relationship between plasma levels and clinical response exists for haloperidol. There may even be a curvilinear relationship between blood level of haloperidol and clinical response such that levels below 4 ng/mL or above 26 ng/mL are associated with poorer clinical response compared with levels within the therapeutic window of 4–26 ng/mL. However, not all studies agree, and clinicians wanting to use this guideline must determine for themselves whether the levels are useful. The other drug for which there may be a clinically useful therapeutic window is clozapine. A number of studies suggest that therapeutic response is correlated with clozapine serum levels above 350 ng/mL (Liu et al. 1996; VanderZwaag et al. 1996). The clinically convincing event occurs when a patient who has not experienced a response improves when a level of antipsychotic that is outside the therapeutic window is adjusted to fall within it. However, in therapeutic drug monitoring of clozapine, serum levels generally do not add much to clinical care. The problem is that there is such great inter-individual variability in clozapine serum levels that they do not adequately predict either response or toxicity.

For a patient whose condition does not appear to be responding to treatment, careful reevaluation for overt and covert side effects is necessary. Adding (or removing) antiparkinsonian drugs or other medications designed to alleviate specific side effects or shifting to another antipsychotic may be helpful. Even having the patient take the whole dose at bedtime may help by decreasing daytime sedation or inertia. Reconsidering diagnosis is also helpful. For some patients who were initially assumed to have schizophrenia, a diagnosis of psychotic depression or bipolar disorder may turn out to be more accurate, and the addition of an antidepressant or lithium may be indicated. Some patients with treatment-resistant DSM-5-TR schizophrenia who have few or no affective symptoms can experience improvement when lithium or valproate is added to an antipsychotic, although this approach rarely results in a full remission. Other augmentation strategies, including the combination of two antipsychotics, may be helpful (see Chapter 9, "Augmentation Strategies for Treatment-Resistant Disorders").

If a patient's psychosis is unremitting and serious and is quite probably either worse or no better while the patient is taking antipsychotic drugs, the clinician should have the patient stop taking all antipsychotics to make sure that their condition is not made worse by them. Moreover, the use of antipsychotics in the face of little apparent response needs to be justified because of the risk of EPS and metabolic side effects. Unfortunately, some patients are simply not responsive to available treatments for psychosis. The lack of response to multiple antipsychotics should prompt a reevaluation of the diagnosis and consideration of comorbidities that might affect response such as active substance abuse.

Maintenance Drug Therapy

For a patient who has recovered from a first psychotic episode, there is no evidence regarding how long to continue antipsychotic therapy. Probably stopping the drug 2 days after the patient appears much better will lead to a return of psychosis, whereas tapering off medication after 3 months might be tolerated by many patients—perhaps 85% of them—without relapse rapidly ensuing. Nonetheless, schizophrenia is a chronic illness characterized by exacerbations and relative remissions, so maintenance pharmacotherapy is almost always required. At some point, the drug action shifts from being directly antipsychotic to preventing relapse. In principle, and generally in practice, patients with schizophrenia reach a stable level of remission—often with residual psychotic symptoms that do not improve with increased medication and that may not worsen when the drug is stopped. In fact, in the short run, some patients feel "better"—more alert and energetic—without medication. However, the risk of relapse is a good deal greater when patients are not taking medication.

Antipsychotic drugs are clearly effective in the prevention of relapse of schizophrenia. Unfortunately, as many as 25%–50% of patients experience a relapse within 2 years despite good compliance with their antipsychotic medication. In one major study, one-half of the antipsychotic-treated schizophrenic patients experienced a relapse by the end of the 2-year study period. About 85% of the placebo-treated patients relapsed over the same period. Recent studies of olanzapine in maintenance treatment suggest that approximately 20% of patients experience a relapse within 1 year while taking the drug, whereas about 70% experience a relapse with placebo treatment (Tran et al. 1998). The rate of relapse with olanzapine in these studies (20%) was better than the rate of relapse with haloperidol (30%) during the same time period. It is clear that antipsychotics are more effective than placebo, but many patients experience a relapse despite adequate drug therapy.

Currently, SGAs are generally the treatment of choice for maintenance therapy of schizophrenia. Reduced risk of tardive dyskinesia, improved cognitive function, and perhaps greater efficacy in treating negative symptoms have resulted in the SGAs being the maintenance treatment of choice for schizophrenia. However, the biggest single drawback to use of second-generation agents in maintenance therapy is their greater proclivity for producing significant weight gain compared with FGA agents (Allison et al. 1999). Weight gain is terribly problematic in patients treated with clozapine or olanzapine. Among the SGAs, risperidone/paliperidone, ziprasidone, aripiprazole, lurasidone, and asenapine appear to have the lowest propensity to cause weight gain, although they all can produce some weight gain. Olanzapine and clozapine tend to have the most weight gain and metabolic issues. In addition, a few patients respond better to first-generation dopamine receptor antagonists than to second-generation agents. For these patients, maintenance with the lowest effective dosage of a first-generation agent is warranted.

Perhaps one-fifth of all patients whose condition is stabilized while taking an antipsychotic medication show signs of increasing psychosis as the drug is tapered—strong evidence that the medication is necessary. For the first-episode patient in full remission, prolonged antipsychotic treatment is not indicated, but generally it has seemed sensible for the patient to continue taking a very gradually decreasing dose of the drug with which they improved. The tapering should last at least 3 months after discharge or from the point of marked improvement. If the patient is expected to be under stress in the next 6–9 months (e.g., completing school, starting a new job, getting divorced), we favor continuing the neuroleptic until the stress point is well past and the patient is generally coping adequately. Recent data suggest that in patients with schizophrenia, maintenance therapy, even after the first episode, could alter the course of the illness in a positive manner. Thus, maintenance therapy is beginning to be used earlier in the course of the illness, even after a single episode.

For patients with a history of two or more psychotic episodes that appear to have occurred after withdrawal of antipsychotics (either by the clinician or by the patient), prolonged maintenance antipsychotic therapy is indicated. Systematic large-scale studies are under way that may modulate our old beliefs. The work of Kane et al. (1983) suggests that as little as about 2.5 mg (0.1 mL) of fluphenazine decanoate every 2 weeks (10% of the fluphenazine decanoate dose at which the patient's condition was clinically stable) is more effective than placebo, although less effective than the full (100%) dose, in preventing relapse. The 10% dose illustrates current problems in weighing the risks and benefits of a low-dose approach: the patients taking this dose appear to feel better and function a bit better than patients on the 100% dose, and their condition is judged to be better by their families. They also develop fewer dyskinetic movements. However, they more often experience relapse into psychosis. Is this outcome "better" or "worse" overall? Several studies suggested that a 20% dose (e.g., about 5 mg every 2 weeks) was as effective as the full dose at preventing relapse for the first year. In the second year, the group receiving the 20% dose had more relapses than did the group receiving the full dose. At this time, for patients with schizophrenia, we favor long-term maintenance at their full antipsychotic dose if possible. Patients who do not tolerate standard doses of classic antipsychotics should be switched to standard doses of SGAs. For patients who are unable to tolerate standard doses, we suggest a gradual taper of the antipsychotic dose over 6–9 months to the lowest dose that controls symptoms.

Among the typical antipsychotics, only fluphenazine and haloperidol are available in long-acting or depot preparations in the United States. Risperidone was the first SGA to also be available in a long-acting form (Risperdal

Consta). This form of risperidone requires injections every 2 weeks but appears to be effective. Some patients in the risperidone long-acting trials at Stanford experienced minor irritation around the injection site, but the drug was remarkably well tolerated by most patients over several years. Since the introduction of long-acting risperidone, several other long-acting SGAs, including olanzapine (Zyprexa Relprevv), paliperidone (Invega Sustenna, Invega Trinza), and aripiprazole (Abilify Maintena), have become available. All of the long-acting SGA injectables may be better tolerated than the first-generation depot antipsychotics, at least in terms of EPS. However, no generic forms of these agents are currently available, and they are substantially more expensive than first-generation agents. For example, a monthly dose of long-acting aripiprazole injectable runs $1,500/month versus about $100/month for haloperidol decanoate. There is no evidence that the long-acting SGA agents are more efficacious than the first-generation agents. A number of other depot drugs (fluspirilene, flupentixol, perphenazine), as well as an oral tablet (penfluridol) that lasts a week, are available in Europe and, in some cases, Canada. Depot fluphenazine and haloperidol are available in the decanoate form.

One of the main reasons antipsychotics do not work is that patients dislike them and refuse to take them; therefore, long-acting injectable antipsychotics have the great advantages that a known amount of drug is administered reliably and that the staff is immediately aware when an injection is missed. However, several controlled studies have failed to show that depot fluphenazine is any more effective than oral fluphenazine in averting psychotic relapse in aftercare patients. Our interpretation of these counterintuitive data is that research studies with dedicated nurses, excellent outreach, weekly medication monitoring, and all patients getting both pills and injections provide an excellent but unrealistic level of aftercare that ensures both pill taking and injection taking. In more typical understaffed aftercare programs, depot fluphenazine injections are likely to be much easier to monitor and to be better monitored than pill taking. More naturalistic studies would probably have shown depot drugs to be more effective at averting relapse, especially in patients with a history of noncompliance. It is not uncommon to find that patients who have repeatedly stopped taking oral antipsychotic medication after hospital discharge and have vociferously objected to taking medication will cooperate faithfully with a depot antipsychotic regimen, presenting themselves for the injection on time, month after month. The reasons for this improved compliance are unclear. One possibility is that patients who stop oral antipsychotic medications feel "better" in a few days as the side effects wear off. Some patients even become transiently euphoric before going on to become grossly psychotic. Stopping oral medication may therefore be reinforcing to the patient, whereas delaying depot injections is not. Intermittent treatment with antipsychotics should be avoided in most patients with schizophrenia.

Other problems in maintenance antipsychotic therapy are evident. First, maintenance therapy reduces relapse in about 50%–75% of the patients on that regimen. Second, it is often very hard to determine whether the patient experienced a relapse because the antipsychotic medication was stopped or whether the patient stopped the medication because they began to experience a relapse. Third, many patients with chronic schizophrenia who are well stabilized in the community become very rigid about their treatment; they become upset (and experience a relapse) if their medication is changed. We have had several long-term aftercare patients who had been taking antipsychotics for more than 5 years who relapsed with as little as a 40% decrease in their antipsychotic dose. In another study, investigators withdrew active medication in patients with schizophrenia who had been stable in the community for 5 years and found an 80% relapse rate over the following year; this finding suggests that low-dose maintenance drug therapy may be necessary for prolonged periods (Hogarty et al. 1995). Again, the newer agents may provide better efficacy and lower risk of tardive dyskinesia. Given the evidence that abrupt stopping of oral antipsychotics may precipitate relapse, more extensive use of depot antipsychotics is indicated for patients with schizophrenia or schizoaffective disorder.

Trials of withdrawing medication to demonstrate continued need for it are not indicated in cases of recurring schizophrenia. However, these trials may be required in order to defend the use of maintenance antipsychotic therapy in patients with intellectual developmental disorder, psychotic depression or other depressive conditions, dementia (in elderly patients), and borderline personality disorder (BPD) or other personality disorders. There is a growing body of evidence that a variety of psychosocial therapies can reduce relapse rates (or, better, postpone relapse) in patients with chronic schizophrenia who also are receiving drug therapy. However, none of these therapies substantially modifies the deficits in interpersonal functioning present in patients with chronic schizophrenia, regardless of whether they are taking medication. Further, these therapies work best in the first year of a long-term study and less well as time progresses. At least part of this problem is that patients seem "better" and push themselves or are pushed into rehabilitation, social programs, or work programs that make demands that are beyond their coping abilities and that lead to relapse (Hogarty et al. 1995).

Use in Other Psychiatric Disorders

Bipolar Disorder

Until the year 2000, virtually all the literature on large-scale studies of prophylactic treatment for patients with bipolar disorder concerned lithium or valproic acid. However, increasing evidence from clinics serving such patients suggests that many of them end up receiving, and probably require, long-term antipsychotic therapy to remain stable in the community (Sernyak and Woods 1993; White et al. 1993). Antipsychotic agents have proved to be more versatile, more rapidly acting, and more reliably effective in the depressed phase of the illness than either lithium or valproate. The SGAs also do not require blood levels as do the mood stabilizers. In addition, a number of the SGAs, including olanzapine, aripiprazole, ziprasidone, risperidone, and quetiapine, are approved in the maintenance treatment of bipolar disorder to prevent relapse. Thus, the SGAs are now among the most common agents used in the treatment of bipolar disorder.

At this time, most of the SGAs have at least two trials supporting their efficacy in treating acute mania. Olanzapine, quetiapine, ziprasidone, asenapine, aripiprazole, and risperidone have FDA approval for this indication. In addition, the SGAs are the only class of agents that have demonstrated clear efficacy in the treatment of bipolar depression. Olanzapine in combination with fluoxetine became the first drug (in a combination capsule, Symbyax) approved for the treatment of bipolar depression. However, even olanzapine alone has notable effects in bipolar depression. Symbyax is available in olanzapine-fluoxetine combinations of 6 mg and 25 mg, 6 mg and 50 mg, 12 mg and 25 mg, and 12 mg and 50 mg. The recommended starting dose is 6 mg and 25 mg, with adjustment as needed. Quetiapine now has demonstrated utility as a monotherapy in the treatment of bipolar depression and has been approved by the FDA for this indication. The approved dosage range is 300–600 mg/day, although there were no differences between 300 mg and 600 mg in efficacy (Endicott et al. 2008; Thase et al. 2006). In 2013, lurasidone became the third agent approved for bipolar depression. The approval of lurasidone for bipolar depression came from two positive registration trials, one that used lurasidone as an adjunctive agent and a second that employed lurasidone as a monotherapy for the treatment of major depression in patients with bipolar I disorder. Both 6-week studies indicated that lurasidone was superior to placebo in reducing depressive symptoms in bipolar patients (Loebel et al. 2014a, 2014b). Both studies used the medication at dosages in the 20–120 mg/day range. We have found that dosages in the 20–60 mg/day range seem to do fine and are better tolerated than the higher dosages. Cariprazine became the fourth agent approved for the treatment of bipolar depression in 2019 and was joined by lumateperone as the fifth agent in 2021.

SGAs already are far more commonly used in the treatment of mood disorders than they are in the treatment of schizophrenia. It is likely that the application of these drugs in the treatment of different phases of bipolar disorder will continue to expand (see Chapter 5).

Unipolar Depression

In psychotic depression, there is good evidence that the combination of perphenazine and amitriptyline is superior to either drug alone. There is no reason to believe that there is anything magical about this pair of drugs; probably any antidepressant plus any antipsychotic would work about as well. Very few studies of psychotic depression have involved SGAs. The initial trials with the combination of fluoxetine and olanzapine compared with olanzapine monotherapy and placebo showed good efficacy for the combination in one trial but a lack of efficacy in a second one (Rothschild et al. 2004). Olanzapine alone failed to separate from placebo. In a National Institute of Mental Health (NIMH)–sponsored trial, the combination did separate from placebo, but it took 6 weeks to see significance (Andreescu et al. 2007). In another NIMH-funded study, Meyers et al. (2009) reported that olanzapine in combination with sertraline was significantly more effective than olanzapine alone. There is limited evidence that amoxapine alone can be useful in the treatment of psychotic depression. Electroconvulsive therapy (ECT) is undeniably effective in treating psychotic depression—perhaps more effective than combinations of a tricyclic antidepressant (TCA) and an antipsychotic. The dosages of antipsychotics used in psychotic depression are often quite high (e.g., 48–72 mg of perphenazine); it is unclear whether such high dosages are necessary. In one double-blind study (Shelton et al. 2001), olanzapine in combination with flu-oxetine was reported to be significantly more effective than placebo. Some analyses have not concluded that the combination of an antipsychotic and an antidepressant is any better than an antidepressant alone (Wijkstra et al. 2005). However, there is little evidence that antipsychotics, including the SGAs, are useful in the monotherapy of psychotic depression (see above).

When FGAs are used in treating depression, the medical record should re-flect the reasons clearly. With continued use for several months, the risks of dyskinesia must be noted and the need for maintenance neuroleptic use must be specifically justified. Many early malpractice suits for tardive dyskinesia in-volved depressed patients who developed dyskinesia while taking typical an-tipsychotics. Data from McLean Hospital suggested that patients with unipolar or bipolar depression, whether psychotic or nonpsychotic, develop dyskinesia twice as early as, and with half the drug exposure of, patients with schizophrenia. There are limited data on rates of tardive dyskinesia in long-term use of SGAs in the adjunctive treatment of major depression. However, the rate of tardive dyskinesia in 1-year open-label treatment with adjunctive aripiprazole for depression was less than 1%. Of the available FGAs, only thi-oridazine is approved by the FDA for use in depression—specifically, moder-ate to marked depression with anxiety or agitation. There are occasional depressed patients who appear to be uniquely responsive to antipsychotics and do not improve while taking more conventional antidepressants.

The use of SGAs in the adjunctive treatment of depression has been in-creasing steadily since 2000. A number of studies now suggest benefit from adding olanzapine, quetiapine, and aripiprazole to antidepressants in the treatment of depression (Berman et al. 2009; Garakani et al. 2008; Marcus et al. 2008; Thase et al. 2006). Aripiprazole was approved for the adjunctive treatment of depression in 2007 at dosages of 2–15 mg/day, and olanzapine in combination with fluoxetine was approved for the treatment of resistant de-pression in 2009. Quetiapine was also approved as an adjunctive treatment for major depression in late 2009. The dosage range of quetiapine studied for de-pression was 150–300 mg/day. Brexpiprazole in doses of 2–4 mg/day has also been shown to be an effective adjunctive agent in the treatment of depression and was approved in 2015. The data indicating efficacy of the SGAs in the treatment of major depression are now more extensive than those for any aug-menting agents used in the treatment of depression. For example, there are more studies of lithium in the augmentation of antidepressant response, but all of the lithium studies combined have a subject enrollment that is a fraction of the number of patients studied with the newer antipsychotics. The advantage of the SGAs over some traditional augmenting agents such as lithium is greater safety (especially in overdose) and more limited blood monitoring.

Because there are no randomized studies to date comparing the SGAs with other common augmenting strategies such as lithium, thyroid hormone, bupropion, and stimulants, it is difficult to compare efficacy among the adjunctive treatments. However, the antipsychotics studies have been fairly consistent in showing adjunctive benefit. Many unanswered questions about adjunctive SGAs in the treatment of major depression remain. For example, it is not clear what the optimal duration of treatment with antipsychotics is or what the long-term safety of these drugs is in a depressed population.

Aripiprazole may have some advantages, at least from a metabolic perspective, over other SGAs in the long-term management of depressed patients. At this time there are not any substantial data supporting the use of SGAs other than aripiprazole, quetiapine, and olanzapine in the adjunctive treatment of depression. To date, only extended-release quetiapine has demonstrated benefit in the monotherapy of major depression. Results from four randomized controlled trials enrolling about 2,000 patients have suggested that quetiapine at dosages averaging 150–300 mg/day is effective in the monotherapy of depression. There may be a select group of patients for whom quetiapine monotherapy might be a reasonable option. Certainly, those depressed patients who might be on the bipolar spectrum are likely candidates for quetiapine monotherapy. In addition, depressed patients with prominent anxiety, agitation, and sleep disturbance might do fine taking a nighttime dose of quetiapine alone. Quetiapine is unlikely to ever be a first-line agent in the treatment of depression because of the weight gain and metabolic concerns, but it could be a second-line agent and is useful as an adjunctive treatment (see Chapter 9).

Anxiety Disorders

Another potential indication for the SGAs is in the treatment of generalized anxiety disorder (GAD). Quetiapine has been studied in controlled trials in the treatment of GAD, and the data were reviewed by an FDA advisory panel in 2009. To date, four trials have shown benefit of quetiapine over placebo and benefit comparable to that of approved GAD drugs, including paroxetine and escitalopram. The trials have typically involved dosages of 50, 150, and 300 mg/day over 8 weeks of treatment. Although the FDA advisory panel agreed that the data supported the efficacy of quetiapine in the treatment of GAD, they recommended against the approval of quetiapine because of safety concerns in this population. Metabolic issues might be an acceptable trade-off in a more serious illness such as bipolar disorder or schizophrenia, but the panel was not convinced this was a reasonable trade-off in GAD.

One advantage over traditional agents for the treatment of GAD, such as the antidepressants, may be a more rapid onset of action. Quetiapine and other SGAs may have rapid benefits for symptoms such as sleep disturbance and agitation. Quetiapine is also a non-habit-forming alternative to the benzodiazepines. On the other hand, quetiapine may carry greater risks of weight gain, EPS, and metabolic issues than the alternatives. As noted in Chapter 3 ("Antidepressants"), TCAs, selective serotonin reuptake inhibitors (SSRIs), and venlafaxine carry less risk and are probably at least as effective as antipsychotic drugs. Recent reviews suggest that both FGAs and SGAs may be effective for a wide range of anxiety problems (see Gao et al. 2005). However, the risks and benefits of all available treatments for GAD should be assessed in a given patient before deciding on a treatment.

We have occasionally used SGAs in the treatment of panic disorder. There are case reports of the utility of olanzapine in the treatment of panic disorder, and we have seen patients who did not respond to or could not tolerate SSRIs or a serotonin-norepinephrine reuptake inhibitor who have done well with olanzapine (Mandalos and Szarek 1999) or quetiapine (Pitchot and Ansseau 2012). Likewise, aripiprazole has been used to augment antidepressants in patients with panic disorder who did not respond to antidepressant monotherapy (Hoge et al. 2008). Of all the SGAs, we have found that quetiapine at dosages of 150–300 mg/day is often well tolerated and effective in the adjunctive treatment of panic disorder that has not responded to an antidepressant alone.

Anxiety frequently accompanies bipolar disorder. The SGAs clearly help mitigate associated symptoms in bipolar patients. For example, Hirschfeld and colleagues (2006) found that quetiapine at 300 and 600 mg/day was significantly better than placebo in improving anxiety symptoms in patients with bipolar I depression.

Obsessive-Compulsive Disorder

An antipsychotic might be particularly useful in treating an anxiety disorder when patients present with OCD plus schizotypal personality or schizophrenia. In such cases, the OCD is reported to show little or no response to standard drug or behavior therapies. It has been suggested that occasional patients do respond when risperidone or an FGA is added, but the situation is far from clear. Some patients with schizophrenia can develop OCD symptoms while taking an SGA, perhaps because of its 5-HT$_2$ antagonism. Adjunctive use of pimozide and other antipsychotics clearly helps with tics associated with OCD and Tourette's disorder. There is evidence that the addition of olanzapine or risperidone to an SSRI helps some patients with OCD. Risperidone has the best track record as an augmenting agent for OCD, but olanzapine is at least as effective as risperidone (Hollander et al. 2003; Koran et al. 2000; Mottard and de la Sablonnière 1999). The most recent work on quetiapine as an augmenter of SSRIs in OCD is mixed (Carey et al. 2012; Vulink et al. 2009). Paliperidone (Storch et al. 2013) and aripiprazole (Sayyah et al. 2012) also have shown benefit in the adjunctive treatment of OCD in small controlled trials. Overall, it appears that about one-third of patients treated with SSRIs benefit from the addition of an antipsychotic (Dold et al. 2013). We have found that lower dosages of many SGAs, such as aripiprazole 5–10 mg/day or quetiapine 100–150 mg/day, added to a standard SSRI appear effective and well tolerated in many patients with OCD.

Posttraumatic Stress Disorder

Antipsychotics have long been used in the treatment of PTSD. At least 25% of combat veterans end up being treated with one or more SGAs for PTSD in the Department of Veterans Affairs. There is no evidence that antipsychotics help much for some of the core symptoms of PTSD, including intrusive ideation and hypervigilance. In fact, the U.S. Department of Veterans Affairs/Department of Defense guidelines for PTSD treatment specifically recommend against the use of antipsychotics. However, antipsychotics can be useful adjunctive agents for the management of agitation, irritable aggression, anxiety, and sleep difficulties in some patients. In addition, PTSD patients seem to benefit from second-generation agents in a reduction of reexperiencing symptoms. Because of the sleep and anti-agitation benefits of olanzapine, we often add 5–10 mg of the drug at night to an SSRI or mood stabilizer. Risperidone

1–3 mg in divided doses also seems very helpful for some combat veterans with irritable aggression (Pivac et al. 2004; States and St Dennis 2003; Wang et al. 2013).

Personality Disorders

Antipsychotics have been employed in the treatment of patients with borderline and schizotypal personality disorders for many years. However, relatively few studies have been done to support this practice. The paucity of studies is due in part to the difficulties of doing pharmacological trials in patients with personality disorders. Comorbidity with major psychiatric disorders is common and complicates the selection of patients for studies and the interpretation of study results.

Schizotypal patients may represent one end of the schizophrenia spectrum and often benefit from antipsychotics. Schizotypal personality in younger patients is often perceived as a prodrome of schizophrenia. The only controlled trial of treating schizotypal personality patients with a second-generation agent, risperidone, reported that a dosage of 0.5–2 mg/day was beneficial (Koenigsberg et al. 2003). Earlier uncontrolled studies with typical antipsychotics also showed benefits.

Until the past 20 years, much of the work with BPD involved typical antipsychotics. A number of open-label and controlled trials suggested that haloperidol can target the impulsive aggression that patients with BPD may exhibit. However, the typical antipsychotics did little to help with the dysphoria and affective instability common to patients with BPD. Long-term treatment with haloperidol generally has been poorly tolerated, often has been discontinued, and has been only modestly helpful (Cornelius et al. 1993).

The SGAs have started to be more comprehensively studied in recent years in the treatment of persons with BPD, and growing evidence suggests that these agents have an important role to play in the treatment of some patients (Ripoll 2012). For example, olanzapine may produce greater global benefits in patients with BPD than does fluoxetine (Zanarini et al. 2004). Furthermore, the addition of olanzapine to dialectical behavior therapy (DBT) in patients with BPD seems to facilitate the rapid reduction of irritability and aggression (Linehan et al. 2008). However, not all placebo-controlled studies of olanzapine in BPD have demonstrated benefits. For example, Schulz and colleagues (2008) did not find olanzapine more effective than placebo in a 12-week study of more than 300 borderline patients. In contrast, in an even larger study, Zanarini and colleagues (2011) concluded that 5–10 mg/day of olanzapine showed a modest advantage over placebo in 451 borderline patients treated for 12 weeks. Smaller trials involving risperidone, aripiprazole, asenapine, and quetiapine have suggested benefits in treating BPD but tend to favor improvement in aggression and impulsivity over improvement of other symptoms. We tend to find that the combination of an SSRI and an SGA is often the optimal pharmacological approach in treating patients with BPD. The SSRI-SGA combination seems to treat dysphoria, mood instability, and impulsivity with good tolerability. Combinations such as paroxetine with risperidone or fluoxetine with olanzapine anecdotally seem well tolerated and effective. The self-identity issues in borderline patients can make weight gain a sensitive issue in prescribing olanzapine, quetiapine, or clozapine. Some data show that risperidone and clozapine are useful in treating self-mutilative behavior and aggression in patients with BPD (Benedetti et al. 1998; Chengappa et al. 1999; Frankenburg and Zanarini 1993). Studies with SGAs have shown more consistent, albeit often modest, effects on treating the core symptoms of BPD. Double-blind studies, although few, have generally suggested benefits of SGAs. For example, in a double-blind trial, aripiprazole was more effective than placebo in treating anxiety, depressive symptoms, and anger in borderline patients (Nickel et al. 2006). Likewise, the addition of olanzapine to DBT was more effective than a placebo added to DBT in addressing core borderline symptoms (Soler et al. 2005).

A reasonable interpretation of these results is that antipsychotics have a stabilizing effect on irritability, mood lability, and impulsivity and that they decrease anxiety. They may have a use in the early stages of a more comprehensive treatment program for patients with BPD such as with DBT. As of this writing, the second-generation agents have shown more consistent benefit in the treatment of borderline symptoms than have the first-generation agents. Thus, given what appears to be a lower long-term risk of some EPS and a broader spectrum of activity for borderline symptoms, the SGAs should generally be used over the FGAs for the treatment of borderline symptoms.

Other States

Antipsychotics are widely used for agitated organic states such as delirium, Alzheimer's dementia, and behavioral dyscontrol associated with intellectual disability, with varying degrees of benefit. Sometimes antipsychotics cause more harm (through side effects) than good, and their use is strictly empirical—valuable only if they help (see Chapter 12, "Pharmacotherapy of Specific Populations"). In conditions such as anxiety, personality disorder, and organic brain syndromes, for which efficacy of these agents is not firmly established, other drug therapies or no drug therapy may be preferable. The use of antipsychotics should never be routine, and their effects and their effectiveness for each particular patient should always be carefully monitored and documented.

Since the SGAs were introduced, there has been a marked increase in their use for dementia. It has been difficult to demonstrate clear benefit of most second-generation drugs in the treatment of psychosis or agitation associated with dementia. One exception has been pimavanserin, which is approved for the treatment of psychosis associated with Parkinson's disease (PD), which is often associated with dementia. Pimavanserin is also being investigated for the treatment of psychosis associated Alzheimer's disease, and preliminary Phase II and Phase III trials suggest that it may be effective, with less of a side effect burden than with other SGAs (Tariot et al. 2021).

The other SGA that has looked promising for the treatment of agitation associated with dementia is brexpiprazole. In two Phase III studies of the treatment of agitation associated with Alzheimer's disease, 2 mg of brexpiprazole appeared more effective than placebo (Grossberg et al. 2020). However, in one of those two trials, the benefit of the 2-mg dose was seen only in a post hoc analysis. Brexpiprazole was well tolerated at dosages of 0.5–2 mg/day, with few adverse events exceeding those seen in the placebo group. Additional studies are under way to determine whether the 2-mg dose can be prospectively shown to be effective for the treatment of agitation in patients with dementia.

On the basis of earlier studies, the FDA placed a class warning around increased mortality in geriatric patients with dementia treated with antipsychotics. When the data are pooled, there is about a 1.7-fold increase in mortality in patients treated with an antipsychotic versus placebo. This mortality appears to be associated with several causes, including cardiovascular events, cerebrovascular accidents (CVAs), and infection-related deaths. That being said, there are few good options or reasonable alternatives to antipsychotics in the treatment of psychosis or agitation associated with dementia. Benzodiazepines, anticonvulsants, and other drugs all have significant limitations in the population of elderly dementia patients. In comparative studies of the SGAs in patients with dementia (Sultzer et al. 2008), the antipsychotics do seem to have better effects than placebo on some symptoms, including anger, aggression, and paranoid ideas. Overall, however, the antipsychotics studied—risperidone, olanzapine, and quetiapine—did not make much of a difference relative to placebo in improving functioning or quality of life. Some greater efficacy was found for risperidone and olanzapine than for quetiapine in this study. We have found that 2.5–7.5 mg of olanzapine given at bedtime is often helpful for treating agitation and insomnia in patients with dementia. We have been less impressed with the as-needed use of olanzapine for achieving rapid improvement in agitation. However, carefully done studies have called into question the efficacy of the SGAs in the treatment of agitation and behavioral dyscontrol associated with dementia (Schneider et al. 2006). Given the black box warning of increased mortality associated with the SGAs in geriatric patients, it is unclear whether the benefits of most SGAs outweigh the risks. However, as new SGAs have emerged, the calculus may be changing. The use of antipsychotics in patients with dementia should be assessed on a case-by-case basis.

Some studies have found a slightly higher rate of CVAs in patients with dementia treated with olanzapine or risperidone. This finding led to an FDA warning, and the risk of CVA is now listed as a potential adverse event in the package inserts of both olanzapine and risperidone. SGAs could conceivably increase the risk of stroke by increasing other risk factors for CVAs, such as obesity and diabetes. However, large-scale analyses of geriatric patients in the community have not found an increased rate of CVAs in patients treated with risperidone or olanzapine (Herrmann et al. 2004). Although the increased risk of CVA associated with SGAs is, at best, small, nonetheless, as with younger patients, monitoring geriatric patients treated with SGAs for changes in weight, glucose levels, and triglyceride levels is worthwhile.

In addition to the treatment of patients with dementia, the SGAs are being applied with some success in patients with other conditions. In 2006, for example, risperidone became the first medication approved for use in treating the irritability associated with pediatric autism (McDougle et al. 2005). Aripiprazole has also been approved for irritability associated with autism spectrum disorders in children since 2009. Previous work with haloperidol in the treatment of autism showed modest benefits but significant EPS. Risperidone appears to be better tolerated. Another potential application of SGAs is in the treatment of anorexia nervosa. No pharmacotherapy has been demonstrated to help anorexia on a consistent basis at this time. However, early open-label trials, case reports, and at least one controlled trial suggest that olanzapine and quetiapine may help reduce the anxiety and obsessiveness around food and body image while contributing to weight gain (Dennis et al. 2006; Mondraty et al. 2005; Powers et al. 2007). In adults, olanzapine has also shown modest benefits in weight gain in anorexia nervosa but not in the psychological symptoms (Attia et al. 2019). However, even modest weight gain in patients with anorexia can be a success. The challenge is convincing a patient with anorexia to start and continue a medication associated with weigh gain.

Second-Generation (Atypical) Antipsychotics

Clozapine

Clozapine (Clozaril) has been available in the United States for about 30 years for use with patients who have treatment-resistant schizophrenia or patients who are unable to tolerate the side effects of FGAs. Clozapine was in many ways the best new development in the treatment of schizophrenia since chlorpromazine was discovered. The drug does have problems and dangers, it does not work for everyone, and patients who are helped substantially may still be far from well. However, it is thus far the only antipsychotic drug that has been shown in controlled studies to be clearly more effective than older antipsychotics in resistant schizophrenia. It is also thus far the only antipsychotic drug that causes essentially no pseudoparkinsonism or dystonia and that is, apparently, unlikely to cause tardive dyskinesia.

Clozapine has been in clinical use in Europe for more than 40 years. It was withdrawn from general use after deaths from agranulocytosis were reported in Finland in the mid-1970s. Over the intervening years, no other antipsychotic with similar properties was found, perhaps because clozapine has an odd mix of pharmacological effects: more dopamine$_1$ (D$_1$) than D$_2$ effects, more effect on cortical and limbic dopaminergic systems than on the basal ganglia, and greater serotonergic (5-HT$_2$), histaminic, and α-adrenergic blocking activity than other available neuroleptics. Evidence from early (pre-1978) multicenter trials showed clozapine to be more effective than haloperidol or chlorpromazine, leading Sandoz Pharmaceuticals to remarket the drug under controlled conditions in some European countries. In the United

Second-generation (dopamine-serotonin antagonist) antipsychotics: overview	
Efficacy	Schizophrenia (FDA approved for all) Treatment-resistant schizophrenia (clozapine) Mania (FDA approved for aripiprazole, asenapine, olanzapine, quetiapine, risperidone, and ziprasidone) Bipolar depression (FDA approved for cariprazine, lurasidone, quetiapine, and Symbyax [olanzapine-fluoxetine]) Depression (FDA approved for adjunctive use for aripiprazole, quetiapine, and brexpiprazole; Symbyax approved for resistant depression)
Side effects	Weight gain Gastrointestinal effects Insulin resistance Sedation Akathisia Orthostatic hypotension Bradykinesia Tachycardia Dizziness $\uparrow$ Triglycerides (except ziprasidone) EPS, NMS (rare) Agranulocytosis (clozapine) (rare) Seizures (clozapine)
Safety in overdose	Seizures with clozapine in overdose. Respiratory depression in combination with other CNS depressants. QT interval changes. Lavage and vital sign support.
Dosage and administration	Clozapine: 12.5–25 mg; then increase dosage 25–50 mg per week, as needed and tolerated, to 300–600 mg/day Risperidone: 0.5–1 mg bid to 3 mg bid by end of first week, as tolerated Olanzapine: 2.5–5 mg hs; increase by 5 mg every week to 20 mg hs Quetiapine: 25 mg bid; increase total daily dose by 50 mg, as needed and tolerated, to 300–600 mg/day Ziprasidone: 20 mg qd or bid; increase by 20–40 mg per week, to a maximum dosage of 80 mg bid Aripiprazole: 15 mg qd; increase up to 30 mg/day after 1 week

Second-generation (dopamine-serotonin antagonist) antipsychotics: overview *(continued)*	
Dosage and administration *(continued)*	Lurasidone: 20–40 mg/day; increase by 20–40 mg/day up to 120–160 mg/day Asenapine: 5–10 mg bid sublingually and then increase by 5 mg/day to a maximum of 10 mg bid Iloperidone: 1 mg po bid day one, 2 mg bid day two, and then increase by 2 mg/day to a target dosage of 6–12 mg/day Brexpiprazole: 1 mg once daily for 4 days; then increase to 2 mg once daily for 3 days; based on response and tolerability, increase to 4 mg/day on day 8. Usual dosage 2–4 mg once daily. Cariprazine: 1.5 mg once daily; 3 mg on day 2 based on response and tolerability; then increase in increments of 1.5 or 3 mg as needed. Usual dosage 3–6 mg once daily. The augmentation in depression may be best at 1.5 mg. Lumateperone: 42 mg/day as the starting and maintenance dosage
	Full benefits in 4 weeks to 6 months
Discontinuation	Mild cholinergic rebound, faster relapse. Taper as slowly as titrated up.
Drug interactions	Fluvoxamine (1A2 inhibitor): ↑ second-generation antipsychotic levels EtOH: ↑ sedation and orthostasis Antihypertensives: may ↑ orthostasis Carbamazepine: ↓ serum levels of olanzapine; ↓ clozapine levels; ↑ hematological adverse events with clozapine CNS depressants: ↑ sedation Ciprofloxacin (Cipro) (potent 1A2 inhibitor): ↑ second-generation antipsychotic levels Potent CYP3A4 inhibitors, such as HIV antivirals (e.g., ritonavir) and azole antifungals (e.g., ketoconazole): may ↑ brexpiprazole and cariprazine levels

Note. CYP = cytochrome P450; EPS = extrapyramidal symptoms; EtOH = ethanol; NMS = neuroleptic malignant syndrome.

States, the FDA insisted that clozapine's efficacy in treating patients with demonstrably treatment-resistant schizophrenia be proved. Such proof was obtained, and the resulting study was published (Kane et al. 1988). Patients with chronic schizophrenia who had experienced at least three adequate neuroleptic trials and had not had a remission in 5 years participated in the study. About one-third of the patients improved after taking clozapine for 4 weeks, compared with 2% of patients who improved after taking chlorpromazine (Kane et al. 1988).

Clozapine may differ from FGAs by modestly reducing negative symptoms (e.g., withdrawal, lack of motivation). However, recent studies such as CATIE and CUtLASS have cast doubt on the real-world effectiveness of second-generation drugs in the treatment of negative symptoms. The debate continues regarding whether typical antipsychotics actually cause negative symptoms or whether such symptoms are an integral part of schizophrenia. In addition, clozapine may also affect other dimensions of schizophrenia, such as suicidality. One large study indicated that patients with schizophrenia or schizoaffective disorder who were treated with clozapine (average dosage = 274 mg/day) were less likely than patients treated with olanzapine to attempt suicide or require emergency intervention for a perceived risk of attempting suicide (Meltzer et al. 2003). The risk of completing suicide was low and not statistically different between drugs. The finding of reduced suicidal behavior led to a unique FDA approval for clozapine for decreasing recurrent suicidal behavior in patients with schizophrenia or schizoaffective disorder. Although other SGAs, such as olanzapine, also appear to reduce suicidal behavior in some patients relative to first-generation agents such as haloperidol, clozapine may have unique properties in reducing suicidal behavior. Clozapine may be better than any of the other SGAs in reducing impulsive aggression, and it is this property that may account for its reported ability to reduce self-aggression, self-mutilation, and suicide attempts. Although the side-effect profile of clozapine will typically prevent its use as a first- or second-line agent, we have seen a number of cases in which clozapine was used effectively to reduce self-destructive behavior in schizophrenia, bipolar disorder, and even patients with BPD.

Clozapine has a tendency to cause serious neutropenia (absolute neutrophil count [ANC] < 500 μL)—affecting as many as 1.2% of all treated patients in the United States. Therefore, it is marketed under a unique system: all patients must be cleared through a national registry before taking clozapine. Currently, numerous pharmaceutical companies are registered with the FDA for marketing clozapine, under either proprietary name or generic label. On December 16, 2016, the individual clozapine patient registries maintained by the different pharmaceutical companies and the National Non-Rechallenge

Master File were replaced by the Clozapine Risk Evaluation and Mitigation Strategy (REMS) program. Under this program, "The requirements to prescribe, dispense, and receive clozapine are incorporated into a single, shared program called the Clozapine Risk Evaluation and Mitigation Strategy (REMS). A REMS is a strategy to manage known or potential risks associated with a drug or group of drugs, and is required by the FDA for clozapine to ensure that the benefits of the drug outweigh the risk of severe neutropenia." The Clozapine REMS program can be accessed at www.clozapinerems.com.

The REMS program requires that patients beginning treatment with clozapine have an ANC (total white blood cell [WBC] count×total percent of neutrophils on differential) of at least >1,500 μL. Approximately 25%–50% of patients of African and Middle Eastern descent may have a benign ethnic neutropenia, and these patients have different requirements for monitoring in the REMS system. For the general population, a complete blood count (CBC) with differential should be done weekly for the first 6 months of treatment, every 2 weeks for the next 6 months, and monthly after 12 months of treatment.

This system of laboratory monitoring contributes to the expense of prescribing clozapine, but generic forms of clozapine have reduced the pill costs considerably. However, because the onset of severe neutropenia is unpredictable—some patients show slow, steady decreases in ANC, whereas others experience an abrupt plunge in ANC, resulting in agranulocytosis—the purpose is to catch all new cases rapidly and to institute medical treatment early to avoid the deaths that were observed in Europe before this adverse effect was recognized. A few deaths have occurred in the United States under weekly monitoring. The agranulocytosis associated with clozapine use is believed to be an autoimmune reaction, not a direct toxic effect on the bone marrow. It is not dose related. Most cases occur in the second through fourth months of treatment, but some reactions have occurred as late as 18 months after the drug was begun. Patients developing agranulocytosis once will rapidly develop it again if the drug is restarted.

Clozapine is available generically in 25-mg, 50-mg, 100-mg, and 200-mg tablets and in 12.5-mg, 25-mg, and 100-mg scored disintegrating tablets, as well as in an oral suspension of 50 mg/mL. The starting dose is 25 mg at bedtime. The manufacturer recommends dosing twice a day, but many patients end up taking the whole dose at bedtime. The dosage should be increased slowly and cautiously from 25 to 200 mg/day over the first 2–3 weeks, then stabilized at that dosage for a few weeks, with further increases as tolerated. Most patients respond well to dosages between 300 and 500 mg/day. If clear improvement has not occurred, the dosage can be gradually increased to 900 mg/day. However, because drug-related grand mal seizures occur quite frequently (in about 15% of patients) at dosages higher than 550 mg/day, anticonvulsants should probably be added. Phenytoin or valproate, in standard anticonvulsant doses, has been used for this purpose at McLean Hospital.

Sedation is one major side effect limiting dosage increases. Many patients develop tolerance to this effect, but some do not. Cardiovascular side effects, both severe orthostatic hypotension and marked tachycardia (up to 130–140 bpm), can occur early in clozapine treatment. These side effects require very slow dose increases and, sometimes, the use of counteractive medications such as modafinil. A few patients develop unpleasant gastrointestinal (GI) distress and flulike symptoms early in treatment and refuse to take the drug again. Drug-induced fevers of around 100°F can occur early in treatment but pass and are not serious. Blood counts should be obtained, but in local experience with more than 300 patients, they have always been normal or elevated. Hypersalivation at night, causing wet pillowcases, is common; clonidine can be helpful in counteracting this side effect. Enuresis occasionally occurs.

Although the manufacturer has strongly urged that other antipsychotics be withdrawn from patients before clozapine is begun, this advice is hard to follow with many psychotic patients. We have almost always added low doses of clozapine to ongoing antipsychotic therapy, then tapered the prior antipsychotic once the clozapine dosage reached 200 mg/day. We have combined clozapine, generally without incident, with benzodiazepines, lamotrigine, lithium, valproic acid, TCAs, trazodone, other SGAs (such as aripiprazole), high-potency first-generation (typical) agents, fluoxetine, and even ECT. Because approximately 40%–70% of patients with resistant schizophrenia will be resistant to clozapine as well, augmenting strategies are often attempted. The evidence to date suggests that augmentation of clozapine with agents such as lamotrigine, amisulpride, and ethyl eicosapentaenoic acid might benefit some patients with resistant schizophrenia (Kontaxakis et al. 2005; Mouaffak et al. 2006). Some patients taking SSRIs and clozapine may develop high clozapine levels and sedation. We recommend periodically checking clozapine levels when the two are combined. Fluvoxamine may be particularly problematic because it is a more potent cytochrome P450 (CYP) 1A2 inhibitor. We have seen several cases of neuroleptic malignant syndrome (NMS) associated with clozapine use, particularly in patients taking concurrent lithium. As indicated earlier, lithium is sometimes thought to predispose patients to NMS. The NMS associated with clozapine may be milder than that associated with first-generation agents and tends not to be characterized by rigidity, fevers, and as high of an elevation in creatine phosphokinase. Rather, the presentation of NMS in clozapine-treated patients may include delirium, autonomic instability, and milder EPS (Hasan and Buckley 1998; Karagianis et al. 1999). Drugs that are known to induce agranulocytosis, such as carbamazepine, should be avoided.

The course of improvement with clozapine treatment is somewhat unpredictable. Patients who clearly show a substantial decrease in psychotic symptoms may do so in the first few weeks of treatment or as late as 3–6 months or more later. Some patients—a third or more in our experience—show marked improvement, although most are not totally free of psychotic residua. Schizoaffective patients may experience more complete improvement than schizophrenic patients, although schizoaffective patients often have better remissions before clozapine treatment. Psychotic and nonpsychotic patients with treatment-resistant mania also usually respond. Patients who take clozapine for 1 or more years may show gradual, continuing improvement. Even minimally improved psychotic patients may be less impulsively angry, violent, or argumentative and may show a gratifying absence of distressing akathisia, parkinsonism, and akinesia. At McLean Hospital, many such patients have continued to be administered clozapine because they are less distressed by their symptoms and are less of a management problem, even though they are still grossly impaired by psychotic symptoms.

Tardive dyskinesia may be unchanged initially by clozapine treatment, but it sometimes fades over time to near the vanishing point. In some patients the dyskinesia improves early, whereas in others it improves only very slowly. It is unclear whether clozapine suppresses dyskinesia or allows it to fade as it might in patients who are no longer taking antipsychotics.

Long-term side effects of maintenance clozapine therapy are not known, although in the United States, a handful of patients have been taking the drug continuously for more than 20 years without known adverse effects (including tardive dyskinesia). With long-term treatment with clozapine, the majority of patients gain weight, whereas a few lose a little weight. There is a controversy about whether clozapine is likely to cause diabetes and ketoacidosis. A consensus development conference on antipsychotic drugs and obesity and diabetes concluded that clozapine appeared to be associated with an increased risk for diabetes (American Diabetes Association et al. 2004). However, this conclusion has not been uniformly adopted.

All the SGAs, especially clozapine, olanzapine, and quetiapine, have been thought to be associated with an increased risk of hyperglycemia and diabetes, and this is now reflected as a warning in the package inserts of all SGAs. Aripiprazole and ziprasidone may carry lesser risks. Risperidone appears to be intermediate in risk between olanzapine and ziprasidone. A number of cases of diabetic ketoacidosis with the use of clozapine and other SGAs have been reported. However, the extent of the enhanced risk of diabetes with the SGAs is much debated. Schizophrenia itself enhances the risk of diabetes, and typical antipsychotics also increase the risk of diabetes. Whatever the extent of the risk, there is little doubt that several of the second-generation agents are associated with considerable weight gain and a risk of obesity. Obesity in turn is thought to be a clear risk factor for insulin resistance, hyperglycemia, and type 2 diabetes. However, cases of diabetes in antipsychotic-treated patients have occurred independently of weight gain, and we have reported that the insulin resistance that occurs with SGAs is not correlated with acute changes in weight. Thus, the disorder and the drug appear to be associated with insulin resistance independently of weight (Meltzer et al. 2005; Reaven et al. 2009), as evidenced by obesity, high blood pressure, and high triglyceride levels. The syndrome generally does not result in diabetes but appears to place subjects at risk for cardiovascular disease. The acute diabetic ketoacidosis appears to be unrelated to the longer-term weight gain and insulin subsensitivity and may be an idiosyncratic reaction.

In the same way as we taught our residents to routinely monitor patients who were taking first-generation antipsychotics for signs of EPS and tardive dyskinesia, we now teach our residents to monitor patients who are taking SGAs for signs of a metabolic syndrome. We agree with the American Psychiatric Association/American Diabetes Association recommendations on screening patients (Table 4–3). A scale and blood pressure cuff are useful pieces of monitoring equipment to keep in the office. The patients most likely to run into trouble with a metabolic syndrome or diabetes are those with the greatest risk factors for these conditions before pharmacotherapy. Thus, it is

Table 4–3. APA/ADA recommendations for screening patients who are taking second-generation antipsychotics

Screen prior to initiating the antipsychotic

　Personal or family history of obesity, diabetes, high cholesterol levels, high blood pressure, or heart disease

　Weight and height (BMI>25)

　Waist circumference (>40 inches in males; >35 inches in females)

　Blood pressure (>130/85)

　Fasting blood glucose levels (>110)

　Fasting cholesterol levels (HDL<40; total>200)

　Fasting triglyceride levels (>175)

Note. Abnormal levels indicated in parentheses. ADA=American Diabetes Association; APA=American Psychiatric Association; HDL=high-density lipoprotein.

important to pay special attention to patients with baseline obesity, dyslipidemias, and a family or personal history of diabetes. If the patient has gained more than 5% of their body weight or has a BMI greater than 30, we may check glucose and lipid levels as frequently as every month until we are convinced that the patient is medically stable. A finger stick is probably more useful than a hemoglobin A1c (HbA1c) unless the patient is already diabetic. The HbA1c is somewhat too global and blunt an assessment to tell us what is happening on a day-to-day basis. A fasting glucose or a finger stick is probably the most useful assessment to obtain in monitoring glucose levels. However, the clinician must keep in mind that patients often maintain fasting glucose levels constant while they become insulin resistant. The resistance may be better monitored by watching for increasing triglyceride or decreasing high-density lipid levels. In addition to screening glucose and lipid levels, we monitor weight and blood pressure and elicit symptoms of diabetes (polydipsia, polyuria, hyperphagia) every few months, and we repeat screening laboratory tests 3 months after the initiation of therapy. Thereafter, we repeat screening labs once a year or as indicated.

　The combined cost of the required weekly CBCs and the drug is somewhat high. However, most insurance carriers may cover all or a portion of the costs; the fiscal cost-benefit ratio for patients in public or private institutions has been determined, and the results favor the use of clozapine. For example, under Medicare Part D, clozapine is covered by most Prescription Drug Plans

(PDPs) under a tiered system, depending on the plan. Now that clozapine is available generically, virtually all county mental health programs are purchasing the generic formulation at great savings over the name brand.

Risperidone

Risperidone (Risperdal) was the second SGA introduced in the United States after clozapine. The drug exerts relatively more D_2 than D_1 antagonism. It also has antagonist effects at $5\text{-}HT_2$ and possibly $5\text{-}HT_1$ receptors. Several multisite collaborative double-blind studies have documented risperidone's apparent effectiveness in treating patients with schizophrenia and its unusual dose-response relationship: 6 mg/day is more effective and associated with fewer side effects than larger dosages, whereas 2 mg/day has been shown to be ineffective. The 6-mg (3 mg bid) dosage is at least as effective as 20 mg of haloperidol. However, the double-blind data regarding side effects are misleading. Although risperidone did not appear to produce much in the way of EPS in comparison to placebo, both "treatments" were associated with more EPS than one might anticipate. Also, a fairer trial would compare 3–6 mg of risperidone with 3.5–7.0 mg of haloperidol because these are the levels at which both drugs block D_2 receptors at 60%–80% efficiency. At these lower doses, it is unclear whether risperidone maintains a significant edge over haloperidol regarding the rates of EPS.

Risperidone is indicated in the treatment of schizophrenia, schizoaffective disorder, acute mania, and mixed states (Hirschfeld et al. 2004). Risperidone was also approved both as a monotherapy and as an adjunctive agent in the treatment of acute mania and is approved in the treatment of irritability and mixed states in autistic patients. The utility of risperidone as a maintenance treatment or a treatment for bipolar depression is as yet unclear. As reported earlier in this chapter, risperidone also has shown benefits in the augmentation treatment of unipolar depression.

In relatively short double-blind studies with healthy patients receiving only risperidone, the dosage could be raised from 1 mg bid to 2 mg bid to 3 mg bid over a few days without adverse effects. In clinical practice, one may need to raise the dosage more slowly. At McLean Hospital, risperidone seemed the ideal drug as a first-line treatment for psychotic patients until worrisome adverse effects such as EPS, orthostatic hypotension, agitation, and oversedation began to be noticed. Orthostasis has been particularly problematic in some patients and occasionally results in syncope and falls. Our experience is that dystonias are somewhat less common with risperidone relative to FGAs. However, bradykinesia and akathisia are often seen with risperidone treatment. Some of these adverse events might have been avoided if the dose had been raised more slowly or more attention had been paid to pharmacokinetic interactions with other drugs, especially SSRIs. We have seen that the combination of an SSRI and risperidone may enhance the orthostatic side effects of the drug. Risperidone appears more likely to raise prolactin levels than does olanzapine. All in all, local enthusiasm at McLean Hospital over risperidone had abated somewhat by the last editions of this manual, although the drug is still widely used nationally.

In addition, the proportion of patients who clearly do much better while taking risperidone than while taking other, typical antipsychotics seems a good deal less impressive than was the case with clozapine. In earlier editions of the manual, we opined that we may have not yet learned how best to use risperidone. Staying low in dose and going slow with everybody, but even lower and slower with older patients or patients taking multiple medications, still seems wise. In elderly patients, starting risperidone at a dosage of 0.5 mg qd or bid and slowly titrating the drug upward appears prudent, and we tend to keep the dosage below 1–2 mg/day for the first 2 weeks in an attempt to limit side effects.

Clozapine has always seemed more effective than older antipsychotics. Risperidone seems more like a somewhat improved haloperidol: it is as effective as haloperidol but has fewer of the side effects typically associated with the latter drug if the dose is kept low. Our impression has been that clinicians who try to switch patients from clozapine to risperidone are often disappointed in the outcome. Still, at least one study has suggested that over a 1-year period, risperidone was equal in efficacy to clozapine and was much better tolerated (Azorin et al. 2001).

Comparative efficacy studies have not found risperidone or other SGAs to have that many advantages over first-generation agents. For example, in CATIE (Lieberman et al. 2005; Stroup et al. 2006), risperidone was about as well tolerated and effective as perphenazine. However, the trial has been criticized for employing doses of risperidone and other agents that may have been too low. In CATIE, many patients were treated with risperidone at dosages (<3 mg/day) that are often considered to be too low. Dosage ranges were selected in part by the manufacturers. The virtues of risperidone seem to disappear when the dosage is increased because the patient is not improving fast enough to suit the insurance company or hospital administration. In affective psychotic patients, risperidone may be more effective for depression and may be more likely to cause mania, whereas clozapine is more effective for mania-like states and may be effective for depression.

Risperidone is a reasonable first-line antipsychotic that may lead to better control of both negative and positive symptoms and may cause somewhat less tardive dyskinesia and NMS. However, compared with other SGAs, risperidone causes more EPS, particularly when the dosage is pushed much beyond 6 mg/day. The cumulative risk of tardive dyskinesia with risperidone treatment for 1 year is around 0.5%–1% in younger patients and perhaps as high as 2.6% in older patients. A long-acting depot formulation, Risperdal Consta, is available for maintenance therapy. Typical dosages range from 25 to 50 mg every 2 weeks.

Weight gain while taking risperidone is generally much less of a problem than it is with clozapine, olanzapine, or quetiapine. Our sense is that weight gain with risperidone is probably more comparable to that seen with aripiprazole and ziprasidone. That said, there have been cases of diabetic ketoacidosis associated with risperidone use, and we employ the same screening methods for all patients taking SGAs at this point.

Some final thoughts about risperidone use:

1. In changing patients from a typical antipsychotic (or clozapine), it is unwise to discontinue the older antipsychotic, wait 2 weeks, and then start risperidone. Phasing in the new drug slowly while phasing out the older drug should lessen the chance of relapse.
2. Adding risperidone to clozapine has already been tried with some benefit, particularly in patients with an incomplete response and/or oversedation while taking clozapine.
3. Dosages of 6 mg/day or less tend to avoid EPS better than do higher dosages.

Paliperidone

In 2006, 9-hydroxyrisperidone (paliperidone [Invega]), the active metabolite of risperidone, was approved in the United States for the acute and maintenance treatment of schizophrenia. Like risperidone, paliperidone is a D_2/5-HT_2 antagonist with some α_1- and α_2-adrenergic and H_1 antagonism as well. An initial application for the use of paliperidone in acute mania was withdrawn because of insufficient data. In 2014, paliperidone received an approved indication as monotherapy or as an adjunct to mood stabilizers or antidepressants for schizoaffective disorder. Paliperidone represents the first drug indicated for the treatment of schizoaffective disorder. In a 6-week randomized controlled trial involving more than 300 patients (Kane et al. 2007), patients treated with 12 mg/day of adjunctive paliperidone extended release (ER) showed significantly greater benefit on the primary outcome measure (Positive and Negative Syndrome Scale [PANSS]) than did those patients receiving placebo. However, both the 6 and 12 mg/day groups experienced greater benefits than did the placebo-treated group on secondary measures, including the Young Mania Rating Scale and the Hamilton Depression Rating Scale. A second 6-week international study (Marder et al. 2007) also demonstrated the efficacy of paliperidone ER in the monotherapy of schizoaffective disorder.

Schizoaffective disorder is in some ways the poor stepchild of schizophrenia, with relatively few carefully controlled studies completed to date. Historically, schizoaffective disorder has been treated with the combination of antipsychotics and mood stabilizers or antidepressants. The paliperidone studies provide additional evidence that a combination strategy is useful but monotherapy with an antipsychotic may be as useful in many schizoaffective patients. The manufacturer of paliperidone received FDA approval in July 2009 for a long-acting injectable formulation of the drug in the maintenance treatment of schizophrenia. Paliperidone palmitate (Invega Sustenna) is a once-a-month injectable that was studied in trials of 9 and 24 weeks' duration. The doses in these studies were 25, 50, and 150 mg per injection. Patients treated with the paliperidone injection showed greater benefit on the PANSS than did subjects receiving placebo. In addition, paliperidone palmitate was more effective than placebo in preventing relapse in the 24-week trial.

The primary advantage of both paliperidone ER and the injectable formulation over risperidone and its formulations is convenience for some patients. Oral risperidone may require twice-daily dosing in some patients versus once-daily for paliperidone. Likewise, paliperidone palmitate is injected once a month versus twice a month for risperidone. The primary disadvantage of paliperidone relative to risperidone is cost. A generic formulation of risperidone was approved by the FDA in 2008, and the cost will come down further as other generic formulations become available. At this time, there are few data to suggest either efficacy or side-effect advantages of the metabolite over its parent drug. Because the long-acting injectable form of risperidone will not be generic, the even longer-acting paliperidone palmitate might be the better choice for many patients.

Iloperidone

Iloperidone (Fanapt) was approved unexpectedly by the FDA in 2009 for the treatment of schizophrenia. Iloperidone was originally developed many years ago by Roussel. Early trials suggested that it was not as effective as haloperidol or risperidone in the treatment of schizophrenia, and the drug was shelved in 1996. The rights to iloperidone were sold to Novartis, then Titan, and finally to Vanda. In 2007, Vanda received a nonapprovable letter from the FDA with both safety and efficacy issues raised about iloperidone. Nonetheless, additional data resulted in Vanda's getting approval for the drug in 2009.

Iloperidone, like other SGAs, is thought to act primarily as a D_2/5-HT_2 antagonist. The drug also has some activity at the α_2, 5-HT_1, D_1, D_2, D_3, D_4, and D_6 receptors. Iloperidone is well absorbed orally and has a peak serum plasma level in 2–4 hours. It has a half-life of around 24–36 hours in most subjects. Iloperidone is a substrate for both CYP2D6 and CYP3A4. Drugs such as fluoxetine can more than double the serum levels of iloperidone, and carbamazepine can substantially reduce serum levels. Thus, adjustments in dosing may be necessary for patients who are concurrently taking drugs that are CYP2D6 or CYP3A4 inhibitors or inducers.

The efficacy of iloperidone was established in two Phase III trials in the United States. In a 6-week trial ($N=706$), iloperidone at either of two dosage ranges (12–16 and 20–24 mg/day) was superior to placebo and equal to an active comparator at the endpoint in the treatment of schizophrenia (Potkin et al. 2008). Likewise, in a 4-week trial ($N=604$), 12 mg bid was superior to placebo in treating both positive and negative symptoms of schizophrenia (Kane et al. 2008).

The most common side effects in the clinical trials were dizziness, dry mouth, fatigue, somnolence, tachycardia, orthostatic hypotension, and weight gain. Tachycardia, dizziness, and weight gain appear to be dose-related, with higher dosages (24 mg/day) causing more problems than lower dosages

(12 mg/day). The weight gain and metabolic effects seem more in line with what has been observed with risperidone than with what has been reported with either olanzapine or clozapine. Across short- and long-term trials, the average weight gain was about 2 kg.

Iloperidone has at least two disadvantages versus other SGAs at this time. One is the slow dosing titration that is required to limit the hypotension seen in clinical trials. About 5% of patients taking iloperidone at a dosage of 24 mg/day experienced hypotension, and more aggressive titration was associated with greater risk of hypotension and syncope. The recommended starting dosage is 1 mg bid, with doubling of the dosage daily to a target dosage of 6–12 mg bid (12–24 mg/day). In the clinical trials, the comparison antipsychotic often seemed to work more rapidly because little titration was required for haloperidol or risperidone. A second disadvantage is that iloperidone can prolong QT intervals. At the higher dosage, there was an increase in QTc intervals by 9 msec. Drugs that inhibit CYP2D6 and CYP3A4 further prolonged the QTc interval. Thus, caution must be exercised in combining iloperidone with CYP450 inhibitors, as well as drugs that are known to prolong QTc intervals, including quinidine, chlorpromazine, and thioridazine.

It is unclear to us exactly where iloperidone is going to fit in the treatment of schizophrenia. It is not going to be a first-line agent because of the dosing and QTc issues. Iloperidone is more expensive than either first-generation drugs or generic SGAs. Patients who cannot tolerate or do not respond to other SGAs might be a candidate for iloperidone.

Olanzapine

Olanzapine (Zyprexa) was introduced to the U.S. market in 1996. Like other SGAs, it has a high binding ratio of 5-HT$_2$ to D$_2$ receptors. The receptor-binding affinities of olanzapine appear to lie somewhere between the very broad receptor effects of clozapine and the more narrow receptor binding of risperidone. Like clozapine, olanzapine is an antagonist of dopamine receptors (D$_1$–D$_4$) and the 5-HT$_2$ receptor. In addition, it is antihistaminic, is anticholinergic, and blocks α_1-adrenergic receptors. Olanzapine is metabolized primarily via the enzymes CYP1A2 and, to a lesser extent, CYP2D6. Olanzapine appears to be at least as effective as haloperidol in the short-term treatment of schizophrenia. It may be better than haloperidol in improving negative symptoms, concurrent depression and suicidality, and cognition. In addition, in premarketing studies, olanzapine 10–20 mg/day was associated with significant improvement in positive symptoms, including delusions, hallucinations, and thought disorder.

Olanzapine is still among the most commonly used second-generation agents even though it is also among the most expensive. CATIE suggested that olanzapine might be somewhat more efficacious overall than other second-generation agents in that it was less likely to be discontinued (Stroup et al. 2006). A full 64% of patients discontinued olanzapine before the 18-month trial was completed, versus 74%–82% of patients discontinuing the comparator antipsychotics. Olanzapine was also more likely than the comparison agents (perphenazine, risperidone, quetiapine, and ziprasidone) to be associated with metabolic side effects.

Olanzapine is now approved for the treatment of a variety of disorders other than schizophrenia. Olanzapine was the first SGA approved for the treatment of acute mania. It probably works faster than and at least as effectively as does lithium or valproate. In addition, olanzapine became the third drug, after lithium and lamotrigine, to show benefit in the prevention of mania and depression in patients with bipolar I disorder. Olanzapine by intramuscular injection has been approved for the acute treatment of agitation in patients with schizophrenia and bipolar disorder. Olanzapine combined with fluoxetine became the first drug approved for the treatment of bipolar depression. As previously reported, olanzapine also appears to have a role in treating psychotic depression and as an augmenting agent in treating unipolar depression (see subsection "Unipolar Depression" earlier in this chapter).

Olanzapine does not appear to be as useful as clozapine in the treatment of refractory schizophrenia. Although comparison studies have generally found the drugs to be equally effective in this context (Bitter et al. 2004; Tollefson et al. 2001), CATIE suggested the superiority of clozapine to olanzapine in treating resistant schizophrenia (McEvoy et al. 2006). Olanzapine is a fairly "dirty" drug in that it affects multiple neurotransmitter systems, but it is not quite as dirty as clozapine. This dirtiness contributes to clozapine's toxicity but may also be important in the efficacy of the drug in more refractory cases.

Head-to-head trials of olanzapine and risperidone in the treatment of refractory depression also suggest that the drugs are probably equally effective but differ in side-effect profiles. Olanzapine is associated with more weight gain and sedation, whereas risperidone is more likely to increase prolactin levels and produce EPS.

Olanzapine has a clear advantage over high-potency typical agents such as haloperidol in that it is associated with fewer EPS. In CATIE (Lieberman et al. 2005), however, the rate of EPS with perphenazine was about the same as it was with the SGAs, including olanzapine. Olanzapine has been shown in multiple studies to produce fewer EPS than does haloperidol. In acute trials, the only extrapyramidal symptom reliably noted at a greater rate than with placebo was akathisia, and the incidence of this effect increases with dose. At least 10% of patients develop akathisia in an acute 6-week trial at dosages of 10–15 mg/day. We have found that propranolol 10 mg bid or tid can help with this problem. However, some patients have a significant worsening of postural hypotension with even small additions of β-blockers, so caution is advised. Dystonic reactions and dyskinesias appear to be somewhat less common with olanzapine at usual dosages. However, patients do tend to report more severe parkinsonian symptoms with increasing dosages of the drug, including feeling stiffer and more slowed down. About 20% of patients will report Parkinson's-type symptoms at dosages above 10 mg/day. Anticholinergic agents clearly help if parkinsonism develops.

The rate of tardive dyskinesia with olanzapine appears to be markedly less than that of first-generation agents but is not zero as it appears to be with clozapine. Tardive dyskinesia occurs at a rate of around 0.5%–1% per year of treatment, which is 10–15 times less frequent than with haloperidol at comparison doses. Even with less aggressive dosing of haloperidol (e.g., 2–5 mg/day) the rates of tardive dyskinesia in olanzapine-treated patients appear to be a fraction of those reported with haloperidol. We recommend periodically assessing patients who are taking any antipsychotic for signs of tardive dyskinesia at regular intervals.

NMS is uncommon but not unheard of with olanzapine use. There are several reports in the literature of olanzapine inducing NMS, including in patients who had previously developed NMS while taking first-generation agents. Our limited experience with NMS in olanzapine-treated patients is that, as with clozapine, the presentation may be atypical, with fewer and less severe EPS than are seen with FGAs.

Anticholinergic side effects such as constipation and dry mouth occur in 5%–10% of patients taking olanzapine at therapeutic dosages. Like risperidone and clozapine, olanzapine produces α-adrenergic blockade, resulting in a dose-related increase in orthostasis and dizziness. We suggest monitoring orthostatic blood pressure, particularly with older patients and those with a history of postural hypotension. Support stockings help orthostasis in older patients. These orthostatic effects are not nearly as dramatic as the effects that can occur with clozapine.

The most problematic side effects with long-term maintenance use of olanzapine are weight gain and sedation. At least 29% of patients gained more than 7% of their body weight in a 6-week trial, and 5.4 kg, or about 12 lb, is the average weight gain with long-term use (Allison et al. 1999). However, we have seen some patients gain 50 lb or more in a year. This weight gain is terribly distressing for many patients. Large weight gains have been thought to be associated with insulin resistance and dyslipidemias, although the former has not been clearly demonstrated. As with other SGAs, patients taking olanzapine should be screened and monitored for metabolic symptoms (see overview of SGAs and Table 4–3 earlier in this chapter).

The weight gain associated with olanzapine appears to be, at least in part, from an increased appetite, and we warn patients that olanzapine can result in a desire to eat more. Most of the weight gain that occurs with olanzapine appears to occur in the first 6 months, with gain then appearing to plateau for up to 3 years. Patients with BMIs < 23 (i.e., thinner patients) have been thought to be most at risk for gaining substantial weight, but this may be an artifact of starting at a lower weight. Obese patients tend to gain much less weight and eventually may actually lose weight. Counting calories or participating in a food monitoring system such as that offered by Weight Watchers and engaging in more rigorous and regular exercise can be very helpful.

Pharmacologically, a number of strategies are worth considering to help with weight gain. The combination pill of olanzapine with the μ opioid receptor antagonist samidorphan (Lybalvi) appears to mitigate some of the risk of weight gain associated with olanzapine. It is approved for the treatment of schizophrenia and bipolar disorder. Almost twice as many patients are likely to gain > 10% of body weight with olanzapine alone (30%) as with the combination with samidorphan (18%) over 24 weeks of treatment (Correll et al. 2020b).

Another combination pill that can help mitigate weight gain associated with a number of different antipsychotics is naltrexone-bupropion (Contrave). This combination pill has been approved for weight management combined with diet in patients with a BMI >30. Although it is not clear that the medication has a prophylactic benefit against olanzapine-associated weight gain, it may be used in conjunction with diet in patients who are struggling with olanzapine-associated weight gain.

An additional medication that has been helpful for some patients with SGA-induced weight gain is topiramate. Topiramate appears to be useful at dosages of 50–100 mg/day as an appetite suppressant.

Metformin has been increasingly used to mitigate antipsychotic-induced weight gain. Although not all studies have shown a benefit of metformin, more than a dozen controlled studies have suggested that concomitant metformin decreases the chance of significant weight gain and can lower BMI in patients taking antipsychotics (de Silva et al. 2016). We have used metformin at dosages of 500 mg bid or tid with mixed success in inducing weight loss or preventing weight gain.

Another class of diabetes medications that holds much promise for mitigating significant weight gain is the glucagon-like-peptide 1 (GLP-1) agonists. These drugs, which include semaglutide (Wegovy) and dulaglutide (Trulicity), are associated with substantial weight loss in type II diabetes. Semaglutide was approved for general weight loss in 2022 in those patients with a BMI>30 or a BMI>27 if associated with at least one weight-related condition such as diabetes, elevated cholesterol, or hypertension. In the studies leading to FDA approval of GLP-1 agonists for the treatment of obesity, more than half of all patients studied lost more than 10% of their body weight. It is probable that many patients with metabolic syndrome associated with SGAs would potentially be candidates for this drug. Semaglutide is once-a-week injectable that starts at 0.25 mg the first month and is increased monthly to a target dose of 2.4 mg at month 5. The most common side effects of the GLP-1 agonists are gastrointestinal, particularly nausea.

Last, data in rodents indicate that mifepristone, a glucocorticoid receptor antagonist, blocks and reverses weight gain due to olanzapine and other antipsychotics (Beebe et al. 2006). Moreover, mifepristone blocks antipsychotic-induced weight gain and weight gain in healthy control subjects (Gross et al. 2009). (Note that the second author [A.F.S.] has a conflict of interest involving mifepristone.)

Olanzapine is very sedating for many patients and should be taken at bedtime if possible. About 40% of patients will report daytime somnolence at a dosage of 15 mg/day. Taking olanzapine on an empty stomach about an hour before bedtime may increase the nighttime sedation and reduce the daytime somnolence. The use of modafinil in doses of 100–200 mg in the morning may help mitigate the somnolence.

There are no reported cases of agranulocytosis, and no blood count monitoring is recommended. Still, some reversible neutropenias and hemolytic anemias have been seen in olanzapine-treated animals. Significant elevations in hepatic transaminases (to greater than three times the upper limit of normal) occur in about 2% of patients, but 5% or more of patients have minor elevations. We are unaware of any serious hepatic problems associated with olanzapine, and monitoring of hepatic enzymes is not indicated.

Olanzapine is usually started at 2.5–5 mg/day, and the dosage is usually increased to 10 mg/day in the first week. Some patients require the usual maximum dosage of 20 mg/day, although we know of some cases in which dosages of 30–40 mg/day have been used successfully. Lieberman has collected a series of patients with refractory conditions in whom responses occurred only when dosages of approximately 60–80 mg/day were used. Some patients complain of somnolence and constipation even at 5 mg/day. In the past, patients often found it difficult to break the tablets, and the manufacturer suggests that doing so breaks the film that protects the active drug from the oxidative effects of exposure to the environment. The result can be that the drug loses its potency if the tablet is broken and not taken within a few hours. However, the drug is now available in 2.5-mg, 5-mg, 7.5-mg, 10-mg, 15-mg, and 20-mg tablets. An intramuscular formulation of olanzapine is available for acute management at dosages of 2.5–10 mg per day. In addition, a long-acting injectable form of olanzapine (Zyprexa Relprevv) is available and is typically dosed at 150–300 mg every 2 weeks or 405 mg every 4 weeks.

Olanzapine appears to be fairly safe in overdose. Up to 1 month's supply (300 mg) has been taken with no ill effects other than drowsiness and slurred speech. Because overdoses often involve multiple drugs, including alcohol, there may be a risk of synergistic central nervous system depression effects, resulting in more serious outcomes, but none have been reported.

Quetiapine

Quetiapine (Seroquel) was released in the United States in 1998 and is now the most commonly prescribed SGA in the United States. Like clozapine, the drug appears to have low affinity for D_1 and D_2 receptors but relatively high affinity for D_4 receptors (Seeman and Tallerico 1999). Clozapine, olanzapine, and quetiapine all seem to have more pronounced effects on mesolimbic dopamine activity than on nigrostriatal pathways, a phenomenon that accounts for their low tendency to produce EPS. Like other SGAs, quetiapine appears to have high affinity for 5-HT_2 receptors. Quetiapine does not appear to have very significant anticholinergic or antihistaminic effects, but it does block α_1-adrenergic receptors to some extent. One potential drawback of the current preparation of quetiapine is its very short half-life—the average half-life is about 2–3 hours—and quetiapine therefore needs to be given at least two times a day. For chronically psychotic patients, this multiple dosing is less than ideal and might result in compliance problems. Fortunately, a sustained-release preparation, quetiapine extended-release tablets, is now available.

Quetiapine has been studied in large groups of schizophrenic patients and has been compared with placebo, chlorpromazine, and haloperidol. In general, quetiapine has been consistently more effective than placebo and at least as effective as comparison drugs in controlling positive symptoms (Gray 1998). After several weeks of treatment, quetiapine also appears to improve negative symptoms. Although quetiapine appears to be a generally effective and well-tolerated antipsychotic, it has not been studied or marketed with the same vigor as have risperidone and olanzapine. Thus, it currently is used much less frequently than either of these drugs, although recently its use has been increasing sharply.

As with other SGAs, quetiapine is effective in the acute treatment of mania and was approved in 2004 for this indication (Ghaemi and Katzow 1999). Adding quetiapine to a mood stabilizer such as lithium is more effective in treating bipolar disorder than using lithium alone (Sachs et al. 2004). There are data suggesting quetiapine at dosages of 300–600 mg/day is an effective treatment for the anxiety component of bipolar depression (Gao et al. 2006). Quetiapine seems to have good antidepressant properties in bipolar depression as well. FDA approval was granted to quetiapine as the first monotherapy for the treatment of the depressed phase of bipolar disorder. It joined Symbyax and now lurasidone, cariprazine, and lumateperone as the treatments for bipolar depression. Additionally, work suggests that quetiapine is a useful maintenance treatment in bipolar disorder. The use of quetiapine as adjunctive treatment and as a monotherapy in the treatment of unipolar depression appears to be effective, but quetiapine was approved only as an adjunctive agent in resistant depression (for discussion, see subsection "Unipolar Depression" earlier in this chapter). Finally, quetiapine has shown efficacy in the treatment of GAD but was not approved secondary to safety concerns raised by the FDA.

Quetiapine has been examined in the treatment of childhood autism but appears to be poorly tolerated and not very effective in this population. Risperidone, which is the only drug approved in the treatment of autism-related behavioral symptoms, appears to be a better choice. Studies are under way to examine the utility of quetiapine in treating psychotic depression and impulsive aggression. At least one study reported success with quetiapine in the treatment of some dimensions of borderline personality (Hilger et al. 2003).

The most common side effects of quetiapine, compared with placebo, are somnolence and dizziness. Quetiapine can produce orthostatic hypotension in about 7% of patients, and 1% may experience frank syncope with rapid titration of the dose. Thus, for outpatients, we tend to use a starting dosage of 50–100 mg/day and increase the dosage in increments of about 100 mg/day, with the goal of achieving a therapeutic dosage of 400–800 mg/day by the end of the second week of treatment. For inpatients, we start at 100 mg and then increase the dose more aggressively, in increments of 100–200 mg, with a target dosage of 400–800 mg/day by day 6 for patients with schizophrenia or bipolar disorder. It is a good idea to check orthostatic blood pressure daily with a more aggressive titration.

Somnolence is experienced by at least 18% of patients taking quetiapine in 6-week clinical trials, but our experience is that as many as 50% of patients complain of somnolence when the dosage is increased above 400 mg/day. Since we have found that most patients with schizophrenia require total daily doses above 300 mg, somnolence is a problem for many patients. We try to shift most of the dose to the evening, so a 400-mg total daily dose is divided into 100 mg in the morning and 300 mg in the evening. This seems to work out for most patients and does not appear to detract from the efficacy of the drug. (Again, modafinil at dosages of 100–200 mg/day can help with the daytime somnolence.) For bipolar depression, the target dosage for quetiapine is 300 mg/day. Although 600 mg/day was also found to be effective, it was no more effective than 300 mg/day and was less well tolerated (Thase et al. 2006).

The weight gain associated with quetiapine seems to be less than that seen with olanzapine and clozapine but more than that seen with other SGAs.

About one-fourth of patients experience an increase in body weight of greater than 7% in 3- to 6-week trials, but this may be an underestimate of what can be expected at higher daily doses. As with other SGAs, monitoring and controlling food intake are the keys to weight management with this drug.

The concern about cataracts in patients treated with quetiapine was overstated. Although dogs did develop cataracts with chronic quetiapine therapy, postmarketing surveillance has not revealed an increased rate of cataract formation in human patients. Infrequent cataract formation has been associated with a number of FGAs and SGAs. The manufacturer recommends ocular examinations every 6 months, but few practitioners follow this recommendation, and we have seen little evidence thus far that it is warranted.

A small percentage of quetiapine-treated patients also exhibit transient and asymptomatic increases in liver enzymes. There have been no reports thus far of hematological abnormalities, but a reversible sinus tachycardia has often been seen.

EPS are not common with quetiapine. As with olanzapine, there have been rare reports of tardive dyskinesia, and these reports are expected to increase as more patients use quetiapine for longer periods of time. Although no clear estimates of the frequency of tardive dyskinesia with quetiapine are available, the frequency is unlikely to be any higher than the low frequency of tardive dyskinesia seen with olanzapine (0.5%–1% per year).

A sustained-release formulation of quetiapine is also currently available. The risk of serious complications from an overdose of quetiapine is small. We are unaware of any fatalities with overdoses up to 10 g.

Ziprasidone

In the year 2000, ziprasidone (Geodon), another SGA, was released to the U.S. market. Ziprasidone is fairly popular in Sweden, where it was released in 1998, and has an efficacy and side-effect profile that will all but ensure a niche for it in the increasingly crowded U.S. market for SGAs.

Ziprasidone, like other SGAs, has a complex pharmacology. It appears to be an agonist at the 5-HT_{1A} receptor and an antagonist of 5-HT_{1D} and 5-HT_{2C} receptors. Ziprasidone has been shown to enhance the release of dopamine in the dorsolateral prefrontal cortex and block the reuptake of both norepinephrine and serotonin (Markowitz et al. 1999). These attributes should make ziprasidone a good antidepressant and anxiolytic as well as an effective antipsychotic. The drug appears to show relatively weak affinity for muscarinic and α-adrenergic receptors.

In studies of schizophrenia and schizoaffective disorder, ziprasidone appeared to be as effective as 15 mg of haloperidol in improving positive psychotic symptoms, as measured by the Brief Psychiatric Rating Scale or the PANSS for schizophrenia (Goff et al. 1998). However, ziprasidone was superior to haloperidol in its effects on negative symptoms and depression. CATIE, on the other hand, did not find advantages in the efficacy of ziprasidone compared with the midpotency agent perphenazine (Lieberman et al. 2005; Stroup et al. 2006). As expected, ziprasidone has been shown to substantially reduce depressive symptoms, as measured by the Montgomery-Åsberg Depression Rating Scale (MADRS), in patients with schizophrenia or schizoaffective disorder. The pharmacology of ziprasidone suggests that it should have antidepressant and anxiolytic effects in nonpsychotic patients as well.

Ziprasidone is an effective antimanic drug and is FDA approved for this indication. Two double-blind trials have demonstrated that ziprasidone at dosages of 80–160 mg/day is effective in the treatment of mania (Keck et al. 2003b). Ziprasidone appears to separate from placebo in mania very early (i.e., within 3 days). Also, preliminary studies indicate that ziprasidone may help in bipolar depression. The intramuscular form of ziprasidone is rapidly effective for treating agitation in psychotic patients, including patients with bipolar mania. Preliminary studies of ziprasidone augmentation of antidepressants have not necessarily shown benefits for the treatment of unipolar depression.

Ziprasidone is generally well tolerated. Most notable is that ziprasidone was at one time unique among the second-generation agents in not being as associated with significant weight gain (Allison et al. 1999). However, many other SGAs, such as lurasidone, lumateperone, aripiprazole, and cariprazine, now also have a lower proclivity for weight gain. As with other SGAs, ziprasidone is associated with a low incidence of EPS, much like with olanzapine and probably better than with risperidone, although head-to-head trials have not been completed.

The most common side effects observed in clinical trials with ziprasidone are drowsiness, dyspepsia, dizziness, constipation, and nausea. Ziprasidone causes weight loss and a decrease in triglycerides (Simpson et al. 2004). There appears to be a dose-related increase in α-adrenergic blockade that can result in dizziness and orthostatic hypotension. Still, these α-adrenergic receptor–blocking effects are much less common than with clozapine and probably are similar to what is seen with risperidone and olanzapine. Concerns regarding conduction effects of the drug have limited its adoption as a first-line therapy in the United States. Ziprasidone is associated with mild to moderate QTc interval prolongation in about 4%–5% of patients taking the drug. The clinical significance of this finding is still unclear, as is the issue of whether it is prudent to follow the electrocardiogram (ECG) in some patients. Postmarketing surveillance has not found a clinically significant effect of QTc prolongation in ziprasidone-treated patients. In general, we tend not to follow ECGs routinely in ziprasidone-treated patients. However, patients with a known history of arrhythmia should have a baseline and repeat ECG.

Ziprasidone has a short half-life (5 hours) that necessitates twice-a-day dosing. The dosage range that appears most effective in clinical studies is 60–80 mg bid or 120–160 mg/day (Keck et al. 1998). The drug should be started at a dosage of 40 mg bid, and the dosage should be increased to 80 mg bid after 1 week. This strategy was used in the mania studies and can now be applied in treating patients with schizophrenia. Earlier experience suggested that initiation of ziprasidone at a dosage of 40 mg/day was not particularly effective. Another major advantage of ziprasidone is that, like olanzapine and aripiprazole, it is available in an intramuscular form. The usual dosage of the intramuscular form is 10 mg every 2 hours as needed, to a maximum dosage of 40 mg/day. In acute emergency situations, SGAs have generally not been preferred because oral dosing requires more time to achieve maximum benefits. Through the intramuscular route, ziprasidone can be administered quickly and reliably. Preliminary reports suggest that intramuscular ziprasidone is as effective as intramuscular haloperidol in treating acute psychosis and agitation but less likely to cause EPS.

Aripiprazole

Aripiprazole (Abilify) is an SGA with a somewhat unique pharmacological profile. It is a partial agonist at D_2 and $5-HT_{1A}$ receptors and also has the $5-HT_2$ properties found with other SGAs. Among the other pharmacological properties of aripiprazole is its affinity as a presynaptic D_2 autoreceptor agonist. Thus, it can enhance as well as inhibit dopamine release in specific regions of the brain. Aripiprazole's pharmacological profile should indicate that it has antipsychotic, antimanic, and antidepressant properties. It was the first adjunctive treatment approved, in 2007, for unipolar major depression.

Aripiprazole is approved for the treatment of schizophrenia and was the latest second-generation agent to be approved in the United States. At least four controlled trials have confirmed the role of aripiprazole in the treatment of schizophrenia. In a meta-analysis of 1,545 patients in placebo-controlled trials, aripiprazole was more effective than placebo and at least as effective as risperidone and haloperidol (Carson et al. 2002). Aripiprazole was the only SGA that was not evaluated in CATIE. Thus, we do not know how it fares in a more real-world setting compared with other SGAs and with perphenazine. In industry-sponsored trials, aripiprazole was superior to haloperidol in the treatment of negative symptoms. Also, aripiprazole was as effective as haloperidol in preventing relapse in 1-year studies of schizophrenia but resulted in a lower dropout rate secondary to a better side-effect profile.

Aripiprazole is one of the only antipsychotics to be approved in the acute and maintenance treatment of adolescents with schizophrenia. There are relatively few controlled trials of antipsychotics in adolescents with schizophrenia. Studies with 13- to 17-year-olds with schizophrenia indicate that aripiprazole is effective at fixed dosages of 10 or 30 mg/day. The higher dosage is not significantly more effective than the lower dosage. The starting dosage in treating adults with schizophrenia is 5–10 mg/day, with a maximum recommended dosage of 30 mg/day. If the patient is activated at a dosage of 10 mg/day, a lower dosage should be tried (e.g., 5 mg/day). In adolescents, the starting dose is 2 mg, with most patients showing benefits at 10 mg/day. The maximum recommended dosage in adolescents with schizophrenia is 30 mg/day.

As of this writing, multiple placebo-controlled trials have shown benefit for aripiprazole in treating acute mania. The antimanic effects of aripiprazole were superior to those of placebo, and the effects were seen within 4 days (Keck et al. 2003a). Aripiprazole appeared to significantly reduce the irritability, lability, and aggressiveness associated with acute mania. Studies have also been completed that indicate that aripiprazole is an effective maintenance treatment in bipolar I disorder. It appears to delay the onset of mania in bipolar I patients. Aripiprazole is thus one of only a handful of agents to have received FDA approval for use in the maintenance treatment of bipolar disorder. In the maintenance trials, aripiprazole clearly delayed time to the next manic episode. The effects of aripiprazole on preventing depression could not be adequately evaluated in these pivotal trials. Aripiprazole is also one of two SGAs, along with risperidone, to be approved in children. Studies in acute bipolar I disorder in patients ages 10–17 years indicate that aripiprazole is effective at dosages of 10 and 30 mg/day. The efficacy of aripiprazole as a maintenance treatment in children with bipolar disorder is not yet established.

Aripiprazole has been evaluated in the treatment of bipolar depression in adults but has not shown reliable benefit in randomized controlled trials, at least as a monotherapy. It is anticipated, but not definitively proven, that aripiprazole should be useful as an adjunctive treatment for bipolar depression just as it is for unipolar depression.

Aripiprazole has a long half-life (about 50–80 hours), so steady state is not achieved for about 2 weeks. The long half-life allows once-a-day dosing. Long-acting depot forms of aripiprazole for maintenance therapy in schizophrenia and short-acting intramuscular forms for acute agitation are available.

The side-effect profile of aripiprazole may be significantly better than that of most other SGAs. The data over 1 year suggest that, like ziprasidone, aripiprazole should be fairly weight-neutral, and aripiprazole lacks any significant effect on QTc intervals. Aripiprazole is one of the few antipsychotics, first- or second-generation, that does not increase prolactin levels and that may even lower these levels. In terms of EPS, there is some question as to whether aripiprazole may have a greater tendency to cause akathisia, but the answer to this question awaits head-to-head comparison trials. Agitation and akathisia certainly seem to occur in some of our aripiprazole-treated patients. The most common side effects seen with aripiprazole in Phase III trials were nausea, tremor, insomnia, headache, and agitation.

The side-effect profile of aripiprazole varies by the age of the patient and the indication for which it is applied. For example, sedation and EPS are much bigger problems in children and adolescents treated with aripiprazole than they are with adults. On the other hand, akathisia is three times more common in depressed adult patients treated with aripiprazole, even at lower doses, than it is in patients with schizophrenia.

In adults with depression, the typical starting adjunctive dosage of aripiprazole is 2–5 mg/day. We have seen patients for whom 2 mg is an adequate dose. On the other hand, we have also seen depressed patients who tolerate and respond to the medication at dosages much higher than the maximum recommended dosage of 15 mg/day. For adults with bipolar disorder, we still tend to start at doses lower than the manufacturer recommends: 5 or 10 mg, with titration to 30 mg as tolerated and needed. The same holds true for adults with schizophrenia. For patients who have a harder time adhering to taking their medication daily and for whom a long-acting injectable is less palatable, oral aripiprazole became available with a sensor (Abilify MyCite) in 2017. This formulation of aripiprazole comes with a tiny ingestible sensor that reacts with stomach acids when swallowed. The patient wears a plastic sensor on the left side of their body, above the lower end of the ribcage. This sensor confirms that the pill was swallowed, and this information can be uploaded to a smartphone app. In addition, the data also can be transmitted automatically to a Web portal for the clinician so that the prescriber can also track the patient's adherence. Although a digital pill is clever, it is probably not ideal for paranoid patients, who may misinterpret the type of monitoring that is occurring. In addition, the aripiprazole digital pill is an expensive option relative to generic aripiprazole. A less expensive and equally effective option, if possible, may be having a family member monitor and administer the oral medication.

Brexpiprazole

Brexpiprazole is an analog of aripiprazole that is approved in the treatment of schizophrenia and is the adjunctive treatment of major depression. Like aripiprazole, it is a partial agonist of the D_2, D_3, and $5\text{-}HT_{1A}$ receptors, while acting as an antagonist of the $5\text{-}HT_{2A}$ receptor.

Brexpiprazole was evaluated in the adjunctive treatment of major depression in two pivotal trials (Thase et al. 2015a, 2015b). These two trials consisted of patients with symptoms that met DSM-IV-TR (American Psychiatric Association 2000) criteria for major depressive disorder (MDD) who had not responded adequately to at least one but no more than three antidepressant trials of adequate dose and duration for the current depressive episode. Subjects were randomly assigned to receive 2 mg/day of adjunctive brexpiprazole or placebo in one trial and 1 or 3 mg/day of adjunctive brexpiprazole or placebo in the other trial. Each trial lasted 6 weeks. The 2 mg/day and 3 mg/day dosages were superior for improving depressive symptoms on the MADRS, but the 1 mg/day dosage did not separate from placebo. Thus, the starting adjunctive dosage of brexpiprazole combined with a standard antidepressant is 0.5–1 mg/day, with a target dosage of 2–3 mg/day.

The efficacy of brexpiprazole in schizophrenia was evaluated in two Phase III studies (Correll et al. 2015; Kane et al. 2015a). Patients who were having an acute exacerbation of schizophrenia were randomly assigned to receive brexpiprazole 2–4 mg/day or placebo for 6 weeks of treatment. In one study, both the 2 mg/day and 4 mg/day dosages of brexpiprazole demonstrated significant improvement over placebo on the PANSS, whereas only the 4 mg/day dosage separated on the primary outcome measure in the second trial. Still, a number of secondary outcome measures were positive with the 2 mg/day dosage. Therefore, most patients with schizophrenia start brexpiprazole at 1 mg/day, and the target dosage is 2–4 mg/day.

Brexpiprazole, like aripiprazole, has a good metabolic side-effect profile relative to other SGAs. That being said, about 7% of patients gained weight while taking various doses of brexpiprazole versus 2% of placebo-treated subjects. The average weight gain was about 1.45 kg with brexpiprazole treatment at 6 weeks versus 0.45 kg with placebo treatment. There are few data from long-term studies to shed light on the risk of significant weight gain with continued use. Akathisia is one of the more common side effects of brexpiprazole and is more likely to occur in depressed patients than in schizophrenic patients. The rate of akathisia was about twice the rate in the depression trials as in the schizophrenia trials (9% vs. 5%, respectively). This higher rate of akathisia was seen in the aripiprazole trials as well. The greater likelihood of akathisia in patients with MDD may be the result of concurrent antidepressant treatment, greater sensitivity to side effects in depressed patients, or some unknown factor. As a general consideration, akathisia in a depressed and suicidal patient would seem problematic. However, brexpiprazole has been studied in the subset of more anxious depressed patients and appeared to be well tolerated (McIntyre et al. 2016).

Brexpiprazole is a substrate for both CYP2D6 and CYP3A4. Thus, dosage adjustment would be indicated in slow metabolizers or those patients taking concurrent strong inhibitors or inducers of those hepatic isoenzymes.

There are no comparative studies as of this writing of brexpiprazole augmentation in major depression with any other augmentation strategy. Brexpiprazole does appear to be a "me-too" drug without clear advantages over using the much less expensive, generic form of aripiprazole. That being said, as with all antipsychotics, there may be patients who respond to, or tolerate better, one drug over the other.

A potential new indication for brexpiprazole is in the treatment of agitation associated with Alzheimer's disease. Although not approved for this indication, brexpiprazole has shown more promise in Phase III clinical trials than other SGAs, with potentially less of a side-effect burden. However, additional trials would be needed for FDA approval.

Lurasidone

Lurasidone has $D_2/5\text{-}HT_2$, $5\text{-}HT_7$ antagonist properties and is also a partial agonist at the $5\text{-}HT_{1A}$ receptor. From this pharmacological profile it would be expected that lurasidone would be useful in both psychotic and mood disorders. Lurasidone was first approved for the treatment of schizophrenia in 2010, and in 2013 it was granted FDA approval for monotherapy and adjunctive treatment of bipolar depression. The efficacy of lurasidone for the treatment of schizophrenia was established primarily by three registration trials known as the Program to Evaluate the Antipsychotic Response of Lurasidone (PEARL) trials (Loebel et al. 2014b; McEvoy et al. 2013; Meltzer et al. 2011). The PEARL studies were large, multicenter randomized controlled trials that evaluated lurasidone relative to placebo alone (PEARL 1) and active comparators olanzapine (PEARL 2) and quetiapine (PEARL 3). The acute trials used lurasidone at dosages of 40–120 mg/day for 6 weeks. In PEARL 1, the 40 mg/day and 120 mg/day, but not 80 mg/day, dosages were more effective than placebo. However, all dosages of lurasidone were effective in the other two PEARL trials, as were olanzapine and quetiapine. Lurasidone appeared rapidly effective, with separation from placebo evident in the first 2 weeks in all three studies.

The efficacy of lurasidone in bipolar depression was established in two controlled 6-week trials. In the monotherapy trial, lurasidone was compared with placebo, and in the adjunctive trial lurasidone or placebo was added to lithium or valproate (Loebel et al. 2013, 2014a). Patients in the monotherapy trial were randomly assigned to receive either lower-dose lurasidone (20–60 mg/day) or higher-dose lurasidone (80–120 mg/day); flexible dosing of 20–120 mg/day was used in the adjunctive trial. In both trials, both the higher and lower dosages were effective in treating bipolar depression as measured by the MADRS and the Clinical Global Impression (CGI) Scale, although higher dosages were not necessarily more effective than the lower dosages. Lurasidone has also been reported to be effective in major depression with mixed features (Suppes et al.

2016). The drug produced great superiority over placebo in patients with mixed features of insomnia and overactivity/agitation.

Lurasidone has generally been well tolerated in clinical trials. Discontinuation rates due to side effects were about the same for both the lurasidone-treated patients and the patients receiving placebo in both the schizophrenia and bipolar depression trials. The most common side effects seen were somnolence, akathisia, EPS, and GI symptoms. The akathisia and EPS appear to be dose related, with higher doses being more poorly tolerated. As with other antipsychotic-induced akathisia, β-blockers and benzodiazepines appear to be helpful. We find that giving the entire dose at bedtime appears to be useful in mitigating daytime somnolence. Taking the drug with food seems to help the GI effects. Lurasidone is less likely to cause weight gain and metabolic effects than olanzapine and quetiapine and seems comparable to aripiprazole in this regard. Elevations in serum glucose and lipid levels appeared to be modest in the clinical trials and comparable to the changes seen in the patients receiving placebo. Thus, lurasidone appears to be better tolerated than many of the SGAs in our experience.

Lurasidone is a substrate for the CYP3A4 isoenzyme and should generally not be used with potent inhibitors of CYP3A4 such as ketoconazole and ritonavir. Likewise, patients should be advised to avoid grapefruit juice because it inhibits the metabolism of lurasidone and increases the likelihood of dose-related side effects such as akathisia. Conversely, strong inducers of CYP3A4, such as rifampin and carbamazepine, reduce the efficacy of lurasidone by dropping serum levels of the drug, and higher lurasidone doses may need to be prescribed.

The recommended starting dosage of lurasidone is 40 mg/day in schizophrenia and 20 mg/day in bipolar depression. The dose may then be increased by 20 mg every day or two. We have found that patients with schizophrenia often seem to do better at dosages in the range of 60–120 mg/day, whereas bipolar patients seem to do fine at dosages of 20–60 mg/day.

Asenapine

Asenapine was approved for the treatment of schizophrenia and manic and mixed states associated with bipolar I disorder in late 2009. As with other SGAs, it is a potent 5-HT$_2$ and D$_2$ antagonist. However, it differs from some of the atypicals in having broad effects on multiple dopamine receptors (D$_1$–D$_4$) and high affinity for many serotonin receptors, including as an antagonist at 5-HT$_1$, 5-HT$_2$, 5-HT$_3$, 5-HT$_5$, and 5-HT$_7$ receptors. Similar to lurasidone, asenapine is a partial agonist at the 5-HT$_{1A}$ receptor. In addition, asenapine is an antagonist at α_1- and α_2-adrenergic receptors and H$_2$ receptors. Thus, asenapine is somewhat more likely than some other members of the class to induce orthostatic hypotension and tends to be sedating.

The efficacy of asenapine in the treatment of schizophrenia appears comparable to that of other SGAs. The three registration trials investigated the utility of asenapine for the treatment of schizophrenia in 6-week fixed-dose studies comparing asenapine with placebo and one of three comparator agents: haloperidol, risperidone, or olanzapine. In two of the three studies, asenapine was superior to placebo and comparable to the active agent. In one study, both olanzapine and asenapine failed to separate from placebo. The dosage of asenapine used in these studies ranged from 5 mg bid to 10 mg bid. Because the effect size for asenapine is somewhat lower than that for other SGAs, some have concluded that asenapine is a weaker agent. However, the effect size for comparator agents was also lower than that seen in earlier studies and might be consistent with the larger placebo effect found in more recent studies (Szegedi et al. 2012). Still, other meta-analyses have concluded that although asenapine is comparable to other SGAs in efficacy, it may be somewhat less effective than more established agents in the treatment of schizophrenia, such as clozapine, olanzapine, and risperidone (Leucht et al. 2013).

Asenapine was evaluated in the treatment of mania and mixed states in two double-blind controlled studies of identical design (McIntyre et al. 2010, 2013). In these trials, 488 patients with bipolar I disorder in a manic or mixed state were randomly assigned to receive asenapine, olanzapine, or placebo for 3 weeks. Both active drugs were more effective than placebo, but the effect size for asenapine was modest (0.45) relative to the effect size for olanzapine. Likewise, in a study of asenapine versus placebo as an add-on treatment with valproate or lithium in treatment of mania or mixed states, asenapine did significantly better than placebo but yielded small effect sizes at weeks 3 and 12 (0.24 and 0.33, respectively) (McIntyre et al. 2010). There was some evidence from the acute and long-term bipolar trials that asenapine might have a role in treating the depressive symptoms of bipolar disorder. Overall, asenapine appears to be one of the weaker antimanic drugs approved for this use. A meta-analysis of the comparative efficacy of approved treatments for mania concluded that the antipsychotics were more effective, as a group, than were mood-stabilizing agents such as lithium or valproate (Cipriani et al. 2011). However, among the antipsychotics, asenapine and ziprasidone were considerably less effective than risperidone, olanzapine, and haloperidol. Because asenapine must be taken as a sublingual tablet, which may not be ideal for many young, acutely manic patients, we find that asenapine is more of a secondary agent in the treatment of acute mania, best reserved for the elderly or patients who cannot swallow pills.

Asenapine is about 95% bound to protein. It has a large volume of distribution and a rapid time to peak plasma levels of about 30–60 minutes. It has less than 1% bioavailability if swallowed, which is why it must be allowed to disintegrate under the tongue. Even then, the bioavailability is only about 35%. Asenapine is available as a transdermal patch, which circumvents some of the problems associated with the sublingual formulation. Asenapine is metabolized primarily by CYP1A2 and then subsequently undergoes glucuronidation. A major dosage adjustment is probably not needed with potent CYP1A2 inhibitors such as fluvoxamine, although the dose of concomitant asenapine might need to be lowered in some cases. Likewise, although asenapine is a weak CYP2D6 inhibitor, it is not likely to inhibit the metabolism of substrates such as paroxetine or desipramine to a significant level.

Asenapine has been generally well tolerated in clinical trials. Among the most reported side effects to occur at greater rates than placebo were somnolence, akathisia, and oral hypoesthesia. About 5% of patients seem to have their tongue and mouth become numb with the sublingual administration of asenapine. Although most patients are able to tolerate this numbness, it was one of the more common reasons patients discontinued the drug in the schizophrenia trials. It is less likely to cause weight gain and increases in blood glucose than either olanzapine or quetiapine. Still, around 15% of patients gained more than 7% of their body weight in the long-term schizophrenia and bipolar trials. The number needed to harm for clinically significant weight gain is 7. Rare but potentially serious hypersensitivity reactions, including angioedema, severe hyponatremia, thrombocytopenia, and QTc prolongation, have also been reported with asenapine.

Although the terminal half-life of asenapine is about 24 hours, the low bioavailability of the drug and high protein binding lend itself to being dosed twice a day. We prefer to have patients start off with a 5-mg dose at bedtime. If they tolerate that dose, we go to 5-mg bid for at least 1 week. Most patients seem to do fine at 10 mg daily, but the dosage can be titrated up to 10 mg bid if needed. The transdermal asenapine patch is usually started at 3.8 mg and may be increased to 5.7 mg after 1 week. The maximum dosage for the patch is 7.6 mg/day, with patches changed every 24 hours. Each day, the patch should be moved to a different site to limit the risk of skin irritation. As with other transdermal patches (selegiline), heat applied to the patch (such as by sunbathing or applying a heating pad) will increase the absorption of the drug and risk more side effects.

Cariprazine

Cariprazine was approved initially in 2015 for the treatment of acute schizophrenia and acute mania. Like aripiprazole, it is a partial agonist of dopamine receptors and serotonin $5-HT_{1A}$ receptors and an antagonist of $5-HT_{2A}$ receptors. Unlike aripiprazole, cariprazine is far more selective for the D_3 than the D_2 receptor. The clinical benefit of D_3 selectivity remains to be seen, but there is some suggestion that the D_3 partial agonism may have procognitive benefits, at least in animal models. In principle, partial dopamine agonists inhibit the receptor when the receptor is being overstimulated and stimulate the receptor when endogenous dopamine levels are low.

Cariprazine was evaluated in three acute pivotal trials in the treatment of schizophrenia (Durgam et al. 2014, 2015a; Kane et al. 2015b). The studies evaluated different cariprazine doses versus placebo over 6 weeks of treatment in schizophrenia patients, ages 18–60, who had an acute exacerbation of their illness. The dosage of cariprazine ranged from 1.5 to 12 mg/day, and the primary outcome measure was symptom improvement on the PANSS. In general, the higher dosages were associated with better response and, not surprisingly, more side effects as well. Cariprazine treatment resulted in a 40%–80% improvement over placebo in the pooling of the three studies. The dosage range of 1.5–6 mg/day seemed to give the best balance of efficacy versus side-effect burden.

Cariprazine was also evaluated in the treatment of bipolar disorder in three randomized controlled trials (Calabrese et al. 2015; Durgam et al. 2015b; Sachs et al. 2015). The three studies in total enrolled just over 1,000 patients with bipolar I acute mania or mixed states. Patients were treated for 3 weeks with cariprazine (3–12 mg/day) or placebo in an inpatient setting. The primary outcome measure was the Young Mania Rating Scale. All three studies showed some benefit of cariprazine, with a 28%–69% improvement over placebo.

The side-effect profile of cariprazine most closely resembles that of aripiprazole, with a low proclivity for increasing prolactin levels and metabolic parameters but with higher rates of akathisia compared with many other SGAs. The rate of akathisia in the bipolar studies was about 20%, which was four times the rate in patients receiving placebo. Likewise, the rates of akathisia among cariprazine-treated patients in the schizophrenia trials were about two to three times those seen among patients receiving placebo. EPS were twice as likely to occur in patients taking cariprazine than in patients receiving placebo in both the schizophrenia and bipolar studies. Because some demographic groups, such as young males, are more susceptible to side effects such as akathisia, additional caution may be warranted. On the other hand, young males may be more sensitive to increases in prolactin levels that will be largely circumvented with cariprazine. Cariprazine is a CYP3A4 substrate, so concomitant use with CYP3A4 inhibitors such as nefazodone will increase serum levels and increase the risk of EPS and akathisia. Conversely, CYP3A4 inducers such as carbamazepine will increase the metabolism of cariprazine and render it less effective.

Cariprazine has been shown to be effective in the monotherapy of bipolar depression and is FDA approved for this indication. The efficacy of cariprazine was established in two Phase III studies in bipolar I depression (Earley et al. 2019, 2020). The 1.5 mg/day dosage was effective in both studies, but the 3 mg dose failed to separate in one of the two studies. The standard starting dose, as with schizophrenia, is 1.5 mg, and most patients seem to respond to this dose. However, the dose may be increased to 3 mg if the patient is not responding to the lower dose and is tolerating the medication. Another indication for cariprazine is in the adjunctive treatment of major depressive disorder; it was approved for this use in December 2022. Although not all studies have been positive, most of the double-blind studies of adjunctive cariprazine have shown a benefit of 1.5–4.5 mg daily combined with a standard antidepressant (Durgam et al. 2016; Fava et al. 2018). We have found that 1.5 mg of cariprazine is at least as effective as other SGAs in the adjunctive treatment of depression and is better tolerated than most.

Pimavanserin

Pimavanserin was approved in 2017 for the treatment of hallucinations and delusions associated with PD. About 60% of PD patients develop chronic psychotic symptoms. Finding options for treating psychotic symptoms in PD has been challenging because all antipsychotics (except clozapine) are potent D_2 antagonists and thus will worsen the motor symptoms of PD. Pimavanserin is a selective inverse agonist of the 5-HT_{2A} receptor and, like other SGAs, is also a 5-HT_{2C} antagonist. However, it is 40 times more selective for the 5-HT_{2A} receptor than for the 5-HT_{2C} receptor (Touma and Touma 2018). A proposed etiology of psychotic symptoms in PD is an upregulation of the 5-HT_{2A} receptor in the prefrontal and visual cortices. An inverse agonist, in contrast to an antagonist, reduces signal transduction rather than blocking the signal. It is likely that other antipsychotics also function in part as inverse agonists of the 5-HT_{2A} receptor. On the other hand, other available antipsychotics are not as selective as pimavanserin on the 5-HT_{2A} receptor.

The efficacy of pimavanserin was established in one Phase II study and one Phase III study. There was a total of three Phase III pivotal trials, but one trial did not show efficacy, and another was terminated early based on the lack of response in the prior Phase III study. The two studies that show benefit of pimavanserin in the treatment of psychotic symptoms in PD are relatively small trials. In the first study, 60 patients with PD were randomly assigned to pimavanserin 20–60 mg/day (mean dosage = 44.8 mg/day) or placebo for 6 weeks (Meltzer et al. 2010). The outcome measure used in the study was the Scale for the Assessment of Positive Symptoms (SAPS), which assesses hallucinations and delusions rather than the negative symptoms common in schizophrenia. Pimavanserin was superior to placebo on a SAPS global severity rating for hallucinations and persecutory delusions. Of note, there was no worsening of the PD symptoms while patients were taking pimavanserin.

In the pivotal Phase III trial, 199 PD patients were randomly assigned to receive 40 mg of pimavanserin or placebo after a 2-week lead-in phase of psychosocial therapy to limit the placebo effect (Cummings et al. 2014). Patients were treated for 6 weeks, and the patients receiving pimavanserin had 37% improvement in psychotic symptoms on the SAPS adapted for PD patients (SAPS-PD) versus only 14% for the patients receiving placebo. Again, there was no worsening of PD symptoms in this study. The most common side effects seen in pimavanserin-treated patients were mostly mild peripheral edema (in 7% of patients), nausea (7%), and a confusional state (6%). Like many antipsychotics, pimavanserin also can prolong QT intervals. Thus, pimavanserin should probably not be used with class 1A antiarrhythmics such as quinidine or with other antipsychotics. Because pimavanserin is also a

CYP3A4 substrate, drugs that inhibit this isoenzyme, like many antiretrovirals, antifungals such as ketoconazole, and nefazodone, could inhibit the metabolism and increase the risk of QT prolongation among other side effects.

As of this writing, pimavanserin is an expensive medication, retailing for more than $50,000/year. There are other strategies for treating psychotic symptoms in patients with PD. Low-dose clozapine (25–50 mg/day) appears to be effective without worsening PD symptoms. At these low dosages, clozapine appears to be reasonably tolerated, even in an elderly population. Quetiapine also appears to be useful at dosages of 25–150 mg/day, but it can worsen PD symptoms. Ziprasidone, olanzapine, and risperidone have all shown variable efficacy in treating psychosis in PD, with some increased risk of worsening motor symptoms.

Pimavanserin is currently being explored for other indications, including as a treatment of psychosis associated with Alzheimer's disease, as an adjunctive treatment for major depression, and for treating negative symptoms of schizophrenia. The typical dosage is 34 mg/day and does not require titration. However, because the drug currently comes only in a 17-mg tablet, it is not unreasonable to start at 17 mg for a few days and, if the medication is tolerated, then go up to the standard 34 mg/day. Pimavanserin is not widely available in retail pharmacies, but specialty pharmacies may order the drug.

Lumateperone

Lumateperone is a butyrophenone SGA first approved for schizophrenia in 2019 and then for bipolar I and II depression in 2021. At this time, it shares with quetiapine the distinction of being the only other drug with a bipolar II depression indication. Relative to other SGAs, lumateperone has a substantially higher ratio of affinity for the 5-HT_{2A} receptor to the D_2 receptor. A typical dose of lumateperone in a healthy individual occupies 80% of 5-HT_{2A} receptors while occupying only 12% of nigrostriatal D_2 receptors. In contrast, a therapeutic dose of most antipsychotics occupies 60%–80% of D_2 receptors. On the D_2 receptor it acts as a presynaptic partial agonist and a postsynaptic antagonist. At the standard dose of 42 mg, lumateperone also acts to block serotonin reuptake and is an indirect D_1 receptor modulator of N-methyl-D-aspartate (NMDA) (Blair 2020).

Lumateperone reaches peak serum levels in 1–2 hours and reaches steady state in about 5 days. It is 97% bound to protein and has a terminal half-life of around 13–21 hours, with many active metabolites. The metabolism of lumateperone is via multiple enzymes, including CYP3A4, CYP1A2, CYP2C8, and uridine diphosphate glucuronosyltransferase 1-1 (UGT1A), but the primary interaction appears to be with CYP3A4. Thus, inducers of CYP3A4 such as carbamazepine can significantly lower lumateperone serum levels, whereas inhibitors of CYP3A4 like fluvoxamine can increase serum levels and side effects.

The approval of lumateperone in schizophrenia was based on two double-blind studies. Each had a small to medium effect size of 0.3–0.4 in reducing psychotic symptoms on the PANSS over 4 weeks of treatment. In one study comparing 28 mg and 42 mg versus placebo, the 42 mg dose but not the 28 mg dose reduced the PANSS score by 4.2 points relative to placebo (Correll et al. 2020a). In the other study, Lieberman and colleagues (2016) randomly assigned 335 patients with schizophrenia to 42–84 mg of lumateperone, 2–4 mg of risperidone, or placebo. Both risperidone and lumateperone were significantly more likely to reduce PANSS scores than was placebo. The effect size for both risperidone and lumateperone was 0.4, but the higher dose of lumateperone did not separate from placebo. Of interest, a post hoc analysis on a small subgroup of patients with more depressive symptoms showed a large effect size (>1) of lumateperone but not risperidone.

Lumateperone has shown good efficacy in the treatment of bipolar I and II depression. In a Phase III study, 377 patients with bipolar depression were randomly assigned to 42 mg of lumateperone or placebo for 6 weeks (Calabrese et al. 2021). The lumateperone-treated patients had a greater improvement in MADRS scores (4.7 points) relative to placebo-treated patients, with noted improvement by day 8. The effect sizes on the MADRS score change from baseline to day 43 were larger in bipolar II than in bipolar I trials (0.49 for bipolar I patients and 0.81 for bipolar II patients).

Lumateperone may have a number of advantages over some of the many SGAs currently available. One important advantage is the ease of dosing. There is only one dose, 42 mg, which is both the starting and the therapeutic dose. Although there is now a 10.5 and a 21 mg dose, most patients tolerate the 42 mg dose fine. Another distinction is the relative lack of EPS. The acute and chronic studies do not reveal a substantial risk of EPS, which would be expected from the low occupancy of nigrostriatal D_2 receptors at therapeutic doses. Lumateperone also seems to be on the low end of risk for causing weight gain and metabolic symptoms relative to other SGAs. One-year data with lumateperone suggest an average weight loss of 2–3 kg in schizophrenic patients and are weight neutral in bipolar patients. The most common side effects in clinical trials have been somnolence/sedation, nausea, dizziness, and dry mouth. Overall, lumateperone appears to be an easy-to-use, well-tolerated SGA with clear efficacy in bipolar depression and more modest efficacy in schizophrenia. The pharmacological profile of lumateperone also suggests that it may be useful in unipolar depression, and studies are under way to examine its efficacy in MDD either as a monotherapy or an adjunctive treatment.

First-Generation (Typical) Antipsychotics

As of this writing, 10 FGAs are still on the U.S. market, with haloperidol being the most commonly prescribed. These drugs differ from the increasingly dominant SGAs in their considerably higher ratio of D_2-to-$5\text{-}HT_2$ antagonism. They may also occupy dopamine receptors for longer periods.

The FGAs continue to have a number of advantages over SGAs. A significant advantage is cost. Most of the FGAs are available generically at a fraction of the cost of newer drugs. Studies such as CATIE and CUtLASS 1 have challenged the idea that the typical agents are less effective or even more poorly tolerated in the treatment of schizophrenia. Finally, the high-potency agents are considerably less likely than most SGAs to cause weight gain. In fact, molindone tends to be associated with less weight gain than other FGAs or SGAs. In some patients, weight gain and its complications may pose a greater long-term risk to the patient than do EPS.

Still, the relatively lower rates of EPS, particularly tardive dyskinesia, and perhaps somewhat better efficacy in treating negative and cognitive symptoms with second-generation agents have made them preferred agents for the long-term management of psychosis. Despite these advantages of SGAs, many patients with schizophrenia remain on FGAs, and this will continue to be the case until we have agents that are clearly superior.

Although there is no evidence that one FGA works any better than another, some patients clearly do take to one agent more than another. As is true for other classes of psychotropic agents, choosing an FGA has more to do with the side-effect profile of the drug than with other factors. Low-potency agents such as chlorpromazine have the advantage of causing less severe EPS but

Typical (D$_2$ antagonist) antipsychotics: overview	
Efficacy	Schizophrenia (positive symptoms) (FDA-approved indication) Tourette's disorder (pimozide; FDA-approved indication) Mania (FDA-approved indication for chlorpromazine only) Psychotic depression (with antidepressant) Drug-induced psychosis Agitation,[a] nausea, hiccups (not FDA approved for these purposes; off-label)
Side effects	EPS (more common in high-potency drugs) NMS (rare) Dry mouth, constipation, urinary retention, sedation, weight gain (more common in low-potency drugs) Skin and eye complications QT interval prolongation (thioridazine)
Dosage and administration	Individualize dosing. 50–150 mg chlorpromazine equivalents (see Table 4–2) to start, with maximum total daily dose of 300–600 mg chlorpromazine equivalents (e.g., 6–12 mg haloperidol).
Safety in overdose	CNS depression, hypotension, ECG changes, EPS. Manage with vital sign support, gastric lavage. Do not induce emesis secondary to aspiration risk.
Drug interactions	CNS depressants: ↑ sedation Antacids: ↓ antipsychotic absorption Carbamazepine: ↓ antipsychotic levels SSRIs: ↑ antipsychotic levels Nicotine: ↓ antipsychotic levels Meperidine: ↑ sedation, hypotension β-Blockers: ↑ hypotension; may ↑ antipsychotic and β-blocker levels TCAs: may ↑ antipsychotic and TCA levels Valproic acid: chlorpromazine may ↑ valproic acid levels

Note.   ECG = electrocardiogram; EPS = extrapyramidal symptoms; NMS = neuroleptic malignant syndrome; SSRI = selective serotonin reuptake inhibitor; TCA = tricyclic antidepressant.
[a]Agitation associated with psychosis: FDA-approved indication for intramuscular olanzapine only.

more sedation, weight gain, and postural hypotension than do higher-potency agents. On the other hand, high-potency antipsychotics such as haloperidol and fluphenazine tend to be preferred over low-potency agents despite their greater proclivity for EPS. The antihistaminic and anticholinergic effects of low-potency agents may be more problematic for the day-to-day functioning of many patients. The art of using these drugs involves choosing the right agent and then managing the inevitable side effects of the drug.

Side Effects

Sedation

Sedation, often accompanied by fatigue, can be useful early in treatment but a liability after the patient has improved. All antipsychotics can be sedating in some patients at some dosages, but chlorpromazine is generally the most sedating. Its sedative effects are often judged to be very unpleasant by non–psychiatrically ill volunteers receiving even 25 mg or 50 mg of the drug in a single dose, but these effects are sometimes accepted or even welcomed by some patients with psychosis or personality disorders. Thioridazine, chlorprothixene, and loxapine are also often relatively sedating, whereas the other high-potency antipsychotics are often less or not at all sedating. In one acute-dosing strategy, the antipsychotic dosage is gradually raised until the psychosis is controlled; at that point the patient develops increased sedation, which then requires dosage reduction. In chronic administration, sedation and fatigue overlap with akinesia, a side effect characterized by inertia, inactivity, and lack of spontaneous movement. Akinesia will often abate when an antiparkinsonian drug is added; it will often abate more slowly when the dosage is lowered. When antipsychotics are used as needed (orally or parenterally), it is likely that sedation is the main effect produced, even though a decrease in psychosis may be desired. As has been discussed, a benzodiazepine (e.g., lorazepam 1–2 mg) may be more appropriate for this purpose. Unfortunately, the short-term (or long-term) utility of as-needed medication of any sort has never been seriously studied.

Autonomic Effects

All antipsychotics can cause postural hypotension, but this problem is presumed to be more common and severe with the low-potency drugs, at least with chlorpromazine and thioridazine, and more dangerous in elderly or medically ill patients. All FGAs also have anticholinergic effects, which are most striking with thioridazine but are also clearly present with chlorpromazine, mesoridazine (no longer available in the United States), and trifluoperazine; they are also present, but to a lesser degree, with the other drugs. Dry mouth, constipation, and urinary hesitancy can occur, as can visual blurring. When antipsychotics are combined with other anticholinergic drugs (antiparkinsonian or TCA drugs), delirium or bowel stasis can occur. Constipation is a milder form of this effect. Retrograde ejaculation is fairly common with thioridazine and can occur with other drugs in this class. This effect can progress to impotence. It is worth inquiring about sexual effects because patients may be upset by such effects but hesitant to mention them spontaneously.

Endocrine Effects

The direct effect of FGA drugs is an increase in blood prolactin level. There is a large and complex literature on this effect because prolactin level has been proposed as an alternative to measuring antipsychotic blood level directly. Attempts to use prolactin level as a guide to adequate dosage in newly hospitalized patients have not been validated to date, but one study suggested that aftercare patients with a low prolactin level were more likely to relapse than were those with a higher level. Hyperprolactinemia can cause breast enlargement and galactorrhea in both female and male patients and may play a role in the impotence in male patients and the amenorrhea in female patients that are occasionally seen with these drugs. To reduce prolactin levels, dopaminergic drugs such as amantadine (200–300 mg/day) or bromocriptine (7.5–15 mg/day) can be tried.

Weight gain, often quite excessive, can occur with all antipsychotic drugs. It is unclear whether it is a result of increased appetite or decreased activity. Molindone is believed to be less likely to cause weight gain and may even cause modest weight loss, again for unknown reasons. Although all antipsychotics except thioridazine are good antiemetics, nausea and vomiting are sometimes seen as side effects, for reasons not yet determined.

Skin and Eye Complications

A variety of allergic skin rashes can occur with antipsychotics (as with all other drugs) but are more common with chlorpromazine. Chlorpromazine with prolonged high-dose administration can cause pigmentation of areas exposed to light and pigment deposits in the eye, chiefly in the back of the cornea and the front of the lens. These deposits almost never affect vision and do not require regular slit lamp examinations. However, patients showing an opaque pupil when a light is shone into the eye should have an ophthalmological evaluation. These deposits probably occur only with chlorpromazine but could conceivably occur with other drugs. Retinal pigmentation occurs only with thioridazine (but has never been reported, so far, with thioridazine's metabolite mesoridazine), and its serious and irreversible effect on vision requires that thioridazine dosage be kept at or below 800 mg/day.

Chlorpromazine often causes skin photosensitivity, manifested as severe sunburn in exposed skin areas after relatively brief (30–60 minutes) exposure to direct sunlight. A sunscreen containing para-aminobenzoic acid (PABA), which screens out ultraviolet rays, will help avoid this effect. Other antipsychotics may cause photosensitivity, and patients taking them are generally advised to wear sunscreen. Sun sensitivity can best be determined by cautious exposure to the sun in gradually increased durations. Many patients will prove able to tolerate the sun normally. Chlorpromazine should be avoided in patients who are likely to spend long periods outdoors at work or for pleasure. Patients taking chlorpromazine for prolonged periods of time can develop a slate-gray to purplish pigmentation of skin areas exposed to sunlight that should fade slowly once the drug is stopped.

Other or Rare Complications

Agranulocytosis has been associated with chlorpromazine and thioridazine and could presumably occur with other FGAs. Its incidence is low—perhaps 1 case in 5,000 patients treated. Agranulocytosis usually appears in the first 3 months of treatment. Monitoring for agranulocytosis does not require frequent or regular blood counts. However, patients developing a sore throat and fever in the first few months of therapy require an emergency WBC count to rule out this rare but serious complication. Leukopenias in the range of 3,000–4,000/mm^3 also occur and are not generally serious, whereas agranulocytosis, often defined as a WBC count of less than 2,000/mm^3 with less than 500/mm^3 of polymorphonuclear leukocytes, is very serious and requires immediate medical attention by a hematologist. Needless to say, clinicians should seriously consider stopping a drug if the WBC count is less than 3,000/mm^3. See the section on clozapine earlier in this chapter for discussion of the particular problem of clozapine-associated agranulocytosis.

A form of allergic obstructive hepatitis was reported relatively frequently in the early days of chlorpromazine use, with an incidence of 2%–3%, but this disease has been much more rarely encountered in recent years. Even when this allergic obstructive hepatitis occurred more frequently, it was a relatively mild, transient disorder that did not lead to hepatic necrosis or permanent liver damage. Liver problems occur so rarely with other antipsychotics as to make one believe that the occasionally abnormal liver function tests seen in patients taking these drugs are due to some intercurrent, unrelated event or drug. Such abnormalities, unless progressive and severe, are not a reason for discontinuing an effective antipsychotic in a patient who needs the drug, although internists tend to blame the antipsychotic, without an adequate basis, when abnormal liver function tests are observed.

Seizures can also occur in patients treated with antipsychotics. Only promazine (no longer used) caused them with any frequency. We know of no good data available on the comparative effects of all antipsychotic drugs on seizure threshold, but our former coauthor Jonathan Cole tended to suspect loxapine and chlorpromazine of being involved in the rare antipsychotic-related seizures seen at McLean Hospital, and we presume that the high-potency drugs are less likely to cause seizures. Certainly, patients with known epilepsy who are receiving anticonvulsants often receive antipsychotics without any obvious effect on seizure frequency. Seizures associated with clozapine use are discussed earlier in this chapter.

Sudden death has been associated with antipsychotic use in healthy young adults. The mechanisms suggested include QTc prolongation, torsades de pointes, ventricular fibrillation, and aspiration of food or vomitus during a grand mal seizure, but no clear etiology has been proved. Several FGAs, including thioridazine, mesoridazine, and droperidol, now contain black box warnings in the package inserts. The use of these drugs has dropped dramatically since these warnings were established. Occasional sudden deaths have been reported among patients in seclusion rooms during summer months. This may be due to the effect of the antipsychotic on heat regulation. However, because sudden, unpredictable deaths occurred in young psychiatric patients before antipsychotic drugs were discovered, their connection with medication remains tenuous. Over the past 30 years we have heard of more sudden deaths associated with thioridazine (four) than with any other antipsychotic, but even with this drug such occurrences are very rare. As a result of a study focusing primarily on QTc prolongation in SGAs, in 2000 thioridazine and its metabolite mesoridazine (Serentil) received a black box warning from the FDA about QTc prolongation. As a result, thioridazine and mesoridazine are unlikely to be used much.

Neurological Effects

Although dopamine receptor blockade in the striatum is the most popular mechanism invoked for all neurological side effects of antipsychotic drugs, and anticholinergic antiparkinsonian drugs are the conventional remedy, the presumed cholinergic-dopaminergic imbalance is probably only a partial explanation.

Dystonia. One of the earliest forms of EPS, dystonia, often manifested by tonic muscle spasm in the tongue, jaw, and neck, usually occurs in the first few hours or days after taking an antipsychotic. It can manifest as a very frightening opisthotonos of the whole body with extensor rigidity or as only mild tongue stiffness. In one small study, dystonia appeared as antipsychotic blood levels were dropping, not rising, making one wonder whether in this case the dystonia might have been a rebound effect as dopamine blockade was waning. In any event, dystonia can be fairly effectively averted by prophylactic antiparkinsonian medication use and rarely occurs with thioridazine. It is more common in younger males but can occur in either sex at any age.

Once present, the dystonia can be rapidly relieved by intravenous antiparkinsonian drugs (only diphenhydramine and benztropine are readily available for parenteral use) or, less rapidly, by intramuscular medication. However, such diverse drugs as diazepam, amobarbital, and caffeine sodium benzoate, and even hypnosis, have been said to relieve it as well. Once the dystonia has resolved and the patient is protected by oral antiparkinsonian medication, the offending antipsychotic can be continued without recurrence of the dystonia. However, patients often feel less apprehensive if a different antipsychotic drug is substituted. Some patients receiving depot fluphenazine develop recurrences of dystonia with succeeding injections. Oculogyric crises, manifested by forced eye rotation, usually upward, are conventionally classified with the dystonias, but they fairly frequently occur—even recur—later in treatment, when more conventional dystonia is rare.

Pseudoparkinsonism.   Sometime in the early stages of treatment, usually between 5 days and 4 weeks, the patient can develop signs of parkinsonism. In contrast to idiopathic Parkinson's disease, pill-rolling tremor is very rare, but muscle stiffness, cogwheel rigidity, stooped posture, masklike facies, and even drooling are quite common. Micrographia occurs and can help differentiate antipsychotic-induced tremor from lithium-induced tremor. Patients rarely develop such severe parkinsonian rigidity that they become incapacitated or even immobilized. When they do, such patients are sometimes misdiagnosed as having catatonia. Patients with such severe rigidity do not respond readily to even massive doses of antiparkinsonian drugs; the condition may require as long as 2 weeks to clear after the antipsychotic drug is stopped. Often, milder degrees of pseudoparkinsonism are seen for prolonged periods in patients taking long-term maintenance medication and can contribute to passive inactivity in such patients.

Akinesia.   Akinesia, a reduction in spontaneous or voluntary movement, can be seen in patients taking maintenance antipsychotic medication in the absence of signs of parkinsonism. Regular coarse tremor can also be seen in the absence of any other parkinsonian signs. Both conditions respond to either administration of antiparkinsonian drugs or reduction in antipsychotic dose.

Akinesia, as well as pseudoparkinsonism and depression, can be confused with the negative symptoms of schizophrenia. One approach to differentiating apathy and alogia due to psychosis from neurological side effects is to institute a therapeutic trial of a drug such as benztropine for 2–4 weeks. If the negative symptoms improve, they were presumably side effects of the antipsychotic, not a result of the psychotic disorder. A trial of an antidepressant can serve the same purpose if depressive symptoms are suspected.

Work at McLean Hospital has suggested that selegiline (Eldepryl), the monoamine oxidase B inhibitor used to treat conventional parkinsonism, is also beneficial at a dosage of 5 mg bid in schizophrenic patients with negative symptoms who are taking antipsychotics. If the selegiline dosage does not exceed 10 mg/day (or 6 mg/day for the transdermal patch), the special diet required with monoamine oxidase inhibitor use is not necessary. A placebo-controlled trial of this use has been completed (Jungerman et al. 1999), and the drug seems to work. If improvement is seen with selegiline, it may be hard to tell whether the drug is effective because it reduces parkinsonian symptoms, reduces depression, or improves negative symptoms directly.

Akathisia.   Akathisia, the inner-driven restlessness caused by antipsychotics, is the least understood and most troublesome of the neurological side effects of these agents. It ranges from an unpleasant subjective feeling of muscular discomfort to an agitated, desperate, markedly dysphoric pacing with hand wringing and weeping. Between these extremes, patients find themselves unable to sit still for long, having to stand up and move around or continually shift their position. Akathisia is sometimes mistaken for psychotic agitation and is treated inappropriately by an increase in antipsychotic dose. It can be experienced even after the first dose of an antipsychotic but can become a clinical problem at any time in the first few weeks of medication use.

Akathisia occurs with thioridazine and olanzapine, as well as with the other older drugs, and may even occur with clozapine and risperidone. It is less responsive to antiparkinsonian drugs than are other neurological side effects and is the bane of maintenance medication, being a common basis for patients' refusing to continue such a regimen. Studies suggest that propranolol at dosages of 30–120 mg/day sometimes suppresses akathisia when neither antiparkinsonian drugs nor benzodiazepines, such as lorazepam, work. Its efficacy casts some doubt on the theory that dopamine receptor blockade is the mechanism underlying akathisia.

Regular, rhythmic leg jiggling—up and down or, less commonly, to and fro—is often seen in patients treated with antipsychotics and is probably, but not certainly, a variant of akathisia, although some consider it a form of tremor. Patients with this phenomenon are often unaware of it or not bothered by it.

The best basis for differential diagnosis of akathisia is to ask the patient whether the restlessness is a muscle feeling or a head feeling—the first being akathisia and the second anxiety. If there is any doubt, it is safer to assume that akathisia exists, because overdosing with antipsychotics is vastly more common than underdosing.

The drug therapy of akathisia often requires polypharmacy. Antiparkinsonian drugs, β-blockers, and benzodiazepines can all be helpful in some patients, but more than one of these agents may be required. Lowering the antipsychotic dosage should also be considered.

Use of Antiparkinsonian Drugs

For decades there have been impassioned arguments pro and con about the prophylactic use of antiparkinsonian drugs (Stanilla and Simpson 1995). Many senior clinicians claim that patients' acceptance of a drug is enhanced and unpleasant side effects are averted by routine administration of antiparkinsonian agents to all patients starting (or restarting) an antipsychotic drug. Others, however, assert that two drugs together (an antipsychotic drug and an antiparkinsonian drug) can be more toxic than an antipsychotic alone and that an antiparkinsonian should be added only when neurological side effects appear.

We believe there is enough evidence that antiparkinsonian drugs avert neurological side effects to use them routinely in treating most acutely psychotic patients younger than age 45 who are starting to take an FGA, unless the anticholinergic side effects are contraindicated. In the less common situation, in which cautious trials of antipsychotics at very low dosages (e.g., haloperidol 1–3 mg/day) are undertaken, prophylactic antiparkinsonian drugs are unnecessary. If routine antiparkinsonian medication is not used prophylactically in the acute treatment of patients, as-needed orders for such patients should be written. After 4 weeks to 6 months of long-term maintenance antipsychotic therapy, the antiparkinsonian drugs can be shifted to an as-needed basis or withdrawn.

A few patients (approximately 15%) will redevelop clear neurological side effects, and even more (approximately 30%) will feel "better" (less anxious or depressed or inert), while continuing to take antiparkinsonian drugs. Some patients with chronic schizophrenia are delighted to stop their antipsychotic but demand to continue their antiparkinsonian drug (Wojcik 1979). Very rarely, patients use trihexyphenidyl or other antiparkinsonian agents to get high, but far more patients taking antipsychotics do better taking antiparkinsonians than not taking them. Rarely, patients develop an anticholinergic delirium or intestinal stasis while taking antiparkinsonian drugs; dry mouth and blurred vision are more common side effects.

Dosage ranges of available antiparkinsonian drugs are given in Table 4–4. If blood level determinations either of the drug itself or of anticholinergic levels by radioreceptor assay were generally available, dosage might be adjusted more rationally. Currently, if a patient has relief from neither neurological side effects nor dry mouth, a cautious increase in dose—even over the maximum

Table 4–4. Antiparkinsonian drugs: names, formulations and strengths, and dosage ranges

Generic name	Brand name	Formulations and strengths	Usual dosage range (mg/day)
Primarily anticholinergic drugs			
Benztropine	Cogentin[a]	Tablets: 0.5, 1, 2 mg Injection: 1 mg/mL (2-mL ampule)	2–6
Diphenhydramine	Benadryl[b]	Tablet: 25 mg Capsules: 25, 50 mg Elixir and syrup: 12.5 mg/5 mL (120-mL and 480-mL bottles) Injection: 50 mg/mL (1-mL single-dose vial; 10-mL multidose vial; 1-mL prefilled syringe)	50–300
Trihexyphenidyl	Arane[b]	Tablets: 2, 5 mg Elixir: 2 mg/5 mL (480-mL bottle)	4–15
Dopaminergic drugs			
Amantadine	Symmetrel[b]	Tablet and capsule: 100 mg Syrup: 50 mg/5 mL (480-mL bottle)	100–300

[a]Tablets only available in generic form.
[b]Available in generic form.

recommended in the *Physicians' Desk Reference*—can be considered, although decreasing the antipsychotic dose may be even more rational.

Most of the antiparkinsonian drugs are assumed to work by their anticholinergic effects and are probably equivalent to one another, although we have seen, in rare cases, syndromes that respond uniquely to the anticholinergic antihistamine diphenhydramine or to ethopropazine. No controlled comparative studies of these drugs exist to guide the clinician. Probably diphenhydramine is more sedating, trihexyphenidyl slightly more stimulating, and biperiden more neutral in this dimension (Table 4–4). Amantadine, which is presumed to work as a dopamine receptor agonist, can be used at dosages of 200–300 mg/day. It is probably as effective as the anticholinergic antiparkinsonian drugs, but it has no proven advantages. Tolerance to its antiparkinsonian effects may also be more of a problem than with anticholinergic antiparkinsonian agents. However, it may be useful when galactorrhea develops because it reduces blood prolactin levels. Although one might expect a dopamine receptor agonist to be a stimulant, patients sometimes find amantadine to be sedating. Bromocriptine, another dopamine receptor agonist, is available for prescription use and has been studied extensively in idiopathic Parkinson's disease. It may well prove useful in treating drug-induced pseudoparkinsonism and probably does not aggravate psychosis in patients whose dosage of antipsychotic has been stabilized. L-dopa has not been systematically studied in pseudoparkinsonism. It probably works too slowly and can sometimes aggravate psychosis. The standard antiparkinsonian drugs generally have no obvious effect on the psychosis; findings from the few controlled studies comparing antipsychotic drugs with and without added antiparkinsonian agents are equivocal.

Anticholinergic effects of the antiparkinsonian drugs can cause cognitive impairment in non–psychiatrically ill subjects and in patients with schizophrenia. The magnitude and clinical importance of this effect are unclear, but it is possible that mild memory problems caused by anticholinergic drug effects might well be overlooked in patients who were already cognitively impaired or sedated. It is well to remember that patients with idiopathic parkinsonism can become delirious at higher dosages of all antiparkinsonian drugs, including amantadine, and these patients should be watched for signs of organicity if these drugs are pushed to higher dosages.

Two newer antiparkinsonian drugs are worth mentioning. Pramipexole (Mirapex) and ropinirole (ReQuip) represent a new class of dopamine receptor agonists. Pramipexole was studied in the treatment of depression and psychosis, but its only FDA-approved indication is for the treatment of PD. Although our experience with these drugs is limited, we have seen patients with schizophrenia who respond to the antiparkinsonian effects of these drugs and do not appear to develop psychotic symptoms at lower dosages (<1 mg/day of pramipexole). There is some evidence that these dopamine receptor agonists may also help with the negative symptoms of schizophrenia. One problem with pramipexole and ropinirole is that they are quite expensive, and third-party payers such as Medicare will typically not cover them for treatment of antipsychotic-induced parkinsonism. Another problem is that dopamine receptor agonists have been associated with visual hallucinations in some patients; about 3% of Parkinson's patients develop visual hallucinations while taking dopamine receptor agonists.

Tardive Dyskinesia

Some patients exposed to antipsychotic drugs develop abnormal, involuntary, irregular choreiform or athetoid movements. These movements most commonly include tongue overactivity (darting, writhing, twisting, or repeated protrusion) and finger movements (choreiform or hand clenching). Chewing or lateral jaw movements, lip puckering, facial grimacing, torticollis or retrocollis, trunk twisting, pelvic thrusting, respiratory grunting, athetoid arm and shoulder movements, and a variety of toe, ankle, and leg movements all occur in a variety of combinations. These are hard to distinguish, at times, from mannerisms associated with schizophrenia and are essentially impossible to distinguish on the basis of phenomenology alone from other, rarer causes of dyskinesia.

Patients with typical movements of the sort described above are still referred to as having *tardive dyskinesia*. Those with major athetoid dystonic movements and sustained postures of the face, neck, arms, or trunk are referred to as having *tardive dystonia*, often a more severe and more incapacitating condition. Athetoid dystonic movements often coexist with the more typical tongue and lip movements of tardive dyskinesia. Tardive dystonia is more likely to be ameliorated by antiparkinsonian drugs than is conventional tardive dyskinesia. *Tardive akathisia*, a syndrome of forced motor restlessness persisting long after antipsychotic drugs have been stopped, can also occur. It is even less common than tardive dystonia. So-called *tardive Tourette's disorder* has also been described.

The severity of tardive dyskinesia ranges from minimal tongue restlessness and finger movements to gross, incapacitating, disfiguring movements. Most identifiable cases are mild and are not noticed by either the patient or the family or are passed off as minor tics or restlessness by both. Even clearly visible dyskinesias are often of little real consequence, but in about 3% of cases the dyskinesia is sufficiently severe to cause social or functional problems. Most patients and families seen in the Tardive Dyskinesia Clinic at McLean Hospital are much more concerned about the possible ultimate consequences of currently very mild dyskinesia than about the minor movements with which the patient presents at the time of consultation.

It is currently impossible to predict which patients will develop dyskinesia, early or late, mild or severe. However, the best available data suggest that there is a rate of development of dyskinesia of about 4%–7% per year over the first 5 years of exposure with first-generation agents and that patients older than age 55 and patients with affective disorders may be at greater risk (Cole et al. 1992; Jeste et al. 1995). In chronically institutionalized psychotic patients, dyskinesia prevalence rates are often on the order of 20%–40%. At the extremes, a few patients develop persistent dyskinesia after only a few weeks of exposure to antipsychotics, but antipsychotic use up to 6 months is generally considered safe. In our experience, about one-half of the patients who develop overt dyskinesia do so while taking the antipsychotic at stable maintenance dosages, whereas about one-quarter first manifest dyskinesia when the antipsychotic is tapered or stopped (covert dyskinesia). Dyskinesia fades away in some patients when their antipsychotics are stopped or weeks, months, or years later. Some patients lose their dyskinesia even while continuing to take medication at a stable maintenance dosage. There is a significant rate of occurrence of dyskinesia in individuals never exposed to antipsychotics—from 1% to 5%, increasing with advancing age; therefore, not all dyskinesias in patients taking antipsychotics are due to the drug. Unfortunately, no one can tell which cases are idiopathic. Neither are there any strong, consistent treatment factors related to dyskinesia. Duration of antipsychotic treatment correlates more commonly with dyskinesia than does total dose.

There is no clear evidence that any one first-generation or typical antipsychotic is less commonly related to tardive dyskinesia development than another. Clozapine appears far less likely to cause tardive dyskinesia; for risperidone, the jury is still out. Basic research data on dopamine receptor overproliferation caused by antipsychotics in laboratory animals have been used to claim that drugs such as thioridazine or molindone should be less likely to cause tardive dyskinesia than other antipsychotics. However, we have seen a number of cases of tardive dyskinesia in patients exposed only, or almost only, to thioridazine and two cases in patients mainly taking molindone. We also saw one patient who had been taking various antipsychotics for years but who developed tardive dyskinesia after a year of taking risperidone alone. In our experience, periods of withdrawal from antipsychotics are not related to tardive dyskinesia development, and lithium exposure does not seem to slow the emergence of dyskinesia.

Antiparkinsonian drug exposure is a more complicated issue. In two cohorts of 100 patients each studied at McLean Hospital because of recent onset of tardive dyskinesia, more months taking antiparkinsonian drugs was significantly correlated with slower onset of the disorder; this finding was replicated in both cohorts. In contrast, Jeste et al. (1995), in an older population in whom antipsychotic drugs were generally avoided, found that the use of antiparkinsonian drugs increased the risk of developing tardive dyskinesia. Kane and McGlashan (1995) found that patients who had severe neurological side effects from antipsychotics tended to be at high risk for development of tardive dyskinesia. Antiparkinsonian drugs are clearly able to exacerbate pre-existing dyskinesia. Our interpretation of this mixture of messages is that prophylactic antiparkinsonian drug use in younger patients is safe and may even be prophylactic against tardive dyskinesia, whereas severe neurological side effects and older age coupled with antiparkinsonian use may make tardive dyskinesia onset more likely. Therefore, the clinician must seriously consider the risks and benefits of extended treatment with antipsychotics in all patients likely to continue taking medication for longer than a few months. This issue must be discussed with the patient and their family unless there are defensible clinical reasons for not doing so. Either way, everything should be documented in the patient's chart, and the process should be redone if signs of dyskinesia are noted. (See Chapter 1, "General Principles of Psychopharmacological Treatment," for further discussion of this issue.)

To date, the available long-term (2- to 10-year) follow-up studies suggest that tardive dyskinesia is not generally a progressive disorder and can improve or vanish over time, even in patients taking antipsychotics. With chronically psychotic patients, the best clinical decision is often to continue the antipsychotic, but this decision must be based on the available facts in each case.

No effective or standard treatment for tardive dyskinesia had been available until the first vesicular monoamine transporter type 2 (VMAT2) drug, valbenazine, was approved in 2017. Valbenazine approval was followed by the approval of deutetrabenazine in 2018. The VMAT2 agents bind selectively to the VMAT2 transporter to decrease dopamine release in a reversible manner. VMAT2 is more selective for dopamine than for other monoamines; thus, blocking the transporter provides relief for the dopamine hypersensitivity that is thought to be the pathophysiological underpinning of tardive dyskinesia. Valbenazine was studied in three randomized controlled trials of 6-week duration with two long-term follow-up studies of 42- and 48-week durations. In the first study, there was no statistical difference on the Abnormal Involuntary Movement Scale (AIMS) scores between a 50- or 100-mg dose and placebo at 6 weeks (Citrome 2017). However, 61% of the 80 subjects who continued in the 42-week open-label study had an average drop of 5.8 points on the AIMS, and the majority (61%) were rated as much or very much improved on the CGI Scale. In the two other Phase III studies (Kinect 2 and 3), there was a drop of 2.4–3.2 in AIMS scores, which reached statistical significance with the 80-mg dose at week 6 in Kinect 3 (Hauser et al. 2017). Discontinuation rates due to side effects were very limited (3% of valbenazine-treated subjects vs. 2% of subjects receiving placebo). Valbenazine appears to be well tolerated. Somnolence is the most common side effect, occurring in about 10% of treated patients, followed by mild anticholinergic effects and headache. Dosing is 40 mg/day for the first week followed by 80 mg/day thereafter. The major advantage of valbenazine over deutetrabenazine may be that it is a once-a-day drug versus twice-a-day for deutetrabenazine.

Deutetrabenazine, which had been previously approved for the treatment of chorea in Huntington's disease, was evaluated in two randomized controlled trials, Aim to Reduce Movements in Tardive Dyskinesia (ARM-TD) 1 and 2, for the treatment of tardive dyskinesia. In the first, deutetrabenazine was titrated from 12 mg/day to 48 mg/day over 6 weeks as tolerated. This was followed by a 6-week maintenance phase and a 1-week washout. Subjects in the deutetrabenazine group had a 3-point reduction on the AIMS versus a 1.6-point drop in the placebo group. In the second study, patients received either

24 mg or 36 mg of the active drug or placebo. The deutetrabenazine groups had a 3.2- to 3.3-point drop on the AIMS versus a 1.4-point drop in the placebo group. In addition, about 40%–50% of subjects were rated as much to very much improved on the CGI Scale. The side-effect profile of deutetrabenazine looks very much like that of valbenazine, with the most common side effects being somnolence, fatigue, and headache. GI side effects and akathisia have been reported with both deutetrabenazine and valbenazine, and both drugs can cause QT prolongation. The usual starting dose of deutetrabenazine is 6 mg given twice daily, with the dosage increased weekly to a target dosage of 12 mg twice daily, to a maximum of 24 mg twice daily.

The VMAT2 inhibitors represent a major advance in the treatment of tardive dyskinesia, but they have one huge downside: cost. Both valbenazine and deutetrabenazine would be perhaps the most expensive drugs prescribed by a psychiatrist, with current daily costs of either drug running in excess of $200 per day as of this writing. Thus, after surveying some of the large national pharmacies, we estimate that the cost of a VMAT2 inhibitor could exceed $70,000 or even reach $100,000 per year depending on the dose. Furthermore, the VMAT2 inhibitors need to be taken for life. Tardive dyskinesia symptoms tend to return within 4 weeks of stopping the medications.

Although no other medications besides the VMAT2 inhibitors have shown convincing efficacy in the treatment of tardive dyskinesia, other strategies may also be worth trying. For example, slowly tapering the antipsychotic dose is often recommended. A shift to a different antipsychotic, particularly clozapine, is also commonly suggested. Findings from a series of positive small studies suggest that vitamin E (400 IU tid) may gradually decrease dyskinesia, particularly if the dyskinesia has been present less than 5 years (Adler et al. 1993; Gardos and Cole 1995). Higher doses of vitamin E tend to cause diarrhea.

Tardive dyskinesia is remarkably heterogeneous in its response to drug therapies. Luckily, most cases of tardive dyskinesia are not serious enough to warrant special treatment. If special treatment is needed, VMAT2 drugs are the most effective treatment but are costly; switching to clozapine is often helpful, but at the cost of many potential side effects and frequent CBC monitoring. Vitamin E seems modestly helpful and benign. Beyond these, the clinician and the patient can often work out a medication regimen unique to the patient, which, over time, seems to help.

Neuroleptic Malignant Syndrome

NMS is a potentially life-threatening complication of antipsychotic drug use. Estimates of its incidence vary from study to study, but a rate of 1% of all psychiatric admissions in which the patients are treated with neuroleptics seems reasonable, although rates as low as 0.07% and as high as 2.4% have been reported. Although criteria for the diagnosis of NMS have fluctuated from article to article, there is general agreement that all patients with NMS have hyperthermia, severe EPS, and autonomic dysfunction. The operational criteria for diagnosis of NMS currently in use at McLean Hospital are presented in Table 4–5, which provides a good description of the range of signs and symptoms that may be present (see also Chapter 10, "Emergency Department Treatment").

Misdiagnosis can obviously occur when patients have both fever caused by infection and pseudoparkinsonism, but the severe muscle rigidity often seen in NMS is rare as an accompanying feature of incidental infection. Serum creatine kinase levels can be increased by intramuscular injections or by violent physical struggling, but rarely to a level as high as 1,000 IU/mL. Neuroleptics can affect temperature-regulating brain centers and can therefore be associated with heatstroke, particularly in hot weather or in hot seclusion rooms, in the absence of other manifestations of NMS. A neuroleptic-induced catatonia, really a severe parkinsonian rigidity, can occur in the absence of fever.

NMS itself usually develops over 1–3 days in patients taking antipsychotics. Many cases develop in the first week, and most within the first month, of treatment with antipsychotics. There is weak evidence that concomitant treatment with lithium may predispose patients to develop NMS. NMS has been observed with essentially all widely used neuroleptics, although thioridazine is perhaps underrepresented. The dose does not seem to be a major factor, although lower doses seem likely to be safer. Depot neuroleptics do not seem to be more likely to cause NMS, but their prolonged duration of action will make the syndrome last about twice as long (Glazer and Kane 1992).

The best treatment is early identification, stopping neuroleptics, and, in moderate to severe cases, rapid transfer to a medical center. The dopamine agonist bromocriptine, at a dosage of 5 mg every 4 hours, can often relieve muscle rigidity and reduce fever. Dantrolene is used in ICUs to reduce muscle spasm. Anticholinergic antiparkinsonian drugs are probably not helpful. Symptomatic treatment (e.g., cooling the body) is helpful.

Table 4–5.   Operational criteria for diagnosis of neuroleptic malignant syndrome

The following three items are all required for a definite diagnosis:
1. Hyperthermia: oral temperature of at least 38.0°C in the absence of another known etiology
2. Severe extrapyramidal symptoms characterized by two or more of the following: lead-pipe muscle rigidity, pronounced cogwheeling, sialorrhea, oculogyric crisis, retrocollis, opisthotonos, trismus, dysphagia, choreiform movements, festinating gait, and flexor-extensor posturing
3. Autonomic dysfunction characterized by two or more of the following: hypertension (at least 20-mm rise in diastolic pressure above baseline), tachycardia (at least 30 bpm), prominent diaphoresis, and incontinence

In retrospective diagnosis, if one of the three items listed above has not been specifically documented, a probable diagnosis is still permitted if the remaining two criteria are clearly met and the patient displays one of the following characteristic signs:
1) Clouded consciousness as evidenced by delirium, mutism, stupor, or coma;
2) leukocytosis (> 15,000 white blood cells/mm^3);
3) serum creatine kinase level greater than 1,000 IU/mL.

The syndrome can recur after it appears to have been brought under control, so patients should be observed carefully for 1 month after the condition is first noted. Neuroleptics should be avoided during that period.

We have successfully used ECT in treating persistently manic patients who have recently experienced an episode of NMS.

In many, but not all, patients, neuroleptics can be restarted cautiously at much lower dosages without the recurrence of NMS. It is not clear whether thioridazine is safer than one-quarter the dosage of the original offending medication. It seems sensible to avoid depot antipsychotics in patients with a history of NMS.

Long-Acting Injectable Antipsychotics

Adherence to a regimen of oral medications is difficult for many patients with schizophrenia and bipolar disorder. In a comparative efficacy trial of CATIE and the Systematic Treatment Enhancement Program for Bipolar Disorder (STEP-BD), more than 75% of patients eventually discontinued their oral medications. Long-acting injectables (LAIs) may be an alternative to daily oral medications for some patients. The primary advantage of injectables is their once- or twice-a-month dosing. On the other hand, disadvantages may include cost, the pain and inconvenience of having to come in regularly for an injection, and the persistence of side effects.

Depot haloperidol is still a commonly used LAI. It has been available as an alternative to depot fluphenazine. It is claimed that depot haloperidol's half-life is long enough that an injection every 4 weeks is adequate. If one assumes that 60–70 mg of orally ingested haloperidol actually survives passage through the gut and the liver to become bioavailable, a monthly injection of 20 times the daily oral dose is indicated. If a patient is treated with 10 mg/day of haloperidol, 200 mg/month of haloperidol decanoate could be given. The comparable conversion figure for fluphenazine is much lower—12.5 mg (0.5 mL) of the decanoate form every 3 weeks for patients taking 10 mg/day of oral fluphenazine. Our guess is that a lower haloperidol decanoate conversion figure will eventually prove adequate.

Dose-ranging studies of haloperidol decanoate suggest that the relapse rates for patients with schizophrenia taking 50 or 100 mg every 4 weeks are only a little higher than the relapse rates for patients taking 200 mg every 4 weeks. The 25-mg dose is clearly inadequate for controlling psychotic symptoms. In the few controlled studies comparing the two depot drugs, haloperidol has tended to be slightly more effective, with slightly fewer EPS. Studies comparing oral with depot haloperidol show fewer side effects for the depot preparation; the opposite is true for the fluphenazine formulations. Clinicians working in a setting where depot antipsychotics are commonly used should probably try depot haloperidol in a few patients and make up their own minds about its utility and consumer acceptance.

Several SGAs are available for use as LAIs. An LAI form of risperidone (Risperdal Consta) was approved in 2003 for the maintenance treatment of schizophrenia. The pivotal trials of the LAI form at 25 mg every 2 weeks for 12 weeks showed that the active drug was almost three times more likely than a placebo injection to lead to improvement on a standard psychosis scale (the PANSS). Since then, a number of controlled trials at doses of 25–75 mg every 2 weeks have shown that the LAI form of risperidone is effective and may have some tolerability advantages over the oral form. For example, the rate of EPS, including tardive dyskinesia, may be lower for the injectable form than for the oral form (Rainer 2008). In 1-year trials, the risperidone injection was associated with a tardive dyskinesia rate of about 1%, which is certainly no higher than, and probably lower than, the rate with the oral medicine. In addition, the rate of tardive dyskinesia with the LAI form of risperidone appears to be considerably lower than the rate reported with haloperidol decanoate or with fluphenazine decanoate. On the other hand, the LAI form of risperidone is much more expensive than the oral generic risperidone and has shown mixed results, compared with oral medications, in some outcome measures, such as decreased time in the hospital and decreasing overall health care costs (Taylor et al. 2009a, 2009b).

An LAI form of paliperidone (Invega Sustenna) was approved by the FDA in July 2009 in the maintenance treatment of schizophrenia. Paliperidone palmitate is a once-a-month injection whose efficacy appears to be similar to that of Risperdal Consta. Administration starts with two injections in the deltoid 1 week apart. The starting dose is typically 234 mg at day 1 and 156 mg at day 8 (Hu 2009). An even longer-lasting form of paliperidone (Invega Trinza) was FDA approved in 2015. Invega Trinza can be given every 3 months and is currently the longest-acting injectable available. Cutting down the need for coming in for an injection from 12 times per year to 4 times per year will be appealing to some patients and their families. Like the once-a-month injection, the longer-acting form comes in prefilled syringes.

The LAI form of olanzapine pamoate (Relprevv) was also approved in late 2009. Injectable olanzapine pamoate has shown efficacy as a once-a-month or twice-a-month injection in the maintenance treatment of schizophrenia. In one 24-week trial, 150 or 300 mg of olanzapine pamoate every 2 weeks or 405 mg every 4 weeks was comparable in efficacy to oral olanzapine 10–20 mg/day. Likewise, a 160-week open-label follow-up reported that the LAI form of olanzapine was significantly different from oral olanzapine in being less likely to be discontinued, less likely to be associated with weight gain >7%, and possibly having lower rates of EPS (Mitchell et al. 2013). The major problem noted in clinical trials with the LAI form of olanzapine has been postinjection delirium and sedation syndrome (PDSS). Accidental injection of olanzapine into the intravascular space may lead to a prolonged oversedation and delirium. In all the olanzapine trials, about 1.4% of patients to date have experienced this syndrome, which can range from mild confusion and gait disturbance to coma. All patients recovered, but in some cases it took days to weeks before full recovery was seen. Special precautions in the injection of olanzapine pamoate may further mitigate the risk of PDSS. Thus, long-acting olanzapine is probably best reserved for patients who need the convenience of a once-a-month injectable and have done best with oral olanzapine or have been unable to tolerate other LAIs.

Aripiprazole (Abilify Maintena) joined other long-acting SGA injectables with FDA approval in March 2013. In Phase III studies evaluating the relapse rate of 403 patients with schizophrenia who were receiving the once-a-month LAI form of aripiprazole or placebo, patients receiving the active drug were four times less likely to relapse over the course of 1 year than were patients receiving placebo (Potkin et al. 2013). Only 10% of patients taking the monthly aripiprazole injection relapsed versus 40% of the patients receiving saline injections. Rates of EPS did not differ significantly between the active drug and placebo groups, but patients in the active drug group were numerically more likely to experience parkinsonism with tremor (8.3%) than were patients in the placebo group (3%). Weight gain was also comparable in the aripiprazole LAI and placebo groups over the course of 1 year. It will take 1–2 weeks for the LAI aripiprazole to reach adequate plasma levels. Thus, when initiating the LAI, we continue oral aripiprazole at the patient's usual dose for the first week after giving an injection of 400 or 300 mg of the LAI. Then we cut the oral dose in half in the second week and discontinue the oral dose at the third week.

The choice of which LAI to use in the management of schizophrenia or bipolar disorder rests primarily on what oral preparation the patient responded to. Thus, patients who responded to and tolerated oral paliperidone and need an LAI because of adherence issues are best kept on LAI paliperidone. Likewise, responders to oral aripiprazole should probably stick with LAI aripiprazole. On the other hand, many patients who use oral risperidone would seem to do fine with LAI paliperidone and require only a once-a-month injection instead of the twice-per-month injection of LAI risperidone. In terms of side effects, particularly EPS, the LAI forms of SGAs seem to be much better tolerated than the depot forms of haloperidol and fluphenazine. However, as mentioned earlier in this chapter, the cost between first-generation LAIs such as haloperidol decanoate and second-generation agents such as LAI paliperidone or olanzapine can easily differ by tenfold or more. Thus, whereas tolerability will generally favor the SGA LAIs, cost will always favor the first-generation agents. There is no clear evidence that the LAI forms of SGAs are superior to the first-generation depot agents in general efficacy or preventing

Table 4–6. Long-acting injectable formulations of second-generation antipsychotics

Generic name	Trade name	Typical dose (mg)	Duration/interval
Risperidone	Risperdal Consta	25–50	2 weeks
Aripiprazole lauroxil	Aristada	441–882	4–6 weeks
Aripiprazole monohydrate	Abilify Maintena	300–400	4 weeks
Olanzapine pamoate	Zyprexa Relprevv	300–405	4 weeks
Paliperidone palmitate	Invega Sustenna	78–234	4 weeks
	Invega Trinza	273–819	12 weeks

relapse in patients with schizophrenia. However, second-generation LAIs do appear less likely to cause EPS. This is an important advantage given that once an extrapyramidal symptom develops with an injectable form, it is likely to persist for the duration of the injection and can be difficult to manage.

Typical doses and durations of LAIs are summarized in Table 4–6.

Adjunctive Treatment of Negative and Cognitive Symptoms

Negative or deficit symptoms contribute significantly to the morbidity associated with schizophrenia. Symptoms such as affective flattening, social withdrawal, executive dysfunction, anhedonia, and poverty of speech and thought content appear to be much more disabling to patients with schizophrenia than are positive symptoms. Although some authors suggest that the negative symptoms are largely related to the negative effects of FGAs, such symptoms were reported in the literature more than 100 years ago, before the availability of neuroleptics.

The pathophysiology of negative symptoms is still unknown. One theory that has gained popularity in recent years is that negative symptoms are related to a relative deficiency of dopamine in the prefrontal cortex. There are reports of levodopa, amphetamine, amantadine, and bromocriptine all being helpful in the negative symptoms of schizophrenia. On the other hand, some investigators have not found these dopamine agonists helpful (Silver and Geraisy 1995). A potential problem with these approaches is the possibility of worsening the psychosis in some patients. However, low doses of stimulants have been used over the years to counteract the sedation and malaise associated with FGAs and clozapine, and these stimulants do not appear to exacerbate psychosis as often as might be expected. Another approach is to use a drug such as selegiline to increase the availability of dopamine generally while also using an FGA. Bodkin et al. (1996) found that selegiline 5 mg bid over 6 weeks significantly improved negative symptoms and EPS in a group of 21 schizophrenia and schizoaffective disorder patients while having no effect on positive symptoms. At these low doses, one would not anticipate significant interactions with second-generation, serotonergic antipsychotics, but caution should be exercised. Finally, low doses of FGAs may actually increase the availability of dopamine synaptically by blocking presynaptic dopamine autoreceptors to release more dopamine. There have been some anecdotal reports of both worsening of positive symptoms and improvement of negative symptoms with low-dose antipsychotics. Amisulpride, a dopamine-blocking benzamide antipsychotic not yet available in the United States, was found in a placebo-controlled study to significantly improve negative symptoms of schizophrenia at low doses (Boyer et al. 1995). At high doses, amisulpride and FGAs may worsen negative symptoms by dampening dopaminergic tone throughout the prefrontal cortex.

The FDA and NIMH have sought to improve treatments for cognitive deficits because these deficits are directly related to the disability seen in schizophrenia. The Measurement and Treatment Research to Improve Cognition in Schizophrenia (MATRICS) initiative seeks to identify the cognitive deficits, develop better measurement tools for assessing cognition in schizophrenia, and encourage clinical trial design for assessing new agents to target these cognitive deficits. A number of potential drug targets are currently being evaluated in the treatment of cognitive deficits in schizophrenia. Among the more promising targets are acetylcholine receptor subtypes. Agonists of the α_7 nicotinic receptor have shown initial promise in improving cognitive deficits. An experimental α_7 agonist, 3-(2,4-dimethoxybenzylidene) anabaseine (DMXB-A), showed significant cognitive benefit in a proof-of-concept study with 12 patients with schizophrenia (Green 2007). Likewise, one acetylcholinesterase inhibitor, galantamine, has shown benefit in some, but not all, studies of treating cognitive deficits in schizophrenia (Gray and Roth 2007). On the other hand, rivastigmine and donepezil have not shown much benefit as adjunctive agents in treating cognitive deficits.

Noradrenergic neurotransmission also appears to be important in cognition. α_2-Adrenergic receptor agonists such as guanfacine and clonidine have shown some benefit in enhancing cognition in small trials (Friedman et al. 2001). Guanfacine continues to be investigated in improving cognition in schizophrenia because it is less likely to induce hypotension than is clonidine.

The role of serotonin in the pathophysiology of positive and negative symptoms gained significant attention with the success of clozapine. As described earlier, all the SGAs have in common a high ratio of 5-HT$_2$-to-D$_2$ affinities relative to FGAs. Certain 5-HT$_2$ agonists such as lysergic acid diethylamide (LSD) can produce hallucinations and other psychotic symptoms, whereas 5-HT$_2$ antagonists seem to improve psychosis. Even though serotonin has a putative effect on dopamine, which can contribute to its favorable effect on positive symptoms and the occasional worsening of EPS, serotonergic agents also appear to help with negative symptoms. All the SGAs share the ability to improve negative symptoms, and this is believed to be due in part to their 5-HT$_2$ antagonism. Of interest is a report that mirtazapine reduced negative symptoms in schizophrenia patients who were taking haloperidol (Berk et al. 2001). In addition, several studies suggested that the SSRIs may improve negative symptoms in schizophrenic patients. For example, in a placebo-controlled study of 34 patients with schizophrenia, Spina et al. (1994) found that adding 20 mg/day of fluoxetine to FGAs substantially improved negative symptoms. Likewise, paroxetine 30 mg/day appears effective in improving negative symptoms (Jockers-Scherübl et al. 2005). However, SSRIs may also increase the toxicity of FGAs and SGAs through competitive inhibition of the enzyme CYP2D6. We have occasionally used sertraline 50–100 mg/day as an adjunctive agent in treating negative symptoms and have found it modestly helpful. A number of other antidepressant treatments, including transdermal selegiline (Bodkin et al. 2005), mirtazapine (Zoccali et al. 2004), and transcranial magnetic stimulation (Jin et al. 2006), have also been suggested to help with negative symptoms of schizophrenia. However, few of these have been subjected to carefully controlled trials. Those that have, including mirtazapine (Berk et al. 2009), have not consistently shown benefit in treating negative symptoms.

Glutamate-specific agents may have a role to play in treating negative and positive symptoms of schizophrenia. NMDA antagonists such as phencyclidine and ketamine produce not only positive psychotic symptoms but also negative symptoms and cognitive symptoms. Thus, drugs that modulate glutamate activity are under investigation for the treatment of cognitive and negative symptoms (Webber and Marder 2008). Among the more promising agents identified by MATRICS are allosteric modulators of α-amino-3-hydroxy-5-methyl-4-isoxazolepropionic acid receptors (ampakines). One ampakine, CX-516, has shown mixed results in treating cognitive symptoms of schizophrenia (Goff et al. 2008). Another type of glutamate agent is one that directly acts on NMDA receptors, including the glycine cosite of the receptor. Agents such as D-cycloserine and glycine have been evaluated for treating cognitive symptoms in schizophrenia. Neither has been all that effective. That being said, glutamate-specific agents continue to be evaluated in the treatment of schizophrenia.

It seems unlikely that we will discover antipsychotics that are profoundly and equally effective at treating both the positive and negative symptoms of schizophrenia. Our understanding of the pathophysiology of schizophrenia, limited as it might be, argues against the likelihood of monotherapies being effective for all symptoms of the disorder. Thus, it appears probable that the treatment of schizophrenia will increasingly depend on a combination of agents that target specific positive and negative symptoms and cognitive symptoms of schizophrenia.

Alternatives to Antipsychotic Therapy

There are currently no reliable, safe, effective drug therapies for schizophrenia and other psychotic disorders that can replace dopamine-blocking antipsychotics. ECT can reverse psychotic excitements and catatonic stupor but has no real value in preventing future episodes of psychosis. Lithium can ameliorate the symptoms of schizophrenia or suppress episodic violence in schizophrenic patients, but it almost never is an adequate drug therapy by itself. Carbamazepine also ameliorates symptoms in some patients with treatment-resistant psychosis when added to a neuroleptic, as a double-blind Israeli study showed (Klein et al. 1984), but it is not by itself an adequate therapy for schizophrenia. Later studies of lithium and anticonvulsants in the adjunctive treatment of schizophrenia have often not supported the earlier trials (Citrome 2009). A trial by Casey and colleagues (2003) found that valproate add-on to risperidone or olanzapine was significantly more effective than placebo add-on in patients with schizophrenia. However, the data on adjunctive use of valproate in schizophrenia appear to be strongest for alleviating aggressive symptoms rather than treating positive or negative symptoms (Schwarz et al. 2008). Diazepam alone has been reported by both Canadian and German groups to rapidly control psychotic symptoms in small numbers of paranoid schizophrenic patients at dosages between 70 and 400 mg/day (the German group used 50-mg tablets). Sedation was not a problem, allegedly, after the first day, and improvement continued for 4 weeks. Neither study reported follow-up data. In one study, high-dose diazepam aggravated schizoaffective symptoms. The findings from these small, brief studies are intriguing, but they do not offer a real and useful pharmacological alternative to the FGAs.

There have been at least seven reports on the use of alprazolam in patients with schizophrenia who were being treated with neuroleptics. Two of the studies involved patients with clear panic attacks as well as chronic psychosis. Both small studies found alprazolam to be useful in suppressing episodes of panic. Several other small studies, mainly in inpatients, found the addition of alprazolam to be beneficial in some patients. The original hypothesis was that alprazolam would be particularly useful in treating negative symptoms, but the studies showed effects of alprazolam on both positive and negative symptoms in some patients. The only large placebo-controlled study involving schizophrenic outpatients yielded completely negative findings (Csernansky et al. 1988); neither diazepam nor alprazolam was more effective than placebo over the course of this 8-week trial. The data from the diverse studies are inconclusive, but a reasonable presumption is that alprazolam might be helpful as an adjunct to neuroleptic treatment in patients with panic attacks or other significant anxiety symptoms.

Propranolol was studied for many years in the treatment of acute and chronic schizophrenia at very high dosages (600–2,000 mg/day) given alone or with a neuroleptic drug. Although Yorkston et al. (1978) reported efficacy in controlled studies, other investigators found equivocal results, with only occasional patients experiencing any benefit. Because two early deaths occurred with this treatment—one death from a silent bleeding peptic ulcer and one sudden death of unknown etiology—this use was not generally recommended. However, subsequent clinical studies of dosages up to 400 mg/day in organically impaired psychiatric patients with impulsive violence or aggression suggested that propranolol might be useful in such patients in controlling temper outbursts, although it did not affect other underlying behavioral organic deficits. If such therapy is attempted, the relevant articles should be reviewed and the dosage should be increased slowly, with blood pressure and pulse monitoring before each dose until the patient is well stabilized at a constant, effective dose. Propranolol has been reported to increase chlorpromazine blood levels and may do so for other antipsychotics as well.

It is possible that carbamazepine, valproate, and lithium also offer more promise in the treatment of disturbed behavior in patients with brain damage, dementia, or intellectual developmental disorder than do the FGAs. Low doses of valproate and SGAs are helpful adjuncts in dementia. However, no antipsychotics or anticonvulsants have proven consistently effective in treating behavioral or psychotic symptoms in dementia, and none have been approved for this indication.

Antipsychotic Drugs in Development

A number of new targets for antipsychotic drug development have shown promise in early randomized trials. One novel target is the trace amine associated receptor 1 (TAAR1). TAAR1 agonists have a variety of indirect effects on monoamines. They inhibit the firing of dopaminergic and serotonergic neurons. In schizophrenia, some research has proposed that the pathophysiology may involve increased capacity for the synthesis of dopamine in striatal areas. TAAR1 agonists interfere with this capacity.

The TAAR1 agonist furthest along in development is ulotaront. Thus far, a Phase II study has been completed that involved 245 patients with an acute relapse of schizophrenia (Koblan et al. 2020). Patients were randomly assigned to 50–75 mg of ulotaront or placebo for 4 weeks. The active group had a very substantial 17.2-point improvement on the PANSS relative to a 9.7-point improvement in the placebo group. In the active group, 65% of patients had a response, defined as >20% improvement on the PANSS, whereas 44% of placebo-treated patients achieved a response. There were no significant differences in EPS, metabolic parameters, or other side effects between the active and placebo groups. This study was followed by a 6-month open-label extension (Correll et al. 2021). In that trial, 90% of patients had a 30% improvement in their PANSS scores from their double-blind baseline, and more than 70% had a 50% improvement from their baseline. As with the acute study, no clinically meaningful changes in EPS, weight, or metabolic parameters were found over

6 months. Ulotaront looks very promising from a safety and efficacy standpoint, and multiple Phase III studies are under way as of this writing.

Another novel class of antipsychotic agents in late development at this time are the muscarine agonists. Xanomeline is one of these cholinergic agonists with affinity for the M_1 and M_4 receptors. In clinical trials, xanomeline has been paired with trospium in a combination called KarXT to limit peripheral muscarine effects, such as nausea and diarrhea. Although xanomeline has little affinity for dopamine receptors, it has indirect antagonist effects on several dopamine receptors in the rodent model. The drug has a half-life of about 4 hours and thus reaches steady state in about 24 hours with repeated dosing.

There have been two published clinical trials with xanomeline in the treatment of schizophrenia to date. The first double-blind study was published in 2008 (Shekhar et al. 2008) and involved 20 patients randomly assigned to either xanomeline titrated from 25 mg tid to a maximum of 75 mg tid or placebo for 4 weeks. Patients in the xanomeline group showed significantly more improvement on the PANSS overall score as well the negative and positive symptom subscales. In a larger randomized trial, xanomeline was well tolerated, with mild to moderate GI side effects being the most commonly seen relative to placebo.

A larger Phase II study involved 182 patients with schizophrenia who were treated with up to 125 mg of xanomeline and 30 mg trospium in two divided doses or placebo for 5 weeks (Brannan et al. 2021). Patients in the active group had significant improvement, with an average drop of 5.9 points more on the PANSS than did the placebo-treated patients. The most common side effects were, again, GI side effects, including constipation, nausea, and vomiting. There were no significant EPS or weight gain/metabolic side effects. In addition, a post hoc analysis of this study showed substantial benefits of xanomeline plus trospium for the treatment of cognitive deficits in this population. Phase III studies have been completed as of this date, and results are pending. Approval for xanomeline plus trospium was filed September 2023.

A number of other antipsychotic agents are available for prescription use in one or more European countries. Some have been available in Europe for years but have never been released in the United States. A few failed to pass the FDA's carcinogenicity screen; we believe this is true of sulpride, amisulpride, and penfluridol. Fluspirilene, an LAI drug, is held in suspension by a chemical that is not approved by the FDA.

Another SGA long available in Europe and Japan is zotepine. Zotepine is a D_2/5-HT_2 antagonist that also has significant effects on other serotonin receptors, including 5-HT_6 and 5-HT_7. In addition, zotepine is a norepinephrine reuptake inhibitor. It has a tricyclic chemical structure and appears to be a reasonable antidepressant. Zotepine appears to be effective in some cases of treatment-resistant schizophrenia, and EPS are quite uncommon with the drug. However, zotepine has two big drawbacks: weight gain and sedation. At least a third of all patients gain a significant amount of weight at dosages of 75–450 mg/day. In addition, many patients have difficulty tolerating the somnolence associated with the drug. As a result, zotepine is not likely to be introduced into the U.S. market.

An active metabolite of clozapine, N-desmethylclozapine (norclozapine) is being actively investigated for the treatment of schizophrenia (Natesan et al. 2007). Norclozapine is a partial agonist at the D_2 receptor and also is a muscarinic receptor agonist. Thus, it is being evaluated for treatment of the cognitive symptoms of schizophrenia. There is some suggestion that norclozapine may be better tolerated and safer than clozapine, but large-scale studies have not been completed to date.

Sulpiride is clearly a second-generation (atypical) antipsychotic in that it differs from the older antipsychotics in its pharmacology. However, it causes pseudoparkinsonism, akathisia, galactorrhea, and tardive dyskinesia to such a degree that its advantages over other neuroleptics more readily available in the United States are unclear. Several drugs available in Europe are clinically and pharmacologically related to sulpiride. One of these, metoclopramide (Reglan), is marketed in the United States for GI diseases but is probably effective in treating psychosis and certainly can cause typical neurological side effects and tardive dyskinesia. Amisulpride has shown antipsychotic as well as antidepressant benefits. Its efficacy appears at least as good in the treatment of schizophrenia as that of other SGAs. Most sulpiride-like drugs are good antiemetics and speed peristalsis, including stomach emptying, making them useful in dyspepsia.

The reason for discussing these drugs in an American psychopharmacology manual is that current FDA and customs policies, influenced by pressures from patients with AIDS, have allowed 3-month supplies of drugs that are not available in the United States to be imported for individual patients with treatment-resistant conditions. It is not clear that any of these drugs are so different and so superior (as was clearly the case with clomipramine in the treatment of OCD) as to impel many psychiatrists to arrange to bring one or more of these drugs to the United States; however, in special situations it might be worth doing. Since September 11, 2001, some patients have at times found importation to be delayed.

Suggested Readings

Alvir JM, Lieberman JA, Safferman AZ, et al: Clozapine-induced agranulocytosis: incidence and risk factors in the United States. N Engl J Med 329(3):162–167, 1993 8515788

Aman MG, Arnold LE, McDougle CJ, et al: Acute and long-term safety and tolerability of risperidone in children with autism. J Child Adolesc Psychopharmacol 15(6):869–884, 2005 16379507

American Psychiatric Association: Diagnostic and Statistical Manual of Mental Disorders, 3rd Edition, Revised. Washington, DC, American Psychiatric Association, 1987

American Psychiatric Association: Diagnostic and Statistical Manual of Mental Disorders, 4th Edition. Washington, DC, American Psychiatric Association, 1994

American Psychiatric Association: Diagnostic and Statistical Manual of Mental Disorders, 4th Edition, Text Revision. Washington, DC, American Psychiatric Association, 2000

Ayd F: Lorazepam update: 1977–1985. Int Drug Ther Newsl 20:33–36, 1985

Baldessarini RJ, Cole JO, Davis JM, et al: Tardive Dyskinesia (Task Force Report No 18). Washington, DC, American Psychiatric Association, 1980

Baldessarini RJ, Cohen BM, Teicher MH: Pharmacological treatment, in Schizophrenia: Treatment of Acute Psychotic Episodes. Edited by Levy ST, Ninan PT. Washington, DC, American Psychiatric Press, 1990, pp 61–118

Baldwin DS, Montgomery SA: First clinical experience with olanzapine (LY 170053): results of an open-label safety and dose-ranging study in patients with schizophrenia. Int Clin Psychopharmacol 10(4):239–244, 1995 8748045

Baptista T, Uzcátegui E, Rangel N, et al: Metformin plus sibutramine for olanzapine-associated weight gain and metabolic dysfunction in schizophrenia: a 12-week double-blind, placebo-controlled pilot study. Psychiatry Res 159(1–2):250–253, 2008 18374423

Barbee JG, Conrad EJ, Jamhour NJ: The effectiveness of olanzapine, risperidone, quetiapine, and ziprasidone as augmentation agents in treatment-resistant major depressive disorder. J Clin Psychiatry 65(7):975–981, 2004 15291687

Beckmann H, Haas S: High dose diazepam in schizophrenia. Psychopharmacology (Berl) 71(1):79–82, 1980 6779328

Benvenga MJ, Leander JD: Olanzapine, an atypical antipsychotic, increases rates of punished responding in pigeons. Psychopharmacology (Berl) 119(2):133–138, 1995 7544900

Berk M, Ichim L, Brook S: Olanzapine compared to lithium in mania: a double-blind randomized controlled trial. Int Clin Psychopharmacol 14(6):339–343, 1999 10565800

Bishop MP, Simpson GM, Dunnett CW, et al: Efficacy of loxapine in the treatment of paranoid schizophrenia. Psychopharmacology (Berl) 51(2):107–115, 1977 14350

Blackwell B: Drug therapy: patient compliance. N Engl J Med 289(5):249–252, 1973 4713764

Bogenschutz MP, George Nurnberg H: Olanzapine versus placebo in the treatment of borderline personality disorder. J Clin Psychiatry 65(1):104–109, 2004 14744178

Brown WA, Laughren T: Low serum prolactin and early relapse following neuroleptic withdrawal. Am J Psychiatry 138(2):237–239, 1981 6109456

Carpenter WT Jr: Serotonin-dopamine antagonists and treatment of negative symptoms. J Clin Psychopharmacol 15(1)(Suppl 1):30S–35S, 1995 7730498

Casey DE: Implications of the CATIE trial on treatment: extrapyramidal symptoms. CNS Spectr 11(7)(Suppl 7):25–31, 2006 16816797

Casey DE, Sands EE, Heisterberg J, et al: Efficacy and safety of bifeprunox in patients with an acute exacerbation of schizophrenia: results from a randomized, double-blind, placebo-controlled, multicenter, dose-finding study. Psychopharmacology (Berl) 200(3):317–331, 2008 18597078

Chouinard G, Jones B, Remington G, et al: A Canadian multicenter placebo-controlled study of fixed doses of risperidone and haloperidol in the treatment of chronic schizophrenic patients. J Clin Psychopharmacol 13(1):25–40, 1993 7683702

Citrome L, Weiden PJ, McEvoy JP, et al: Effectiveness of lurasidone in schizophrenia or schizoaffective patients switched from other antipsychotics: a 6-month, open-label, extension study. CNS Spectr 16:1–10, 2013 24330868

Cohen BM: The clinical utility of plasma neuroleptic levels, in Guidelines for the Use of Psychotropic Drugs. Edited by Stancer H. New York, Spectrum, 1984, pp 245–260

Cole JO: Antipsychotic drugs: is more better? McLean Hospital Journal 7:61–87, 1982

Cole JO, Gardos G: Alternatives to neuroleptic drug therapy. McLean Hospital Journal 10:112–127, 1985

Cole JO, Yonkers KA: Non-benzodiazepine anxiolytics, in The American Psychiatric Press Textbook of Psychopharmacology. Edited by Schatzberg AF, Nemeroff CB. Washington, DC, American Psychiatric Press, 1995, pp 231–244

Cole JO, Gardos G, Gelernter J, et al: Supersensitivity psychosis. McLean Hospital Journal 9:46–72, 1984

Comaty JE, Janicak PG: Depot neuroleptics. Psychiatr Ann 17:491–496, 1987

Creese I: Dopamine and antipsychotic medications, in Psychiatry Update: The American Psychiatric Association Annual Review, Vol 4. Edited by Hales RE, Frances AJ. Washington, DC, American Psychiatric Press, 1985, pp 17–36

Dando TM, Keating GM: Quetiapine: a review of its use in acute mania and depression associated with bipolar disorder. Drugs 65(17):2533–2551, 2005 16296876

Davis JM: Overview: maintenance therapy in psychiatry I: schizophrenia. Am J Psychiatry 132(12):1237–1245, 1975 914

Davis RJ, Cummings JL: Clinical variants of tardive dyskinesia. Neuropsychiatry Neuropsychol Behav Neurol 1:31–38, 1988

De Deyn PP, Rabheru K, Rasmussen A, et al: A randomized trial of risperidone, placebo, and haloperidol for behavioral symptoms of dementia. Neurology 53(5):946–955, 1999 10496251

De Deyn PP, Carrasco MM, Deberdt W, et al: Olanzapine versus placebo in the treatment of psychosis with or without associated behavioral disturbances in patients with Alzheimer's disease. Int J Geriatr Psychiatry 19(2):115–126, 2004 14758577

Delva NJ, Letemendia FJ: Lithium treatment in schizophrenia and schizoaffective disorders. Br J Psychiatry 141:387–400, 1982 6129016

Dixon L, Weiden PJ, Frances AJ, et al: Alprazolam intolerance in stable schizophrenic outpatients. Psychopharmacol Bull 25(2):213–214, 1989 2602514

Donaldson SR, Gelenberg AJ, Baldessarini RJ: The pharmacologic treatment of schizophrenia: a progress report. Schizophr Bull 9(4):504–527, 1983 6140750

Douyon R, Angrist B, Peselow E, et al: Neuroleptic augmentation with alprazolam: clinical effects and pharmacokinetic correlates. Am J Psychiatry 146(2):231–234, 1989 2563211

Ferreri MM, Loze JY, Rouillon F, et al: Clozapine treatment of a borderline personality disorder with severe self-mutilating behaviours. Eur Psychiatry 19(3):177–178, 2004 15158928

Finnerty RJ, Goldberg HL, Nathan L, et al: Haloperidol in the treatment of psychoneurotic anxious outpatients. Dis Nerv Syst 37(11):621–624, 1976 791602

Fluvoxamine for obsessive-compulsive disorder. Med Lett Drugs Ther 37(942):13–14, 1995 7845314

Fluvoxamine gains approval for obsessive-compulsive disorder. Am J Health Syst Pharm 52(4):355, 1995 7757852

Galbrecht CR, Klett CJ: Predicting response to phenothiazines: the right drug for the right patient. J Nerv Ment Dis 147(2):173–183, 1968 5677325

Gardos G, Casey D: Tardive Dyskinesia and Affective Disorders. Washington, DC, American Psychiatric Press, 1984

Gardos G, Perenyi A, Cole J: Polypharmacy revisited. McLean Hospital Journal 5:178–195, 1980

Garza-Treviño ES, Hollister LE, Overall JE, et al: Efficacy of combinations of intramuscular antipsychotics and sedative-hypnotics for control of psychotic agitation. Am J Psychiatry 146(12):1598–1601, 1989 2686478

Gelenberg AJ (ed): Risperidone and mania. Biological Therapies in Psychiatry Newsletter 17:45, 1994

Gelenberg AJ, Mandel MR: Catatonic reactions to high-potency neuroleptic drugs. Arch Gen Psychiatry 34(8):947–950, 1977 889419

Gerson SL: G-CSF and the management of clozapine-induced agranulocytosis. J Clin Psychiatry 55(Suppl B):139–142, 1994 7525542

Gilbert PL, Harris MJ, McAdams LA, et al: Neuroleptic withdrawal in schizophrenic patients: a review of the literature. Arch Gen Psychiatry 52(3):173–188, 1995 7872841

Goff DC, Sullivan LM, McEvoy JP, et al: A comparison of ten-year cardiac risk estimates in schizophrenia patients from the CATIE study and matched controls. Schizophr Res 80(1):45–53, 2005 16198088

Greendyke RM, Schuster DB, Wooton JA: Propranolol in the treatment of assaultive patients with organic brain disease. J Clin Psychopharmacol 4(5):282–285, 1984 6490964

Hamner MB, Faldowski RA, Ulmer HG, et al: Adjunctive risperidone treatment in post-traumatic stress disorder: a preliminary controlled trial of effects on comorbid psychotic symptoms. Int Clin Psychopharmacol 18(1):1–8, 2003 12490768

Hayes PE, Schulz SC: The use of beta-adrenergic blocking agents in anxiety disorders and schizophrenia. Pharmacotherapy 3(2 Pt 1):101–117, 1983 6134273

Hillebrand JJ, van Elburg AA, Kas MJ, et al: Olanzapine reduces physical activity in rats exposed to activity-based anorexia: possible implications for treatment of anorexia nervosa? Biol Psychiatry 58(8):651–657, 2005 16018979

Hogarty GE: Treatment and the course of schizophrenia. Schizophr Bull 3(4):587–599, 1977 22929

Hogarty GE, Ulrich RF: Temporal effects of drug and placebo in delaying relapse in schizophrenic outpatients. Arch Gen Psychiatry 34(3):297–301, 1977 190970

Hyttel J, Arnt J, Costall B, et al: Pharmacological profile of the atypical neuroleptic sertindole. Clin Neuropharmacol 15(Suppl 1 Pt A):267A–268A, 1992 1354033

Hyttel J, Nielsen JB, Nowak G: The acute effect of sertindole on brain 5-HT2, D2 and alpha 1 receptors (ex vivo radioreceptor binding studies). J Neural Transm (Vienna) 89(1–2):61–69, 1992 1329856

Inoue A, Seto M, Sugita S, et al: Differential effects on D2 dopamine receptor and prolactin gene expression by haloperidol and aripiprazole in the rat pituitary. Brain Res Mol Brain Res 55(2):285–292, 1998 9582438

Jandl M, Bittner R, Sack A, et al: Changes in negative symptoms and EEG in schizophrenic patients after repetitive transcranial magnetic stimulation (rTMS): an open-label pilot study. J Neural Transm (Vienna) 112(7):955–967, 2005 15517429

Jefferson J, Greist J: Haloperidol and lithium: their combined use and the issue of their compatibility, in Haloperidol Update, 1958–1980. Edited by Ayd F. Baltimore, MD, Ayd Medical Communications, 1980

Kane JM, Woerner M, Weinhold P, et al: A prospective study of tardive dyskinesia development: preliminary results. J Clin Psychopharmacol 2(5):345–349, 1982 6127353

Katz IR, Jeste DV, Mintzer JE, et al: Comparison of risperidone and placebo for psychosis and behavioral disturbances associated with dementia: a randomized, double-blind trial. J Clin Psychiatry 60(2):107–115, 1999 10084637

Keck PE Jr, Caroff SN, McElroy SL: Neuroleptic malignant syndrome and malignant hyperthermia: end of a controversy? J Neuropsychiatry Clin Neurosci 7(2):135–144, 1995 7626956

Keepers GA, Clappison VJ, Casey DE: Initial anticholinergic prophylaxis for neuroleptic-induced extrapyramidal syndromes. Arch Gen Psychiatry 40(10):1113–1117, 1983 6138011

Khouzam HR, Donnelly NJ: Remission of self-mutilation in a patient with borderline personality during risperidone therapy. J Nerv Ment Dis 185(5):348–349, 1997 9171814

Klein DF: False suffocation alarms, spontaneous panics, and related conditions: an integrative hypothesis. Arch Gen Psychiatry 50(4):306–317, 1993 8466392

Kordon A, Wahl K, Koch N, et al: Quetiapine addition to serotonin reuptake inhibitors in patients with severe obsessive-compulsive disorder: a double-blind, randomized, placebo-controlled study. J Clin Psychopharmacol 28(5):550–554, 2008 18794652

Lawler CP, Prioleau C, Lewis MM, et al: Interactions of the novel antipsychotic aripiprazole (OPC-14597) with dopamine and serotonin receptor subtypes. Neuropsychopharmacology 20(6):612–627, 1999 10327430

Lee PE, Gill SS, Freedman M, et al: Atypical antipsychotic drugs in the treatment of behavioural and psychological symptoms of dementia: systematic review. BMJ 329(7457):75, 2004 15194601

Levenson JL: Neuroleptic malignant syndrome. Am J Psychiatry 142(10):1137–1145, 1985 2863986

Lieberman JA, Kane JM, Johns CA: Clozapine: guidelines for clinical management. J Clin Psychiatry 50(9):329–338, 1989 2670914

Lindenmayer JP: New pharmacotherapeutic modalities for negative symptoms in psychosis. Acta Psychiatr Scand Suppl 388:15–19, 1995 7541598

Lingjaerde O: Benzodiazepines in the treatment of schizophrenia, in The Benzodiazepines: From Molecular Biology to Clinical Practice. Edited by Costa E. New York, Raven, 1983, pp 369–381

Lipinski JF Jr, Zubenko GS, Cohen BM, et al: Propranolol in the treatment of neuroleptic-induced akathisia. Am J Psychiatry 141(3):412–415, 1984 6142657

Lobo MC, Whitehurst TS, Kaar SJ, et al: New and emerging treatments for schizophrenia: a narrative review of their pharmacology, efficacy and side effect profile relative to established antipsychotics. Neurosci Biobehav Rev 132:324–361, 2022 34838528

Loebel A, Cucchiaro J, Xu J, et al: Effectiveness of lurasidone vs. quetiapine XR for relapse prevention in schizophrenia: a 12-month, double-blind, noninferiority study. Schizophr Res 147(1):95–102, 2013 23583011

Luby E: Reserpine-like drugs—clinical efficacy, in Psychopharmacology: A Review of Progress, 1957–1967. Edited by Efron D. Washington, DC, U.S. Government Printing Office, 1968, pp 1077–1082

Marder SR, Van Putten T: Who should receive clozapine? Arch Gen Psychiatry 45(9):865–867, 1988 2901253

Marder SR, Hubbard JW, Van Putten T, et al: Pharmacokinetics of long-acting injectable neuroleptic drugs: clinical implications. Psychopharmacology (Berl) 98(4):433–439, 1989 2570430

Mason AS, Granacher RP: Clinical Handbook of Antipsychotic Drug Therapy. New York, Brunner/Mazel, 1978

May PRA: Treatment of Schizophrenia: A Comparative Study of Five Treatment Methods. New York, Science House, 1968

McEvoy JP, Hogarty GE, Steingard S: Optimal dose of neuroleptic in acute schizophrenia: a controlled study of the neuroleptic threshold and higher haloperidol dose. Arch Gen Psychiatry 48(8):739–745, 1991 1883257

Meltzer HY, Elkis H, Vanover K, et al: Pimavanserin, a selective serotonin (5-HT)2A-inverse agonist, enhances the efficacy and safety of risperidone, 2mg/day, but does not enhance efficacy of haloperidol, 2mg/day: comparison with reference dose risperidone, 6mg/day. Schizophr Res 141(2–3):144–152, 2012 22954754

Menaster M: Use of olanzapine in anorexia nervosa. J Clin Psychiatry 66(5):654–655, author reply 655–656, 2005 15889956

Meyer JM, Nasrallah HA, McEvoy JP, et al: The Clinical Antipsychotic Trials of Intervention Effectiveness (CATIE) Schizophrenia Trial: clinical comparison of subgroups with and without the metabolic syndrome. Schizophr Res 80(1):9–18, 2005 16125372

Monnelly EP, Ciraulo DA, Knapp C, et al: Low-dose risperidone as adjunctive therapy for irritable aggression in posttraumatic stress disorder. J Clin Psychopharmacol 23(2):193–196, 2003 12640221

Moore NA, Tye NC, Axton MS, et al: The behavioral pharmacology of olanzapine, a novel "atypical" antipsychotic agent. J Pharmacol Exp Ther 262(2):545–551, 1992 1354253

Morrison JA, Cottingham EM, Barton BA: Metformin for weight loss in pediatric patients taking psychotropic drugs. Am J Psychiatry 159(4):655–657, 2002 11925306

Nasrallah HA, Silva R, Phillips D, et al: Lurasidone for the treatment of acutely psychotic patients with schizophrenia: a 6-week, randomized, placebo-controlled study. J Psychiatr Res 47(5):670–677, 2013 23421963

Nemeroff CB: Use of atypical antipsychotics in refractory depression and anxiety. J Clin Psychiatry 66(Suppl 8):13–21, 2005 16336032

Nosè M, Cipriani A, Biancosino B, et al: Efficacy of pharmacotherapy against core traits of borderline personality disorder: meta-analysis of randomized controlled trials. Int Clin Psychopharmacol 21(6):345–353, 2006 17012981

Owen RR Jr, Cole JO: Molindone hydrochloride: a review of laboratory and clinical findings. J Clin Psychopharmacol 9(4):268–276, 1989 2671060

Owen RR Jr, Beake BJ, Marby D, et al: Response to clozapine in chronic psychotic patients. Psychopharmacol Bull 25(2):253–256, 1989 2602519

Papakostas GI, Petersen TJ, Nierenberg AA, et al: Ziprasidone augmentation of selective serotonin reuptake inhibitors (SSRIs) for SSRI-resistant major depressive disorder. J Clin Psychiatry 65(2):217–221, 2004 15003076

Papakostas GI, Petersen TJ, Kinrys G, et al: Aripiprazole augmentation of selective serotonin reuptake inhibitors for treatment-resistant major depressive disorder. J Clin Psychiatry 66(10):1326–1330, 2005 16259548

Patkar AA, Peindl K, Mago R, et al: An open-label, rater-blinded, augmentation study of aripiprazole in treatment-resistant depression. Prim Care Companion J Clin Psychiatry 8(2):82–87, 2006 16862232

Perrella C, Carrus D, Costa E, et al: Quetiapine for the treatment of borderline personality disorder; an open-label study. Prog Neuropsychopharmacol Biol Psychiatry 31(1):158–163, 2007 17045720

Phillips KA, McElroy SL, Keck PE Jr, et al: A comparison of delusional and nondelusional body dysmorphic disorder in 100 cases. Psychopharmacol Bull 30(2):179–186, 1994 7831453

Pini S, Abelli M, Cassano GB: The role of quetiapine in the treatment of bipolar disorder. Expert Opin Pharmacother 7(7):929–940, 2006 16634715

Pisciotta AV: Agranulocytosis induced by certain phenothiazine derivatives. JAMA 208(10):1862–1868, 1969 4890332

Potenza MN, Wasylink S, Longhurst JG, et al: Olanzapine augmentation of fluoxetine in the treatment of refractory obsessive-compulsive disorder (letter). J Clin Psychopharmacol 18(5):423–424, 1998 9790164

Potkin SG, Cohen M, Panagides J: Efficacy and tolerability of asenapine in acute schizophrenia: a placebo- and risperidone-controlled trial. J Clin Psychiatry 68(10):1492–1500, 2007 17960962

Ram A, Cao Q, Keck PE Jr, et al: Structural change in dopamine D2 receptor gene in a patient with neuroleptic malignant syndrome. Am J Med Genet 60(3):228–230, 1995 7573176

Rapaport MH, Gharabawi GM, Canuso CM, et al: Effects of risperidone augmentation in patients with treatment-resistant depression: results of open-label treatment followed by double-blind continuation. Neuropsychopharmacology 31(11):2505–2513, 2006 16760927

Robertson MM, Trimble MR: Major tranquillisers used as antidepressants: a review. J Affect Disord 4(3):173–193, 1982 6127357

Rocca P, Marchiaro L, Cocuzza E, et al: Treatment of borderline personality disorder with risperidone. J Clin Psychiatry 63(3):241–244, 2002 11926724

Roy-Byrne P, Gerner R, Liston E, et al: ECT for acute mania: a forgotten treatment modality. J Psychiatr Treat Eval 3:83–86, 1981

Sachs GS, Lafer B, Truman CJ, et al: Lithium monotherapy: miracle, myth, and misunderstanding. Psychiatr Ann 24:299–306, 1994

Salam SA, Kilzieh N: Lorazepam treatment of psychogenic catatonia: an update. J Clin Psychiatry 49(12)(suppl):16–21, 1988 3058684

Saltz BL, Kane JM, Woerner MG, et al: Prospective study of tardive dyskinesia in the elderly. Psychopharmacol Bull 25(1):52–56, 1989 2772118

Salzman C: The use of ECT in the treatment of schizophrenia. Am J Psychiatry 137(9):1032–1041, 1980 6107048

Shelton RC: Treatment options for refractory depression. J Clin Psychiatry 60(Suppl 4):57–61, discussion 62–63, 1999 10086483

Silver J, Yudofsky S: Propranolol for aggression: literature review and clinical guidelines. Int Drug Ther Newsl 20:9–12, 1985

Siris SG, Morgan V, Fagerstrom R, et al: Adjunctive imipramine in the treatment of postpsychotic depression: a controlled trial. Arch Gen Psychiatry 44(6):533–539, 1987 3555386

Skarsfeldt T: Comparison of short-term administration of sertindole, clozapine and haloperidol on the inactivation of midbrain dopamine neurons in the rat. Eur J Pharmacol 254(3):291–294, 1994 7912200

Solmi M, Pigato G, Kane JM, et al: Treatment of tardive dyskinesia with VMAT-2 inhibitors: a systematic review and meta-analysis of randomized controlled trials. Drug Des Devel Ther 12:1215–1238, 2018 29795977

Soloff PH, Cornelius J, George A, et al: Efficacy of phenelzine and haloperidol in borderline personality disorder. Arch Gen Psychiatry 50(5):377–385, 1993 8489326

Soloff PH, Lis JA, Kelly T, et al: Risk factors for suicidal behavior in borderline personality disorder. Am J Psychiatry 151(9):1316–1323, 1994 8067487

Stigler KA, Mullett JE, Erickson CA, et al: Paliperidone for irritability in adolescents and young adults with autistic disorder. Psychopharmacology (Berl) 223(2):237–245, 2012 22549762

Stoppe G, Brandt CA, Staedt JH: Behavioural problems associated with dementia: the role of newer antipsychotics. Drugs Aging 14(1):41–54, 1999 10069407

Suzuki T, Misawa M: Sertindole antagonizes morphine-, cocaine-, and methamphetamine-induced place preference in the rat. Life Sci 57(13):1277–1284, 1995 7674819

Szigethy EM, Schulz SC: Risperidone in comorbid borderline personality disorder and dysthymia (letter). J Clin Psychopharmacol 17(4):326–327, 1997 9241018

Teicher MH, Glod CA, Aaronson ST, et al: Open assessment of the safety and efficacy of thioridazine in the treatment of patients with borderline personality disorder. Psychopharmacol Bull 25(4):535–549, 1989 2631134

Thase ME, Corya SA, Osuntokun O, et al: A randomized, double-blind comparison of olanzapine/fluoxetine combination, olanzapine, and fluoxetine in treatment-resistant major depressive disorder. J Clin Psychiatry 68(2):224–236, 2007 17335320

Tollefson GD, Sanger TM, Lu Y, et al: Depressive signs and symptoms in schizophrenia: a prospective blinded trial of olanzapine and haloperidol. Arch Gen Psychiatry 55(3):250–258, 1998 9510219

Tuason VB, Escobar JI, Garvey M, et al: Loxapine versus chlorpromazine in paranoid schizophrenia: a double-blind study. J Clin Psychiatry 45(4):158–163, 1984 6370967

Tzeng TB, Stamm G, Chu SY: Sensitive method for the assay of sertindole in plasma by high-performance liquid chromatography and fluorimetric detection. J Chromatogr B Biomed Appl 661(2):299–306, 1994 7894670

Vieta E, Herraiz M, Fernández A, et al: Group for the Study of Risperidone in Affective Disorders (GSRAD): efficacy and safety of risperidone in the treatment of schizoaffective disorder: initial results from a large, multicenter surveillance study. J Clin Psychiatry 62(8):623–630, 2001 11561935

Weiss EL, Potenza MN, McDougle CJ, et al: Olanzapine addition in obsessive-compulsive disorder refractory to selective serotonin reuptake inhibitors: an open-label case series. J Clin Psychiatry 60(8):524–527, 1999 10485634

Wolfgang SA: Olanzapine in whole, not half, tablets for psychosis from Alzheimer's dementia. Am J Health Syst Pharm 56(21):2245–2246, 1999 10565707

Wolkowitz OM, Breier A, Doran A, et al: Alprazolam augmentation of the antipsychotic effects of fluphenazine in schizophrenic patients: preliminary results. Arch Gen Psychiatry 45(7):664–671, 1988 3289524

Wu RR, Zhao JP, Guo XF, et al: Metformin addition attenuates olanzapine-induced weight gain in drug-naive first-episode schizophrenia patients: a double-blind, placebo-controlled study. Am J Psychiatry 165(3):352–358, 2008 18245179

Zanarini MC, Frankenburg FR: Olanzapine treatment of female borderline personality disorder patients: a double-blind, placebo-controlled pilot study. J Clin Psychiatry 62(11):849–854, 2001 11775043

Zanarini MC, Schulz SC, Detke H, et al: Open-label treatment with olanzapine for patients with borderline personality disorder. J Clin Psychopharmacol 32(3):398–402, 2012 22544004

Zhou DD, Zhou XX, Li Y, et al: Augmentation agents to serotonin reuptake inhibitors for treatment-resistant obsessive-compulsive disorder: a network meta-analysis. Prog Neuropsychopharmacol Biol Psychiatry 90:277–287, 2019 30576763

References

Adler LA, Peselow E, Rotrosen J, et al: Vitamin E treatment of tardive dyskinesia. Am J Psychiatry 150(9):1405–1407, 1993 8102511

Allison DB, Mentore JL, Heo M, et al: Antipsychotic-induced weight gain: a comprehensive research synthesis. Am J Psychiatry 156(11):1686–1696, 1999 10553730

American Diabetes Association; American Psychiatric Association; American Association of Clinical Endocrinologists, et al: Consensus development conference on antipsychotic drugs and obesity and diabetes. Diabetes Care 27(2):596–601, 2004 14747245

American Psychiatric Association: Diagnostic and Statistical Manual of Mental Disorders, 2nd Edition. Washington, DC, American Psychiatric Association, 1968

American Psychiatric Association: Diagnostic and Statistical Manual of Mental Disorders, 4th Edition, Text Revision. Washington, DC, American Psychiatric Association, 2000

American Psychiatric Association: Diagnostic and Statistical Manual of Mental Disorders, 5th Edition. Arlington, VA, American Psychiatric Association, 2013

Amminger GP, Schäfer MR, Papageorgiou K, et al: Long-chain omega-3 fatty acids for indicated prevention of psychotic disorders: a randomized, placebo-controlled trial. Arch Gen Psychiatry 67(2):146–154, 2010 20124114

Andreescu C, Mulsant BH, Peasley-Miklus C, et al: Persisting low use of antipsychotics in the treatment of major depressive disorder with psychotic features. J Clin Psychiatry 68(2):194–200, 2007 17335316

Attia E, Steinglass JE, Walsh BT, et al: Olanzapine versus placebo in adult outpatients with anorexia nervosa: a randomized clinical trial. Am J Psychiatry 176(6):449–456, 2019 30654643

Azorin JM, Spiegel R, Remington G, et al: A double-blind comparative study of clozapine and risperidone in the management of severe chronic schizophrenia. Am J Psychiatry 158(8):1305–1313, 2001 11481167

Baldessarini RJ, Viguera AC: Neuroleptic withdrawal in schizophrenic patients. Arch Gen Psychiatry 52(3):189–192, 1995 7872842

Beebe KL, Block T, Debattista C, et al: The efficacy of mifepristone in the reduction and prevention of olanzapine-induced weight gain in rats. Behav Brain Res 171(2):225–229, 2006 16782211

Benedetti F, Sforzini L, Colombo C, et al: Low-dose clozapine in acute and continuation treatment of severe borderline personality disorder. J Clin Psychiatry 59(3):103–107, 1998 9541151

Berk M, Ichim C, Brook S: Efficacy of mirtazapine add on therapy to haloperidol in the treatment of the negative symptoms of schizophrenia: a double-blind randomized placebo-controlled study. Int Clin Psychopharmacol 16(2):87–92, 2001 11236073

Berk M, Gama CS, Sundram S, et al: Mirtazapine add-on therapy in the treatment of schizophrenia with atypical antipsychotics: a double-blind, randomised, placebo-controlled clinical trial. Hum Psychopharmacol 24(3):233–238, 2009 19330802

Berman RM, Fava M, Thase ME, et al: Aripiprazole augmentation in major depressive disorder: a double-blind, placebo-controlled study in patients with inadequate response to antidepressants. CNS Spectr 14(4):197–206, 2009 19407731

Bitter I, Dossenbach MR, Brook S, et al: Olanzapine versus clozapine in treatment-resistant or treatment-intolerant schizophrenia. Prog Neuropsychopharmacol Biol Psychiatry 28(1):173–180, 2004 14687871

Blair HA: Lumateperone: first approval. Drugs 80(4):417–423, 2020 32060882

Bodkin JA, Cohen BM, Salomon MS, et al: Treatment of negative symptoms in schizophrenia and schizoaffective disorder by selegiline augmentation of antipsychotic medication: a pilot study examining the role of dopamine. J Nerv Ment Dis 184(5):295–301, 1996 8627275

Bodkin JA, Siris SG, Bermanzohn PC, et al: Double-blind, placebo-controlled, multicenter trial of selegiline augmentation of antipsychotic medication to treat negative symptoms in outpatients with schizophrenia. Am J Psychiatry 162(2):388–390, 2005 15677608

Bosanac P, Hollander Y, Castle D: The comparative efficacy of intramuscular antipsychotics for the management of acute agitation. Australas Psychiatry 21(6):554–562, 2013 23996795

Boyer P, Lecrubier Y, Puech AJ, et al: Treatment of negative symptoms in schizophrenia with amisulpride. Br J Psychiatry 166(1):68–72, 1995 7894879

Brannan SK, Sawchak S, Miller AC, et al: Muscarinic cholinergic receptor agonist and peripheral antagonist for schizophrenia. N Engl J Med 384(8):717–726, 2021 33626254

Calabrese JR, Keck PE Jr, Starace A, et al: Efficacy and safety of low- and high-dose cariprazine in acute and mixed mania associated with bipolar I disorder: a double-blind, placebo-controlled study. J Clin Psychiatry 76(3):284–292, 2015 25562205

Calabrese JR, Durgam S, Satlin A, et al: Efficacy and safety of lumateperone for major depressive episodes associated with bipolar I or bipolar II disorder: a Phase 3 randomized placebo-controlled trial. Am J Psychiatry 178(12):1098–1106, 2021 34551584

Campillo A, Castillo E, Vilke GM, et al: First-generation antipsychotics are often prescribed in the emergency department but are often not administered with adjunctive medications. J Emerg Med 49(6):901–906, 2015 26433424

Carbon M, Hsieh CH, Kane JM, et al: Tardive dyskinesia prevalence in the period of second-generation antipsychotic use: a meta-analysis. J Clin Psychiatry 78(3):e264–e278, 2017 28146614

Carey PD, Lochner C, Kidd M, et al: Quetiapine augmentation of serotonin reuptake inhibitors in treatment-refractory obsessive-compulsive disorder: is response to treatment predictable? Int Clin Psychopharmacol 27(6):321–325, 2012 22859064

Carpenter WT Jr, Heinrichs DW: Early intervention, time-limited, targeted pharmacotherapy of schizophrenia. Schizophr Bull 9(4):533–542, 1983 6140752

Carpenter WT Jr, Hanlon TE, Heinrichs DW, et al: Continuous versus targeted medication in schizophrenic outpatients: outcome results. Am J Psychiatry 147(9):1138–1148, 1990 1974743

Carson WH, Stock E, Saha AR, et al: Meta-analysis of the efficacy of aripiprazole in schizophrenia. Eur Psychiatry 17(Suppl 1):105, 2002

Casey DE, Daniel DG, Wassef AA, et al: Effect of divalproex combined with olanzapine or risperidone in patients with an acute exacerbation of schizophrenia. Neuropsychopharmacology 28(1):182–192, 2003 12496955

Chang WC, Kwong VWY, Lau ESK, et al: Sustainability of treatment effect of a 3-year early intervention programme for first-episode psychosis. Br J Psychiatry 211(1):37–44, 2017 28385705

Chengappa KN, Ebeling T, Kang JS, et al: Clozapine reduces severe self-mutilation and aggression in psychotic patients with borderline personality disorder. J Clin Psychiatry 60(7):477–484, 1999 10453803

Cipriani A, Barbui C, Salanti G, et al: Comparative efficacy and acceptability of antimanic drugs in acute mania: a multiple-treatments meta-analysis. Lancet 378(9799):1306–1315, 2011 21851976

Citrome L: Adjunctive lithium and anticonvulsants for the treatment of schizophrenia: what is the evidence? Expert Rev Neurother 9(1):55–71, 2009 19102669

Citrome L: Valbenazine for tardive dyskinesia: a systematic review of the efficacy and safety profile for this newly approved novel medication: what is the likelihood to be helped or harmed? Int J Clin Pract 71(7):e12964, 2017 28497864

Cole JO, Gardos G, Boling LA, et al: Early dyskinesia—vulnerability. Psychopharmacology (Berl) 107(4):503–510, 1992 1603892

Cornelius JR, Soloff PH, Perel JM, et al: Continuation pharmacotherapy of borderline personality disorder with haloperidol and phenelzine. Am J Psychiatry 150(12):1843–1848, 1993 8238640

Correll CU, Skuban A, Ouyang J, et al: Efficacy and safety of brexpiprazole for the treatment of acute schizophrenia: a 6-week randomized, double-blind, placebo-controlled trial. Am J Psychiatry 172(9):870–880, 2015 25882325

Correll CU, Davis RE, Weingart M, et al: Efficacy and safety of lumateperone for treatment of schizophrenia: a randomized clinical trial. JAMA Psychiatry 77(4):349–358, 2020a 31913424

Correll CU, Newcomer JW, Silverman B, et al: Effects of olanzapine combined with samidorphan on weight gain in schizophrenia: a 24-week phase 3 study. Am J Psychiatry 177(12):1168–1178, 2020b 32791894

Correll CU, Koblan KS, Hopkins SC, et al: Safety and effectiveness of ulotaront (SEP-363856) in schizophrenia: results of a 6-month, open-label extension study. NPJ Schizophr 7(1):63, 2021 34887427

Csernansky JG, Riney SJ, Lombrozo L, et al: Double-blind comparison of alprazolam, diazepam, and placebo for the treatment of negative schizophrenic symptoms. Arch Gen Psychiatry 45(7):655–659, 1988 3289523

Cummings J, Isaacson S, Mills R, et al: Pimavanserin for patients with Parkinson's disease psychosis: a randomised, placebo-controlled phase 3 trial. Lancet 383(9916):533–540, 2014 24183563

Davis JM, Chen N, Glick ID: A meta-analysis of the efficacy of second-generation antipsychotics. Arch Gen Psychiatry 60(6):553–564, 2003 12796218

Delay J, Deniker P, Harl JM: Therapeutic use in psychiatry of phenothiazine of central elective action (4560 RP) (in French). Ann Med Psychol (Paris) 110(21):112–117, 1952 12986408

Dennis K, Le Grange D, Bremer J: Olanzapine use in adolescent anorexia nervosa. Eat Weight Disord 11(2):e53–e56, 2006 16809970

de Silva VA, Suraweera C, Ratnatunga SS, et al: Metformin in prevention and treatment of antipsychotic induced weight gain: a systematic review and meta-analysis. BMC Psychiatry 16(1):341, 2016 27716110

Dold M, Aigner M, Lanzenberger R, et al: Antipsychotic augmentation of serotonin reuptake inhibitors in treatment-resistant obsessive-compulsive disorder: a meta-analysis of double-blind, randomized, placebo-controlled trials. Int J Neuropsychopharmacol 16(3):557–574, 2013 22932229

Durgam S, Starace A, Li D, et al: An evaluation of the safety and efficacy of cariprazine in patients with acute exacerbation of schizophrenia: a Phase II, randomized clinical trial. Schizophr Res 152(2–3):450–457, 2014 24412468

Durgam S, Cutler AJ, Lu K, et al: Cariprazine in acute exacerbation of schizophrenia: a fixed-dose, phase 3, randomized, double-blind, placebo- and active-controlled trial. J Clin Psychiatry 76(12):e1574–e1582, 2015a 26717533

Durgam S, Starace A, Li D, et al: The efficacy and tolerability of cariprazine in acute mania associated with bipolar I disorder: a phase II trial. Bipolar Disord 17(1):63–75, 2015b 25056368

Durgam S, Earley W, Guo H, et al: Efficacy and safety of adjunctive cariprazine in inadequate responders to antidepressants: a randomized, double-blind, placebo-controlled study in adult patients with major depressive disorder. J Clin Psychiatry 77(3):371–378, 2016 27046309

Earley W, Burgess MV, Rekeda L, et al: Cariprazine treatment of bipolar depression: a randomized double-blind placebo-controlled Phase 3 study. Am J Psychiatry 176(6):439–448, 2019 30845817

Earley WR, Burgess MV, Khan B, et al: Efficacy and safety of cariprazine in bipolar I depression: a double-blind, placebo-controlled Phase 3 study. Bipolar Disord 22(4):372–384, 2020 31628698

Emsley R, Nuamah I, Gopal S, et al: Relapse after antipsychotic discontinuation in schizophrenia as a withdrawal phenomenon vs illness recurrence: a post hoc analysis of a randomized placebo-controlled study. J Clin Psychiatry 79(4):17m11874, 2018 29924507

Endicott J, Paulsson B, Gustafsson U, et al: Quetiapine monotherapy in the treatment of depressive episodes of bipolar I and II disorder: improvements in quality of life and quality of sleep. J Affect Disord 111(2–3):306–319, 2008 18774180

Fava M, Durgam S, Earley W, et al: Efficacy of adjunctive low-dose cariprazine in major depressive disorder: a randomized, double-blind, placebo-controlled trial. Int Clin Psychopharmacol 33(6):312–321, 2018 30045066

Frankenburg FR, Zanarini MC: Clozapine treatment of borderline patients: a preliminary study. Compr Psychiatry 34(6):402–405, 1993 8131384

Friedman JI, Adler DN, Temporini HD, et al: Guanfacine treatment of cognitive impairment in schizophrenia. Neuropsychopharmacology 25(3):402–409, 2001 11522468

Gao K, Gajwani P, Elhaj O, et al: Typical and atypical antipsychotics in bipolar depression. J Clin Psychiatry 66(11):1376–1385, 2005 16420074

Gao K, Muzina D, Gajwani P, et al: Efficacy of typical and atypical antipsychotics for primary and comorbid anxiety symptoms or disorders: a review. J Clin Psychiatry 67(9):1327–1340, 2006 17017818

Garakani A, Martinez JM, Marcus S, et al: A randomized, double-blind, and placebo-controlled trial of quetiapine augmentation of fluoxetine in major depressive disorder. Int Clin Psychopharmacol 23(5):269–275, 2008 18703936

Gardos G, Cole JO: The evaluation and treatment of neuroleptic-induced movement disorders. Harv Rev Psychiatry 3(3):130–139, 1995 9384940

Ghaemi SN, Katzow JJ: The use of quetiapine for treatment-resistant bipolar disorder: a case series. Ann Clin Psychiatry 11(3):137–140, 1999 10482123

Glazer WM, Kane JM: Depot neuroleptic therapy: an underutilized treatment option. J Clin Psychiatry 53(12):426–433, 1992 1362569

Goff DC, Posever T, Herz L, et al: An exploratory haloperidol-controlled dose-finding study of ziprasidone in hospitalized patients with schizophrenia or schizoaffective disorder. J Clin Psychopharmacol 18(4):296–304, 1998 9690695

Goff DC, Lamberti JS, Leon AC, et al: A placebo-controlled add-on trial of the Ampakine, CX516, for cognitive deficits in schizophrenia. Neuropsychopharmacology 33(3):465–472, 2008 17487227

Gray JA, Roth BL: Molecular targets for treating cognitive dysfunction in schizophrenia. Schizophr Bull 33(5):1100–1119, 2007 17617664

Gray R: Quetiapine: a new atypical antipsychotic for the treatment of schizophrenia. Ment Health Care 1(5):163–164, 1998 9791402

Green AI, Faraone SV, Brown WA: Prolactin shifts after neuroleptic withdrawal. Psychiatry Res 32(3):213–219, 1990 1975101

Green MF: Stimulating the development of drug treatments to improve cognition in schizophrenia. Annu Rev Clin Psychol 3:159–180, 2007 17716052

Gross C, Blasey CM, Roe RL, et al: Mifepristone treatment of olanzapine-induced weight gain in healthy men. Adv Ther 26(10):959–969, 2009 19888560

Grossberg GT, Kohegyi E, Mergel V, et al: Efficacy and safety of brexpiprazole for the treatment of agitation in Alzheimer's dementia: two 12-week, randomized, double-blind, placebo-controlled trials. Am J Geriatr Psychiatry 28(4):383–400, 2020 31708380

Gründer G, Hippius H, Carlsson A: The "atypicality" of antipsychotics: a concept re-examined and re-defined. Nat Rev Drug Discov 8(3):197–202, 2009 19214197

Hasan S, Buckley P: Novel antipsychotics and the neuroleptic malignant syndrome: a review and critique. Am J Psychiatry 155(8):1113–1116, 1998 9699705

Hauser RA, Factor SA, Marder SR, et al: KINECT 3: a Phase 3 randomized, double-blind, placebo-controlled trial of valbenazine for tardive dyskinesia. Am J Psychiatry 174(5):476–484, 2017 28320223

Herrmann N, Mamdani M, Lanctôt KL: Atypical antipsychotics and risk of cerebrovascular accidents. Am J Psychiatry 161(6):1113–1115, 2004 15169702

Herz MI, Szymanski HV, Simon JC: Intermittent medication for stable schizophrenic outpatients: an alternative to maintenance medication. Am J Psychiatry 139(7):918–922, 1982 6124133

Herz MI, Glazer WM, Mostert MA, et al: Intermittent vs maintenance medication in schizophrenia: two-year results. Arch Gen Psychiatry 48(4):333–339, 1991 1672588

Hilger E, Barnas C, Kasper S: Quetiapine in the treatment of borderline personality disorder. World J Biol Psychiatry 4(1):42–44, 2003 12582977

Hirschfeld RM, Keck PE Jr, Kramer M, et al: Rapid antimanic effect of risperidone monotherapy: a 3-week multicenter, double-blind, placebo-controlled trial. Am J Psychiatry 161(6):1057–1065, 2004 15169694

Hirschfeld RM, Weisler RH, Raines SR, et al: Quetiapine in the treatment of anxiety in patients with bipolar I or II depression: a secondary analysis from a randomized, double-blind, placebo-controlled study. J Clin Psychiatry 67(3):355–362, 2006 16649820

Hogarty GE, Kornblith SJ, Greenwald D, et al: Personal therapy: a disorder-relevant psychotherapy for schizophrenia. Schizophr Bull 21(3):379–393, 1995 7481569

Hoge EA, Worthington JJ III, Kaufman RE, et al: Aripiprazole as augmentation treatment of refractory generalized anxiety disorder and panic disorder. CNS Spectr 13(6):522–527, 2008 18567977

Hollander E, Baldini Rossi N, Sood E, et al: Risperidone augmentation in treatment-resistant obsessive-compulsive disorder: a double-blind, placebo-controlled study. Int J Neuropsychopharmacol 6(4):397–401, 2003 14604454

Hu RJ: What is the optimal dosing for atypical antipsychotics? A practical guide based on available evidence. Prim Psychiatry 16:43–49, 2009

Jeste DV, Caligiuri MP, Paulsen JS, et al: Risk of tardive dyskinesia in older patients: a prospective longitudinal study of 266 outpatients. Arch Gen Psychiatry 52(9):756–765, 1995 7654127

Jin Y, Potkin SG, Kemp AS, et al: Therapeutic effects of individualized alpha frequency transcranial magnetic stimulation (alphaTMS) on the negative symptoms of schizophrenia. Schizophr Bull 32(3):556–561, 2006 16254067

Jockers-Scherübl MC, Bauer A, Godemann F, et al: Negative symptoms of schizophrenia are improved by the addition of paroxetine to neuroleptics: a double-blind placebo-controlled study. Int Clin Psychopharmacol 20(1):27–31, 2005 15602113

Jones PB, Barnes TR, Davies L, et al: Randomized controlled trial of the effect on quality of life of second- vs first-generation antipsychotic drugs in schizophrenia: Cost Utility of the Latest Antipsychotic Drugs in Schizophrenia Study (CUtLASS 1). Arch Gen Psychiatry 63(10):1079–1087, 2006 17015810

Jungerman T, Rabinowitz D, Klein E: Deprenyl augmentation for treating negative symptoms of schizophrenia: a double-blind, controlled study. J Clin Psychopharmacol 19(6):522–525, 1999 10587287

Kane JM, McGlashan TH: Treatment of schizophrenia. Lancet 346(8978):820–825, 1995 7545770

Kane JM, Rifkin A, Woerner M, et al: Low-dose neuroleptic treatment of outpatient schizophrenics I: preliminary results for relapse rates. Arch Gen Psychiatry 40(8):893–896, 1983 6347119

Kane J, Honigfeld G, Singer J, et al: Clozapine for the treatment-resistant schizophrenic: a double-blind comparison with chlorpromazine. Arch Gen Psychiatry 45(9):789–796, 1988 3046553

Kane JM, Davis JM, Schooler N, et al: A multidose study of haloperidol decanoate in the maintenance treatment of schizophrenia. Am J Psychiatry 159(4):554–560, 2002 11925292

Kane J, Canas F, Kramer M, et al: Treatment of schizophrenia with paliperidone extended-release tablets: a 6-week placebo-controlled trial. Schizophr Res 90(1–3):147–161, 2007 17092691

Kane JM, Lauriello J, Laska E, et al: Long-term efficacy and safety of iloperidone: results from 3 clinical trials for the treatment of schizophrenia. J Clin Psychopharmacol 28(2)(Suppl 1):S29–S35, 2008 18334910

Kane JM, Skuban A, Ouyang J, et al: A multicenter, randomized, double-blind, controlled phase 3 trial of fixed-dose brexpiprazole for the treatment of adults with acute schizophrenia. Schizophr Res 164(1–3):127–135, 2015a 25682550

Kane JM, Zukin S, Wang Y, et al: Efficacy and safety of cariprazine in acute exacerbation of schizophrenia: results from an international, Phase III clinical trial. J Clin Psychopharmacol 35(4):367–373, 2015b 26075487

Kapur S, Zipursky RB, Remington G: Clinical and theoretical implications of 5-HT2 and D2 receptor occupancy of clozapine, risperidone, and olanzapine in schizophrenia. Am J Psychiatry 156(2):286–293, 1999 9989565

Karagianis JL, Phillips LC, Hogan KP, et al: Clozapine-associated neuroleptic malignant syndrome: two new cases and a review of the literature. Ann Pharmacother 33(5):623–630, 1999 10369628

Keck P Jr, Buffenstein A, Ferguson J, et al: Ziprasidone 40 and 120 mg/day in the acute exacerbation of schizophrenia and schizoaffective disorder: a 4-week placebo-controlled trial. Psychopharmacology (Berl) 140(2):173–184, 1998 9860108

Keck PE Jr, Marcus R, Tourkodimitris S, et al: A placebo-controlled, double-blind study of the efficacy and safety of aripiprazole in patients with acute bipolar mania. Am J Psychiatry 160(9):1651–1658, 2003a 12944341

Keck PE Jr, Versiani M, Potkin S, et al: Ziprasidone in the treatment of acute bipolar mania: a three-week, placebo-controlled, double-blind, randomized trial. Am J Psychiatry 160(4):741–748, 2003b 12668364

Kishimoto T, Hagi K, Nitta M, et al: Effectiveness of long-acting injectable vs oral antipsychotics in patients with schizophrenia: a meta-analysis of prospective and retrospective cohort studies. Schizophr Bull 44(3):603–619, 2018 29868849

Klein E, Bental E, Lerer B, et al: Carbamazepine and haloperidol v placebo and haloperidol in excited psychoses: a controlled study. Arch Gen Psychiatry 41(2):165–170, 1984 6365015

Koblan KS, Kent J, Hopkins SC, et al: A non-D2-receptor-binding drug for the treatment of schizophrenia. N Engl J Med 382(16):1497–1506, 2020 32294346

Koenigsberg HW, Reynolds D, Goodman M, et al: Risperidone in the treatment of schizotypal personality disorder. J Clin Psychiatry 64(6):628–634, 2003 12823075

Kontaxakis VP, Ferentinos PP, Havaki-Kontaxaki BJ, et al: Randomized controlled augmentation trials in clozapine-resistant schizophrenic patients: a critical review. Eur Psychiatry 20(5–6):409–415, 2005 16171655

Koran LM, Ringold AL, Elliott MA: Olanzapine augmentation for treatment-resistant obsessive-compulsive disorder. J Clin Psychiatry 61(7):514–517, 2000 10937610

Leucht S, Arbter D, Engel RR, et al: How effective are second-generation antipsychotic drugs? A meta-analysis of placebo-controlled trials. Mol Psychiatry 14(4):429–447, 2009a 18180760

Leucht S, Corves C, Arbter D, et al: Second-generation versus first-generation antipsychotic drugs for schizophrenia: a meta-analysis. Lancet 373(9657):31–41, 2009b 19058842

Leucht S, Komossa K, Rummel-Kluge C, et al: A meta-analysis of head-to-head comparisons of second-generation antipsychotics in the treatment of schizophrenia. Am J Psychiatry 166(2):152–163, 2009c 19015230

Leucht S, Cipriani A, Spineli L, et al: Comparative efficacy and tolerability of 15 antipsychotic drugs in schizophrenia: a multiple-treatments meta-analysis. Lancet 382(9896):951–962, 2013 23810019

Lieberman JA, Tollefson G, Tohen M, et al: Comparative efficacy and safety of atypical and conventional antipsychotic drugs in first-episode psychosis: a randomized, double-blind trial of olanzapine versus haloperidol. Am J Psychiatry 160(8):1396–1404, 2003 12900300

Lieberman JA, Stroup TS, McEvoy JP, et al: Effectiveness of antipsychotic drugs in patients with chronic schizophrenia. N Engl J Med 353(12):1209–1223, 2005 16172203

Lieberman JA, Davis RE, Correll CU, et al: ITI-007 for the treatment of schizophrenia: a 4-week randomized, double-blind, controlled trial. Biol Psychiatry 79(12):952–961, 2016 26444072

Linehan MM, McDavid JD, Brown MZ, et al: Olanzapine plus dialectical behavior therapy for women with high irritability who meet criteria for borderline personality disorder: a double-blind, placebo-controlled pilot study. J Clin Psychiatry 69(6):999–1005, 2008 18466045

Liu HC, Chang WH, Wei FC, et al: Monitoring of plasma clozapine levels and its metabolites in refractory schizophrenic patients. Ther Drug Monit 18(2):200–207, 1996 8721285

Loebel A, Cucchiaro J, Sarma K, et al: Efficacy and safety of lurasidone 80 mg/day and 160 mg/day in the treatment of schizophrenia: a randomized, double-blind, placebo- and active-controlled trial. Schizophr Res 145(1–3):101–109, 2013 23415311

Loebel A, Cucchiaro J, Silva R, et al: Lurasidone as adjunctive therapy with lithium or valproate for the treatment of bipolar I depression: a randomized, double-blind, placebo-controlled study. Am J Psychiatry 171(2):169–177, 2014a 24170221

Loebel A, Cucchiaro J, Silva R, et al: Lurasidone monotherapy in the treatment of bipolar I depression: a randomized, double-blind, placebo-controlled study. Am J Psychiatry 171(2):160–168, 2014b 24170180

Mandalos GE, Szarek BL: New-onset panic attacks in a patient treated with olanzapine. J Clin Psychopharmacol 19(2):191, 1999 10211927

Marcus RN, McQuade RD, Carson WH, et al: The efficacy and safety of aripiprazole as adjunctive therapy in major depressive disorder: a second multicenter, randomized, double-blind, placebo-controlled study. J Clin Psychopharmacol 28(2):156–165, 2008 18344725

Marder SR, Kramer M, Ford L, et al: Efficacy and safety of paliperidone extended-release tablets: results of a 6-week, randomized, placebo-controlled study. Biol Psychiatry 62(12):1363–1370, 2007 17601495

Markowitz JS, Brown CS, Moore TR: Atypical antipsychotics part I: pharmacology, pharmacokinetics, and efficacy. Ann Pharmacother 33(1):73–85, 1999 9972387

McDougle CJ, Scahill L, Aman MG, et al: Risperidone for the core symptom domains of autism: results from the study by the Autism Network of the Research Units on Pediatric Psychopharmacology. Am J Psychiatry 162(6):1142–1148, 2005 15930063

McEvoy JP, Lieberman JA, Stroup TS, et al: Effectiveness of clozapine versus olanzapine, quetiapine, and risperidone in patients with chronic schizophrenia who did not respond to prior atypical antipsychotic treatment. Am J Psychiatry 163(4):600–610, 2006 16585434

McEvoy JP, Citrome L, Hernandez D, et al: Effectiveness of lurasidone in patients with schizophrenia or schizoaffective disorder switched from other antipsychotics: a randomized, 6-week, open-label study. J Clin Psychiatry 74(2):170–179, 2013 23473350

McGlashan TH, Zipursky RB, Perkins D, et al: Randomized, double-blind trial of olanzapine versus placebo in patients prodromally symptomatic for psychosis. Am J Psychiatry 163(5):790–799, 2006 16648318

McIntyre RS, Cohen M, Zhao J, et al: Asenapine for long-term treatment of bipolar disorder: a double-blind 40-week extension study. J Affect Disord 126(3):358–365, 2010 20537396

McIntyre RS, Tohen M, Berk M, et al: DSM-5 mixed specifier for manic episodes: evaluating the effect of depressive features on severity and treatment outcome using asenapine clinical trial data. J Affect Disord 150(2):378–383, 2013 23712026

McIntyre RS, Weiller E, Zhang P, et al: Brexpiprazole as adjunctive treatment of major depressive disorder with anxious distress: results from a post-hoc analysis of two randomised controlled trials. J Affect Disord 201:116–123, 2016 27208498

Meltzer HY: Treatment-resistant schizophrenia—the role of clozapine. Curr Med Res Opin 14(1):1–20, 1997 9524789

Meltzer HY, Bastani B, Kwon KY, et al: A prospective study of clozapine in treatment-resistant schizophrenic patients I: preliminary report. Psychopharmacology (Berl) 99(suppl):S68–S72, 1989 2813667

Meltzer HY, Alphs L, Green AI, et al: Clozapine treatment for suicidality in schizophrenia: International Suicide Prevention Trial (InterSePT). Arch Gen Psychiatry 60(1):82–91, 2003 12511175

Meltzer HY, Chen Y, Jayathilake K: Effect of risperidone and olanzapine on measures associated with the insulin resistance syndrome. Neuropsychopharmacology 30(Suppl 1):S138, 2005

Meltzer HY, Mills R, Revell S, et al: Pimavanserin, a serotonin(2A) receptor inverse agonist, for the treatment of Parkinson's disease psychosis. Neuropsychopharmacology 35(4):881–892, 2010 19907417

Meltzer HY, Cucchiaro J, Silva R, et al: Lurasidone in the treatment of schizophrenia: a randomized, double-blind, placebo- and olanzapine-controlled study. Am J Psychiatry 168(9):957–967, 2011 21676992

Meyers BS, Flint AJ, Rothschild AJ, et al: A double-blind randomized controlled trial of olanzapine plus sertraline vs olanzapine plus placebo for psychotic depression: the Study of Pharmacotherapy of Psychotic Depression (STOP-PD). Arch Gen Psychiatry 66(8):838–847, 2009 19652123

Miller DD, McEvoy JP, Davis SM, et al: Clinical correlates of tardive dyskinesia in schizophrenia: baseline data from the CATIE schizophrenia trial. Schizophr Res 80(1):33–43, 2005 16171976

Mitchell M, Kothare P, Bergstrom R, et al: Single- and multiple-dose pharmacokinetic, safety, and tolerability profiles of olanzapine long-acting injection: an open-label, multicenter, nonrandomized study in patients with schizophrenia. Clin Ther 35(12):1890–1908, 2013 24184052

Mondraty N, Birmingham CL, Touyz S, et al: Randomized controlled trial of olanzapine in the treatment of cognitions in anorexia nervosa. Australas Psychiatry 13(1):72–75, 2005 15777417

Mottard JP, de la Sablonnière JF: Olanzapine-induced obsessive-compulsive disorder. Am J Psychiatry 156(5):799–800, 1999 10327925

Mouaffak F, Tranulis C, Gourevitch R, et al: Augmentation strategies of clozapine with antipsychotics in the treatment of ultraresistant schizophrenia. Clin Neuropharmacol 29(1):28–33, 2006 16518132

Natesan S, Reckless GE, Barlow KB, et al: Evaluation of N-desmethylclozapine as a potential antipsychotic—preclinical studies. Neuropsychopharmacology 32(7):1540–1549, 2007 17164815

Nickel MK, Muehlbacher M, Nickel C, et al: Aripiprazole in the treatment of patients with borderline personality disorder: a double-blind, placebo-controlled study. Am J Psychiatry 163(5):833–838, 2006 16648324

Nuttall GA, Eckerman KM, Jacob KA, et al: Does low-dose droperidol administration increase the risk of drug-induced QT prolongation and torsade de pointes in the general surgical population? Anesthesiology 107(4):531–536, 2007 17893447

Pantelis C, Yücel M, Wood SJ, et al: Early and late neurodevelopmental disturbances in schizophrenia and their functional consequences. Aust N Z J Psychiatry 37(4):399–406, 2003 12873323

Perkins DO, Gu H, Boteva K, et al: Relationship between duration of untreated psychosis and outcome in first-episode schizophrenia: a critical review and meta-analysis. Am J Psychiatry 162(10):1785–1804, 2005 16199825

Pitchot W, Ansseau M: Efficacy of quetiapine in treatment-resistant panic disorder: a case report. Asian J Psychiatr 5(2):204–205, 2012 22813673

Pivac N, Kozaric-Kovacic D, Muck-Seler D: Olanzapine versus fluphenazine in an open trial in patients with psychotic combat-related post-traumatic stress disorder. Psychopharmacology (Berl) 175(4):451–456, 2004 15064916

Posselt CM, Albert N, Nordentoft M, Hjorthøj C: The Danish OPUS early intervention services for first-episode psychosis: a Phase 4 prospective cohort study with comparison of randomized trial and real-world data. Am J Psychiatry 178(10):941–951, 2021 34315283

Potkin SG, Litman RE, Torres R, et al: Efficacy of iloperidone in the treatment of schizophrenia: initial phase 3 studies. J Clin Psychopharmacol 28(2)(Suppl 1):S4–S11, 2008 18334911

Potkin SG, Raoufinia A, Mallikaarjun S, et al: Safety and tolerability of once monthly aripiprazole treatment initiation in adults with schizophrenia stabilized on selected atypical oral antipsychotics other than aripiprazole. Curr Med Res Opin 29(10):1241–1251, 2013 23822566

Powers PS, Bannon Y, Eubanks R, et al: Quetiapine in anorexia nervosa patients: an open label outpatient pilot study. Int J Eat Disord 40(1):21–26, 2007 16927383

Rainer MK: Risperidone long-acting injection: a review of its long term safety and efficacy. Neuropsychiatr Dis Treat 4(5):919–927, 2008 19183782

Reaven GM, Lieberman JA, Sethuraman G, et al: In search of moderators and mediators of hyperglycemia with atypical antipsychotic treatment. J Psychiatr Res 43(11):997–1002, 2009 19268968

Remington G, Kapur S: D2 and 5-HT2 receptor effects of antipsychotics: bridging basic and clinical findings using PET. J Clin Psychiatry 60(Suppl 10):15–19, 1999 10340683

Ripoll LH: Clinical psychopharmacology of borderline personality disorder: an update on the available evidence in light of the Diagnostic and Statistical Manual of Mental Disorders–5. Curr Opin Psychiatry 25(1):52–58, 2012 22037092

Rothschild AJ, Williamson DJ, Tohen MF, et al: A double-blind, randomized study of olanzapine and olanzapine/fluoxetine combination for major depression with psychotic features. J Clin Psychopharmacol 24(4):365–373, 2004 15232326

Sachs G, Chengappa KN, Suppes T, et al: Quetiapine with lithium or divalproex for the treatment of bipolar mania: a randomized, double-blind, placebo-controlled study. Bipolar Disord 6(3):213–223, 2004 15117400

Sachs GS, Greenberg WM, Starace A, et al: Cariprazine in the treatment of acute mania in bipolar I disorder: a double-blind, placebo-controlled, Phase III trial. J Affect Disord 174:296–302, 2015 25532076

Sayyah M, Sayyah M, Boostani H, et al: Effects of aripiprazole augmentation in treatment-resistant obsessive-compulsive disorder (a double blind clinical trial). Depress Anxiety 29(10):850–854, 2012 22933237

Schneider LS, Tariot PN, Dagerman KS, et al: Effectiveness of atypical antipsychotic drugs in patients with Alzheimer's disease. N Engl J Med 355(15):1525–1538, 2006 17035647

Schulz SC, Zanarini MC, Bateman A, et al: Olanzapine for the treatment of borderline personality disorder: variable dose 12-week randomised double-blind placebo-controlled study. Br J Psychiatry 193(6):485–492, 2008 19043153

Schwarz C, Volz A, Li C, Leucht S: Valproate for schizophrenia. Cochrane Database Syst Rev (3):CD004028, 2008 18646098

Seeman P, Tallerico T: Rapid release of antipsychotic drugs from dopamine D2 receptors: an explanation for low receptor occupancy and early clinical relapse upon withdrawal of clozapine or quetiapine. Am J Psychiatry 156(6):876–884, 1999 10360126

Sernyak MJ, Woods SW: Chronic neuroleptic use in manic-depressive illness. Psychopharmacol Bull 29(3):375–381, 1993 7907185

Shekhar A, Potter WZ, Lightfoot J, et al: Selective muscarinic receptor agonist xanomeline as a novel treatment approach for schizophrenia. Am J Psychiatry 165(8):1033–1039, 2008 18593778

Shelton RC, Tollefson GD, Tohen M, et al: A novel augmentation strategy for treating resistant major depression. Am J Psychiatry 158(1):131–134, 2001 11136647

Silver H, Geraisy N: No difference in the effect of biperiden and amantadine on negative symptoms in medicated chronic schizophrenic patients. Biol Psychiatry 38(6):413–415, 1995 8547463

Simpson GM, Glick ID, Weiden PJ, et al: Randomized, controlled, double-blind multicenter comparison of the efficacy and tolerability of ziprasidone and olanzapine in acutely ill inpatients with schizophrenia or schizoaffective disorder. Am J Psychiatry 161(10):1837–1847, 2004 15465981

Soler J, Pascual JC, Campins J, et al: Double-blind, placebo-controlled study of dialectical behavior therapy plus olanzapine for borderline personality disorder. Am J Psychiatry 162(6):1221–1224, 2005 15930077

Spina E, De Domenico P, Ruello C, et al: Adjunctive fluoxetine in the treatment of negative symptoms in chronic schizophrenic patients. Int Clin Psychopharmacol 9(4):281–285, 1994 7868850

Stanilla JK, Simpson GM: Drugs to treat extrapyramidal side effects, in The American Psychiatric Press Textbook of Psychopharmacology. Edited by Schatzberg AF, Nemeroff CB. Washington, DC, American Psychiatric Press, 1995, pp 281–299

States JH, St Dennis CD: Chronic sleep disruption and the reexperiencing cluster of posttraumatic stress disorder symptoms are improved by olanzapine: brief review of the literature and a case-based series. Prim Care Companion J Clin Psychiatry 5(2):74–79, 2003 15156234

Storch EA, Goddard AW, Grant JE, et al: Double-blind, placebo-controlled, pilot trial of paliperidone augmentation in serotonin reuptake inhibitor-resistant obsessive-compulsive disorder. J Clin Psychiatry 74(6):e527–e532, 2013 23842022

Stroup TS, Lieberman JA, McEvoy JP, et al: Effectiveness of olanzapine, quetiapine, risperidone, and ziprasidone in patients with chronic schizophrenia following discontinuation of a previous atypical antipsychotic. Am J Psychiatry 163(4):611–622, 2006 16585435

Sultzer DL, Davis SM, Tariot PN, et al: Clinical symptom responses to atypical antipsychotic medications in Alzheimer's disease: Phase 1 outcomes from the CATIE-AD effectiveness trial. Am J Psychiatry 165(7):844–854, 2008 18519523

Sun SX, Liu GG, Christensen DB, et al: Review and analysis of hospitalization costs associated with antipsychotic nonadherence in the treatment of schizophrenia in the United States. Curr Med Res Opin 23(10):2305–2312, 2007 17697454

Suppes T, Baldessarini RJ, Faedda GL, et al: Discontinuation of maintenance treatment in bipolar disorder: risks and implications. Harv Rev Psychiatry 1(3):131–144, 1993 9384841

Suppes T, Silva R, Cucchiaro J, et al: Lurasidone for the treatment of major depressive disorder with mixed features: a randomized, double-blind, placebo-controlled study. Am J Psychiatry 173(4):400–407, 2016 26552942

Szegedi A, Verweij P, van Duijnhoven W, et al: Meta-analyses of the efficacy of asenapine for acute schizophrenia: comparisons with placebo and other antipsychotics. J Clin Psychiatry 73(12):1533–1540, 2012 23290326

Tariot PN, Cummings JL, Soto-Martin ME, et al: Trial of pimavanserin in dementia-related psychosis. N Engl J Med 385(4):309–319, 2021 34289275

Taylor DM, Fischetti C, Sparshatt A, et al: Risperidone long-acting injection: a prospective 3-year analysis of its use in clinical practice. J Clin Psychiatry 70(2):196–200, 2009a 19026261

Taylor D, Fischetti C, Sparshatt A, et al: Risperidone long-acting injection: a 6-year mirror-image study of healthcare resource use. Acta Psychiatr Scand 120(2):97–101, 2009b 19207128

Thase ME, Macfadden W, Weisler RH, et al: Efficacy of quetiapine monotherapy in bipolar I and II depression: a double-blind, placebo-controlled study (the BOLDER II study). J Clin Psychopharmacol 26(6):600–609, 2006 17110817

Thase ME, Youakim JM, Skuban A, et al: Adjunctive brexpiprazole 1 and 3 mg for patients with major depressive disorder following inadequate response to antidepressants: a Phase 3, randomized, double-blind study. J Clin Psychiatry 76(9):1232–1240, 2015a 26301771

Thase ME, Youakim JM, Skuban A, et al: Efficacy and safety of adjunctive brexpiprazole 2 mg in major depressive disorder: a Phase 3, randomized, placebo-controlled study in patients with inadequate response to antidepressants. J Clin Psychiatry 76(9):1224–1231, 2015b 26301701

Titus-Lay EN, Ansara ED, Isaacs AN, et al: Evaluation of adherence and persistence with oral versus long-acting injectable antipsychotics in patients with early psychosis. Ment Health Clin 8(2):56–62, 2018 29955546

Tollefson GD, Birkett MA, Kiesler GM, et al: Double-blind comparison of olanzapine versus clozapine in schizophrenic patients clinically eligible for treatment with clozapine. Biol Psychiatry 49(1):52–63, 2001 11163780

Touma KTB, Touma DC: Pimavanserin (Nuplazid) for the treatment of Parkinson disease psychosis: a review of the literature. Ment Health Clin 7(5):230–234, 2018 29955528

Tran PV, Dellva MA, Tollefson GD, et al: Oral olanzapine versus oral haloperidol in the maintenance treatment of schizophrenia and related psychoses. Br J Psychiatry 172:499–505, 1998 9828990

VanderZwaag C, McGee M, McEvoy JP, et al: Response of patients with treatment-refractory schizophrenia to clozapine within three serum level ranges. Am J Psychiatry 153(12):1579–1584, 1996 8942454

Van Putten T: Why do schizophrenic patients refuse to take their drugs? Arch Gen Psychiatry 31(1):67–72, 1974 4151750

Vulink NC, Denys D, Fluitman SB, et al: Quetiapine augments the effect of citalo-pram in non-refractory obsessive-compulsive disorder: a randomized, double-blind, placebo-controlled study of 76 patients. J Clin Psychiatry 70(7):1001–1008, 2009 19497245

Wang R, Wang L, Li Z, et al: Latent structure of posttraumatic stress disorder symp-toms in an adolescent sample one month after an earthquake. J Adolesc 36(4):717–725, 2013 23849666

Webber MA, Marder SR: Better pharmacotherapy for schizophrenia: what does the fu-ture hold? Curr Psychiatry Rep 10(4):352–358, 2008 18627675

White E, Cheung P, Silverstone T: Depot antipsychotics in bipolar affective disorder. Int Clin Psychopharmacol 8(2):119–122, 1993 8102150

Wijkstra J, Lijmer J, Balk F, et al: Pharmacological treatment for psychotic depression. Cochrane Database Syst Rev (4):CD004044, 2005 16235348

Wojcik J: Antiparkinson drug use. Biological Therapies in Psychiatry Newsletter 2:5–7, 1979

Yorkston N, Zaki S, Havard C: Some practical aspects of using propranolol in the treatment of schizophrenia, in Propranolol and Schizophrenia. Edited by Roberts E, Amacher P. New York, Alan R Liss, 1978, pp 83–97

Zanarini MC, Frankenburg FR, Parachini EA: A preliminary, randomized trial of flu-oxetine, olanzapine, and the olanzapine-fluoxetine combination in women with borderline personality disorder. J Clin Psychiatry 65(7):903–907, 2004 15291677

Zanarini MC, Schulz SC, Detke HC, et al: A dose comparison of olanzapine for the treatment of borderline personality disorder: a 12-week randomized, double-blind, placebo-controlled study. J Clin Psychiatry 72(10):1353–1362, 2011 21535995

Zoccali R, Muscatello MR, Cedro C, et al: The effect of mirtazapine augmentation of clozapine in the treatment of negative symptoms of schizophrenia: a double-blind, placebo-controlled study. Int Clin Psychopharmacol 19(2):71–76, 2004 15076014

5

Mood Stabilizers

The term *mood stabilizer* was first reported in relation to lithium salts when it became clear that they were effective not only in alleviating mania but also as a prophylaxis against both manic and depressive cycles. Since the introduction of lithium to the United States in 1969, relatively few drugs have been approved as overall mood stabilizers (Table 5–1). However, in more recent years, drugs such as lamotrigine, olanzapine, olanzapine plus samidorphan, quetiapine, risperidone, ziprasidone, and aripiprazole have been approved for the maintenance treatment of bipolar disorder. In addition, many medications have been approved for the acute treatment of mania, and the first drugs for the acute treatment of bipolar depression have now also been approved. It is somewhat less clear that any of the anticonvulsants currently used in treating bipolar affective disorder are as deserving of the term *mood stabilizer* as is lithium. On the other hand, the second-generation antipsychotics (SGAs) with clear benefits in the acute treatment and prevention of both mania and depression do appear deserving of such designation.

A derivative of valproic acid, divalproex sodium, was approved in 1994 by the FDA for the treatment of acute mania. Since that time, it has surpassed

Table 5–1. Non-SGA mood stabilizers: names, formulations, and strengths

Generic name	Brand name[a]	Formulations and strengths
Carbamazepine	Carbamazepine	Chewable tablets: 100, 200 mg Tablets: 100, 200, 300, 400 mg
	Carbatrol	Capsules (extended release): 100, 200, 300 mg
	Epitol	Chewable tablets: 100 mg
	Tegretol	Suspension: 100 mg/5 mL Tablets: 200 mg
	Tegretol-XR	Tablets: 100, 200, 400 mg
Divalproex sodium	Depakote	Capsules (delayed release): 125 mg Tablets (delayed release): 125, 250, 500 mg
	Depakote ER	Tablets: 250, 500 mg
Gabapentin	Gabapentin	Tablets: 100, 300, 400, 600, 800 mg
	Neurontin	Capsules: 100, 300, 400 mg Solution: 250 mg/5 mL Tablets: 600, 800 mg
Gabapentin enacarbil	Horizant	Tablets (extended release): 300, 600 mg
Lamotrigine	Lamictal	Tablets: 25, 100, 150, 200 mg
	Lamictal CD	Tablets (for suspension): 2, 5, 25 mg
	Lamictal ODT	Tablets: 25, 50, 100, 200 mg
	Lamictal XR	Tablets: 25, 50, 100, 200, 250, 300 mg
	Lamotrigine	Tablets: 25, 50, 100, 150, 200, 250 mg
Lithium carbonate	Lithium carbonate	Capsules: 150, 300, 600 mg Tablets (extended release): 300, 450 mg Tablets: 300 mg

Table 5–1. Non-SGA mood stabilizers: names, formulations, and strengths *(continued)*

Generic name	Brand name[a]	Formulations and strengths
Lithium carbonate *(continued)*	Lithobid	Tablets (extended release): 300 mg
Lithium citrate	Lithium citrate	Solution: 8 mEq/5 mL
Oxcarbazepine	Oxtellar XR	Tablets: 150, 300, 600 mg
	Trileptal	Suspension: 300 mg/5 mL
		Tablets: 150, 300, 600 mg
Phentermine hydrochloride+topiramate	Qsymia	Capsules (extended release): 3.75 mg/23 mg; 7.5 mg/46 mg; 11.25 mg/69 mg; 15 mg/92 mg
Tiagabine hydrochloride	Gabitril	Tablets: 2, 4, 12, 16 mg
Topiramate	Eprontia	Solution: 25 mg/mL
	Qudexy XR	Capsules: 25, 50, 100, 150, 200 mg
	Topamax	Capsules: 15, 25 mg
		Tablets: 25, 50, 100, 200 mg
	Trokendi XR	Capsules: 25, 50, 100, 200 mg
Valproic acid	Valproic acid	Capsules: 250 mg
		Syrup: 250 mg/5 mL
Valproate sodium	Valproic sodium	Injection: 100 mg/mL

Note. CR=controlled release; ER=extended release; ODT=orally disintegrating tablet; XR=extended release.
[a]Where the brand name is the same as the generic name, the brand-name products may be no longer available.

lithium in the treatment of bipolar disorder in the United States. Divalproex sodium offers the advantages over lithium of a superior therapeutic index and generally less toxicity. Although divalproex sodium clearly alleviates manic symptoms, the efficacy in preventing manic episodes with this drug is less well established than with lithium. Still, it appears to prevent manic and depressive episodes in clinical practice. Valproate may also have a wider range of efficacy in subtypes of bipolar disorder that are less responsive to lithium, including rapid cycling and mixed states.

The anticonvulsant lamotrigine became only the second drug approved for use in the maintenance treatment of bipolar disorder. Although results from initial studies of lamotrigine in the treatment of acute mania were disappointing, findings from subsequent studies of lamotrigine in delaying the time to onset of a new mood episode were quite convincing. Lithium is more robust in preventing mania than in preventing depression, but the converse may be true for lamotrigine. Because most patients with bipolar disorder live in the depressed phase of the illness, lamotrigine was a welcome option for clinicians treating bipolar patients.

Carbamazepine has been used for many years in the treatment of bipolar disorder, despite the lack of an FDA-approved indication for this purpose. An extended-release formulation of carbamazepine (Equetro) was first approved in the United States for the treatment of mania in 2004. In recent years, carbamazepine has become a third-line agent after lithium, valproate, and the SGAs. The less preferred status of carbamazepine has been due in part to its complex pharmacokinetic interactions and lower therapeutic index, which make it somewhat more difficult to use in combination with many medications. In addition, the studies supporting its utility in bipolar disorder had, until recently, been much smaller and less rigorous than the studies that were completed with divalproex sodium and lithium. A related, newer compound, oxcarbazepine, does not appear to induce liver enzymes quite as much as carbamazepine does and may be better tolerated. As of this writing, it is not being actively studied in large-scale monotherapy trials but is being used by practitioners.

A variety of other anticonvulsants have been studied in bipolar disorder. These include gabapentin, pregabalin, topiramate, tiagabine, ethosuximide, zonisamide, and levetiracetam. At the time of this writing, none of these drugs have convincing controlled data supporting their use as a monotherapy in any phase of bipolar disorder. Nonetheless, drugs like topiramate have shown benefits in counteracting weight gain associated with traditional mood stabilizers such as lithium or divalproate.

The SGAs have played a growing role in the treatment of bipolar disorder and are now among the most common agents used in its treatment. Olanzapine, which had been approved for the treatment of acute mania in 2000, became the first antipsychotic also approved in the maintenance treatment of bipolar I disorder. Like lithium, it probably does a better job preventing mania than it does preventing depression. At this time, all of the SGAs, with the exception of clozapine and iloperidone, are approved in the treatment of mania. The popularity of the SGAs stems in no small part from their rapid onset of action relative to other treatments for bipolar disorder and their versatility in the treatment of both poles as well as maintenance treatment.

There have been literally thousands of controlled studies of antidepressant drugs in the treatment of unipolar depression in the past 50 years, but far fewer studies have been completed on the treatment of bipolar depression. The general assumption had been that an antidepressant should be effective whether treating bipolar or unipolar depression. As we know from our clinical experience, however, this assumption appears to be wrong. Bipolar depressions may not respond to, or may be worsened by, standard antidepressants. Five medications are currently approved for bipolar depression: olanzapine plus fluoxetine combination, quetiapine, lurasidone, cariprazine, and lumateperone. In this chapter, we consider the range of potential mood stabilizers currently used in clinical practice. In addition, more investigational agents are considered. (See Table 5–1 for a listing of mood stabilizers and their formulations and strengths.)

General Treatment Approaches

Acute Mania

In some respects, the treatment of acute mania is among the least problematic components of treating bipolar disorder. Patients with bipolar disorder spend much less time in mania, hypomania, or mixed states than they do in depression. In addition, there are many effective treatments for mania but few for maintenance treatment or treatment of bipolar depression. In bipolar I disorder, the ratio of depression to mania is approximately 3 to 1, and it is as much as 40 to 1 in bipolar II disorder. Four classes of medications are effective in the treatment of acute mania: first-generation antipsychotics (FGAs), SGAs, anticonvulsants, and lithium. The pharmacotherapy of mania often requires combinations of these agents.

Currently, the SGAs are among the most used agents in acute mania. The advantages over other classes of agents include a more rapid onset of action than lithium or the anticonvulsants, fewer extrapyramidal symptoms (EPS) than the FGAs, and greater evidence of efficacy in the subsequent maintenance treatment and treatment of bipolar depression than other classes of agents. Monotherapy trials with quetiapine, asenapine, cariprazine, olanzapine, risperidone, ziprasidone, and aripiprazole have consistently shown benefit over placebo in the treatment of acute mania, and all are FDA approved for this indication. In one meta-analysis, the SGAs averaged a 53% response rate on the Young Mania Rating Scale, compared with 30% for placebo (Perlis et al. 2006). The addition of most SGAs to a mood stabilizer such as lithium or divalproex also has shown superiority over the addition of placebo (Scherk et al. 2007). Thus, for patients not responding to an SGA alone, the addition of a mood stabilizer appears to be a useful strategy.

FGAs probably work as well as SGAs in the treatment of acute mania. In 1974, thorazine was the second drug approved in the United States for the treatment of acute mania. Unlike in the Clinical Antipsychotic Trials of Intervention Effectiveness (CATIE), there have been no comparisons of first-generation drugs and SGAs in terms of the efficacy in the treatment of mania. Cost generally is a benefit of the FGAs, although many SGAs are now available as generics. The concerns about EPS, particularly in a population of bipolar patients, are a factor in first-generation drugs being used less frequently than the SGAs.

The classic mood stabilizers—lithium, divalproex, and carbamazepine—clearly are beneficial both in monotherapy and as combination agents in the treatment of acute mania. Their primary limitation is the time it takes for these agents to be effective. Whereas benefits from antipsychotics are often seen in the first days of treatment, it often takes 1 week or longer to see the antimanic benefits of lithium, divalproex, and carbamazepine. This delay of action is due in no small part to the need to titrate up the dose of these agents. In the current environment, where rapid stabilization is needed to reduce the number of hospital days, delays can be quite expensive. Beyond this, of course, patients in acute mania may be suffering tremendously, and interventions that can rapidly limit the manic episode are obviously desirable.

Thus, given the available data, it may make sense to start the treatment of acute mania with an SGA or possibly an FGA. Patients who are unresponsive to a therapeutic dose of an antipsychotic after 3–7 days often respond to the addition of a mood stabilizer. Benzodiazepines, which are discussed later in this chapter, might also be reasonable adjunctive agents to start with to target sleep, anxiety, and agitation in an acutely manic patient.

Acute Bipolar Depression

Depression is the predominant mood state in bipolar disorder. Patients with bipolar I disorder who were followed over 13 years spent about 32% of their lives in a depressed state versus 9% in mania and 6% mixed or cycling (Judd et al. 2003). In patients with bipolar II disorder, the disparity between poles is even more dramatic; about 1% of time is spent in hypomania versus 50% in the depressed state. Unfortunately, the depressed state is also the more difficult pole to treat. Although we have many good medications to limit mania and hypomania, we have very few proven strategies for bipolar depression.

The long-standing belief that standard antidepressants work in bipolar depression has been increasingly challenged. Sachs and colleagues (2007) have completed what is among the most rigorous studies to date evaluating antidepressant efficacy in bipolar patients. As part of the Systematic Treatment Enhancement Program for Bipolar Disorder (STEP-BD) program, patients with bipolar disorder who were taking a standard mood stabilizer and experiencing a major depressive episode were randomly assigned to adjunctive bupropion, paroxetine, or placebo. Durable recovery, defined as at least 8 consecutive weeks of euthymia, was slightly more likely in the placebo group (27%) than in the antidepressant group (23%). On the other hand, switches into mania were no more likely while taking the antidepressant than while taking the placebo. Likewise, in a prospective evaluation of switch rates when venlafaxine, bupropion, or sertraline was added to a standard mood stabilizer, Altshuler and colleagues (2006) found a relatively low rate of switching into mania and achievement of efficacy (as defined by a reduction in symptoms by ≥50%) about 50% of the time with each of the antidepressants. Venlafaxine was more likely than the other antidepressants to induce a switch into mania. This finding is consistent with earlier data suggesting that the tricyclic antidepressants were somewhat more likely to induce switching than other classes of medications. In a follow-up study of acute responders to antidepressants, Altshuler and colleagues (2009) found that the vast majority of acute responders to antidepressants (69%) maintained response at 1-year follow-up. The switch rate was no higher than that seen with mood stabilizers alone.

As of this writing, only five medications have been approved for the treatment of bipolar depression. The first was the combination of fluoxetine and olanzapine (Symbyax). Tohen and colleagues (2003b) found that relative to placebo, the combination of fluoxetine and olanzapine was superior in improving depressive symptoms at all time points over an 8-week trial. In addition, the combination was superior to olanzapine alone. The second drug to be approved for bipolar depression was quetiapine. Two pivotal placebo-controlled trials have confirmed the efficacy of quetiapine monotherapy at dosages of 300 and 600 mg/day. The higher dosage was somewhat more efficacious than 300 mg/day, but more side effects were seen with the higher dosage. In 2013, lurasidone was approved as a monotherapy and an adjunctive treatment in bipolar depression. The PREVAIL studies demonstrated the efficacy of lurasidone adjunctively with lithium or valproate and as a monotherapy in the treatment of bipolar I depression (Loebel et al. 2014). In addition, lurasidone monotherapy has been reported to be very effective in treating major depression with mixed features (Suppes et al. 2016).

Cariprazine was approved in the treatment of schizophrenia and for acute mania and was subsequently approved for the treatment of bipolar I depression in 2020. Two Phase II and two Phase III studies established the efficacy of cariprazine in bipolar depression (Do et al. 2021). In one of these 3-week trials, the 1.5 mg/day dosage was more efficacious than the 3 mg/day dosage. The number needed to treat in the four studies ranged from 5 to 11, and patients usually responded in the first 4–7 days of treatment. Akathisia and nausea were the most common side effects in the bipolar depression studies. The biggest advantages of cariprazine relative to other SGAs in bipolar depression are its low proclivity for weight gain and straightforward dosing of 1.5–3 mg/day.

Lumateperone became the fifth agent approved in the treatment of bipolar I depression and the second agent, after quetiapine, approved for the treatment of bipolar II depression. Lumateperone demonstrated efficacy in two Phase III studies both as a monotherapy and in conjunction with lithium or valproate. The standard dosage of 42 mg daily reduced Montgomery-Åsberg Depression Rating Scale scores by 4.6 points relative to placebo over 6 weeks in an outpatient study of 381 patients (Calabrese et al. 2021). The most common side effects seen in the bipolar studies were somnolence and nausea. EPS rates were similar to those seen in the placebo group, and there were minimal weight gain or metabolic side effects. Only 1.1% of patients in the lumateperone group gained more than 7% of their body weight, versus no patients in the placebo group.

Several other medications have some support for an efficacy claim in bipolar depression, but the data are not overwhelming. For example, lamotrigine appeared efficacious in the treatment of bipolar depression in one placebo-controlled trial (Calabrese et al. 1999b). However, four subsequent trials failed to show benefit. In very small trials, both modafinil and pramipexole have shown benefit in the treatment of bipolar depression. Armodafinil has been more extensively studied in bipolar depression. Although an initial controlled trial was positive (Calabrese et al. 2010), the adjunctive use of armodafinil failed to statistically separate from placebo in three subsequent randomized controlled Phase III trials. Lithium has long been used in bipolar depression but has not been particularly effective as an acute monotherapy.

Given the available data, patients with bipolar depression should first be taking a mood stabilizer or an SGA. Patients who cycle into depression despite taking adequate doses of one mood stabilizer should be considered for another. For example, a bipolar patient taking lithium who has a depressive episode might benefit from addition of an SGA such as quetiapine and vice versa. Likewise, a patient who is already receiving maintenance treatment with olanzapine and cycles into a depressive episode might be expected to benefit from the addition of lithium or lamotrigine. A lack of response to two mood-stabilizing agents for an acute depressive episode, which is quite common, might prompt consideration of a third agent, such as an antidepressant, armodafinil, modafinil, pramipexole, or yet another mood stabilizer. All too many patients with bipolar depression do not get adequate relief from three or more psychotropic agents. The tendency is to continue adding more agents in an increasingly desperate attempt to provide relief for a suffering patient. Unfortunately, we have very few empirical data to guide our decision beyond the combination of two agents. Ultimately, finding the optimal regimen for a bipolar patient may be a time-consuming trial-and-error process. However, many patients do find a regimen that, while not perfect, offers substantial benefit.

Maintenance Therapy

As with recurrent depression, each subsequent episode of mania or depression may predispose the patient to yet other recurrences and is associated with greater disability and a poorer prognosis. Because bipolar disorder, by definition, is a recurrent illness, maintenance treatment, with the goal of preventing or reducing the number of subsequent cycles, is a standard part of treatment. A mood stabilizer has long been considered the cornerstone of maintenance therapy. Although many agents are used in maintenance therapy, only a handful have convincing evidence supporting their use.

Lithium was the first maintenance medication approved for bipolar disorder (in 1974). In multiple randomized controlled trials done since then, lithium has been consistently effective as a maintenance therapy (see section "Lithium" later in this chapter). However, it is more effective in preventing mania than depression. In addition, many patients still relapse while taking the drug. For example, Geddes and colleagues (2004) found that although the relapse rate did drop in bipolar patients when lithium was used, 40% of the patients still relapsed. Furthermore, lithium is difficult to tolerate for many patients, and the dropout rate is high.

Lamotrigine was the second drug approved, in 2003, for the maintenance treatment of bipolar disorder. Unlike the other approved maintenance treatments, lamotrigine appears to have greater efficacy in preventing depression recurrence than in preventing mania. It also distinguishes itself from other maintenance treatments in not being associated with much weight gain or sedation. Lamotrigine's primary disadvantages are its slow titration schedule and its risk of rash (see section "Lamotrigine" later in this chapter).

The SGAs have become increasingly used in maintenance treatment of bipolar disorder. Olanzapine was approved as a maintenance treatment for bipolar disorder in 2004, followed by aripiprazole in 2005, quetiapine in 2008, and ziprasidone, as well as the long-acting injectable form of risperidone, in 2009. Like lithium, the SGAs are probably more effective in preventing mania than depression. Advantages of SGAs over other approved maintenance treatments include rapid and easy titration, relative safety in overdose, and demonstrated benefits of these agents in treating mania and, at least in the case of olanzapine and quetiapine, depressive symptoms as well. Unfortunately, adverse events associated with SGAs, such as weight gain, metabolic effects, and sedation, often limit adherence and present long-term problems.

Other mood stabilizers, such as divalproex and carbamazepine, are still commonly used as maintenance treatments but do not have as consistent evidence supporting their use as do the FDA-approved maintenance treatments. That being said, many patients find the approved treatments to be ineffective, and clinicians may find divalproex or carbamazepine a reasonable alternative.

Given the data, it makes sense to start maintenance treatment in bipolar patients with a monotherapy, understanding that single agents may well prove to be insufficient. We still think lithium is as good a choice as any to start with. Lamotrigine may be the best tolerated of the approved maintenance treatments and may be a better choice in patients whose primary difficulty is depression recurrence. Among the SGAs, aripiprazole may have some long-term advantages over other SGAs in terms of weight gain and sedation. When a monotherapy fails to prevent a recurrence, combinations of agents are used, but these are not well studied. Ketter (2008) reported that combining an SGA with a standard mood stabilizer such as lithium may improve the outcome of maintenance treatment. This makes good sense, and, clinically, such combinations are common.

Over the previous decade, a number of studies have explored the effectiveness of various combinations in maintenance therapy. The Bipolar Affective Disorder: Lithium/Anti-Convulsant Evaluation (BALANCE) trial compared open-label lithium, valproate, and the combination over a 2-year period. Lithium and lithium plus valproate were significantly more effective than valproate alone (BALANCE investigators and collaborators et al. 2010). In contrast, lithium added to optimized personalized therapy was not superior to optimized personal therapy alone over 6 months (Nierenberg et al. 2013), and in the Bipolar Choice Study, lithium plus optimalized personal therapy was similar to quetiapine plus optimalized therapy (Nierenberg et al. 2016). Overall, these data suggest lithium can add benefit to patients treated with anticonvulsants.

Rapid-Cycling Bipolar Disorder

Rapid-cycling bipolar disorder is characterized in DSM-5-TR (American Psychiatric Association 2022) as having four or more mood episodes in the previous 12 months that meet the criteria for manic, hypomanic, or major depressive episode. The prevalence of rapid cycling in bipolar patients ranges from 14% to 50%, with 20% of STEP-BD patients meeting criteria for rapid cycling at entry. It is unclear whether rapid cycling constitutes a transitory phenomenon or a persistent subtype of bipolar disorder. In most patients, rapid cycling appears to be transitory, but some patients have persistent rapid cycling. As with other forms of the illness, depression tends to be the predominant mood state in rapid cycling.

Although the pathophysiology of rapid cycling is not fully understood, a number of agents are thought to potentially promote rapid cycling in bipolar patients. These include antidepressants, stimulants, steroids, and possibly sympathomimetics and caffeine. Other potential triggers include shift work, sleep disruption, stresses, substance abuse, hypothyroidism, and other hormonal abnormalities.

The first step in treatment is to identify possible triggers and eliminate or minimize them as feasible. For example, antidepressants should be tapered, as opposed to suddenly discontinued, to minimize discontinuation effects and prevent sudden worsening of mood instability. Thyroid status should be evaluated and treated if necessary. Attempts should be made to control the intake of illicit substances and alcohol.

After potential precipitating factors have been dealt with, the next step in the treatment of bipolar disorder is to apply pharmacotherapy. Unfortunately, very few randomized controlled trials exist in the treatment of rapid-cycling bipolar disorder. One of the features of rapid-cycling bipolar disorder has been a greater resistance to lithium. However, the response to lithium does seem to improve substantially if offending agents such as antidepressants are removed and thyroid status is stabilized. In addition, the evidence to date would suggest that lithium is probably about as effective as the anticonvulsants (Fountoulakis et al. 2013). Still, successful treatment with lithium often manifests with a sharp reduction in hypomanic and manic cycles but a continuation of depressive cycles. Many studies suggest that rapid-cycling patients who do not respond to lithium are often responsive to divalproex. As with lithium, divalproex often proves much more successful in reducing manic cycles than depressive episodes. Lamotrigine would seem like a logical choice to add on or substitute for another mood stabilizer because its primary efficacy is seen in preventing depressive cycles. However, the track record for lamotrigine in the treatment of rapid cycling has also been mixed. Lamotrigine appears to be more successful in treating rapid cycling in bipolar II patients than in bipolar I patients. The SGAs, including clozapine, have shown somewhat more consistent benefits in treating rapid-cycling bipolar disorder than have other agents. Controlled studies with olanzapine-fluoxetine combination, olanzapine alone, aripiprazole, and quetiapine have all suggested probable efficacy in reducing both depressive and manic episodes in patients with rapid-cycling bipolar disorder. Nonetheless, many patients are poorly responsive to SGAs.

Successful treatment of rapid cycling, then, involves identifying and mitigating triggers and using combinations of agents because monotherapy response often proves to be less than adequate. SGAs often appear to be helpful in controlling rapid cycling, so we often start there. Addition of lamotrigine or divalproex in patients with rapid-cycling bipolar disorder who are taking another mood stabilizer is often helpful. Clozapine should be considered in patients whose disorder is refractory to standard SGA–mood stabilizer combinations.

Mixed States

Mixed states in bipolar disorder can represent a formidable diagnostic and treatment challenge. The DSM-5-TR mixed features specifier can be applied to bipolar I disorder, bipolar II disorder, and major depression. Rather than requiring that the full criteria for both mania and depression be met, which was quite rare in clinical practice, a mixed state currently requires meeting the full criteria for one mood state while meeting three of the criteria for another. For example, mixed states might include all of the symptom criteria for hypomania as well as several depressive symptoms. In addition to the combination of manic/hypomanic and depressive features, there are often other associated symptoms, including psychosis, severe anxiety, agitation, and lability of mood. At least 30% of acute episodes of bipolar disorder have mixed features. Mixed states may represent a transition from one pole to another, the late stage of a manic episode, or a consistent hybrid of symptoms seen in some patients. Mixed features are more common in hypomania/mania than in major depression.

Relatively few studies have looked at treatment response specifically for mixed states (Krüger et al. 2005). Rather, treatment studies of mania often include patients with mixed states, but these patients represent a minority of the studied population. In the few studies to date that target mixed states specifically, the results are inconclusive. However, divalproex has perhaps been more consistently effective in treating mixed states than has lithium. In fact, in some crossover studies, patients with mixed states that had not responded to lithium appeared to do much better while taking divalproex. Also, elevated depressive symptoms in mixed states might predict better response to valproate than to lithium. Carbamazepine may also be useful in treating mixed states. However, there may be greater evidence of the prophylactic benefit of carbamazepine in preventing mixed states than in acute treatment. Lamotrigine has proven to be useful in patients with treatment-refractory bipolar disorder, including in some small open-label studies in mixed states. However, the necessity of a slow titration limits the utility of lamotrigine in treating any acute states.

There are perhaps more data on the utility of SGAs in the treatment of mixed states than for other agents. At least four double-blind studies of olanzapine have included patients with mixed states. Baker et al. (2003) analyzed the response specifically in patients with mixed features and found that olanzapine, relative to placebo, improved both depressive and manic symptoms in mixed states more within the first week of treatment. However, the improvement in depressive symptoms might have been driven by an improvement in symptoms such as insomnia and paranoia rather than an improvement in mood. There is at least one double-blind study examining the efficacy of quetiapine, ziprasidone, and clozapine, and the data suggest some efficacy for all of these agents in lessening both manic and depressed symptoms in patients in mixed states. As of this writing, there are no published prospective studies of any agents for the treatment of DSM-5-TR major depression with mixed features. However, two prospective studies have used criteria similar to DSM-5 (American Psychiatric Association 2013) criteria (two rather than three mixed symptoms). Both lurasidone (Suppes et al. 2016) and ziprasidone (Patkar et al. 2012) have shown efficacy in mixed depression.

From the limited available data, the use of an SGA monotherapy or adjunctive use with another agent seems reasonable as first-line therapy for mixed states. Given the complexity of symptoms in mixed states, it is unlikely that monotherapies will provide sufficient relief. The combination of divalproex and an SGA should be considered when monotherapy is ineffective. The addition of lamotrigine or lithium might be considered if the combination of an SGA and valproate is ineffective. Antidepressants should generally be avoided, but benzodiazepines are often helpful in targeting sleep, anxiety, and agitation.

In summary, mixed states are challenging to treat. The empirical data are not sufficient to provide clear guidelines. However, there is evidence that certain strategies may help more than others, and these strategies should be tried first.

Lithium therapy: overview	
Efficacy	Bipolar mania and prophylaxis (FDA indicated) Depression augmentation
Side effects	Tremor Polyuria Polydipsia Weight gain Cognitive slowing Hypothyroidism ↓ Renal function Dermatological side effects Memory problems
Safety in overdose	Frequently lethal in blood levels above 3.0 mEq/L and toxic above 1.5 mEq/L. Maintain fluid/ electrolyte balance. Gastric lavage; mannitol diuresis vs. hemodialysis for higher blood levels.
Dosage and administration	Start at 300 mg bid or tid and increase total daily dosage by up to 300 mg, as needed and tolerated, to blood level of 0.6–1.2 mEq/L for bipolar mania and 0.4–0.8 mEq/L for augmentation.
Discontinuation	Sudden discontinuation associated with ↑ risk of relapse. Taper over 3 months for bipolar mania if feasible.
Drug interactions	Antipsychotics: may ↑ lithium toxicity Bupropion: may ↑ seizure risk Carbamazepine: neurotoxicity (rare) Diuretics: ↑ lithium levels Iodide salts: ↑ hypothyroidism Neuromuscular blockers: respiratory depression NSAIDs: ↑ lithium levels SSRIs: serotonin syndrome (rare) Theophylline: ↓ lithium levels Urinary alkalinizers: ↓ lithium levels Verapamil: ↑ or ↓ lithium levels

Note.   NSAID = nonsteroidal anti-inflammatory drug; SSRI = selective serotonin reuptake inhibitor.

Lithium

History and Indications

Lithium, usually as the carbonate and occasionally as the citrate salt, is still widely used in American psychiatry. However, the use of valproate for the treatment of mood disorders now surpasses that of lithium. Lithium is approved by the FDA for the treatment of acute mania and as maintenance therapy to prevent or diminish the intensity of "subsequent episodes in those manic-depressive patients with a history of mania." As discussed in this section, lithium is often used in patients with a variety of recurrent episodic illnesses, with or without prominent affective features. It is also used adjunctively in patients with mood lability, with impulsive or episodic violence or anger, or even with premenstrual dysphoria, alcoholism, borderline personality disorder (BPD), or chronic schizophrenia. Further, it is used as a potentiating agent in a variety of treatment-resistant disorders.

The use of lithium salts in psychiatry was initiated by John Cade, an Australian state hospital superintendent, in 1949, and it proved to be an effective, though somewhat toxic, treatment (Cade 1949). The addition of serum level monitoring made the treatment safe and provided the first general use of blood level monitoring for a psychiatric drug. The use of lithium in psychiatry increased worldwide, although the United States was slow to participate because of an earlier disastrous experience in that country with the unmonitored use of lithium chloride as a salt substitute, which had led to severe toxic reactions, some of which were fatal. Schou (1978) was the first to report compelling evidence that lithium carbonate dramatically reduced the incidence and duration of serious affective episodes in bipolar patients. Since that time, a large number of controlled, double-blind studies have confirmed that lithium is clearly effective in reducing recurrences in both bipolar and unipolar affective disorders, as well as being more effective than placebo in treating acute mania.

Pharmacological Effects

Much has been learned in the past 30 years about the possible mechanism of lithium in the treatment of bipolar disorder. However, we are still some way from defining the key factors of lithium's efficacy. It has become clearer that the pharmacology of lithium is tremendously complex. Lithium may affect different parts of the brain differently at different times. It is evident that lithium's antibipolar effects are probably the result of complex actions on at least three systems. Lithium appears to modulate the balance between excitatory and inhibitory effects of various neurotransmitters such as serotonin (5-hydroxytryptamine; 5-HT), norepinephrine, glutamate, GABA, and dopamine. Lithium also affects neural plasticity through its effects on glycogen synthetase kinase-3β, cyclic adenosine moniphosphate–dependent kinase, and protein kinase C. Finally, lithium adjusts signaling activity via effects on second-messenger activity (Jope 1999).

Lithium appears to enhance serotonergic transmission in a number of ways. For example, lithium appears to increase synthesis of serotonin by increasing tryptophan reuptake in synaptosomes after even short-term use. With long-term use (2–3 weeks), lithium appears to enhance the release of 5-HT from neurons in the parietal cortex and the hippocampus. Furthermore, the chronic administration of lithium appears to cause a downregulation in serotonin$_{1A}$ (5-HT$_{1A}$), serotonin$_{1B}$, and serotonin$_2$ (5-HT$_2$) receptor subtypes (Massot et al. 1999).

Lithium also affects a number of other monoamine neurotransmitters. Initially, lithium appears to increase the rate of synthesis of norepinephrine in some parts of the brain. It reduces the excretion of norepinephrine in patients with mania but increases the excretion of norepinephrine metabolites in patients with depression. These effects are consistent with lithium's beneficial actions in both mania and depression. Likewise, lithium appears to block postsynaptic dopamine receptors' supersensitivity, in keeping with the clinical data that lithium is effective in controlling mania even when psychotic features are present.

In recent years, the effect of lithium on second-messenger systems has been of particular interest. Because lithium affects a variety of neurotransmitters, some investigators have speculated that the principal action of the drug may be on the postsynaptic signal that a number of neurotransmitters generate. The so-called G proteins have been of particular interest in lithium research because they function as signal transducers for a number of receptor types. The G proteins appear to be quite important in coordinating a balance among various neurotransmitters in the brain. Some preliminary evidence suggests that lithium may have a direct or indirect effect on G proteins that mediates their actions.

The role of the phosphatidylinositol (PtdIns) system, another second-messenger system, in the actions of lithium remains unclear. Lithium appears to inhibit a number of enzymes in the Ptdlns system, including inositol monophosphatase. It is believed that the Ptdlns system affects the receptor activity of many neurotransmitter systems, including the serotonergic, cholinergic, and noradrenergic systems. The role of the Ptdlns second-messenger system in lithium's actions is the subject of continued investigation.

Clinical Indications

Lithium use can be divided into four main clinical areas:

1. To control rapidly acute, overt psychopathology as in mania or agitation
2. To attempt to modify milder, ongoing, or frequent but episodic clinical symptoms such as chronic depression or episodic irritability
3. To establish a prophylactic maintenance regimen to avert future mood episodes
4. To enhance the effect of antidepressants in patients with major depressive episodes (see Chapter 3, "Antidepressants," and Chapter 9, "Augmentation Strategies for Treatment-Resistant Disorders")

Acute Mania

No final, conclusive statement about the use of lithium as a sole or primary drug treatment for acute mania is possible. The initial approval of lithium in the treatment of acute mania was based on three small double-blind studies completed before 1971. A later study addressing the question of lithium for acute mania (Lambert and Venaud 1992) found that half of 36 acutely manic patients who completed a 3-week trial responded to lithium and that this was about twice the rate seen with placebo. These results were similar to those found in a larger, multicenter-based study comparing lithium, valproate, and placebo in the treatment of acute mania (Bowden et al. 1994). In that study, both lithium and valproate were twice as likely as placebo to produce a marked reduction in manic symptoms over a 3-week period.

Lithium alone is clearly more effective than placebo and is probably as effective as an antipsychotic in treating patients with less severe mania. It is probably less effective and slower acting than an antipsychotic in disturbed, psychotic manic, schizoaffective, or very hyperactive patients.

Given the delayed onset of action of lithium (7–14 days), most clinicians do not initiate treatment with lithium alone in acute mania. It is common practice to begin by administering patients an antipsychotic, on the assumption that it will produce the most rapid control of psychopathology or aid in patient management. Many clinicians then add lithium—either on the first day of drug therapy or after the mania has begun to respond to antipsychotics—to stabilize the patient on both drugs. When the patient is clearly much improved, some clinicians gradually taper the antipsychotic over several months so that the patient will be taking lithium alone at the end of the episode. In patients whose hospitalizations are brief, both medications will be in use at discharge, and the antipsychotic will be tapered when the patient is back in the community. Some early studies on antipsychotic use indicated that more than 50% of the patients were still taking antipsychotics at 6-month follow-up. Currently, most patients who have an SGA started for acute mania likely continue it as a maintenance therapy.

An alternative strategy that has long been popular is to initiate treatment of the acutely manic patient with both lithium and a benzodiazepine such as lorazepam or clonazepam (Lenox et al. 1992). This strategy allows the clinician to immediately address the insomnia and hyperactivity without the potentially toxic effects of an antipsychotic. However, using only a benzodiazepine with lithium may not be ideal in the treatment of the acutely psychotic manic patient. In such patients, triple therapy—a benzodiazepine, an antipsychotic, and lithium—allows smaller doses of the first two agents to be used for the acute episode while lithium is initiated for long-term treatment.

The problem of severe neurotoxicity, reported mainly with the combined use of haloperidol or another high-potency antipsychotic and lithium, deserves comment here. In the 1970s there was considerable concern about the possibility of serious drug interactions between lithium and haloperidol, a concern based almost exclusively on anecdotal reports. When the possible interaction was reviewed more recently, no significant interaction between lithium and neuroleptics was detected beyond merely additive adverse effects (Kessel et al. 1992). Neurotoxicity, including delirium and other mental status changes, may occur with lithium alone even at therapeutic dosages in elderly and organically compromised patients. More recent experience suggests that patients who developed neurotoxicity on the combination either were lithium toxic (often at toxic levels) or had a neuroleptic malignant syndrome. In general, the combination of antipsychotics and lithium appears to be safe and efficacious.

Bipolar Maintenance Treatment

The evidence that lithium is effective in the prophylaxis of recurrent bipolar episodes is far more substantial than the evidence of lithium's efficacy in treating acute mania. Until olanzapine received a similar approval, lithium was the only drug with an FDA-approved indication for the maintenance treatment of bipolar disorder. At least 10 double-blind studies suggested that the relapse rate for bipolar patients is two to three times higher with placebo than with lithium. Among the best lithium studies have been those completed using lithium as an active control in the lamotrigine maintenance studies (Goodwin et al. 2004). These studies confirmed the utility of lithium in the maintenance treatment of bipolar disorder. In addition, lithium is clearly effective in preventing suicide attempts and completions in bipolar patients (Baldessarini et al. 2006). However, the rapid discontinuation of lithium in some of the earlier trials probably affected the relapse rates. A recent Swedish national registry study reported that suicide-related events were significantly lower (14%) when bipolar patients were treated with lithium than when they were taking valproate (Song et al. 2017). The prophylactic effects of lithium appear more pronounced in preventing manic than depressive recurrences, but both are positively affected. However, only half, or perhaps fewer than half, of lithium-treated patients have complete suppression of all episodes, even with excellent medication compliance. Furthermore, at least some of the patients who have manic recurrences while taking maintenance lithium are blamed for noncompliance unjustifiably: the noncompliance is probably secondary to a recurrence of mania rather than vice versa. In addition, some patients respond to lithium with suppression of mania but with continuing episodes of depression; others show only a partial reduction in severity in both phases.

We have seen a number of patients who had been taking lithium for several years but continued to have episodes of mania and depression; they were judged to be lithium nonresponders, but their condition was clearly even worse when lithium therapy was abandoned as ineffective. Patients with rapid-cycling and mixed-state types of bipolar disorder generally do less well while taking lithium than do patients with less frequent or purely manic episodes. However, even some of the former can have the severity of their episodes ameliorated. In addition, patients who tend to develop severe stage III manic episodes with psychotic disorganization do more poorly with lithium treatment alone.

In initiating maintenance prophylactic lithium therapy, both the patient and (when available) a spouse or a significant other need careful instruction about the purposes and requirements of lithium therapy, including its side effects and complications. There is evidence that continuing involvement of bipolar patients and their spouses in couples groups or of single patients in lithium support groups is helpful in maintaining drug compliance and in helping patients deal with past, current, and future problems.

Many bipolar patients, when contemplating maintenance lithium therapy, ask, "Will I have to take lithium forever?" There are two issues in this area. One is whether patients ever stop having recurrent manic and depressive episodes once several episodes have occurred, and the other is whether abruptly stopping lithium will trigger an affective episode that might not have otherwise occurred. The evidence from placebo substitution and lithium discontinuation studies involving patients whose condition was already stabilized successfully with lithium maintenance is that relapses occur with considerable frequency: about half the patients relapsed within 6 months. In other, uncontrolled studies, which involved small series of patients, patients relapsed floridly within a few days. We suspect that the latter consequence is unusual but may actually occur with some patients; it may account for some of the florid relapses seen in patients taking maintenance lithium who experiment with stopping (or forget to take) their medication for a few days. In our experience, however, stopping lithium abruptly for 2 or 3 days in patients who have developed uncomfortable symptoms of lithium toxicity has never led to a florid relapse.

The area of lithium discontinuation is not well understood, but most clinicians assume that essentially all bipolar patients whose condition is stable with lithium need to continue the medication indefinitely. Data confirm that abrupt discontinuation of lithium after long-term treatment significantly increases the rate and speed of relapse (Faedda et al. 1993). More gradual discontinuation of lithium in bipolar patients over several months appears to mitigate this risk substantially (Suppes et al. 1993). Discontinuation of lithium can be associated with increased risk for suicide (Tondo et al. 2001).

One wonders, however, whether withdrawal from lithium could be worth a trial for patients who have really stabilized both their illness and their life circumstances for several years and in whom there is some evidence that prior episodes were precipitated by stressors that are no longer present. Such trials of withdrawal from lithium need to be discussed in detail with patients and their families, with all parties taking into account that about 90% of patients with mania will have a recurrence at some time. Given the occasional rapid relapses observed with sudden discontinuation, slowly tapering the drug in monthly 300-mg decrements would be indicated. Post and colleagues (1992) reported that some patients who discontinued their lithium did not experience a response when readministered lithium for a recurrence of the disorder. These data suggest that it may be prudent to err on the side of continuing lithium maintenance for longer rather than shorter periods. However, a later prospective, naturalistic study demonstrated that patients with a recurrence of mania who had previously had a response to lithium generally appear to have a response to rechallenge with the drug (Coryell et al. 1998).

Schizophrenia Spectrum Illnesses

There is some evidence that lithium, at serum levels in the range of 0.8–1.1 mEq/L, is useful in combination with an antipsychotic in treating patients with schizoaffective disorder. Early reports suggested that many of these patients benefit from the addition of lithium to a regimen of antipsychotics. In the few controlled studies in which lithium was added to an antipsychotic in schizophrenic patients with or without manic symptoms, lithium was often more effective, on average, than placebo. However, monotherapy with lithium appears much less efficacious than treatment with an antipsychotic alone in the treatment of schizophrenia. Furthermore, more recent studies of the efficacy of adjunctive lithium in the treatment of schizophrenia have not consistently demonstrated the beneficial effects of lithium seen in earlier studies (Citrome 2009a). In some chronically impaired schizophrenic patients with no more than the usual amount of affective overlay, lithium produces useful but limited additional improvement when added to an antipsychotic regimen. This effect occurs often enough to make a trial of lithium easily justifiable for any patient with treatment-resistant schizophrenia or schizoaffective disorder, although perhaps only one in five will show clinical improvement. Also, for a subgroup of chronically schizophrenic patients with brief, episodic angry outbursts, lithium appears to act by decreasing impulsive anger rather than by reducing the level of psychosis. In addition, the anti-suicidal properties of lithium may be useful in some suicidal patients with schizophrenia (Filaković and Erić 2013). However, in patients with chronic, treatment-resistant psychotic illness, drug treatments are often added and continued for months or years, even if no obvious clinical response or only a trivial improvement has occurred, in the hope that the extra drugs might be helping. There seems little justification for continuing such a use of lithium for longer than 6 months if no clinical benefit is apparent.

Depressive Disorders

Some depressive episodes improve with lithium alone. In fact, a number of controlled studies suggest that lithium may be as effective as tricyclic antidepressants (TCAs) in the treatment of major depression. The response time, however, often lags behind that of standard antidepressants. For recurrent unipolar depression, maintenance treatment with lithium appears to be as effective as long-term treatment with imipramine in preventing recurrences (Prien et al. 1984). A number of studies also suggest that adding lithium to a TCA, a selective serotonin reuptake inhibitor (SSRI), or a monoamine oxidase inhibitor in a patient who has not responded to the antidepressant after 3–6 weeks may lead to a clear favorable response (see Chapters 3 and 9).

In recurrent unipolar depression, the evidence from large-scale studies on the exact prophylactic potential of lithium is mixed; some studies showed lithium and imipramine to be equally effective, whereas other studies showed imipramine to be superior to lithium and both drugs to be superior to placebo. The combination of imipramine and lithium was not superior to imipramine alone. In bipolar II depression, a 16-week trial compared lithium alone, sertraline alone, and the combination. The three were equal, and the switch rates seen were about 15% (Altshuler et al. 2017). Thus, clinicians may choose to use lithium alone to prevent recurrence of depression in bipolar patients.

Just as lithium is known to have antisuicide properties in patients with bipolar disorder, emerging evidence also suggests that lithium is an equally effective prophylaxis in patients with unipolar depression. Guzzetta and colleagues (2007) evaluated suicide attempts and risks in patients with recurrent major depressive disorder who had participated in long-term trials in which lithium was used. The investigators estimated that the risk of completed suicides and suicide attempts was 90% greater when the patients were not treated with adjunctive lithium than when they were taking the drug. Subsequently, meta-analyses have revealed that lithium appears to reduce suicidal behavior in patients with major depressive disorder and bipolar disorder (Cipriani et al. 2013a; Del Matto et al. 2020). A large multicenter prospective trial to evaluate the efficacy of lithium in reducing the risk of suicide in patients with treatment-resistant depression who had made a recent suicide attempt (Cipriani et al. 2013a) has not yet to our knowledge been published. However, a recent, relatively large study on lithium preventing suicide in Department of Veterans Affairs patients with bipolar disorder or major depression who had recently attempted suicide failed to show efficacy in comparison to placebo (Katz et al. 2022). Thus, although meta-analyses do indicate efficacy of lithium in preventing suicide, questions remain regarding how effective it actually is.

Lithium is among the better studied augmenters of antidepressant response. Although most studies of lithium augmentation involved augmentation of TCAs, lithium has proved useful in the augmentation of a variety of antidepressants (Bschor and Bauer 2006). One of the larger randomized, albeit open, trials of lithium augmentation was in the Sequenced Treatment Alternatives for Resistant Depression (STAR*D) trial. In that study, patients who had experienced two previous failed medication trials were randomly assigned to lithium or triiodothyronine (T_3; Cytomel) augmentation. Approximately 16% of patients achieved remission when lithium was added versus 25% of patients who were randomly assigned to T_3 augmentation (Nierenberg et al. 2006a). The difference was not statistically significant, but lithium was more poorly tolerated than the T_3. Although it is clear that lithium is an effective augmenter of antidepressants, there are far more choices for augmentation now than there were 30 years ago, and lithium's popularity in resistant depression has waned.

Rage and Irritability

There is a reasonable clinical literature, mainly but not exclusively, placebo controlled, that supports the proposition that some patients with episodic uncontrolled outbursts of violent rage have a response to lithium. The drug certainly is not always effective in such cases, but these predominantly nonpsychotic behavior disorders often present such appalling clinical problems that any drug with a chance of helping substantially deserves a trial. We concur with Tupin's classic position that in populations such as violent prisoners, lithium controls outbursts of rage that are nontriggered or are triggered instantaneously by minor stimuli, but it does not affect premeditated aggressive behavior (Tupin 1975). The drug is helpful in some patients with organic disorders or intellectual developmental disorders who display episodic angry outbursts. Lithium has also shown some utility in the treatment of children with episodic aggressive outbursts and in mitigating the self-destructive behavior of some patients with BPD. It should be noted that there have been a few case reports of lithium causing increased aggressive behavior in patients with temporal lobe spike activity on the electroencephalogram (EEG). The use of anticonvulsants and antipsychotics has largely supplanted lithium use in the management of hostility, impulse control, and aggression in a variety of disorders (Goedhard et al. 2006).

Side Effects

Neuromuscular and Central Nervous System Effects

Among the most common side effects in lithium therapy is tremor, principally noticed in the fingers (Table 5–2). It is faster than pseudoparkinsonian tremor and resembles intentional, coffee-induced, or familial tremor. When tremor is severe enough to affect handwriting, the writing is usually jagged and irregular but not micrographic as in parkinsonism. Tremor sometimes is worse at peak lithium blood level and can be ameliorated by dosage rearrangement. Dosage reduction can often be used to bring the blood level low enough to make tremor either absent or mild and inconspicuous. If there is good reason to maintain a serum lithium level that causes a disturbing degree of tremor, propranolol at dosages ranging from 10 to 160 mg/day can be used to reduce the tremor.

Some patients taking lithium also develop cogwheeling and mild signs of parkinsonism, and naturally occurring parkinsonism can be aggravated. With toxic lithium levels, gross tremulousness and ataxia with dysarthria occur: the patient appears to have gross neurological disorder and, often, to be confused or, less often, to be delirious at the same time. Seizures occur rarely with severe lithium toxicity.

Some patients taking lithium complain of slowed mentation and forgetfulness and, on testing, show a memory deficit. In addition, some patients may experience drowsiness and fatigue, which may further exacerbate the feeling of being slowed down. Pooled data on side effects of lithium therapy suggest that memory problems are perhaps the leading cause of noncompliance and the third most common side effect overall (Goodwin and Jamison 1990). Although such patients are often suspected or accused of "using" these symptoms

Table 5–2. Toxicology of mood stabilizers

System	Lithium	Valproate	CBZ	Gabapentin	Lamotrigine	Topiramate	Tiagabine
CNS	Tremor Ataxia Cognitive slowing	Sedation Tremor Ataxia	Sedation Dizziness Ataxia	Somnolence Dizziness Ataxia	Dizziness Ataxia Somnolence	Dizziness Ataxia Speech problems Cognitive slowing	Dizziness Somnolence Difficulty concentrating
GI	Dyspepsia Weight gain Diarrhea	Dyspepsia LFT increases Weight gain Hepatic failure (rare) Pancreatitis	Dyspepsia	Dyspepsia (rare)	Nausea Vomiting	Nausea Dyspepsia Abdominal pain	Nausea Abdominal pain
Dermatological	Rash Hair loss Acne	Rash Hair loss	Rash	Pruritus (rare)	Rash Acne	Rash (rare) Pruritis (rare)	Rash (rare) Alopecia
Renal/urogenital	NDI Nephropathy	Minimal	SIADH	None	Vaginitis Urinary tract infection	Dysmenorrhea Metabolic acidosis[a]	None
Cardiac	T wave changes Sinoatrial block	Minimal Risk of polycystic ovary syndrome	Arrhythmia	None	Palpitations (rare) Hypotension (rare)	BP changes (rare)	Hypertension Palpitations
Hematological	Leukocytosis	Thrombocytopenia	Thrombocytopenia	Leukopenia (rare)	None	Leukopenia	None

Table 5–2. Toxicology of mood stabilizers *(continued)*

System	Lithium	Valproate	CBZ	Gabapentin	Lamotrigine	Topiramate	Tiagabine
							Drug
Hematological *(continued)*		Coagulation defect	Aplastic anemia (rare)				
Endocrine	Hypothyroidism	Minimal	Lower levels of T$_3$, T$_4$	None	Hypothyroidism (rare)	Weight decrease	Goiter (rare)

Note. BP = blood pressure; CBZ = carbamazepine; GI = gastrointestinal; LFT = liver function test; NDI = nephrogenic diabetes insipidus; SIADH = syndrome of inappropriate antidiuretic hormone; T$_3$ = triiodothyronine; T$_4$ = thyroxine.
[a]Secondary to hyperchloremia.

to avoid necessary lithium therapy, our impression is that these complaints are real and constitute a basis for lowering the dosage or trying another therapy.

Some patients worry that they may become less creative while taking lithium. However, Schou (1979), a pioneer in lithium therapy, has asserted that 75% of patients note no change or an improvement in their creativity with lithium therapy. The bipolar patients who have the most prominent neuropsychological effects of lithium tend to be younger, depressed patients with higher lithium serum levels (Kocsis et al. 1993). Patients who complain that lithium is affecting their cognition or creativity might do well at a somewhat lower dosage.

With all the above neurological symptoms, stopping lithium will lead to a disappearance of the side effects, but the symptoms and signs may persist for 2–5 days, longer than one would expect it to take to clear the offending lithium from the body.

Gastrointestinal Effects

Chronic nausea and watery diarrhea can occur together or separately as signs of lithium toxicity. Episodic nausea occurring only after each dose may be due to local gastric irritation and may be relieved by taking lithium with food. Shifting to a different lithium preparation may also be helpful. For example, in cases of upper gastrointestinal (GI) distress, sustained-release preparations may be beneficial. In contrast, patients with diarrhea who are on sustained-release preparations may benefit from a switch to the shorter-release forms.

Weight Gain and Endocrine Effects

Some patients gain weight progressively while taking lithium, and this side effect is second only to cognitive side effects as a reason that patients stop taking the medication. The mechanisms underlying this side effect are unclear. However, lithium appears to have an insulin-like action that may result in relative hypoglycemia (Jefferson et al. 1987). This hypoglycemia may in turn promote eating and subsequent weight gain. More commonly, increased appetite with resulting weight gain is the problem, and attempting to control weight with dietary regulation is often very difficult for the patient. Weight gain is greater in patients who are overweight to begin with and is probably greater in patients with polydipsia, perhaps because they drink caloric fluids. A few patients have overt edema and/or lose several pounds rapidly when lithium is stopped.

Most patients show a transitory decrease in thyroid levels early in lithium therapy, and a very few show goiter with normal thyroid studies except for elevated thyroid-stimulating hormone (TSH) levels. Some clinicians add thyroid supplements at this point. However, we recommend using exogenous thyroid hormone primarily in patients with marked goiter or in those with associated anergia.

Up to 20% of patients, more commonly women, develop clinical hypothyroidism on lithium therapy, and 30% develop elevated TSH levels (Jefferson et al. 1987).

In our clinic, we will typically obtain a TSH level before initiating lithium and then repeat it at 6 months and annually thereafter.

Renal Effects

Lithium causes polyuria with secondary polydipsia to a noticeable degree in some (perhaps roughly one out of five) patients. In a few patients this effect may extend to severe renal diabetes insipidus, with urine volume up to 8 L/day and difficulty in concentrating urine and maintaining adequate lithium serum levels. This range of renal effects is due to a decrease in the resorption of fluid from the distal tubules of the kidney. It can be treated, obviously, by lowering the dose of lithium or stopping the drug. In most, but not all, cases the renal effect wears off days or weeks after lithium is stopped.

An alternative strategy with patients in whom lithium is clearly necessary and the polyuria is distressing is to add a loop or thiazide diuretic. It is well documented that hydrochlorothiazide at a dosage of 50 mg/day decreases lithium clearance by about 50% and therefore increases lithium plasma levels. Thus, one can rationally add 50 mg/day of hydrochlorothiazide and then reduce the lithium dosage by 50% and carefully restabilize the desired lithium level. This maneuver is sometimes effective, as it is in naturally occurring nephrogenic diabetes insipidus, and can be used in milder but troublesome cases of polyuria. At the time of our first edition, amiloride (Midamor) had recently been reported to decrease lithium-induced polyuria without, allegedly, affecting either potassium excretion or lithium serum levels. However, we have seen some patients who showed increased lithium levels when amiloride was added. If this strategy is tried, one should check lithium levels carefully while assessing amiloride's effectiveness in improving renal resorption of fluid and decreasing urine volume. There is renewed interest in the use of amiloride for renal side effects (Kamali et al. 2017).

The prohibition in the *Physicians' Desk Reference* (PDR) against combining lithium with diuretics, particularly of the thiazide type, is much overstated. It is true that harm can occur if a patient is stabilized on lithium at a clinically useful blood level (e.g., 0.8 mEq/L) and a thiazide diuretic is added in ignorance: the lithium level can double, and the patient may suddenly develop signs of lithium toxicity. This increase can also occur with other drugs, most notably nonsteroidal anti-inflammatory drugs such as ibuprofen, naproxen, and indomethacin. However, we see no problem in starting lithium therapy in a patient already stabilized on a thiazide diuretic; even patients undergoing dialysis have been successfully treated with lithium. Renal impairment before lithium therapy means the clinician should raise the dosage very slowly and cautiously, monitoring serum levels carefully.

A different and potentially more serious renal problem is interstitial nephritis, first reported by Danish workers in 1977. It is characterized by renal scarring and destruction. Currently, the problem no longer seems as threatening as it did initially. Major renal impairment manifested by seriously decreased creatinine clearance appears to be quite rare. In a review, Gitlin (1993) suggested that up to 5% of lithium-treated patients developed some renal insufficiency, but these changes were generally not clinically significant. In a later review, polyuria secondary to lithium-induced decreases in renal tubular function appeared to be progressive in many patients, whereas changes in glomerular function were not (Gitlin 1999). Patients exposed to multiple periods of lithium toxicity may be at greater risk for developing renal insufficiency. However, some patients with chronic affective disorders who have never taken lithium show renal pathology, and not all kidney dysfunction in patients taking lithium is necessarily caused by the drug.

Still, it is worth checking kidney function every 6–12 months in patients on maintenance lithium. The "best" way would be to measure creatinine clearance periodically, but logistical problems and doubts about patient reliability in 24-hour urine collection have caused this procedure to be generally disfavored. Serum creatinine itself offers a reasonable indicator of kidney function because creatinine production is a function of muscle mass and is not affected by diet. We typically obtain a serum creatinine level before initiating lithium and repeat it annually thereafter or as clinically indicated. Lithium serum level at constant intake is also a function of glomerular filtration. Watching both measures periodically should allow detection of early changes in glomerular function. Some practitioners check the patients' reactive ability to concentrate their urine. If the lithium dosage requirement gradually decreases and serum creatinine is persistently elevated (above 1.6 mg/100 mL), a nephrology consultation is indicated. Even if renal impairment appears to exist, the decision whether to stop lithium therapy should be based on the total picture. Patients who obtain major benefits from maintenance lithium and have either a mild renal deficit or a kidney problem that may not be lithium related can continue taking lithium, but more frequent monitoring of kidney function is required.

Cardiovascular Effects

Lithium can produce a variety of benign effects on the electrocardiogram (ECG), including T wave flattening and inversion. A few cases have been reported in which a sick sinus node syndrome has been brought on by lithium. This complication is very rare and probably not predictable unless the condition antedates the lithium therapy. Some patients have developed problems with sinus node conduction after concurrent use of antiarrhythmic drugs (Jefferson et al. 1987). Baseline ECGs are desirable in older patients or patients with a history of any cardiac dysfunction. Some caution should also be exercised in using lithium in patients with particularly low heart rates at baseline.

Dermatological Effects

A wide variety of diverse rashes from lithium have been described. Acne is perhaps the most common dermatological effect of lithium use and has been reported to be helped by topical retinoic acid. Aggravation of preexisting or dormant psoriasis is well documented, and a dry, noninflamed papular eruption is relatively common with maintenance lithium. Both zinc sulfate and tetracycline have been tried as treatments for rashes, with variable success. Other rashes—of an itchy, presumably allergic nature, less typical with lithium—can occur and often disappear if the specific lithium brand being used is changed. Presumably, these are allergic reactions to some ingredient in the capsule or tablet other than the lithium itself. Alopecia can occur in patients taking lithium, but the hair often regrows, either with or without lithium.

Preparations

Lithium is available in the United States in several formulations (see Table 5–1). The standard and least expensive form is the carbonate in 300-mg capsules or scored tablets. Sustained-release preparations of the carbonate are also available, as is a liquid preparation of lithium citrate; one teaspoonful of the liquid has the equivalent in ion content of 300 mg of the carbonate (8 mEq). Other preparations, including the sulfate, and other dosage strengths are used in Europe. Despite more than 50 years of clinical experience with lithium, it is not entirely clear whether any of the formulations have definite superiority for any purpose, aside from relieving GI side effects. Lithium citrate is obviously useful in patients who dislike or cannot swallow pills.

The sustained-release preparations result in lower peak serum lithium levels after ingestion and probably result in the release of less lithium ion in the stomach and more in the small intestine. If lithium irritation of the stomach mucosa is causing nausea after each dose, the sustained-release preparation may reduce gastric irritation. If diarrhea is a problem (and is not due to an elevated serum lithium level), the citrate may cause even faster absorption in the upper GI tract and may reduce the diarrhea. However, we have seen patients who have diarrhea with standard lithium carbonate whose diarrhea lessened when they took sustained-release lithium. The basic problem is that it is still unclear which lithium side effects are related to peak serum level and which are related to steady-state serum level. Clinically, any side effect that occurs mainly 1–2 hours after each oral dose of the standard preparation might be improved by the sustained-release form. For example, nausea may be caused by gastric irritation from lithium or by an elevated serum level. The former causes transient nausea after each dose, whereas the latter causes persistent nausea.

It was believed that sustained-release lithium would, in general, have fewer side effects and might, in particular, have less effect on the concentrating ability of the renal tubules, leading to less polyuria and polydipsia. This belief does not seem to be the case, and it may even be that massing the total daily dose of lithium at bedtime may cause fewer renal effects. One major European center (Copenhagen) has routinely been using once-a-day lithium dosing for many years, suggesting that this dosage scheme is feasible and effective.

Dosage and Administration

Lithium dosage is titrated to achieve both therapeutic response and adequate plasma levels. The general presumption is that levels of about 0.7–1.0 mEq/L are appropriate for maintenance therapy or the treatment of conditions other than manic or psychotic excitement, whereas levels up to 1.5 mEq/L are sometimes needed in treating acute mania. Levels should be obtained about 12 hours after the last dose, at which time the vagaries of absorption after drug ingestion are well past and a relative steady state has been achieved (see the subsection on blood levels in the section "Tricyclic and Tetracyclic Antidepressants" in Chapter 3). These "ideal" levels are, of course, not carved in stone and must be interpreted in the clinical context. Someone who has marked tremor, oversedation, vomiting, and ataxia at a level of 0.8 mEq/L either cannot tolerate that level or has some other medical condition causing the symptoms; lithium intolerance is the more likely possibility. Other patients receiving maintenance therapy appear to have averted affective episodes for years at levels as low as 0.4–0.6 mEq/L, and patients with daily symptoms such as irritability and anger report clinical improvement at very low plasma levels. It is very hard to prove that these are or are not "real" drug responses. It is our belief that many patients can be successfully maintained at relatively low plasma levels, particularly when the lithium is combined with another agent. Occasionally, for a patient whose mania is still uncontrolled despite a level of 1.5 mEq/L for several days and who has no side effects, a higher level can be cautiously tried.

Expedient establishment of high, adequate plasma levels of lithium (e.g., 0.8–1.2 mEq/L) is desired for acute mania. An initial regimen of 300 mg bid to qid is indicated in healthy adolescent or adult patients; plasma levels should initially be obtained every 3 or 4 days to ensure early detection of toxic lithium levels. The dosage should be titrated up (or down) as necessary to achieve a level of approximately 1.0 mEq/L. In patients older than 60 or those with possible renal impairment, the lower starting dose is indicated. In some elderly patients, we initiate lithium at 150 mg bid. Several articles have described techniques for predicting the optimal dosage of lithium from a loading dose followed by several determinations of levels over the next 24 hours. These techniques can be used, but they do not seem to us to offer benefit over clinical titration. Response in acutely manic states may require 7–14 days, even with adequate plasma levels. As plasma levels stabilize, the frequency of testing may be decreased to two times a week initially, and eventually to once a week, as both plasma levels and the clinical condition level out. If inadequate clinical response occurs within 4 weeks, it is safe to assume that lithium monotherapy will not be effective for the acute episode. At this point, or earlier, addition of a second mood stabilizer should be considered.

With patients who are in remission and are being stabilized with lithium to avert future affective episodes, one can begin at even lower dosages (one or two 300-mg doses per day); weekly plasma levels are often sufficient during dosage adjustment. Again, the goal is to find a well-tolerated plasma level as close to 0.8 mEq/L as possible. It seems reasonable that higher plasma levels should be associated with better prophylaxis. In one major collaborative study sponsored by the National Institute of Mental Health (NIMH), patients whose lithium was maintained at 0.8 mEq/L and above had consistently fewer recurrences than patients stabilized at lower levels (0.6 mEq/L or below) but had more side effects. The efficacy data in this study generated considerable controversy because when patients were initially randomly assigned to low plasma level groups, the dose may have been decreased so rapidly as to enhance the likelihood of relapse. Once a patient on maintenance lithium is stabilized adequately with weekly plasma levels for a few weeks, monthly levels are sufficient, and after 6–12 months of stability, testing the levels every 6 months or as clinically indicated may suffice.

Once a patient has a stable daily dosage, it can be spread over the day in any suitable regimen. Usually, twice a day—morning and bedtime—is convenient and well tolerated, and doses are less likely to be forgotten or overlooked. It has been suggested, but not proved, that once-a-day dosing enhances compliance and may be associated with less polyuria. We have found that once-a-day dosing at bedtime is often effective, but some patients feel drugged or dazed in the morning. Gastric irritation after each dose is the major reason for use of divided doses. Smaller, more frequent doses are common (and logistically easy) among hospitalized patients, but the patients are sometimes inadvertently discharged on these regimens when a simpler regimen would suffice and might be taken more reliably after the patient returns home.

For other target symptoms, when the situation is less urgent, an initial dosage of 300 mg bid seems adequate. Some patients who end up benefiting from lithium have presented with histories of marked lithium intolerance that appears to have been caused by overaggressive initial dosing. In these less acute situations, a plasma level of 0.5–0.8 mEq/L is probably adequate, and less frequent plasma level monitoring may be needed. It is also important to remember that you are treating the patient, not the plasma level, and that both clinical status and adverse effects need frequent and careful monitoring. Some patients report clear symptom relief at levels around 0.5 mEq/L; it seems unwarranted to push them to higher levels unless they break through with symptoms at lower levels. Similarly, keeping a patient chronically nauseated, mentally dulled, and grossly tremulous just to maintain an "adequate" plasma level is counterproductive in almost all situations. In general, we advise aiming for lower levels (<0.6 mEq/L) in elderly patients. For patients with chronic disorders manifesting overt, current target psychopathology—depression, schizophrenia, and cyclothymia—a trial of about 4 weeks at adequate blood levels (or the highest tolerated levels) is usually sufficient to determine whether lithium will be clinically useful.

If a patient has responded to lithium in the past but has stopped the drug for weeks or months, and if there is no reason to believe that kidney function has changed in the interim, it is clinically reasonable to immediately reinstate the drug at the prior dosage without retitrating. However, some patients require gradual dose escalation to allow optimal dosing. Frequent blood level monitoring should be reinstituted.

Use in Pregnancy

At one time, lithium was the only psychoactive nonanticonvulsant, nonbenzodiazepine drug that was thought to be associated with a specific birth defect, Ebstein's anomaly. This serious cardiac abnormality is not common in children born to mothers taking lithium (4.5–7.6/1,000 live births/10,000 births), but the defect is more common in these children than in the population at large (Gentile 2012). These estimates are much lower than earlier estimates, and some reviews have called into question whether there is a valid association of Ebstein's anomaly and lithium use (Giles and Bannigan 2006). The risk of a major birth defect needs to be discussed with patients taking lithium who either are planning to become pregnant or are already pregnant because the risk appears to exist primarily with first-trimester use (see Chapter 12, "Pharmacotherapy of Specific Populations"). The general risk of a major birth defect appears to be two to three times greater with lithium use than in the general population (Cohen et al. 1994). An Israeli report noted elevated rates of cardiovascular anomalies and recommended fetal echocardiography and fetal ultrasound to check for the presence of cardiac abnormalities in patients exposed to lithium during cardiogenesis (Diav-Citrin et al. 2014). Perhaps the most definitive report is the 2017 report by Patorno et al. They explored more than 1 million births over 10 years from 2000 through 2010 in a Medicaid database. The risk of cardiac abnormalities with first-term exposure was elevated (risk ratio = 1.65), with a prevalence of Ebstein's anomaly of 0.6 per 100 live births versus 0.18 in unexposed fetuses. The absolute reported numbers were lower than previous numbers, but the risk was clearly elevated (Patorno et al. 2017).

Another risk of lithium use, particularly in the third trimester, is large gestational weight infants. Higher birth weights have been reported for some time in mothers exposed to lithium. The long-term significance of these higher birth weights in infants is not established, but higher birth weight is not necessarily associated with poorer health outcomes.

Bipolar disorder itself increases the risk of adverse events in pregnancy and after birth. For example, women with bipolar disorder, whether or not they are treated, are more likely than women who do not have bipolar disorder to deliver by C-section, experience preterm labor, have smaller gestational birth children, and have infants born with low serum glucose levels (Bodén et al. 2012). Thus, the risk for poor outcomes in pregnancy is not limited to the risk associated with lithium or other treatments for bipolar disorder.

There is likely a fetal "dose" of lithium that is more likely to be associated with teratogenic effects. Using a pharmacokinetic model of fetal exposure to lithium, Horton and colleagues (2012) estimated that the maximum safe dosing of lithium in a pregnant woman to limit the risk of teratogenic effects is 400 mg three times daily. Although this estimate is based on pharmacokinetic modeling, it does make sense to limit the exposure to lithium, if possible. On the other hand, other mood-stabilizing agents such as valproate and carbamazepine are known to pose even greater teratogenic risks. The antipsychotics may be a safer choice, at least from the perspective of teratogenic risk, than are any of the mood stabilizers.

Table 5–3. Anticonvulsant dosages in bipolar illness

Medication	Usual dosage range	Serum level (μg/mL)
Valproate	15–60 mg/kg/day	50–125
Carbamazepine	200–1,600 mg/day	6–10
Lamotrigine	50–200 mg/day	NA
Gabapentin	900–3,600 mg/day	NA
Oxcarbazepine	600–2,400 mg/day	NA

Note. NA=not applicable.

Anticonvulsants

In the past four decades, increasing attention has been paid to the use of anticonvulsant medications in psychiatry, mainly to promote mood stabilization (Table 5–3). The application of these agents stems from a number of observations on the psychiatric sequelae of temporal lobe epilepsy, including hallucinations, angry outbursts, and religiosity. These observations spurred on the use of phenytoin in psychiatric patients in the 1950s—with, at best, equivocal results, although a controlled trial found phenytoin to be effective in the treatment of mania (Mishory et al. 2000). In more recent years, several groups have further suggested that psychiatric symptoms could emanate from limbic seizures and that kindling phenomena could play a major role in the development of psychoses and psychiatric disorders.

Understandably, then, a number of reports have emerged that other anticonvulsant agents (e.g., carbamazepine and valproic acid), which act preferentially on temporal lobe or limbic systems, are effective in patients with bipolar disorder, particularly in acute mania. Three compounds, valproic acid, carbamazepine, and lamotrigine, have received the lion's share of attention (for chemical structures of the thymoleptic anticonvulsants, see Figure 5–1), although several of the available anticonvulsants could eventually prove useful in treating mood disorders.

Valproate

In contrast to almost all other drugs used in psychiatry, valproic acid has no rings. (Carbamazepine is tricyclic; valproic acid could be said to be acyclic.) The drug is available in the United States in the following forms: immediate-

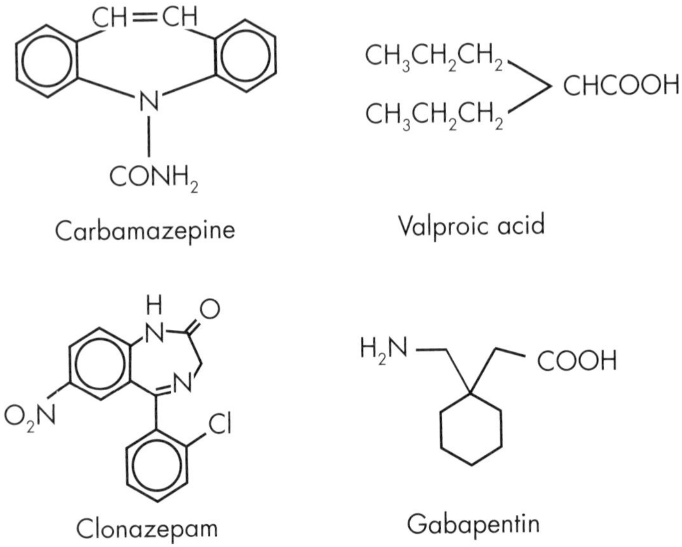

Figure 5–1.   Chemical structures of thymoleptic anticonvulsants.

release valproic acid (Depakene) and sodium valproate (Depakene syrup); delayed-release divalproex sodium (Depakote and Depakote Sprinkle), containing equal molar of valproic acid and sodium valproate; an extended-release formulation of divalproex (Depakote ER), approved for migraines and bipolar mania; and an injectable form (Depacon). The amide of valproic acid (valpromide [Dépamide]) is used in Europe. All these preparations convert to valproic acid in the plasma.

Valproate may be the most convenient general term to encompass all these formulations. Valproate is FDA approved in epilepsy for use in simple and complex absence attacks, partial seizures, and migraine prophylaxis. Valproate was given FDA approval for the treatment of acute mania in 1994, followed by approval for Depakote ER in 2005. Valproate is still among the most commonly used drugs in the treatment of bipolar disorder in American psychiatry. In addition, valproate continues to be employed in treating many other kinds of symptoms, including aggression, agitation, and impulsivity in patients with a variety of disorders.

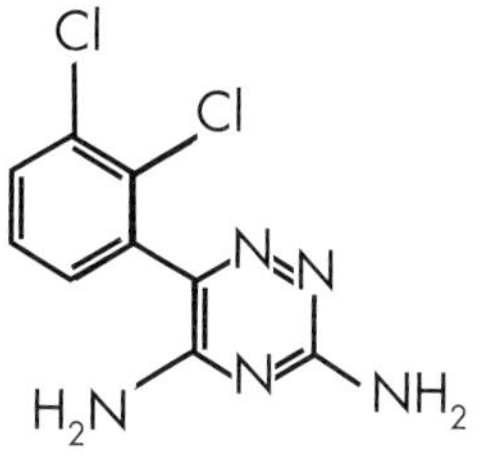

Lamotrigine

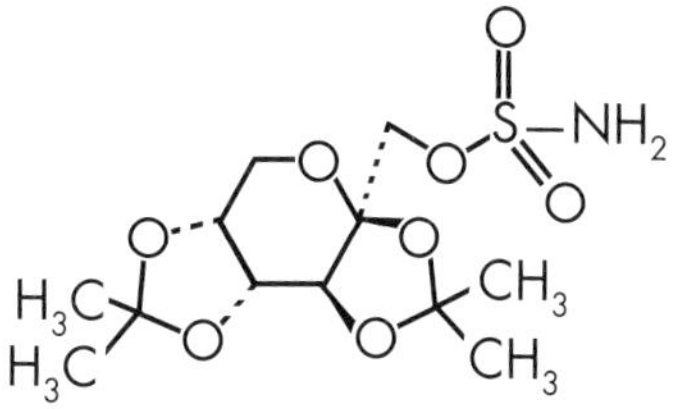

Topiramate

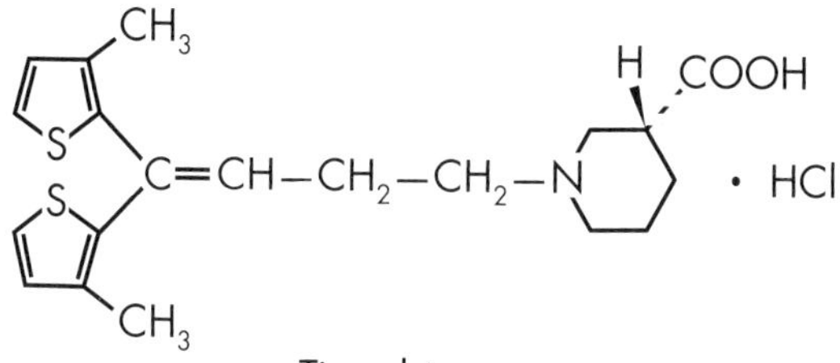

Tiagabine

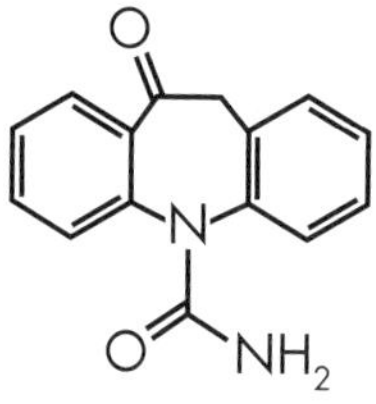

Oxcarbazepine

Figure 5–1. Chemical structures of thymoleptic anticonvulsants *(continued).*

Clinical Indications

Early work in the late 1960s by Lambert in France identified valproate as effective in a wide range of patients with mania and schizoaffective mania when added to a wide variety of other drugs. Lambert's group reported on more than 100 patients but did not describe the patients in detail. In their study, which involved mainly patients with treatment-resistant schizoaffective disorder with

Valproate therapy: overview	
Efficacy	Acute mania (FDA approved) Bipolar prophylaxis (may be effective) Mixed, rapid-cycling bipolar disorder Seizure disorders (FDA approved)
Side effects	Weight gain Sedation GI upset
Safety in overdose	Serious effects notable mostly at 20 times normal serum level. Symptoms include nausea, vomiting, CNS depression, and seizures. Manage with gastric lavage, forced emesis, and assisted ventilation.
Dosage and administration	Start IR formulation at 15 mg/kg/day and ER formulation at 25 mg/kg/day in divided doses, up to a maximum of 60 mg/kg. Achieve serum levels of 50–100 µg/mL.
Discontinuation	Rapid discontinuation increases the risk of rapid relapse in bipolar disorder. Otherwise, discontinuation symptoms are uncommon.

Drug interactions	Drugs that ↑ valproate serum levels include
	  Cimetidine
	  Erythromycin
	  Phenothiazines
	  Fluoxetine
	  Aspirin
	  Ibuprofen
	Drugs that ↓ valproate serum levels include
	  Rifampin
	  Carbamazepine
	  Phenobarbital
	  Ethosuximide

Note. ER=extended-release; GI=gastrointestinal; IR=immediate-release.

mania, moderate improvement was reported in more than half of the patients. In those patients with acute mania without prior drug therapy, 10 of 14 improved. These results agree with the findings of a study of valproate by Pope and colleagues (1991) at McLean Hospital and with other local clinical experience. In Pope et al.'s study, there was a 54% improvement in a standard mania rating score in the valproate group, compared with only a 5% improvement in this score in the placebo group. Interestingly, the antimanic effects of valproate were often observed in the first few days of treatment.

Since the Pope study, a number of double-blind studies have been completed attesting to the efficacy of valproate in treating acute mania. Among the largest of these, a double-blind, placebo-controlled study of 179 patients found that lithium and valproate were equivalent in effectiveness in treating acute mania and twice as effective as placebo (Bowden and McElroy 1995). In addition, there is evidence that a loading dose strategy, typically using about 20 mg/kg/day of valproate, may reduce the onset of action to 5 days or less (Keck et al. 1993a; McElroy et al. 1993). Using a 30 mg/kg loading dose to start, with a reduction to 20 mg/kg after a few days, has also been suggested. The current data suggest that valproate is at least as well studied and as effective as lithium in the treatment of acute mania. However, both lithium and valproate appear to be slower acting than the atypical antipsychotics in the treatment of acute mania.

Valproate may be particularly useful in patients with mixed-state or rapid-cycling types of bipolar disorder. Freeman et al. (1992) found that valproate showed good efficacy relative to lithium in the acute and long-term management of mixed states. Bowden and colleagues (Bowden and Singh 2005; Bowden et al. 1994) noted that valproate was more effective than lithium in treating bipolar patients with mixed states and irritable features and was also effective in treating bipolar patients with rapid cycling. A number of other small open-label studies suggested that valproate may be quite useful in treating mixed and manic states but somewhat less useful in preventing depressive episodes in bipolar patients with rapid cycling. Patients with a history of EEG abnormalities in conjunction with bipolar disorder appear to be good candidates for valproate treatment. Other predictors of response to valproate include lack of psychotic episodes in patients with concurrent BPD (Calabrese et al. 1993). Still, even the combination of valproate and lithium or lamotrigine is often ineffective in many patients with rapid-cycling bipolar disorder (Kemp et al. 2012), and more effective treatments for this disorder are needed.

Several open-label studies have suggested that valproate is an effective prophylactic agent in the treatment of bipolar disorder. Most of these studies suggested that valproate may be somewhat more effective in preventing manic than depressive episodes. In a double-blind longitudinal study, Lambert and Venaud (1992) found that valproate was better tolerated than, and as effective as, lithium in preventing subsequent bipolar episodes over a 2-year period. A large multicenter study involving more than 300 patients failed, however, to demonstrate the efficacy of valproate over placebo in the prevention of mania (Bowden et al. 2000). A priori selection of primary outcome measures appeared to interfere with demonstrating the effectiveness of divalproex in the prophylaxis of mania. However, clinical experience with the drug still suggests that it is effective in the maintenance treatment of bipolar disorder.

The efficacy of valproate in treating acute unipolar or bipolar depression is largely untested. The one controlled study to date of extended-release valproate in patients with bipolar depression did suggest that valproate-treated subjects were twice as likely as patients receiving placebo to achieve remission after 6 weeks of treatment (Muzina et al. 2011). Several uncontrolled studies and case reports suggested that valproate may have modest antidepressant efficacy in bipolar depression.

We have reported that valproate may be useful in the treatment of agitation associated with major depression (DeBattista et al. 2005). There are also case reports suggesting that valproate may have a role in treating refractory major depression. Bowden and colleagues' maintenance study suggested that divalproex prevented depressive episodes better than placebo in bipolar patients even though it failed to show similar effects in mania (Bowden et al. 2000). Low-dose valproate has been successfully used to treat cyclothymia (Jacobsen 1993).

Some case reports and open-label studies have suggested that valproate may be useful in treating panic disorder, particularly when the disorder is complicated by substance abuse and there is concern about using a benzodiazepine (Baetz and Bowen 1998; Keck et al. 1993b; Ontiveros and Fontaine 1992; Woodman and Noyes 1994). We have generally not found valproate to be that useful in treating anxiety disorders.

A study compared 4 weeks of valproate with placebo as an add-on to risperidone or olanzapine in decompensating schizophrenic patients. Valproate add-on was significantly more effective than placebo in reducing positive symptoms (Casey et al. 2001). There is also some evidence that valproate might speed response to antipsychotics in schizophrenia.

Valproate has been used for many years in the treatment of agitation. A number of open-label trials have reported that valproic acid is effective in treating agitation associated with dementia and brain injury (Herrmann 1998; Hilty et al. 1998; Kunik et al. 1998; Lott et al. 1995). We have found that agitated patients with dementia often respond to dosages as low as 125 mg/day, although higher dosages are often tolerated and sometimes needed in these patients. Controlled trials have suggested that low-dose valproate is often ineffective but higher doses are often associated with high rates of discontinuation secondary to side effects (Lonergan et al. 2004). The most recent study (Tariot et al. 2011) was consistent with this observation—that is, valproate failed to separate from placebo in reduction of agitation and was associated with considerable side effects. Our group has also been interested in the use of divalproex sodium as an adjunctive agent in the treatment of agitation associated with depression (DeBattista et al. 2005). In a 4-week open trial, we found that an average dose of about 750 mg of divalproex significantly diminished agitation in depressed patients.

Valproate is also increasingly being used to control aggression, particularly in patients with brain injuries. Several open studies reported that valproate helps control impulsivity, explosive outbursts, physical aggression, and self-destructiveness in patients with brain injuries or intellectual developmental disorder (Geracioti 1994; Ruedrich et al. 1999; Wroblewski et al. 1997). Some evidence suggests that valproate may attenuate disruptive behavior in aggressive adolescents (Donovan et al. 1997). In juvenile offenders, valproate appeared to decrease aggressive outbursts (Steiner et al. 2003). In addition, adolescents who are at risk for developing bipolar disorder and who also have problems with aggression tend to be less aggressive while taking valproate (Saxena et al. 2006). Not all patterns of aggression in adolescents respond equally well to valproate. Padhy and colleagues (2011) found that in premeditated aggression in teens, valproate was effective in reducing aggression. However, valproate was not particularly effective in preventing spontaneous aggressive outbursts in methadone-treated patients (Zarghami et al. 2013).

Valproate has been studied in the treatment of the impulsivity, affective instability, and self-destructiveness of BPD. Borderline personality symptoms are sometimes thought to overlap with those of bipolar II disorder, and it makes some sense to apply valproate to the treatment of patients with BPD. Most studies have been small and uncontrolled (Hirschman et al. 1997; Stein et al. 1995; Wilcox 1995). However, in a more recent, larger trial, valproate did appear to be significantly more effective than placebo in patients with Cluster B personality disorders (Hollander et al. 2005). Valproate does appear to be an important adjunctive agent for controlling some symptoms in many patients with

BPD. It has the advantage of being less toxic than lithium and most other anti-convulsants in this population with self-destructive behavior. Furthermore, the addition of omega-3 fatty acids (eicosapentaenoic acid [EPA] 1.2 g/day and docosahexaenoic acid [DHA] 0.8 g/day) to valproate might improve its efficacy in controlled anger outbursts and impulsivity (Bellino et al. 2014).

Dosage and Administration

The plasma half-life of valproate is on the order of 10–15 hours. A drug such as carbamazepine, phenobarbital, or phenytoin, given concurrently, will induce hepatic enzymes and shorten valproate's half-life by speeding its metabolism. In contrast to carbamazepine, valproate is a modest hepatic enzyme inhibitor. Once an adequate blood level has been attained, it is likely to remain adequate if intake remains constant. Blood levels should be taken about 12 hours after the last dose.

The usual starting dosage of valproate in the immediate-release (IR) formulation is 15 mg/kg/day in two divided doses. Thus, the average 75-kg male might be started on 500 mg bid. In less acute settings, we tend to recommend a starting dose of 250–500 mg the first day, and that dose, if tolerated, is titrated upward. Some clinicians employ once-a-day dosing of valproate for the IR formulation in an effort to enhance compliance. Given the pharmacokinetics of IR valproate, twice-a-day dosing is probably ideal. In addition, the large peaks in plasma levels with once-a-day dosing often produce GI side effects, and this strategy tends to be poorly tolerated. Still, attaining high levels of this highly bound, hydrophilic agent could allow more effective delivery into the CNS. The extended-release formulation of divalproex sodium (Depakote ER) was approved for use in the treatment of acute mania or mixed episodes in bipolar disorder. The ER form is not bioequivalent to the IR form—it appears to produce a serum level that is 10%–20% lower than with Depakote—which suggests some need for increasing the dose (by about one-third) when converting patients to the ER formulation. The ER formulation may be somewhat less associated with side effects such as weight gain. Preliminary studies have indicated that switching from the delayed-release Depakote DR to the even-slower-release ER formulation of Depakote in bipolar patients was well tolerated and maintained stability. The dosage can be increased each week by 10 mg/kg/day until an adequate therapeutic level is achieved, or to a maximum dosage of 60 mg/kg/day.

As described earlier, loading doses in the range of 20 mg/kg seem to speed the onset of action in treating acute mania. Intravenous loading of divalproex sodium also appears to help stabilize mixed states and rapid cycling but may have little effect on bipolar depression (Grunze et al. 1999a). Patients with mania tolerate medication side effects better than do those with depression. Thus, loading strategies are generally avoided in the latter.

In manic patients, levels greater than 45 μg/mL seem to be required for antimanic effect, and levels up to 100 μg/mL are well tolerated. Sometimes, levels as high as 125 μg/mL are required for optimal efficacy of valproate in the treatment of acute mania. Most data suggest that blood levels should probably be between 85 μg/mL and 125 μg/mL in the treatment of patients with mania or mixed states. Higher levels appear to be associated with side effects, including thrombocytopenia, weight gain, and sedation (Bowden and Singh 2005). In beginning valproate therapy, the enteric-coated divalproex sodium is generally less likely to cause GI distress than are the other formulations. Initial dosages of 250 mg bid are common; the higher daily dosage should be reserved for actively manic patients. Valproic acid plasma levels should be obtained every few days until a level greater than 50 μg/mL is reached. There is some suggestion that clinicians should push the dose to achieve levels greater than 75 μg/mL in patients who are not responding. There is considerable variability in levels obtained depending on the time since last dose. Over time, blood levels should be collected in a similar relationship to last dose. As with other drugs with which dosage is titrated to reach a specified blood level, the final daily dosage could vary widely, anywhere from 750 to 3,000 mg/day. Some improvement may be evident within 4 days and should be seen within 2 weeks of attaining a therapeutic blood level. If improvement has not occurred, higher doses and levels can be tried for another 2 weeks, but side effects may prove limiting. Sedation and GI distress are the likeliest limiting side effects early in therapy, but only sedation is common, and valproate seems generally better tolerated than lithium carbonate.

When a patient acutely improves while taking valproate, one assumes that the drug can be continued as a maintenance therapy at the same dosage and level, watching for any toxicity. This may, in fact, be a wise course. However, many patients undergoing a trial of valproate are already taking various other drugs (e.g., lithium, a neuroleptic, carbamazepine, an antidepressant, clonazepam). Once valproate is working, the other drugs can be gradually withdrawn one at a time to determine whether they are needed. Some may prove unnecessary, but tapering and stopping others may invite a relapse. Only one-third of patients experience adequate response to monotherapy, so combination treatment is now the rule rather than the exception. Valproic acid levels can be monitored weekly until stable and presumably adequate levels are achieved, and then monthly or less often during prolonged maintenance therapy. The level should be rechecked if new side effects occur or if the clinical condition worsens.

Side Effects

When valproate was initially introduced, as an antiepileptic, a major concern was the risk of severe, sometimes fatal, hepatotoxicity (Table 5–2). Fatal cases have all been in neonates receiving multiple anticonvulsants, particularly barbiturates. Children younger than 2 years appear at greatest risk for severe hepatotoxicity. The risk of hepatotoxicity makes the task of monitoring psychiatric patients taking valproate a risk-benefit conundrum. One could order liver function tests every month or so because no one is sure whether severe hepatocellular toxicity will occur. On the other hand, the available data support the position that frequent liver function tests are unnecessary and that patients and/or relatives should be told of the remote risk and informed about early symptoms of liver disease (e.g., anorexia, jaundice, nausea, lethargy). We recommend liver function tests every 6–12 months at most. If liver function tests are done, minor elevations of hepatic enzyme levels up to three times the normal limit should not necessarily lead to stopping the drug. Balancing the apparent clinical benefit to the patient with the abnormality of the liver function tests is reasonable. The better the patient's response, the more one persists in giving valproate in the face of progressively abnormal liver function tests.

Pancreatitis can occur with divalproex sodium after varying lengths of exposure. We have had one case of pancreatitis that occurred after the patient had been taking the drug for more than 1 year. The patient presented with abdominal pain and had elevated serum amylase levels. The reaction abated with drug cessation. The side effect is rare but does occur at a high enough incidence for the clinician to consider.

Weight gain is the most common reason patients discontinue valproate. As many as half of the patients who use valproate chronically experience significant weight gain. Maintaining an adequate diet and exercise regimen is clearly necessary for patients taking valproate. Despite their best efforts, however, many patients find it difficult to control their weight. We have found that the addition of topiramate at dosages of 50–200 mg/day has been an effective anorexiant for many patients and may help with mood stabilization.

Thrombocytopenia and platelet dysfunction have been reported in patients taking valproate. Patients should be advised to report easy bruising or bleeding. Platelet levels can be checked periodically, but generally, counts above 75,000/cc do not require anything other than monitoring.

Sedation is among the most common side effects of valproate therapy. As with other medications, shifting more of the dose closer to bedtime will mitigate daytime sedation.

GI upset, the second most common side effect of valproate after weight gain, can take the form of nausea, cramps, emesis, and diarrhea and is dose related. Enteric-coated tablets or divalproex sprinkle capsules help, as do histamine$_2$ blockers (e.g., famotidine [Pepcid] at 20 mg bid). Tremor and ataxia can also occur.

Another side effect, alopecia, is thought to be due to valproate's interference with zinc and selenium deposition. Some clinicians instruct patients to take multivitamins fortified with these two metals; Centrum Silver is a vitamin supplement commonly used for this purpose. If significant alopecia occurs, the valproate should be discontinued. Hair regrowth may take several months.

Coma and death are rare when valproate is taken with suicidal intent. The drug can be removed by hemodialysis. There is also one report that valproate coma was reversed by naloxone.

Another, more recent concern has been the observation that valproic acid may be associated with the development of polycystic ovaries in women. A study of 238 epileptic women found that 43% of patients taking valproic acid had polycystic ovaries and 17% had elevated testosterone levels (Isojärvi et al. 1993). Among the women who started valproic acid before age 20, 80% had polycystic ovaries. Because more than 50% of women taking valproic acid were also obese, and because obesity is associated with polycystic ovaries, it is unclear whether valproic acid's effects on the high rate of polycystic ovaries were a direct result of the drug or an indirect effect of contributing to obesity. However, in STEP-BD, women with polycystic ovary syndrome (PCOS) who discontinued their valproate appeared to have significant improvement in PCOS symptoms despite the fact that there was no significant change in weight (Joffe et al. 2006). This suggests that valproate may have a direct contribution to PCOS independent of obesity. In addition, some forms of epilepsy appear to be associated with polycystic ovaries, independent of anticonvulsant use. Independent replication of valproate as a cause of polycystic ovaries has not been reported despite hundreds of thousands of patients having been treated. Two small surveys suggest rates of about 8%–10% in women treated with the drug, which are slightly higher than the rates in the general population (4%–7%; Joffe and Cohen 2004). Some child psychiatrists have suggested caution in treating adolescent female bipolar patients with valproate, given the available data on polycystic ovaries (Eberle 1998). Some studies involving women with bipolar disorder who were taking divalproex also have not shown an association with PCOS (Rasgon 2004). There has been, however, a suggestion of a relationship to increased testosterone levels in women with bipolar disorder (Rasgon et al. 2005). Most recently, women who were treated with valproate demonstrated significantly more common PCOS and ovulatory dysfunction than did women treated with lamotrigine (Morrell et al. 2008). It is best to monitor females who are taking valproate for the development of weight gain, hirsutism, menstrual irregularities, and acne.

Drug Interactions

Serious drug interactions are uncommon with valproate. However, the metabolism of valproate is approximately 25% dependent on the cytochrome P450 (CYP) system. A number of drugs that competitively inhibit various enzymes of the CYP system—including cimetidine, the SSRIs, and erythromycin— may be associated with an increase in valproate levels (Table 5–4). Additionally, many nonsteroidal anti-inflammatory agents, including aspirin, may increase free valproate levels. Other drugs, such as carbamazepine and rifampin, have been associated with reducing valproate levels.

Valproate has been associated with an increase in the serum levels of a variety of drugs, including carbamazepine, warfarin, and tolbutamide. These interactions are generally not clinically significant but may require reduced doses of the concurrent medications. Valproate can double the level of concurrent lamotrigine and increase the risk of rashes. When these two agents are used together, lamotrigine doses are increased very gradually. In rare cases, valproate therapy has been associated with hyperammonemia, with or without

Table 5–4. Drug interactions of anticonvulsant mood stabilizers

Anticonvulsant	Drugs that may ↑ anticonvulsant levels	Drugs that may ↓ anticonvulsant levels	Drugs whose blood levels ↓ with concurrent anticonvulsant use
Valproate	Aspirin Cimetidine Clarithromycin Erythromycin Fluoxetine Fluvoxamine Ibuprofen Phenothiazines Topiramate Troleandomycin	Carbamazepine Ethosuximide Oxcarbazepine Phenobarbital Phenytoin Primidone Rifampin	Zonisamide Clinically significant metabolic induction by other drugs with valproate not reported
Carbamazepine	Cimetidine Ciprofloxacin Clarithromycin Diltiazem Doxycycline Erythromycin Fluconazole Fluoxetine Fluvoxamine Grapefruit juice Isoniazid Itraconazole	Felbamate Phenobarbital Rifampin	Atypical antipsychotics Benzodiazepines Doxycycline Ethosuximide Fentanyl Glucocorticoids Methadone Neuroleptics Oral contraceptives Phenytoin Protease inhibitors TCAs (?)

Table 5–4.   Drug interactions of anticonvulsant mood stabilizers *(continued)*

Anticonvulsant	Drugs that may ↑ anticonvulsant levels	Drugs that may ↓ anticonvulsant levels	Drugs whose blood levels ↓ with concurrent anticonvulsant use
	Ketoconazole Nefazodone Norfloxacin Prednisolone Propoxyphene Protease inhibitors (e.g., ritonavir, indinavir) TCAs Troleandomycin Valproate Verapamil Warfarin		Theophylline
Lamotrigine	Valproate	Carbamazepine Ethosuximide Oral contraceptives Oxcarbazepine Phenobarbital Phenytoin Primidone	Valproate
Oxcarbazepine			Ethinyl estradiol Levonorgestrel
Topiramate			Oral contraceptives

Note.   TCAs=tricyclic antidepressants; ↑=increase; ↓=decrease.

encephalopathy, which may occur despite normal hepatic function tests. Concomitant administration of topiramate and valproate may raise this risk. In the package insert, a precaution is issued of the associated risk of hyperammonemia with topiramate use. Moreover, valproate is contraindicated in patients with known urea cycle disorder (e.g., ornithine transcarbamylase deficiency).

Use in Pregnancy

When valproate is taken during the first trimester of pregnancy, neural tube defects (e.g., spina bifida, anencephaly) can occur. Thus, valproate should generally be discontinued before anticipated pregnancies. However, if it is necessary to continue valproate because of the significant risk of a disruptive relapse of bipolar illness during pregnancy, the patient should be started on folate, 1 mg/day, early in the pregnancy, and an ultrasound should be ordered at 18–20 weeks to assess for fetal abnormalities. During the last 6 weeks of the pregnancy, vitamin K should also be prescribed to decrease the risk of excessive bleeding. Given the risk of relapse in the postpartum period, valproate should generally be restarted after delivery to reduce the risk.

Reports of lower IQ in children exposed in utero to valproate continue to be published (Meador et al. 2009, 2013; Vinten et al. 2005) and are very troubling. Therefore, we currently recommend avoiding use of the drug during pregnancy whenever possible or in patients likely to become pregnant. A recent paper on valproate provides a useful review of the issues involved (Andrade 2018).

Carbamazepine

Carbamazepine was originally synthesized in 1957 and was introduced into the European market in the early 1960s as a treatment for epilepsy, particularly epilepsy involving the temporal lobes. Subsequently, it became widely used as a treatment for tic douloureux—trigeminal neuralgia. Its use for bipolar disorder stems from the early 1970s, when Japanese researchers reported it was effective in many patients with manic-depressive illness, including patients whose condition was refractory to lithium. Ballenger and Post later reported that carbamazepine was effective in a double-blind crossover trial in patients with acute bipolar disorder (Ballenger and Post 1980). Since that time, many other controlled studies have documented the utility of carbamazepine for acute mania. Kishimoto et al. (1983) reported that it was also effective in maintenance therapy, and a number of controlled studies have subsequently confirmed this finding. However, carbamazepine had never been FDA approved for the treatment of any aspect of bipolar disorder until an ER form of the drug (Equetro) was approved in 2005 for the treatment of acute mania. We tend to regard carbamazepine as a less good initial choice than either valproate, lithium, or an SGA in the treatment of bipolar disorder because of the propensity for pharmacokinetic interactions with carbamazepine.

Carbamazepine has drug interaction and side-effect profiles that make it more cumbersome to use, and although well studied, it is still less well studied than either lithium or valproate. Still, many patients who do not have an adequate response to valproate or lithium do well with carbamazepine, and the combination of carbamazepine and another mood stabilizer or atypical antipsychotic is often helpful.

Clinical Indications

There are now multiple controlled studies of carbamazepine in the treatment of acute mania and additional controlled studies on its use as a mood stabilizer in the maintenance treatment of bipolar disorder. The FDA approval of Equetro for the treatment of acute mania and mixed states was based on data from controlled trials (Owen 2006; Weisler et al. 2006). Many of the earlier studies have been compromised by concurrent neuroleptic or other drug use. Enough clinical evidence exists to justify using carbamazepine in patients with bipolar disorder, with a reasonable expectation that a proportion of them—about 50%—will show clear clinical benefit. However, some patients who derive benefit from carbamazepine have residual symptoms. The drug may work more rapidly than lithium but less rapidly than antipsychotics in acute mania.

Some patients who respond to carbamazepine improve or stabilize with the drug alone; others do better with carbamazepine plus another mood stabilizer or antipsychotic (see Chapter 9). The major problem in assessing the clinical value of a drug like carbamazepine, which is used mainly in treating seriously symptomatic psychiatric patients in whom more standard treatments have failed, is that all other medications are rarely discontinued before the carbamazepine is added. Later, if the patient does well, other preexisting drugs may or may not be tapered and stopped. Clinically, it is often hard to be sure

Carbamazepine therapy: overview

Efficacy	Acute mania (FDA approved for Equetro only) Mixed, rapid-cycling bipolar (not FDA approved) Seizure disorders (FDA approved)
Side effects	Sedation Dizziness Fatigue and nausea Ataxia
Safety in overdose	Serious symptoms may occur at 10–20 times normal serum levels. Symptoms include nausea, vomiting, CNS depression, respiratory depression, and seizures. Management includes gastric lavage, forced emesis, assisted ventilation.
Dosage and administration	For the XR form: 200 mg bid, to therapeutic range of 800–1,200 mg/day. Follow serum levels to 6–10 μg/mL.
Discontinuation	Carbamazepine has not been associated with a withdrawal syndrome with rapid discontinuation. However, as with other mood stabilizers, rapid discontinuation is associated with an increased risk of rapid relapse. In bipolar patients, decrease dose over 6 months. In nonbipolar patients, dose may be decreased by 25% every 3 days.
Drug interactions	Drugs that may ↑ carbamazepine levels include cimetidine, ciprofloxacin, diltiazem, fluvoxamine, fluoxetine, doxycycline, erythromycin, fluconazole, grapefruit juice, isoniazid, ketoconazole, macrolide antibiotics (erythromycin, clarithromycin, troleandomycin), nefazodone, norfloxacin, prednisolone, propoxyphene, protease inhibitors (e.g., ritonavir), TCAs, valproate, verapamil, and warfarin Drugs whose blood levels are ↓ by coadministration with carbamazepine include atypical antipsychotics, benzodiazepines, doxycycline, ethosuximide, fentanyl, glucocorticoids, haloperidol, methadone, oral contraceptives, phenothiazines, phenytoin, sertraline, TCAs, and theophylline

Note.   TCAs = tricyclic antidepressants; XR = extended-release.

when carbamazepine itself is really working and when prior therapy may finally have begun to work.

Some evidence suggests that carbamazepine works better than lithium in producing stability in rapid-cycling bipolar patients (those with four or more affective episodes a year). Even though there is some preliminary evidence of carbamazepine's superiority to lithium in rapid cycling, it is clear that this bipolar subtype is difficult to treat with any agent. In one major study, patients without rapid-cycling bipolar illness were much more likely to respond to carbamazepine alone than were patients with rapid-cycling bipolar illness (Okuma 1993). Likewise, carbamazepine may be more effective than lithium in the maintenance treatment of patients with mixed episodes or rapid cycling (Greil et al. 1998). Some evidence suggests that carbamazepine is preferentially effective in more severe, paranoid, and angry manic patients than in euphoric, overactive, overtalkative, or overfriendly manic patients. Other potential indications for the drug include continuous-cycling bipolar illness, in which there are no periods of euthymia between bipolar episodes. Overall, the data on predictors of carbamazepine response have been mixed.

Carbamazepine has not been well studied in the treatment of major depression. Several small studies suggested that carbamazepine may be useful in the treatment of bipolar depression, particularly when lithium is added to the regimen. In general, carbamazepine does not appear to be nearly as effective in acute depression as in acute mania. Likewise, some case reports suggest that carbamazepine is effective in the treatment of panic disorder, but there are much better antipanic drugs than carbamazepine, and the only controlled trial yielded negative findings.

A complicating factor in adding carbamazepine to an antipsychotic is that carbamazepine induces liver enzymes and speeds metabolism of some other drugs. Haloperidol levels are clearly lowered substantially. Likewise, carbamazepine is known to induce the metabolism of a number of atypical agents, including olanzapine, risperidone, and clozapine. Levels of other antipsychotics can be checked before and 2–4 weeks after carbamazepine is added to see whether they have changed. Worsening in some patients (and improvement in others) could be attributed to lowering of the neuroleptic blood level rather than to the direct effects of carbamazepine. Similarly, carbamazepine may lower TCA and other antidepressant plasma levels, making such combinations difficult.

Pilot studies of carbamazepine show some promise for this drug in treating violent nonpsychotic patients and patients undergoing alcohol or benzodiazepine withdrawal.

An intriguing study by Cowdry and Gardner (1988) involved patients with BPD who had histories of frequent impulsive acts. In this small, double-blind study, carbamazepine was notable for substantially decreasing impulsivity. The patients' therapists all judged the patients to be much better. The patients, however, did not feel the drug was very effective. In the same study, the patients felt better—but were much more impulsive—while taking alprazolam. Thus, there may be a role for carbamazepine in treating patients with BPD. However, valproate also appears to be helpful in treating patients with BPD and may be easier to use. Similarly, oxcarbazepine may also be effective in reducing impulsivity and anger outbursts in borderline patients (Bellino et al. 2005).

Other psychiatric disorders may also be characterized by impulsivity, aggressive outbursts, and affective instability. Studies in aggression and impulsivity have been mixed (Huband et al. 2010). Patients with PTSD sometimes have these difficulties, and a number of open-label studies suggest that carbamazepine is useful in treating some of these patients. Carbamazepine has demonstrated utility in the treatment of agitation and violent outbursts associated with dementia. It is possible that carbamazepine is helpful in nephrogenic diabetes insipidus because it increases vasopressin release. Unfortunately, carbamazepine's ability to effect such an increase is blocked by lithium, making carbamazepine ineffective in lithium-induced polyuria and polydipsia. Carbamazepine can, but rarely does, cause hyponatremia and water intoxication.

Dosage and Administration

Blood levels of carbamazepine should be monitored at least weekly throughout the first 8 weeks of treatment because the drug induces liver enzymes, which then speed the drug's own metabolism. The blood level established at 3 weeks may decrease by one-third at 6 weeks, even when the carbamazepine dosage is held constant. Starting with 100 mg (one half-tablet) at bedtime is suggested to see whether the patient is oversedated. If the drug is well tolerated, it should be given at a dosage of 100 mg bid on the second day, followed by 200 mg bid for the next few days. A sustained-release form of carbamazepine, Tegretol XR, is often taken once a day. Serum levels should be obtained twice a week in the first 2 weeks when possible—always about 12 hours after the last dose.

The dose should be adjusted to maintain a serum level of 4–12 µg/mL. Higher levels are generally not more effective and are often difficult to attain because of hepatic induction. We generally aim for levels in the range of 6–10 µg/mL. Adjusting levels upward means more risk of side effects. The most common signs of excessive carbamazepine blood levels are diplopia, malcoordination, and sedation. Tolerance will also often develop. Moving all or most of the daily dose to bedtime may help mitigate problems with sedation.

Carbamazepine ER (Equetro) is usually started at 400 mg/day in divided doses, and the dosage is then increased by 200 mg/day to a target dosage of about 600–1,200 mg/day. In the pooled bipolar trials, the mean dosage was 707 mg/day. The maximum studied dosage is 1,600 mg/day.

Side Effects

The major concern with the clinical use of carbamazepine is the threat of agranulocytosis or aplastic anemia, both potentially lethal conditions. As is usual with very rare, serious adverse drug reactions, estimates of incidence vary widely, in this cases from 1 in 10,000 patients treated to a more recently estimated 1 in 125,000. There is a growing consensus that frequent monitoring of blood counts is of limited value for patients receiving carbamazepine therapy. Aplastic anemia, thrombocytopenia, and agranulocytosis occur so rapidly that a daily blood count would be required to detect them. Thus, some experts have taken the position that regular blood counts are unnecessary and that warning the patient and/or significant others to watch for overt symptoms of bone marrow suppression (e.g., fever, bruising, bleeding, sore throat, petechiae) is more cost-effective.

Clinical practice with respect to carbamazepine has long been to avoid regular blood counts. However, although the rate of agranulocytosis with carbamazepine (about 1%–2%) is less than that with clozapine, the FDA has demanded weekly counts. Obviously, no compelling recommendation is possible with respect to carbamazepine. One compromise would be to get a complete blood count with every carbamazepine blood level.

Serious dermatological reactions, including toxic epidermal necrolysis and Stevens-Johnson syndrome, have been reported with carbamazepine and appear as a black box warning for this drug. Generally, the risk is 1–6 per 10,000 patients newly started on carbamazepine in the white population, but it may be 10 times higher in select Asian populations, especially among individuals of Chinese ancestry. The risk of this reaction with carbamazepine may be strongly associated with an inherited allelic variant of the *HLA-B* gene, the *HLA-B*1502* (Yip et al. 2012).

Once patients have started taking carbamazepine, a surprising number of them show a relative leukopenia, with or without a drop in erythrocytes, during the first few weeks. Approximately 7% of adult patients and 12% of children develop leukopenias while taking carbamazepine (Sobotka et al. 1990). Patients who run low white blood cell counts (WBCs) at baseline appear to be at particular risk for developing significant leukopenias. Drops in WBC (in cells/mm^3) to the low 3,500s are not uncommon. If the differential is normal (more than 1,000 polymorphonuclear leukocytes) and the patient seems to be benefiting from the treatment, carbamazepine can be continued. However, high-risk patients should be monitored frequently in the first 3 months of therapy. After observing a WBC under 3,000 cells/mm^3, the clinician will almost certainly feel a need to get counts more frequently. The availability of consultation with a friendly, interested, helpful hematologist is an asset to clinicians working with drugs such as carbamazepine and clozapine.

The most common side effects of carbamazepine are sedation, fatigue, nausea, and dizziness. At higher doses, ataxia, diplopia, muscle incoordination, and nystagmus may be evident. Overdose of carbamazepine may result in stupor progressing to coma and death.

Carbamazepine also can occasionally cause elevations in liver enzymes, but serious hepatotoxicity is quite rare. γ-Glutamyl transferase, an index of hepatic activity, is frequently increased (up to 100%) and is typically not a cause for concern unless the level is more than three times the normal level. Carbamazepine shares with TCAs the ability to slow cardiac conduction. Rashes with carbamazepine are probably a bit more common than with other psychiatric drugs; one review estimated a 5% incidence during the initiation of carbamazepine therapy.

Drug Interactions

Carbamazepine can influence the metabolism of a variety of drugs (see Table 5–4), a feature that complicates its clinical use. Quite frequently, it is difficult to assess the effect of carbamazepine on concurrent drug therapy.

Carbamazepine is metabolized mostly by the CYP3A3/4 enzyme and can be increased by drugs that inhibit this enzyme, including erythromycin, ketoconazole, fluvoxamine, fluoxetine, and calcium channel blockers. Serum carbamazepine levels should be monitored closely with concurrent use of these medications. In turn, carbamazepine induces the hepatic metabolism of many drugs that are metabolized via the CYP3A3/4 enzyme , including steroids, oral contraceptives, TCAs, sertraline, benzodiazepines, and calcium channel blockers. This interaction reduces the serum levels of these drugs and may decrease their efficacy. For some drugs, such as the TCAs, blood levels can be monitored. For most other drugs, monitoring serum levels is not helpful. Little information is available about carbamazepine's effects on SSRI levels. There have been cases of oral contraceptive failure with concurrent carbamazepine use, and patients may need higher doses of benzodiazepines or antipsychotics if carbamazepine is used concurrently.

There have been some reports of CNS toxicity associated with the combination of carbamazepine and lamotrigine (Besag et al. 1998). Symptoms have included dizziness and diplopia and appear to be related to changes in the serum level of lamotrigine. Adding lamotrigine to carbamazepine appears to be more problematic than vice versa. The use of clozapine in combination with carbamazepine is probably ill-advised. Although it is unclear whether the combination substantially increases the risks of leukopenias, other options should be exercised before carbamazepine and clozapine are used together.

Use in Pregnancy

In the past, carbamazepine was believed to be the safest of the anticonvulsants and the mood stabilizers for use during pregnancy. However, it has become evident that carbamazepine is associated with the occurrence of fetal abnormalities of the type seen with hydantoin: an increased incidence of craniofacial defects, fingernail hypoplasia, neural tube defects, and developmental delay. In addition, there is some evidence that in utero carbamazepine exposure may be associated with low infant IQ, although the evidence is not nearly as strong as it is for valproate (Banach et al. 2010). Therefore, carbamazepine should be discontinued, if possible, during the first trimester of pregnancy. As with divalproex sodium, folate supplements may reduce the risk of some of the neural tube effects of carbamazepine.

Carbamazepine does enter breast milk, and the serum concentrations in the infant may be as high as 15% of the maternal serum level (Brent and Wisner 1998). Although it is unclear what effect this serum level has on a developing infant, breastfeeding should be discouraged unless no reasonable alternative exists.

Lamotrigine

Lamotrigine (Lamictal) had been used for a number of years in Europe before being introduced in the United States. Lamotrigine has an FDA-approved indication for the treatment of partial complex and generalized seizures. In the early 1990s, lamotrigine began to be investigated as a treatment for bipolar disorder when epileptic patients reported an improvement in their general sense of well-being independent of seizure control. Although early controlled trials focusing on acute mania failed to show benefit, subsequent trials in the maintenance treatment of bipolar disorder demonstrated that lamotrigine delays the time to a next depressive or manic episode. These trials led to lamotrigine's FDA approval in 2003 as only the second drug, after lithium, indicated for the maintenance treatment of bipolar I disorder to delay the time to occurrence of mood episodes.

Lamotrigine has a variety of pharmacodynamic effects that may explain its mood-stabilizing properties. For example, in addition to decreasing glutamate release, lamotrigine also appears to modulate the reuptake of serotonin and generally blocks the reuptake of monoamines, including dopamine (Xie and Hagan 1998). Despite the evidence that lamotrigine has a profile that may confer antidepressant effects in addition to anticycling effects, the switch rate appears very low in bipolar patients treated with lamotrigine. In fact, the pivotal maintenance trials of lamotrigine in bipolar disorder did not suggest any higher rate of switching than with placebo.

Clinical Indications

Lamotrigine is indicated to delay the onset of new mood episodes in the maintenance treatment of bipolar disorder. Two pivotal studies, involving more than 500 bipolar I patients, provided evidence of the efficacy of lamotrigine in maintenance treatment. The first started with patients who were hypomanic or manic, whereas the second started with patients in the depressed phase of the illness. Once the patients' acute mood symptoms had resolved, they were randomly assigned to receive either lamotrigine or placebo for 12 months. What these studies demonstrated was that patients receiving the lamotrigine did better longer than did the patients receiving placebo. The time to a new episode of depression or mania was delayed in the lamotrigine-treated patients—sometimes as much as twofold—relative to placebo, and this delay was most pronounced for depressive episodes.

Lamotrigine may be useful in other aspects of bipolar disorder. For example, several open-label trials suggested that lamotrigine is effective as an add-on or as monotherapy in patients who had no response to traditional trials of lithium, often in combination with other mood stabilizers (Calabrese et al. 1999a, 1999b; Fogelson and Sternbach 1997; Koek and Yerevanian 1998; Kotler and Matar 1998; Kusumakar and Yatham 1997a, 1997b). Case studies suggest that lamotrigine may be effective in treating rapid-cycling and mixed presentations of bipolar disorder (Fatemi et al. 1997; Kusumakar and Yatham 1997a). However, controlled studies have not consistently demonstrated efficacy of the addition of lamotrigine to the medication regimen of rapid-cycling patients who have not responded to lithium or valproate (Kemp et al. 2012).

In a larger open trial (N=75) involving bipolar patients, Calabrese and colleagues (1999b) found that 48% of patients in a depressive episode had marked improvement in symptoms, and 20% had moderate improvement. In patients in a hypomanic or manic state, 81% had marked improvement while taking lamotrigine. However, in controlled studies, lamotrigine has not proved effective for the treatment of mania.

There is some evidence that lamotrigine may also be effective in the treatment of bipolar depression. In a study by Calabrese and colleagues (1999b), 175 patients with bipolar depression were randomly assigned to receive either 200 mg of lamotrigine, 50 mg of lamotrigine, or placebo for 7 weeks. Despite the promise of this early trial, four subsequent studies of lamotrigine monotherapy in the treatment of depression failed to show benefit. However, there may be benefit from adding lamotrigine to lithium in treating bipolar depression. In one study, van der Loos and colleagues (2009) added lamotrigine or placebo to lithium in patients with bipolar depression and found that lamotrigine was superior to placebo in reducing overall Montgomery-Åsberg Depression Rating Scale scores as well as in achieving a 50% reduction in symptoms. Unfortunately, controlled trials have not shown consistent benefit in the treatment of bipolar depression.

Lamotrigine has been compared with olanzapine-fluoxetine combination (OFC; Symbyax) in the treatment of bipolar depression. In one trial, lamotrigine monotherapy did not appear as effective as OFC in improving acute bipolar depression (Brown et al. 2006). On the other hand, it was much better tolerated than OFC. In addition, augmenting mood stabilizer plus antidepressant combinations with lamotrigine also appeared to be of some benefit relative to adding either risperidone or inositol in one STEP-BD analysis of refractory bipolar depression (Nierenberg et al. 2006b). Finally, as reported earlier in this chapter, lamotrigine is also effective in delaying recurrence of depression and mania in bipolar patients. Thus, in 2003 lamotrigine became the second drug approved for the maintenance treatment of bipolar disorder. In addition, lamotrigine is not associated with a significant switch to mania or hypomania.

Lamotrigine has been used as an augmenting agent in the treatment of resistant unipolar depression with mixed results. In some case reports and small open-label studies, lamotrigine has been useful when added to a standard antidepressant (Solmi et al. 2016). However, in the only controlled study to date, lamotrigine at dosages up to 400 mg/day added to paroxetine failed to separate from placebo in unipolar depression (Barbee et al. 2011). Lamotrigine augmentation may make the most sense in those patients with resistant depression who have not experienced a response to other augmenting strategies or who might possibly be on the bipolar spectrum.

Another role for lamotrigine may be in the treatment of rapid-cycling bipolar disorder. In a crossover study of patients with refractory (mainly) rapid-cycling disorder, lamotrigine (52% response rate), but not gabapentin (26% response rate), was more effective than placebo (23% response rate) in reducing symptoms (Frye et al. 2000).

Preliminary evidence suggests that in addition to its potential use in treating bipolar disorder, lamotrigine may have a role in treating related conditions. Case reports suggest that lamotrigine may be effective in cyclothymia, resistant unipolar depression, schizoaffective disorder (Erfurth et al. 1998a, 1998b), and even BPD (Pinto and Akiskal 1998).

Side Effects

Lamotrigine, when dosed conservatively, appears to be generally well tolerated by most patients. In fact, compared with other available approved maintenance treatments in bipolar disorder, lamotrigine is the least likely to be associated with weight gain (Sachs et al. 2006) or cognitive side effects. However, a black box warning in the PDR indicates that lamotrigine is associated with an increased risk of rash in up to 10% of patients. More concerning is the risk of serious skin reactions, which occur in 1 in 1,000 adults and 1 in 100 children. These serious rashes, which include Stevens-Johnson syndrome, may be fatal. Our general recommendation is that patients be well informed about the risk of rashes. We provide patients with a list of antigen precautions. For example, in the first 3 months of treatment, we recommend avoiding new food or new deodorants, detergents, cosmetics, fabric softeners, and so forth. Also, patients should be advised to avoid excessive sun exposure early in treatment. Furthermore, anyone with a rash accompanied by systemic symptoms such as fever or discomfort in the mouth, eye, or bladder should be instructed to discontinue the lamotrigine and go to the emergency department for evaluation. Patients without systemic symptoms should be advised to see a dermatologist immediately. The risk of rash appears to be increased when the dose of lamotrigine is titrated too rapidly or when lamotrigine is added to valproate, which doubles the serum level of lamotrigine. In addition, patients who develop a rash while taking lamotrigine may well have a recurrence of the rash when rechallenged with the drug (Buzan and Dubovsky 1998).

Common side effects include (in order of frequency) dizziness, headache, double vision, unsteadiness, sedation, and uncomplicated rash. These symptoms occur in more than 10% of treated patients, appear to be dose related, and may improve over time. There have been reports that lamotrigine may, perhaps because of its serotonergic properties, decrease libido and delay orgasm in both men and women. It is unclear whether any of the antidotes regarding SSRIs reported in Chapter 3 will help with lamotrigine-induced sexual dysfunction. Weight gain appears less common with lamotrigine than with lithium or valproate.

Overdoses can be serious and have been associated with the ingestion of 5 g or more of lamotrigine at one time. Symptoms of overdose can include delirium, periorbital edema, generalized erythema, hepatitis, and renal failure (Briassoulis et al. 1998; Mylonakis et al. 1999). The management of overdose includes gastric lavage and supportive care.

Dosage and Administration

Lamotrigine is typically started at 25 mg/day for the first week, and the dosage is typically increased by 25–50 mg every 2 weeks. If the patient is currently taking valproate, the lamotrigine should be started at 12.5 mg/day and increased to 25 mg/day by the end of the third week. Thereafter, the dosage should be increased by no more than 12.5–25 mg every 2 weeks. Starter kits are available for both generic and name-brand lamotrigine for patients concurrently taking valproate. These blue starter kits take out the guesswork for patients in titrating up their lamotrigine dose. Alternative green starter kits are available for patients taking concurrent carbamazepine or other anticonvulsants but not valproate. Most of the bipolar disorder studies have had a target dosage of around 200 mg/day. We have certainly seen patients with either bipolar or unipolar depression who appear to do well with dosages of 50–100 mg/day. However, maximum dosage for lamotrigine may be as high as 500 mg/day.

No clear association between serum levels of lamotrigine and response exists. Thus, routine monitoring of serum levels is not advised. However, in one small case series involving lamotrigine in treating schizoaffective disorder, serum levels greater than 10 mg/L were associated with a greater response than were lower levels.

Like all mood stabilizers, lamotrigine should be gradually tapered rather than abruptly discontinued if possible. Although no discontinuation syndromes have been reported to date with lamotrigine, seizures are occasionally reported with the abrupt discontinuation of any anticonvulsant.

Drug Interactions

As noted earlier, the primary interactions with lamotrigine are a doubling of serum levels with the addition of valproate and a reduction of at least 25% of serum levels in conjunction with carbamazepine. Likewise, phenobarbital and primidone decrease serum levels of lamotrigine by about 40%. Thus, higher doses of lamotrigine may be needed with carbamazepine, primidone, and phenobarbital, whereas the dose of lamotrigine should be cut in half with concurrent valproate. In addition, lamotrigine appears to reduce serum levels of valproate by about 25%.

Valproate appears to increase lamotrigine levels; thus, the more conservative dosing strategy is recommended when a patient is taking valproate. One report indicated that sertraline can substantially increase lamotrigine levels and lead to lamotrigine toxicity (Kaufman and Gerner 1998). Sertraline's inhibition of lamotrigine glucuronidation was suspected in that report, and lamotrigine levels were increased by 25% with just 25 mg of sertraline. At this time, it is advisable to adjust the starting and maintenance doses of lamotrigine downward with concurrent use of sertraline.

Alcohol theoretically can exacerbate the sedation associated with lamotrigine. Interactions with over-the-counter drugs are not known.

Use in Pregnancy

Lamotrigine is an FDA category C drug in pregnancy. Animal studies suggest the possibility of fetal abnormalities, but human studies do not exist. As with other agents, the known risks of discontinuing the drug for a pregnant patient should be assessed along with the unknown risk of continuing taking it. At this time, most patients would be advised to discontinue the drug before conception if possible. In the Medicaid pregnancy database study noted earlier (Patorno et al. 2017), lithium had a significantly elevated risk ratio for cardiac abnormalities compared with lamotrigine.

Other Anticonvulsants

Several other anticonvulsants have become available in recent years that, as with valproate, carbamazepine, and lamotrigine, are being explored in treating bipolar disorder and other psychiatric conditions (Table 5–5). Gabapentin has been well studied in bipolar disorder and generally has been an ineffective albeit benign treatment. In addition, preliminary studies have been done on oxcarbazepine, topiramate, and tiagabine in the treatment of bipolar disorder, with variable results. In contrast, at the time of this writing almost no data exist on the psychiatric benefits of anticonvulsants such as ethosuximide, levetiracetam, and zonisamide.

Gabapentin and Pregabalin

Gabapentin (Neurontin) was released in the United States in 1994 as an adjunctive treatment for focal seizures. In animal models, gabapentin appeared to have anxiolytic properties, and, as with other anticonvulsants, it began to be examined in the treatment of bipolar disorder. The mechanism of action for gabapentin was once thought to be via increasing GABA levels in the brain, but the mode by which it accomplishes this increase, if it does so, is still not elucidated. Gabapentin does seem to affect calcium channels, and this may be important in its anticonvulsant and analgesic properties. Gabapentin and its chemical cousin pregabalin have been more promising in the treatment of anxiety disorders than in the treatment of mood disorders. Both pregabalin and gabapentin are known to bind to the α_2-δ subunit of a voltage-gated cal-

Table 5–5. Other anticonvulsants

	Pregabalin (Lyrica)	Oxcarbazepine (Trileptal)	Gabapentin (Neurontin)	Lamotrigine (Lamictal)	Topiramate (Topamax)	Tiagabine (Gabitril)
Serum plasma level, ng/mL	NA	NA	NA	NA	NA	1–234
Adult dosage, mg/day	150–600 300–450 given in divided doses (for fibromyalgia) 150–300 given in divided doses (for neuropathic pain)	600–2,400	900–2,400 (for seizure maintenance treatment)	300–500 (for seizure maintenance treatment) 200 (for bipolar disorder monotherapy) 100 (concurrently with valproate for bipolar disorder)	200–400 (for seizure maintenance treatment) 100 given in two divided doses (for migraine prophylaxis)	4–32

Table 5–5. Other anticonvulsants *(continued)*

	Pregabalin (Lyrica)	Oxcarbazepine (Trileptal)	Gabapentin (Neurontin)	Lamotrigine (Lamictal)	Topiramate (Topamax)	Tiagabine (Gabitril)
Adult dosage, mg/day *(continued)*				400 (concurrently with carbamazepine or other enzyme-inducing drugs [and without valproate] for bipolar disorder)		
Protein binding	—	40% bound	Minimally bound (<3%)	55% bound	20% bound	96% bound
Half-life, hours	—	2–9	5–7	25–32	20–30	7–9
Metabolic pathway	—	Hepatic CYP3A enzyme	Drug not appreciably metabolized hepatically	Glucuronidation/ conjugation	20% metabolized hepatically	Oxidation/glu-curonidation
Routes of elimination	—	Renal (95%); fecal (5%)	Renal	Renal	Renal	Urinary (25%); fecal (63%)

Table 5–5. Other anticonvulsants (continued)

	Pregabalin (Lyrica)	Oxcarbazepine (Trileptal)	Gabapentin (Neurontin)	Lamotrigine (Lamictal)	Topiramate (Topamax)	Tiagabine (Gabitril)
Common drug interactions	No significant drug interactions are known; antacids decrease absorption and bioavailability of pregabalin	Induces metabolism of CYP3A3/4-dependent drugs (weaker than carbamazepine); decreases levels of phenobarbital, phenytoin, sex steroids, haloperidol, valproic acid, calcium channel blockers, and others (see Table 5–4)	No significant drug interactions are known; antacids decrease bioavailability of gabapentin by 20%; cimetidine decreases renal clearance by 13%	Valproate doubles serum levels; carbamazepine decreases serum levels by 50%; phenytoin decreases serum levels by 50%	Phenobarbital decreases serum levels by 40%; carbamazepine decreases topiramate levels by 50%–60%; valproate decreases topiramate levels by 15%; phenytoin decreases topiramate levels by 48%	Carbamazepine decreases tiagabine levels; phenytoin decreases tiagabine levels; tiagabine decreases valproate levels

Table 5–5.   Other anticonvulsants *(continued)*

	Pregabalin (Lyrica)	Oxcarbazepine (Trileptal)	Gabapentin (Neurontin)	Lamotrigine (Lamictal)	Topiramate (Topamax)	Tiagabine (Gabitril)
Common adverse effects	Somnolence, dizziness, ataxia, fatigue	Dizziness, drowsiness, ataxia, weight gain	Somnolence, dizziness, fatigue, ataxia	Rash: 1 in 10 (serious rashes, such as Stevens-Johnson syndrome: 1 in 1,000), dizziness, ataxia, nausea, vomiting	Psychomotor slowing, decreased concentration, somnolence, fatigue, anorexia, kidney stone formation	Dizziness, depression, asthenia, nervousness, tremors, somnolence, cognitive deficits
Indications (FDA approved)	Partial seizures Postherpetic neuralgia Fibromyalgia Neuropathic pain associated with diabetic neuropathy	Partial complex seizures	Partial seizures Postherpetic neuralgia	Partial seizures Maintenance treatment of bipolar I disorder	Epilepsy Prophylaxis of migraine headaches	Epilepsy

Note.   CYP = cytochrome P450; NA = not applicable.
Source.   Adapted for the most part from 2002 black book.

cium channel in the brain and spinal cord. The result is to reduce the flow of calcium into the axon during depolarization and thus to reduce neurotransmitter release from that neuron. Pregabalin has been approved in the treatment of epilepsy, fibromyalgia, and neuropathic pain and at one time was under review for the treatment of generalized anxiety disorder (GAD). The studies showing benefit of pregabalin in GAD appear compelling, and pregabalin might ultimately be approved for this anxiety disorder. Pregabalin's advantage is that it has more predictable absorption and, thus, more predictable blood levels than does gabapentin.

Clinical indications.   As with all the anticonvulsants used in psychiatry except divalproex sodium and lamotrigine, the only FDA-approved indication for gabapentin and pregabalin had been adjunct treatment of patients with complex partial seizures. Both drugs are approved for use in pain conditions, with pregabalin being the first treatment approved for fibromyalgia and both drugs demonstrating efficacy in the treatment of neuropathic pain.

Soon after its release, however, reports began to emerge that gabapentin might be useful for a variety of psychiatric and nonpsychiatric conditions. Much of the psychiatric investigation of gabapentin over the past decade has focused on its role in the treatment of bipolar disorder. The very benign side-effect and drug interaction profiles of gabapentin made it a potentially attractive alternative to other mood stabilizers. However, much of the data on gabapentin in bipolar disorder are anecdotal, and more rigorous studies suggested that gabapentin has modest mood-stabilizing effects.

A number of open-label studies, most of which were small, suggested a modest role for gabapentin in bipolar disorder. These studies suggested that gabapentin, typically in dosages of 900–2,700 mg/day, may help with bipolar depression, mixed states, mania, and hypomania (Letterman and Markowitz 1999).

Data from double-blind studies are much more limited. One study at NIMH (Frye et al. 2000) examined the efficacy of gabapentin in a small group of patients with treatment-resistant bipolar disorder; over 6 weeks, 26% of the patients taking gabapentin, compared with 23% of the patients receiving placebo, had a response. Unfortunately, more definitive controlled studies of gabapentin as an add-on to lithium or valproic acid done by Parke-Davis demonstrated that gabapentin was no more effective than placebo (Pande et al. 1999). Upward adjustment of the lithium dose in the placebo group may have obscured an effect for the drug.

What one can draw from the gabapentin studies to date is that the mood-stabilizing effects of gabapentin are modest to negligible. Gabapentin may help somewhat with the depressive and manic phases of bipolar disorder, and it tends to be well tolerated. However, the use of gabapentin as a monotherapy for the treatment of mania or rapid cycling does not appear to be justified. A lawsuit against the manufacturer of gabapentin for off-label marketing in the treatment of bipolar disorder, as well as the lack of studies demonstrating efficacy, resulted in a substantial decrease in the use of gabapentin for the management of bipolar disorder (Chace et al. 2012).

As with gabapentin, the evidence supporting pregabalin in the treatment of bipolar disorder is mostly limited to small, open-label studies (Schaffer et al. 2013) and case studies (Conesa et al. 2012). Pregabalin may also help with akathisia induced by agents such as aripiprazole (De Berardis et al. 2013).

The role of gabapentin in treating anxiety disorders may be greater than its role in treating bipolar disorder. Case reports and double-blind studies support a possible role for gabapentin in anxiety disorders, particularly social phobia and panic disorder. In a randomized controlled trial, Pande and colleagues (1999) found that gabapentin at dosages of 900–3,600 mg/day was superior to placebo in the treatment of 69 patients with social phobia. However, the difference in response to gabapentin relative to placebo, although statistically significant, was not dramatic. Still, gabapentin appears to be a well-tolerated option for some patients with social anxiety disorder. Gabapentin may also prove to be a useful add-on for patients getting only a partial response to antidepressants in the treatment of social phobia.

Pregabalin at dosages ranging from 150 to 600 mg/day appears to be as effective as a benzodiazepine in the treatment of GAD but without the risk of dependence (Frampton and Foster 2006). There have been at least eight studies to date suggesting that pregabalin is effective in the monotherapy and adjunctive treatment of GAD (Wensel et al. 2012). It may be particularly helpful as an adjunctive treatment to SSRIs in the treatment of GAD (Both et al. 2014). One of us (C.D.) commonly uses pregabalin at dosages of 150–300 mg/day in patients with GAD who have not responded to an SSRI alone. Anecdotally, it seems to be more potent than gabapentin in the treatment of GAD, but there are no comparison studies. Pregabalin is also being investigated in other anxiety disorders such as social anxiety disorder.

Another psychiatric use of gabapentin may be in the treatment of neuroleptic-induced movement disorders. Hardoy et al. (1999) found that 14 of 16 patients with various mood disorders who had tardive dyskinesia improved with the addition of gabapentin at dosages above 900 mg/day. Blepharospasms and oral mandibular dyskinesias appeared to improve with the addition of gabapentin.

Finally, small case series have suggested that gabapentin might help mitigate symptoms of withdrawal from cocaine and alcohol (Chatterjee and Ringold 1999; Letterman and Markowitz 1999; Myrick et al. 1998). More recently, Mason et al. (2014) reported that 900 mg/day and 1,800 mg/day of gabapentin were effective in reducing alcohol consumption. The higher dosage was more effective than 900 mg/day. In addition, Mason et al. (2012) had also reported a pilot study indicating that gabapentin was effective in treating cannabis abuse.

Gabapentin and pregabalin are now commonly used in the treatment of neuropathic pain conditions. A number of studies, including several double-blind studies, attest to the efficacy of gabapentin in improving pain associated with trigeminal neuralgia (Carrazana and Schachter 1998), postherpetic neuralgia (Colman and Stadel 1999; Rowbotham et al. 1998), and diabetic neuropathy (Backonja et al. 1998; Gorson et al. 1999; Morello et al. 1999). It has also been suggested that gabapentin is helpful in migraine prophylaxis (D'Andrea et al. 1999; Lampl et al. 1999).

In 2007, pregabalin became the first drug approved for the treatment of fibromyalgia (duloxetine was subsequently approved). Studies of pregabalin in the treatment of fibromyalgia suggested that the drug improves pain, sleep, and anxiety but not depressed mood in these patients (Häuser et al. 2009). In another multicenter trial, pregabalin was found to be significantly more effective than placebo in reducing symptoms of anxiety and depression in depressed patients with fibromyalgia who were taking antidepressants (Arnold et al. 2015).

Side effects.   Gabapentin and pregabalin are generally well tolerated. The most common side effects of both gabapentin and pregabalin leading to discontinuation of these medications are somnolence and dizziness. The extent of these symptoms can be mitigated by administering a larger percentage of the drug at night.

Other possible adverse effects associated with both gabapentin and pregabalin include ataxia, tremor, nausea, double vision, and headache. Pregabalin appears to be associated with more weight gain than does gabapentin. It is our experience that these side effects tend to be dose related, mild, and manageable. If possible, a lower dose should be attempted before the drug is discontinued. The headache often responds to nonsteroidal anti-inflammatory drugs and tends to improve with time. Patients can gain weight while taking gabapentin, but, apparently, weight gain is much less than with most other potential mood stabilizers. Sexual side effects appear to be uncommon.

Neither gabapentin nor pregabalin is appreciably metabolized by the liver, and both are excreted largely unchanged. Thus, both drugs can be used by patients with advanced liver disease.

No completed suicides have been reported to date with gabapentin or pregabalin doses alone. Overdoses have not typically been associated with significant adverse effects other than somnolence.

Drug interactions.   No serious drug interactions have been reported with gabapentin or pregabalin. Neither gabapentin nor pregabalin appears to inhibit CYP enzymes to any degree, and the drugs do not appear to alter the kinetics of lithium or additional anticonvulsants. Antacids can reduce the bioavailability of gabapentin and pregabalin by 20%, so these agents should not be taken simultaneously with gabapentin. Alcohol and other CNS depressants, theoretically, can increase the somnolence and cognitive effects associated with gabapentin and pregabalin.

Use in pregnancy.   Gabapentin and pregabalin are category C drugs, and their teratogenic effects in pregnancy have not been well studied. In rats exposed to much higher relative doses than are typically used in patients, gabapentin appeared to inhibit bone ossification in fetal pups. Neural tube defects do not appear to be common. As with all anticonvulsants, the risks of discontinuing the gabapentin have to be weighed against the largely unknown risk of continuing to take the drug during pregnancy. When possible, gabapentin should be discontinued before conception or in the first trimester in most patients until additional data are available on the safety of the drug in pregnancy.

Dosage and administration.   Gabapentin is usually started at 300 mg taken at night. If tolerated, the dose can be increased to 300 mg bid the next day. For some anxiety conditions, we start at 300 mg bid or tid. If the patient complains of excessive somnolence or dizziness, most of the dose can be given at night, to a maximum dose of 1,200 mg taken at one time. Doses higher than 1,200 mg at one time are not well absorbed. To maximize compliance, we suggest sticking with bid dosing up to 1,200 mg bid. Thereafter, tid dosing is necessary up to dosages of 3,600 mg/day. Some patients do quite well at dosages in the range of 900–2,400 mg/day. For patients being treated for pain, the dosage is often titrated up to as high as 3,600 mg/day.

Pregabalin is usually started at a dosage of 75 mg twice daily, and the dosage is increased to a maximum of 450 mg/day in divided doses (bid or tid regimen). After a week, the dosage may be increased to 150 mg twice daily. The target dosage of 300–450 mg/day is the same for GAD as it is for epilepsy and fibromyalgia. Dosages up to 600 mg/day have been studied but are not necessarily more effective than lower dosages. Patients with postherpetic neuralgia and neuropathic pain associated with diabetes often benefit from 150–300 mg/day.

Topiramate

Topiramate was FDA approved in 1998 and has the unique property among potential mood stabilizers of being associated with weight loss rather than weight gain in 20%–50% of patients. A few preliminary reports suggest that topiramate may have mood-stabilizing effects as an adjunctive therapy in bipolar disorder, cyclothymia, and schizoaffective disorder (Gordon and Price 1999; Stephen et al. 1998). Unfortunately, none of the four double-blind trials conducted showed any benefit of topiramate in the treatment of mania, mixed states, or any other aspect of bipolar disorder (Kushner et al. 2006). Open trials and case series have suggested that the addition of topiramate to a standard mood stabilizer might help in the treatment of rapid cycling and comorbid alcohol abuse and comorbid aggression in bipolar patients. Topiramate may also help with substance abuse problems independent of bipolar disorder.

Perhaps the most common use of topiramate in current clinical practice is as an anorexiant to mitigate weight gain associated with other mood-stabilizing agents such as olanzapine. In one prospective study, the addition of topiramate to olanzapine for 1 year seemed to mitigate the expected weight gain from olanzapine (Vieta et al. 2004). Another controlled trial has suggested that patients with bipolar disorder and concurrent binge-eating disorder benefit from the addition of topiramate to lithium (Kotwal et al. 2006). Topiramate may also mitigate lithium-induced weight gain in children and adolescents (Mahmoudi-Gharaei et al. 2012). Even in nonpsychiatric patients, topiramate seems to promote weight loss. Weight loss of up to 25 kg in 6 months has been reported in patients who started topiramate in addition to their mood stabilizer. In our experience, 50 mg/day is often an optimal dosage of topiramate to help with weight loss.

The most common side effects of topiramate are somnolence, paresthesias, dizziness, vision problems, anorexia, and cognitive problems. The cognitive side effects are the most troublesome, with some patients reporting dullness or memory problems. These effects generally occur at dosages greater than 100 mg/day, but we have seen them persist in an older patient even with a dosage reduction to 25 mg/day. In such cases, the side effects of the drug remit with cessation. Discontinuation of topiramate occurs most commonly secondary to psychomotor slowing, memory problems, fatigue, and sedation. There is an increased risk of kidney stone formation with topiramate, particularly when the patient is on a ketogenic diet and/or taking a carbonic anhydrase inhibitor. Patients should be instructed to drink plenty of water.

Hyperchloremic metabolic acidosis is also a theoretical side effect that we have not observed. The risk of developing this condition may be enhanced by concomitant use of carbonic anhydrase inhibitors (e.g., acetazolamide), renal disease, diarrhea, and other causes. Monitoring of serum bicarbonate during topiramate treatment is recommended.

Drugs with which topiramate interacts include carbamazepine and valproate, which reduce topiramate blood levels by 50% and 15%, respectively. Conversely, topiramate can lower valproate levels by about 15%. Alcohol appears to potentiate the somnolence and ataxia associated with topiramate.

Topiramate is usually initiated at a dosage of 12.5–25 mg/day, and the dosage is usually increased by 25 mg per week. Dosages as low as 50 mg/day have anecdotally been added to standard mood stabilizers or olanzapine to counteract weight gain associated with these agents. We have found this to be a helpful strategy at 50–150 mg/day. For mood effects, the average dosages have been 100–200 mg/day given in divided doses. The usual maximum dosage of topiramate is 400 mg/day.

Tiagabine

Tiagabine was FDA approved for the treatment of epilepsy in 1998 and appears to have GABA reuptake blocking properties. It may have anxiolytic properties in animal models. However, Phase III trials conducted by Cephalon in patients with GAD failed to show benefit of tiagabine in this population. In one small case series, the addition of tiagabine appeared to help three patients with treatment-resistant bipolar disorder (Kaufman and Gerner 1998). In another open study of acute mania, tiagabine was rapidly loaded and was found to be ineffective and poorly tolerated (Grunze et al. 1999b). In this small series, one patient had a seizure that was probably related to the higher starting dose of tiagabine. Likewise, in an open case series of tiagabine in refractory bipolar disorder, tiagabine was poorly tolerated and not particularly effective (Suppes et al. 2002). At this time, there does not appear to be much evidence supporting the utility of tiagabine in either acute treatment of manic symptoms or maintenance treatment of bipolar disorder (Vasudev et al. 2011a, 2012; Young et al. 2006a, 2006b). In addition, the tolerability of tiagabine has been problematic.

Common side effects of tiagabine include dose-related somnolence, dizziness, syncope, and nausea. There have also been reports of tiagabine inducing seizures.

Tiagabine is usually started at a dosage of 4 mg/day, and the dosage is increased by 4–8 mg per week. The maximum dosage of tiagabine is 56 mg/day given in two to four divided doses.

Oxcarbazepine

Oxcarbazepine (Trileptal) is chemically related to carbamazepine and was introduced in the United States in 2000. Oxcarbazepine had been used in Europe for many years, and its use in treating bipolar disorder dates at least to the early 1980s. However, few studies have examined the efficacy of oxcarbazepine in bipolar disorder. Controlled studies in pediatric bipolar populations have not found oxcarbazepine particularly efficacious (MacMillan et al. 2006; Wagner et al. 2006). The few small studies and case reports available suggest that oxcarbazepine is effective as an add-on therapy in the treatment of acute mania and perhaps other aspects of bipolar disorder (Emrich 1990; Pratoomsri et al. 2005). Randomized comparison trials of oxcarbazepine added to lithium suggest that oxcarbazepine is about as effective as valproate add-on (Suppes et al. 2007) and may be better tolerated than carbamazepine (Juruena et al. 2009). However, limited placebo-controlled studies have not demonstrated clear efficacy of oxcarbazepine in bipolar disorder (Vasudev et al. 2008, 2011b; Vieta et al. 2008). We have used oxcarbazepine in treating bipolar patients who could not tolerate carbamazepine or with whom we were concerned about drug interactions. As with carbamazepine, we have sometimes used oxcarbazepine to treat agitation.

The primary advantages of oxcarbazepine over its chemical analog, carbamazepine, may be that it is better tolerated, does not tend to autoinduce its own metabolism, and has somewhat less significant drug interactions. Importantly, oxcarbazepine has not had a significant tendency to induce the blood dyscrasias, such as aplastic anemia, that are occasionally reported with carbamazepine. However, there is one case report of an oxcarbazepine-related neutropenia (Hsiao et al. 2010).

Oxcarbazepine is often a milder inducer of the CYP3A3/4 enzyme compared with carbamazepine. Still, oxcarbazepine can render oral contraceptives less effective and reduce serum levels of valproate, phenytoin, and other drugs. Thus, it is important to advise patients who are taking oral contraceptives that they may need to switch to a higher-potency oral contraceptive or to supplement the pill with a barrier method.

Oxcarbazepine is usually initiated at around 300 mg bid, and the dosage is increased gradually up to 2,400 mg/day. In the clinical trials of oxcarbazepine in bipolar disorder, the average dosage in most studies was 600–1,200 mg/day. Our experience is that the dosages of oxcarbazepine required to treat psychiatric symptoms are about 50% higher than those for carbamazepine.

An investigational agent related to oxcarbazepine and carbamazepine, eslicarbazepine, has been thought to have a role in the treatment of bipolar disorder (Nath et al. 2012). However, two double-blind Phase II studies in acute mania failed to demonstrate efficacy. There was some suggestion that eslicarbazepine could provide benefit in maintenance therapy (Grunze et al. 2015). Eslicarbazepine was approved in 2015 for the treatment of partial-onset seizures.

Levetiracetam, Zonisamide, and Ethosuximide

With the sudden availability of many anticonvulsants on the market, there has been an interest in the potential role of these newer agents in bipolar and other psychiatric disorders. Levetiracetam is a rather benign anticonvulsant with a good side-effect profile. At the highest doses, some patients experience somnolence and fatigue, but levetiracetam appears to be fairly weight neutral and has not been associated with much in the way of cognitive or sexual side effects. Dosages of 500–1,500 mg bid have been said to be effective in a few case reports and a small open study in the treatment of mania and depression, with few side effects (Post et al. 2005). However, there is no convincing evidence of the drug's utility in bipolar disorder at this time, and our limited clinical experience with the drug has not been consistent with robust benefits. Controlled studies of levetiracetam in the treatment of bipolar depression have not been positive (Saricicek et al. 2011), and the Canadian Network for Mood and Anxiety Treatments currently advises against the use of levetiracetam in bipolar depression on the basis of a lack of evidence (McIntyre et al. 2012).

Zonisamide at dosages of 100–600 mg/day has been reported to improve manic and depressive symptoms as an adjunctive treatment (Ghaemi et al. 2006, 2008). In addition, zonisamide, like topiramate, may have utility as an adjunctive treatment to control weight gain in bipolar patients (Wang et al. 2008). We have also found that zonisamide 200–400 mg/day, like topiramate, can facilitate weight loss in bipolar patients. However, zonisamide has been associated with worsening mood symptoms in some patients (McElroy et al. 2005). In fact, the only controlled trial in the literature to date did not demonstrate efficacy of zonisamide as an add-on treatment for mania or mixed states (Dauphinais et al. 2011). Zonisamide might also have a role as an anorexiant and has been shown to mitigate olanzapine-induced weight gain in bipolar patients and patients with schizophrenia (McElroy et al. 2012). However, the cognitive side effects of zonisamide may limit its utility at doses required to suppress weight gain.

To date, there are no studies of ethosuximide in the published literature demonstrating efficacy in bipolar disorder. Like zonisamide, ethosuximide has been used as an anorexiant. There have been reports of ethosuximide associated with psychosis, suicidal ideation, and mania induction (Chien 2011). Thus, it is not clear that there is any role for ethosuximide in the treatment of bipolar disorder at this time.

Antipsychotics

Antipsychotic drugs have long been recognized as important agents in treating acute mania (see Chapter 4). Chlorpromazine was the second drug approved for acute mania after lithium. Because all the standard mood stabilizers (lithium, valproate, carbamazepine) require monitoring, have slow onsets of action, and are not as helpful during the depressed phase of the illness, the atypical antipsychotics are becoming more commonly used as mood stabilizers. In fact, much of the use of atypical antipsychotics is already in the treatment of mood disorders. Olanzapine has more FDA indications in the treatment of bipolar disorder than does lithium. Olanzapine has long been approved for acute mania and was more recently approved for use in the maintenance treatment of bipolar disorder and (in combination with fluoxetine) in the acute treatment of bipolar depression. Compared with lithium and carbamazepine, antipsychotics tend to work more rapidly in controlling the excitement, agitation, thought disorder, and psychosis that may accompany acute mania. However, even in contexts in which psychotic symptoms are not present, the antipsychotics work at least as well as, and perhaps even better than, lithium in acute mania. As with olanzapine, the other SGAs are also proving to be more versatile than agents such as lithium and valproate in treating different aspects of bipolar disorder.

Olanzapine was FDA approved for the treatment of acute mania in 2000 and for maintenance therapy in 2003. For several years, there were case reports suggesting that olanzapine is effective in mixed states (Ketter et al. 1998; Zullino and Baumann 1999), bipolar depression (Weisler et al. 1997), and acute mania (Ravindran et al. 1997). A pivotal double-blind study involving 139 patients with bipolar mania indicated that 48% of patients responded to olanzapine, whereas only half that number responded to placebo (Tohen et al. 1999). Olanzapine was well tolerated in these patients. There are now multiple positive trials of olanzapine in acute mania. There are two comparison trials with valproate in acute mania (Tohen et al. 2003a; Zajecka et al. 2002). In both, olanzapine produced better efficacy, although only in the larger study (Tohen et al. 2003a) did the difference reach statistical significance. Olanzapine appeared to produce more side effects. Sporadic reports suggest that olanzapine may induce hypomania or mania in some patients (Lindenmayer and Klebanov 1998; Reeves et al. 1998). However, it has become evident that olanzapine and other atypicals probably do not commonly result in switching to mania and have a role to play in the long-term maintenance of bipolar disorder. Olanzapine alone also appears to do better than placebo in treating bipolar depression, but the combination with fluoxetine is even more effective (Tohen et al. 2003b). The combination of olanzapine and an SSRI is more effective than olanzapine alone (see Chapter 9).

Virtually all of the current SGA agents except clozapine and iloperidone have had at least two double-blind studies (e.g., Keck et al. 2003a, 2003b) that indicated the drugs were effective in the treatment of acute mania. Quetiapine, ziprasidone, risperidone, asenapine, lurasidone, cariprazine, and aripiprazole are all approved for the treatment of acute mania. Although olanzapine appears to be effective in delaying the time to a new mood episode in patients with bipolar I disorder, some patients do not tolerate chronic treatment with olanzapine. Weight gain or metabolic concerns are an issue for some patients. Aripiprazole and quetiapine have also demonstrated efficacy in the maintenance treatment of bipolar disorder and are alternatives to olanzapine for some patients. In addition, several SGAs are now approved in bipolar depression.

Olanzapine was first approved in combination with fluoxetine for the treatment of bipolar depression, and in 2006, quetiapine obtained approval as a monotherapy for the treatment of acute bipolar depression. More recently, OFC was approved for the treatment of resistant unipolar depression (see Chapter 3). Both ziprasidone and aripiprazole continue to be explored in the treatment of bipolar depression, and it would not be particularly surprising if both of these drugs prove equal to quetiapine and olanzapine in this regard. Likewise, virtually all of the atypicals are being investigated in the maintenance treatment of bipolar disorder. It is evident that the atypical antipsychotics will play an increasingly large role in the treatment of bipolar disorder relative to the anticonvulsants or other classes of agents.

Although clozapine is without pivotal trials in bipolar disorder, it should be considered in the treatment of some bipolar patients. Clozapine appears to be effective in the treatment of patients with more refractory bipolar disorder, including the rapid-cycling subtype and bipolar disorder accompanied by psychosis (Green et al. 2000; Kimmel et al. 1994; Suppes et al. 1994). The toxicity of clozapine relegates it to use as a third-line treatment when standard agents have failed.

Among the newer SGAs, asenapine was approved in 2009 for the treatment of acute mania and mixed states in adults with bipolar I disorder (see Chapter 4). Two 3-week randomized placebo-controlled studies indicated superiority of asenapine over placebo (Citrome 2009b). There is no evidence of asenapine's having superior efficacy relative to other SGAs. However, it does cause less weight gain than do clozapine and quetiapine. Another option is lurasidone, which had been approved for the treatment of acute mania and then received an additional indication in the monotherapy of bipolar depression in 2013. Lurasidone also has the advantage of being less likely to cause weight gain and metabolic issues when compared with olanzapine and quetiapine.

Another agent approved since the last edition of this manual is cariprazine (see Chapter 4). Phase II and III trials suggested that cariprazine appears effective in the treatment of schizophrenia and bipolar mania and depression and in treatment-resistant depression as an add-on to standard antidepressants. However, cariprazine can be quite sedating and has more metabolic side effects than many other SGAs. For unclear reasons, the drug is better tolerated in bipolar patients than in patients with schizophrenia. The drug has been approved for the treatment of schizophrenia as well as for acute mania and mixed states (Sachs et al. 2015). The dosage in bipolar studies has been 3–12 mg/day, with an average of about 4–5 mg/day. In addition, it has been studied in bipolar I depression, in which at 1.5 mg/day (but not at 0.75 or 3.0 mg/day) it was significantly more effective than placebo (Durgam et al. 2016).

Benzodiazepines

Several benzodiazepines, chiefly clonazepam and lorazepam, have been reported to be useful in the adjunctive treatment of acute mania. It was initially believed that clonazepam might have antimanic properties unique among the benzodiazepines. However, it has become increasingly clear that this is probably not the case. All the benzodiazepines appear to have a role in treating the hyperkinesis, agitation, and insomnia associated with acute mania. Chouinard and associates in Montreal had done much of the key work with clonazepam in mania (see, e.g., Chouinard et al. 1983). Reports suggested that clonazepam might be useful as an adjunct to lithium or neuroleptics in the treatment of acute mania. However, Bradwejn and colleagues (1990) found that clonazepam did not appear to be efficacious in the treatment of acute mania and was inferior to lorazepam in this regard. Salzman and colleagues (1991) reported that lorazepam 2 mg IM was as effective in reducing aggression and agitation in psychotic patients as haloperidol 5 mg IM. Lorazepam's effects appeared to be independent of its sedative properties. Lorazepam was better tolerated than was haloperidol. No evidence up to this time has supported the use of a benzodiazepine alone for the maintenance treatment of bipolar disorder. The one study that used clonazepam alone for prophylaxis was stopped early because all of the enrolled subjects relapsed within 3 months while taking the medication.

Experience with clonazepam in the treatment of acute mania has been that it tends to lead to sedated manic patients whose mania is unchanged when the sedation wears off. We have not been impressed with the antimanic versus sedating properties of clonazepam. When a bipolar patient requires an agent for sleep, anxiety, or catatonia, clonazepam or the other benzodiazepines should be considered.

The dosages of clonazepam typically employed are 1–6 mg/day, although much higher dosages were used in the original studies. Lorazepam dosages are similar, ranging from 1.5 to 8 mg/day.

The side effects of clonazepam and lorazepam are those of all current benzodiazepines: sedation, ataxia, and malcoordination. With any sedative drug, in rare cases patients become disinhibited and agitated. Patients with a history of ADHD in childhood may be at particular risk for sedative-induced angry agitation. We have seen occasional bipolar patients who reported feeling angrier after taking clonazepam. No prospective data on this potential side effect are available.

Management of Acute Agitation in Bipolar Disorder

The combination of antipsychotics and benzodiazepines has long been used to manage agitation in acute mania. Several antipsychotic formulations have been specifically approved for the treatment of agitation in bipolar disorder and/or schizophrenia. These include intramuscular formulations of olanzapine and ziprasidone and the intranasal formulation of loxapine. The use of these drugs in emergency is discussed further in Chapter 9.

Beyond the first- and second-generation antipsychotics and benzodiazepines, dexmedetomidine is a different class of medication approved in 2022 for the acute treatment of agitation in bipolar disorder and schizophrenia. Dexmedetomidine is a potent α_2-adrenergic agonist previously used in anesthesia procedures. It is a rapidly acting sublingual medication with effects typically seen within 20–30 minutes. Preskorn and colleagues (2022) found that 120–180 µg of dexmedetomidine was more effective than placebo at improving agitation within 2 hours in 380 bipolar patients as measured in by the Positive and Negative Syndrome Scale–Excited Component. The drug was well tolerated, with the most common side effects being somnolence, dry mouth, hypotension, and dizziness. Like intranasal loxapine, dexmedetomidine requires a fairly cooperative agitated patient. The medication is administered on a thin film under the tongue or in the buccal area. As with other sublinguals such as asenapine, swallowing the film or consuming food or drink within 15 minutes after administration will decrease or eliminate the effectiveness of the drug. The drug causes a dose-related increase in orthostatic hypotension, and taking dexmedetomidine with benzodiazepines, antipsychotics, or hypnotics within 4 hours significantly increases the risk of orthostasis and bradycardia. A distinct advantage of dexmedetomidine is that it will not cause the EPS that are a significant risk of intramuscular antipsychotics. Dexmedetomidine is probably more potent than a benzodiazepine in treating agitation (although comparison studies have not been done). It appears less likely than a benzodiazepine to worsen delirium and in fact has been used in the treatment of delirium. Thus, for some agitated bipolar patients, dexmedetomidine might be a better choice than an antipsychotic or benzodiazepine. The drug is usually dosed at 120–180 μg given sublingually in the buccal area outside the bite and may be repeated every 2 hours, with up to three total doses. Blood pressure should be monitored, especially in older patients.

Calcium Channel Blockers

The calcium channel blockers, which include verapamil, nifedipine, diltiazem, and a number of newer agents, are used primarily in the treatment of hypertension, angina, and supraventricular arrhythmias. Dysregulation of intracellular calcium may be involved in some affective disorders, and this notion prompted Dubovsky and colleagues to begin studying the efficacy of calcium channel blockers in treating bipolar patients (Dubovsky et al. 1982). Since then, a number of studies have suggested that calcium channel blockers may have antimanic properties. Most of these studies were uncontrolled and small, and interpretation of their findings was complicated by other drug use. The greatest rationale for retrying these agents stems from large-scale genetic studies that point to an alteration in a calcium channel gene as being associated with increased risk for bipolar disorder (Cipriani et al. 2016).

There is no evidence that patients whose condition is resistant to lithium or the anticonvulsants are any more likely to respond to the calcium channel blockers. On the contrary, patients who are unresponsive to the standard agents appear likely to be unresponsive to calcium channel agents as well. However, there may be instances in which the calcium channel blockers are worth considering in the treatment of a bipolar patient. For example, bipolar patients with cardiovascular problems (e.g., supraventricular arrhythmias, hypertension) that may be helped by a calcium channel blocker might be assessed for antimanic effect while taking these drugs to determine whether they could be substituted for standard mood-stabilizing agents. Likewise, a calcium channel blocker may be worth trying with a pregnant bipolar patient because the teratogenic risk of this category of drugs appears to be substantially lower than that of any of the standard agents. The most common side effects of the calcium channel blockers are dizziness, headache, and nausea.

More serious side effects, which are rare, include malignant arrhythmias, hepatotoxicity, and severe hypotension and syncope. The calcium channel blockers can produce orthostasis in elderly patients and may have an additive hypotensive effect when used with other antihypertensive drugs. At high doses, anergy and somnolence are sometimes reported.

Dosing for the calcium channel blockers in treating bipolar illness is not well defined. Most investigators have used the typical doses used for cardiovascular indications. Verapamil has been the most studied agent in its class. The usual starting dosage in treating hypertension is 80 mg bid or tid, up to a maximum dosage of 480 mg/day. An alternative strategy is to start with a half or a full 240-mg slow-release tablet and titrate the dosage upward to the maximum dosage as tolerated. It is important to monitor blood pressure and pulse regularly as the dose is being titrated. Given the risk of arrhythmias, a baseline ECG is also advised. Blood levels have never been correlated with efficacy or toxicity for any indication of a calcium channel antagonist. Some investigators believe that the novel biochemical profile of nimodipine and other dihydropyridines may confer greater brain penetrance and more efficacy in the treatment of bipolar disorder. Controlled trials are currently under way.

Although combining the standard mood stabilizers in difficult cases of bipolar illness is supported by the literature, there is no substantial evidence that adding a calcium channel blocker to lithium or other agents is advantageous. In fact, there are reports of enhanced neurotoxicity when verapamil was added to lithium and carbamazepine. In general, it appears prudent to avoid these combinations until we better understand the risks and benefits. There is, however, recent renewed interest in these agents because allelic variants for a gene that encodes for a subunit of calcium channel have been reported to connote risk for bipolar disorder (Szczepankiewicz 2013).

Omega-3 Fatty Acids

Omega-3 and omega-6 fatty acids are the building blocks of fats in the same way that amino acids are the building blocks of proteins. A number of reports have suggested that affective illness may be associated with deficiencies of some omega-3 fatty acids. For example, there appears to be some correlation between a higher ratio of arachidonic acid and EPA in more severely depressed patients than in less severely depressed patients. Other studies have suggested that there may be lower levels of omega-3 fatty acids in the membranes of red blood cells in depressed patients than in healthy control subjects. Furthermore, there is limited evidence suggesting that omega-3 fatty acids may impact signal transduction in a manner analogous to the way lithium affects it. The lower rates of depression in some Asian countries may be due to greater amounts of fish consumed in regular diets.

A double-blind study reported that adding supplemental omega-3 fatty acids to the drug regimens of bipolar patients improved their outcomes (Stoll et al. 1999). In this study, 30 bipolar patients were randomly assigned to receive either 9.6 g/day of omega-3 supplements or olive oil (as a control) for 4 months. They continued taking standard mood stabilizers. The patients treated with omega-3 experienced longer remission and more complete resolution of symptoms than did the placebo-treated patients.

Since the Stoll study, there have been several controlled trials of omega-3 fatty acids in the treatment of depression and bipolar disorder. The data supporting the efficacy of omega-3 fatty acids in the treatment of bipolar disorder have been mixed. For example, two other controlled trials of omega fatty acids (up to 6 g/day of EPA) in bipolar disorder failed to show benefit (Keck et al. 2006; Post et al. 2003). However, in perhaps the most rigorous controlled trial to date, Frangou and colleagues (2006) found that the addition of both 1 and 2 g/day of EPA to a standard mood stabilizer was superior to adjunctive placebo in reducing Hamilton Depression Rating Scale scores and Global Impression of Illness scores in bipolar patients. The EPA did not show benefit in improving manic symptoms, and 2 g/day was no more effective than 1 g/day.

In unipolar depression, the data on omega-3 fatty acids are also unclear. For example, some studies of omega-3 fatty acids in perinatal depression (Freeman et al. 2006) and pediatric depression (Nemets et al. 2006) have suggested benefits, whereas other controlled studies have failed to show any advantage of supplementing omega-3 fatty acids in adult depressed patients (Marangell et al. 2003). Most studies have used 1–6 mg/day of EPA, and others have used DHA. A few reports mentioned use of the combination of EPA and DHA.

The role of omega-3 fatty acid supplements in the treatment of affective illness remains uncertain. Studies thus far suggest a more reliable effect of omega-3 fatty acids in some forms of unipolar depression than in bipolar maintenance. In addition, the data to date are more indicative of a benefit in treating depressive symptoms in bipolar disorder than in treating or preventing manic symptoms. However, the correct dose, duration of treatment, and form of omega-3 fatty acids remain to be established. Because these fatty acids are fairly benign and may have other health benefits, some clinicians are supplementing mood-stabilizing or antidepressant regimens with omega-3 fatty acids. The most commonly reported side effects are belching and a fishy aftertaste. Given the available data that suggest that omega-3 fatty acids may be beneficial in some patients and have few side effects, the American Psychiatric Association (APA) has endorsed the use of EPA and DHA in patients with mood, impulse-control, and psychotic disorders. The APA recommends at least 1 g/day of EPA/DHA.

Suggested Readings

Abou-Saleh MT: Who responds to prophylactic lithium therapy? Br J Psychiatry Suppl (21):20–26, 1993 8217063

Abraham G, Delva N, Waldron J, et al: Lithium treatment: a comparison of once- and twice-daily dosing. Acta Psychiatr Scand 85(1):65–69, 1992 1546552

Altesman R, Cole JO: Lithium therapy: a practical review, in Psychopharmacology Update. Edited by Cole JO. Lexington, MA, Collamore, 1980, pp 3–18

Ayd F: Carbamazepine for aggression, schizophrenia and nonaffective syndromes. Int Drug Ther Newsl 19:9–12, 1984

Bahk WM, Shin YC, Woo JM, et al: Topiramate and divalproex in combination with risperidone for acute mania: a randomized open-label study. Prog Neuropsychopharmacol Biol Psychiatry 29(1):115–121, 2005 15610953

Baldessarini RJ, Tondo L: Lithium and suicidal risk. Bipolar Disord 10(1):114–115, 2008 18199250

Baldessarini RJ, Tondo L: Suicidal risks during treatment of bipolar disorder patients with lithium versus anticonvulsants. Pharmacopsychiatry 42(2):72–75, 2009 19308882

Barzman DH, Delbello MP: Topiramate for co-occurring bipolar disorder and disruptive behavior disorders. Am J Psychiatry 163(8):1451–1452, 2006 16877668

Benedetti A, Lattanzi L, Pini S, et al: Oxcarbazepine as add-on treatment in patients with bipolar manic, mixed or depressive episode. J Affect Disord 79(1–3):273–277, 2004 15023507

Biederman J, Lerner Y, Belmaker RH: Combination of lithium carbonate and haloperidol in schizoaffective disorder: a controlled study. Arch Gen Psychiatry 36(3):327–333, 1979 369472

Bowden CL: Predictors of response to divalproex and lithium. J Clin Psychiatry 56(3)(Suppl 3):25–30, 1995 7883739

Bruno A, Micò U, Pandolfo G, et al: Lamotrigine augmentation of serotonin reuptake inhibitors in treatment-resistant obsessive-compulsive disorder: a double-blind, placebo-controlled study. J Psychopharmacol 26(11):1456–1462, 2012 22351381

Calabrese JR, Delucchi GA: Spectrum of efficacy of valproate in 55 patients with rapid-cycling bipolar disorder. Am J Psychiatry 147(4):431–434, 1990 2107762

Calabrese JR, Markovitz PJ, Kimmel SE, et al: Spectrum of efficacy of valproate in 78 rapid-cycling bipolar patients. J Clin Psychopharmacol 12(1)(suppl):53S–56S, 1992 1541718

Calabrese JR, Keck PE Jr, Starace A, et al: Efficacy and safety of low- and high-dose cariprazine in acute and mixed mania associated with bipolar I disorder: a double-blind, placebo-controlled study. J Clin Psychiatry 76(3):284–292, 2015 25562205

Calvert NW, Burch SP, Fu AZ, et al: The cost-effectiveness of lamotrigine in the maintenance treatment of adults with bipolar I disorder. J Manag Care Pharm 12(4):322–330, 2006 16792438

Chen CK, Shiah IS, Yeh CB, et al: Combination treatment of clozapine and topiramate in resistant rapid-cycling bipolar disorder. Clin Neuropharmacol 28(3):136–138, 2005 15965313

Conway CR, Chibnall JT, Nelson LA, et al: An open-label trial of adjunctive oxcarbazepine for bipolar disorder. J Clin Psychopharmacol 26(1):95–97, 2006 16415718

Daban C, Martínez-Arán A, Torrent C, et al: Cognitive functioning in bipolar patients receiving lamotrigine: preliminary results. J Clin Psychopharmacology 26(2):178–181, 2006 16633148

Davanzo P, Nikore V, Yehya N, et al: Oxcarbazepine treatment of juvenile-onset bipolar disorder. J Child Adolesc Psychopharmacol 14(3):344–345, 2004 15650489

Deandrea D, Walker N, Mehlmauer M, et al: Dermatological reactions to lithium: a critical review of the literature. J Clin Psychopharmacol 2(3):199–204, 1982 6212599

Deicken RF: Verapamil treatment of bipolar depression. J Clin Psychopharmacol 10(2):148–149, 1990 2341592

Deltito JA: The effect of valproate on bipolar spectrum temperamental disorders. J Clin Psychiatry 54(8):300–304, 1993 8253697

Delva NJ, Letemendia FJ: Lithium treatment in schizophrenia and schizo-affective disorders. Br J Psychiatry 141:387–400, 1982 6129016

Denicoff KD, Meglathery SB, Post RM, et al: Efficacy of carbamazepine compared with other agents: a clinical practice survey. J Clin Psychiatry 55(2):70–76, 1994 8077157

Di Costanzo E, Schifano F: Lithium alone or in combination with carbamazepine for the treatment of rapid-cycling bipolar affective disorder. Acta Psychiatr Scand 83(6):456–459, 1991 1882698

Dilsaver SC, Swann AC, Shoaib AM, et al: The manic syndrome: factors which may predict a patient's response to lithium, carbamazepine and valproate. J Psychiatry Neurosci 18(2):61–66, 1993 8461283

Dwight MM, Keck PE Jr, Stanton SP, et al: Antidepressant activity and mania associated with risperidone treatment of schizoaffective disorder. Lancet 344(8921):554–555, 1994 7520110

Evans RW, Gualtieri CT: Carbamazepine: a neuropsychological and psychiatric profile. Clin Neuropharmacol 8(3):221–241, 1985 2994882

Frankenburg FR, Tohen M, Cohen BM, et al: Long-term response to carbamazepine: a retrospective study. J Clin Psychopharmacol 8(2):130–132, 1988 3372707

Gelenberg AJ, Carroll JA, Baudhuin MG, et al: The meaning of serum lithium levels in maintenance therapy of mood disorders: a review of the literature. J Clin Psychiatry 50(suppl):17–22, discussion 45–47, 1989 2689433

Gelenberg AJ, Kane JM, Keller MB, et al: Comparison of standard and low serum levels of lithium for maintenance treatment of bipolar disorder. N Engl J Med 321(22):1489–1493, 1989 2811970

Gerner RH, Stanton A: Algorithm for patient management of acute manic states: lithium, valproate, or carbamazepine? J Clin Psychopharmacol 12(1)(suppl):57S–63S, 1992 1541719

Ghaemi SN, Schrauwen E, Klugman J, et al: Long-term lamotrigine plus lithium for bipolar disorder: one year outcome. J Psychiatr Pract 12(5):300–305, 2006 16998417

Gobbi G, Gaudreau PO, Leblanc N: Efficacy of topiramate, valproate, and their combination on aggression/agitation behavior in patients with psychosis. J Clin Psychopharmacol 26(5):467–473, 2006 16974186

Goodnick PJ: Verapamil prophylaxis in pregnant women with bipolar disorder. Am J Psychiatry 150(10):1560, 1993 8379565

Goodwin GM: Recurrence of mania after lithium withdrawal: implications for the use of lithium in the treatment of bipolar affective disorder. Br J Psychiatry 164(2):149–152, 1994 8173817

Guscott R, Taylor L: Lithium prophylaxis in recurrent affective illness: efficacy, effectiveness and efficiency. Br J Psychiatry 164(6):741–746, 1994 7952980

Himmelhoch JM, Poust RI, Mallinger AG, et al: Adjustment of lithium dose during lithium-chlorothiazide therapy. Clin Pharmacol Ther 22(2):225–227, 1977 884923

Huguelet P, Morand-Collomb S: Effect of topiramate augmentation on two patients suffering from schizophrenia or bipolar disorder with comorbid alcohol abuse. Pharmacol Res 52(5):392–394, 2005 16009565

Joffe RT, Post RM, Roy-Byrne PP, et al: Hematological effects of carbamazepine in patients with affective illness. Am J Psychiatry 142(10):1196–1199, 1985 4037133

Jones KL, Lacro RV, Johnson KA, et al: Pattern of malformations in the children of women treated with carbamazepine during pregnancy. N Engl J Med 320(25):1661–1666, 1989 2725616

Keck PE Jr, McElroy SL, Vuckovic A, et al: Combined valproate and carbamazepine treatment of bipolar disorder. J Neuropsychiatry Clin Neurosci 4(3):319–322, 1992 1498585

Kenna HA, Jiang B, Rasgon NL: Reproductive and metabolic abnormalities associated with bipolar disorder and its treatment. Harv Rev Psychiatry 17(2):138–146, 2009 19373621

Ketter TA, Pazzaglia PJ, Post RM: Synergy of carbamazepine and valproic acid in affective illness: case report and review of the literature. J Clin Psychopharmacol 12(4):276–281, 1992 1527232

Lenox RH, Watson DG: Lithium and the brain: a psychopharmacological strategy to a molecular basis for manic depressive illness. Clin Chem 40(2):309–314, 1994 8313612

Li PP, Young LT, Tam YK, et al: Effects of chronic lithium and carbamazepine treatment on G-protein subunit expression in rat cerebral cortex. Biol Psychiatry 34(3):162–170, 1993 8399809

Lin YH, Liu CY, Hsiao MC: Management of atypical antipsychotic-induced weight gain in schizophrenic patients with topiramate. Psychiatry Clin Neurosci 59(5):613–615, 2005 16194268

Lipinski JF, Pope HG Jr: Possible synergistic action between carbamazepine and lithium carbonate in the treatment of three acutely manic patients. Am J Psychiatry 139(7):948–949, 1982 6807113

Marcotte D: Use of topiramate, a new anti-epileptic as a mood stabilizer. J Affect Disord 50(2–3):245–251, 1998 9858083

Marcus WL: Lithium: a review of its pharmacokinetics, health effects, and toxicology. J Environ Pathol Toxicol Oncol 13(2):73–79, 1994 7884646

McCoy L, Votolato NA, Schwarzkopf SB, et al: Clinical correlates of valproate augmentation in refractory bipolar disorder. Ann Clin Psychiatry 5(1):29–33, 1993 8348196

McElroy SL, Keck PE Jr: Treatment guidelines for valproate in bipolar and schizoaffective disorders. Can J Psychiatry 38(3)(Suppl 2):S62–S66, 1993 8500081

McElroy SL, Keck PE Jr, Pope HG Jr: Sodium valproate: its use in primary psychiatric disorders. J Clin Psychopharmacol 7(1):16–24, 1987 3102563

Mitchell P, Withers K, Jacobs G, et al: Combining lithium and sodium valproate for bipolar disorder. Aust N Z J Psychiatry 28(1):141–143, 1994 8067959

Modell JG, Lenox RH, Weiner S: Inpatient clinical trial of lorazepam for the management of manic agitation. J Clin Psychopharmacol 5(2):109–113, 1985 3988969

Mørk A, Geisler A, Hollund P: Effects of lithium on second messenger systems in the brain. Pharmacol Toxicol 71(Suppl 1):4–17, 1992 1336196

Murray JB: Lithium maintenance therapy for bipolar I patients: possible refractoriness to reinstitution after discontinuation. Psychol Rep 74(2):355–361, 1994 8197273

Nilsson A, Axelsson R: Lithium discontinuers II: therapeutic outcome. Acta Psychiatr Scand 84(1):78–82, 1991 1681682

Okuma T, Yamashita I, Takahashi R, et al: Comparison of the antimanic efficacy of carbamazepine and lithium carbonate by double-blind controlled study. Pharmacopsychiatry 23(3):143–150, 1990 1973844

Pande AC, Crockatt JG, Janney CA, et al: Gabapentin in bipolar disorder: a placebo-controlled trial of adjunctive therapy. Bipolar Disord 2(3 Pt 2):249–255, 2000 11249802

Pazzaglia PJ, Post RM: Contingent tolerance and reresponse to carbamazepine: a case study in a patient with trigeminal neuralgia and bipolar disorder. J Neuropsychiatry Clin Neurosci 4(1):76–81, 1992 1627967

Pazzaglia PJ, Post RM, Ketter TA, et al: Preliminary controlled trial of nimodipine in ultra-rapid cycling affective dysregulation. Psychiatry Res 49(3):257–272, 1993 8177920

Post RM, Rubinow DR, Ballenger JC: Conditioning and sensitisation in the longitudinal course of affective illness. Br J Psychiatry 149:191–201, 1986 3535979

Post RM, Uhde TW, Roy-Byrne PP, et al: Correlates of antimanic response to carbamazepine. Psychiatry Res 21(1):71–83, 1987 2885878

Pratoomsri W, Yatham LN, Bond DJ, et al: Oxcarbazepine in the treatment of bipolar disorder: a review. Can J Psychiatry 51(8):540–545, 2006 16933591

Prettyman R: Lithium neurotoxicity at subtherapeutic serum levels. Br J Psychiatry 164(1):123, 1994 7907921

Price LH, Heninger GR: Lithium in the treatment of mood disorders. N Engl J Med 331(9):591–598, 1994 8047085

Prien RF, Caffey EM Jr: Long-term maintenance drug therapy in recurrent affective illness: current status and issues. Dis Nerv Syst 38(12):981–992, 1977 412649

Sachs GS, Rosenbaum JF, Jones L: Adjunctive clonazepam for maintenance treatment of bipolar affective disorder. J Clin Psychopharmacol 10(1):42–47, 1990 2106533

Sachs GS, Weilburg JB, Rosenbaum JF: Clonazepam vs. neuroleptics as adjuncts to lithium maintenance. Psychopharmacol Bull 26(1):137–143, 1990 1973545

Schatzberg AF, DeBattista C: Phenomenology and treatment of agitation. J Clin Psychiatry 60(Suppl 15):17–20, 1999 10418809

Schatzberg AF, DeBattista CB, DeGolia S: Valproate in the treatment of agitation associated with depression. Psychiatr Ann 26(7):S470–S473, 1996

Schou M: Lithium treatment during pregnancy, delivery, and lactation: an update. J Clin Psychiatry 51(10):410–413, 1990 2211538

Sheard MH, Marini JL, Bridges CI, et al: The effect of lithium on impulsive aggressive behavior in man. Am J Psychiatry 133(12):1409–1413, 1976 984241

Silvers KM, Woolley CC, Hamilton FC, et al: Randomised double-blind placebo-controlled trial of fish oil in the treatment of depression. Prostaglandins Leukot Essent Fatty Acids 72(3):211–218, 2005 15664306

Simhandl C, Denk E, Thau K: The comparative efficacy of carbamazepine low and high serum level and lithium carbonate in the prophylaxis of affective disorders. J Affect Disord 28(4):221–231, 1993 8227758

Small JG, Klapper MH, Milstein V, et al: Carbamazepine compared with lithium in the treatment of mania. Arch Gen Psychiatry 48(10):915–921, 1991 1929761

Strömgren LS: The combination of lithium and carbamazepine in treatment and prevention of manic-depressive disorder: a review and a case report. Compr Psychiatry 31(3):261–265, 1990 2187656

Suppes T, Baldessarini RJ, Faedda GL, et al: Risk of recurrence following discontinuation of lithium treatment in bipolar disorder. Arch Gen Psychiatry 48(12):1082–1088, 1991 1845226

Teratogenic effects of carbamazepine. N Engl J Med 321(21):1480–1481, 1989 2811966

Tilkian AG, Schroeder JS, Kao JJ, et al: The cardiovascular effects of lithium in man: a review of the literature. Am J Med 61(5):665–670, 1976 790953

Tohen M, Castillo J, Cole JO, et al: Thrombocytopenia associated with carbamazepine: a case series. J Clin Psychiatry 52(12):496–498, 1991 1752850

Tohen M, Castillo J, Pope HG Jr, et al: Concomitant use of valproate and carbamazepine in bipolar and schizoaffective disorders. J Clin Psychopharmacol 14(1):67–70, 1994 8151006

Uhde T, Post R, Ballenger J, et al: Carbamazepine in the treatment of neuropsychiatric disorders, in Anticonvulsants in Affective Disorders (Excerpta Medica International Congress Series, No 626). Edited by Emrich H, Okuma T, Muller A. Amsterdam, Excerpta Medica, 1984, pp 111–131

Valproate and carbamazepine join lithium as primary treatments for bipolar disorder. Am J Health Syst Pharm 52(4):358, 361, 1995 7757856

Valproate and mood disorders: perspectives. Summit conferences on the Treatment of Bipolar Disorders, July 27–28, 1990, Colorado Springs, Colorado and January 24–27, 1991, Snowmass, Colorado. J Clin Psychopharmacol 12(1)(suppl):1S–68S, 1992 1347299

Valproate for bipolar disorder. Med Lett Drugs Ther 36(929):74–75, 1994 8047048

Vendsborg PB, Bech P, Rafaelsen OJ: Lithium treatment and weight gain. Acta Psychiatr Scand 53(2):139–147, 1976 1251759

Wang Z, Gao K, Kemp DE, et al: Lamotrigine adjunctive therapy to lithium and divalproex in depressed patients with rapid cycling bipolar disorder and a recent substance use disorder: a 12-week, double-blind, placebo-controlled pilot study. Psychopharmacol Bull 43(4):5–21, 2010 21240149

Williams AL, Katz D, Ali A, et al: Do essential fatty acids have a role in the treatment of depression? J Affect Disord 93(1–3):117–123, 2006 16650900

Wright BA, Jarrett DB: Lithium and calcium channel blockers: possible neurotoxicity (letter). Biol Psychiatry 30(6):635–636, 1991 1932412

Zarate CA Jr, Tohen M, Banov MD, et al: Is clozapine a mood stabilizer? J Clin Psychiatry 56(3):108–112, 1995 7883728

References

Altshuler LL, Suppes T, Black DO, et al: Lower switch rate in depressed patients with bipolar II than bipolar I disorder treated adjunctively with second-generation antidepressants. Am J Psychiatry 163(2):313–315, 2006 16449487

Altshuler LL, Post RM, Hellemann G, et al: Impact of antidepressant continuation after acute positive or partial treatment response for bipolar depression: a blinded, randomized study. J Clin Psychiatry 70(4):450–457, 2009 19358785

Altshuler LL, Sugar CA, McElroy SL, et al: Switch rates during acute treatment for bipolar II depression with lithium, sertraline, or the two combined: a randomized double-blind comparison. Am J Psychiatry 174(3):266–276, 2017 28135846

American Psychiatric Association: Diagnostic and Statistical Manual of Mental Disorders, 5th Edition. Arlington, VA, American Psychiatric Association, 2013

American Psychiatric Association: Diagnostic and Statistical Manual of Mental Disorders, 5th Edition, Text Revision. Washington, DC, American Psychiatric Association, 2022

Andrade C: Valproate in pregnancy: recent research and regulatory responses. J Clin Psychiatry 79(3):18f12351, 2018 29873961

Arnold LM, Sarzi-Puttini P, Arsenault P, et al: Efficacy and safety of pregabalin in patients with fibromyalgia and comorbid depression taking concurrent antidepressant medication: a randomized, placebo-controlled study. J Rheumatol 42(7):1237–1244, 2015 26034150

Backonja M, Beydoun A, Edwards KR, et al: Gabapentin for the symptomatic treatment of painful neuropathy in patients with diabetes mellitus: a randomized controlled trial. JAMA 280(21):1831–1836, 1998 9846777

Baetz M, Bowen RC: Efficacy of divalproex sodium in patients with panic disorder and mood instability who have not responded to conventional therapy. Can J Psychiatry 43(1):73–77, 1998 9494751

Baker RW, Milton DR, Stauffer VL, et al: Placebo-controlled trials do not find association of olanzapine with exacerbation of bipolar mania. J Affect Disord 73(1–2):147–153, 2003 12507747

BALANCE investigators and collaborators; Geddes JR, Goodwin GM, et al: Lithium plus valproate combination therapy versus monotherapy for relapse prevention in bipolar I disorder (BALANCE): a randomized open-label trial. Lancet 375(9712):385–395, 2010 20092882

Baldessarini RJ, Pompili M, Tondo L: Suicide in bipolar disorder: risks and management. CNS Spectr 11(6):465–471, 2006 16816785

Ballenger JC, Post RM: Carbamazepine in manic-depressive illness: a new treatment. Am J Psychiatry 137(7):782–790, 1980 7386656

Banach R, Boskovic R, Einarson T, et al: Long-term developmental outcome of children of women with epilepsy, unexposed or exposed prenatally to antiepileptic drugs: a meta-analysis of cohort studies. Drug Saf 33(1):73–79, 2010 20000869

Barbee JG, Thompson TR, Jamhour NJ, et al: A double-blind placebo-controlled trial of lamotrigine as an antidepressant augmentation agent in treatment-refractory unipolar depression. J Clin Psychiatry 72(10):1405–1412, 2011 21367355

Bellino S, Paradiso E, Bogetto F: Oxcarbazepine in the treatment of borderline personality disorder: a pilot study. J Clin Psychiatry 66(9):1111–1115, 2005 16187767

Bellino S, Bozzatello P, Rocca G, et al: Efficacy of omega-3 fatty acids in the treatment of borderline personality disorder: a study of the association with valproic acid. J Psychopharmacol 28(2):125–132, 2014 24196948

Besag FM, Berry DJ, Pool F, et al: Carbamazepine toxicity with lamotrigine: pharmacokinetic or pharmacodynamic interaction? Epilepsia 39(2):183–187, 1998 9577998

Bodén R, Lundgren M, Brandt L, et al: Risks of adverse pregnancy and birth outcomes in women treated or not treated with mood stabilisers for bipolar disorder: population based cohort study. BMJ 345:e7085, 2012 23137820

Both C, Kojda G, Lange-Asschenfeldt C: Pharmacotherapy of generalized anxiety disorder: focus and update on pregabalin. Expert Rev Neurother 14(1):29–38, 2014 24308277

Bowden CL, McElroy SL: History of the development of valproate for treatment of bipolar disorder. J Clin Psychiatry 56(3)(Suppl 3):3–5, 1995 7883740

Bowden CL, Singh V: Valproate in bipolar disorder: 2000 onwards. Acta Psychiatr Scand Suppl 426(426):13–20, 2005 15833096

Bowden CL, Brugger AM, Swann AC, et al: Efficacy of divalproex vs lithium and placebo in the treatment of mania (erratum: JAMA 271:1830, 1994). JAMA 271(12):918–924, 1994 8120960

Bowden CL, Calabrese JR, McElroy SL, et al: A randomized, placebo-controlled 12-month trial of divalproex and lithium in treatment of outpatients with bipolar I disorder. Arch Gen Psychiatry 57(5):481–489, 2000 10807488

Bradwejn J, Shriqui C, Koszycki D, et al: Double-blind comparison of the effects of clonazepam and lorazepam in acute mania. J Clin Psychopharmacol 10(6):403–408, 1990 2126794

Brent NB, Wisner KL: Fluoxetine and carbamazepine concentrations in a nursing mother/infant pair. Clin Pediatr (Phila) 37(1):41–44, 1998 9475699

Briassoulis G, Kalabalikis P, Tamiolaki M, et al: Lamotrigine childhood overdose. Pediatr Neurol 19(3):239–242, 1998 9806147

Brown EB, McElroy SL, Keck PE Jr, et al: A 7-week, randomized, double-blind trial of olanzapine/fluoxetine combination versus lamotrigine in the treatment of bipolar I depression. J Clin Psychiatry 67(7):1025–1033, 2006 16889444

Bschor T, Bauer M: Efficacy and mechanisms of action of lithium augmentation in refractory major depression. Curr Pharm Des 12(23):2985–2992, 2006 16918427

Buzan RD, Dubovsky SL: Recurrence of lamotrigine-associated rash with rechallenge (letter). J Clin Psychiatry 59(2):87, 1998 9501897

Cade JF: Lithium salts in the treatment of psychotic excitement. Med J Aust 2(10):349–352, 1949 18142718

Calabrese JR, Woyshville MJ, Kimmel SE, et al: Predictors of valproate response in bipolar rapid cycling. J Clin Psychopharmacol 13(4):280–283, 1993 8376616

Calabrese JR, Bowden CL, McElroy SL, et al: Spectrum of activity of lamotrigine in treatment-refractory bipolar disorder. Am J Psychiatry 156(7):1019–1023, 1999a 10401445

Calabrese JR, Bowden CL, Sachs GS, et al: A double-blind placebo-controlled study of lamotrigine monotherapy in outpatients with bipolar I depression: Lamictal 602 Study Group. J Clin Psychiatry 60(2):79–88, 1999b 10084633

Calabrese JR, Ketter TA, Youakim JM, et al: Adjunctive armodafinil for major depressive episodes associated with bipolar I disorder: a randomized, multicenter, double-blind, placebo-controlled, proof-of-concept study. J Clin Psychiatry 71(10):1363–1370, 2010 20673554

Calabrese JR, Durgam S, Satlin A, et al: Efficacy and safety of lumateperone for major depressive episodes associated with bipolar I or bipolar II disorder: a Phase 3 randomized placebo-controlled trial. Am J Psychiatry 178(12):1098–1106, 2021 34551584

Carrazana EJ, Schachter SC: Alternative uses of lamotrigine and gabapentin in the treatment of trigeminal neuralgia. Neurology 50(4):1192, 1998 9566432

Casey DE, Tracy KA, Daniel D, et al: Divalproex sodium enhances anti-psychotic-induced improvement in schizophrenia, in Abstracts of the 40th Annual Meeting of the American College of Neuropsychopharmacology, Waikoloa, HI, 2001, p 281

Chace MJ, Zhang F, Fullerton CA, et al: Intended and unintended consequences of the gabapentin off-label marketing lawsuit among patients with bipolar disorder. J Clin Psychiatry 73(11):1388–1394, 2012 23146199

Chatterjee CR, Ringold AL: A case report of reduction in alcohol craving and protection against alcohol withdrawal by gabapentin. J Clin Psychiatry 60(9):617, 1999 10520981

Chien J: Ethosuximide-induced mania in a 10-year-old boy. Epilepsy Behav 21(4):483–485, 2011 21689989

Chouinard G, Young SN, Annable L: Antimanic effect of clonazepam. Biol Psychiatry 18(4):451–466, 1983 6407539

Cipriani A, Girlanda F, Agrimi E, et al: Effectiveness of lithium in subjects with treatment-resistant depression and suicide risk: a protocol for a randomised, independent, pragmatic, multicentre, parallel-group, superiority clinical trial. BMC Psychiatry 13:212, 2013a 23941474

Cipriani A, Hawton K, Stockton S, et al: Lithium in the prevention of suicide in mood disorders: updated systematic review and meta-analysis. BMJ 346:f3646, 2013b 23814104

Cipriani A, Saunders K, Attenburrow MJ, et al: A systematic review of calcium channel antagonists in bipolar disorder and some considerations for their future development. Mol Psychiatry 21(10):1324–1332, 2016 27240535

Citrome L: Adjunctive lithium and anticonvulsants for the treatment of schizophrenia: what is the evidence? Expert Rev Neurother 9(1):55–71, 2009a 19102669

Citrome L: Asenapine for schizophrenia and bipolar disorder: a review of the efficacy and safety profile for this newly approved sublingually absorbed second-generation antipsychotic. Int J Clin Pract 63(12):1762–1784, 2009b 19840150

Cohen LS, Friedman JM, Jefferson JW, et al: A reevaluation of risk of in utero exposure to lithium (erratum: JAMA 271:1485, 1994). JAMA 271(2):146–150, 1994 8031346

Colman E, Stadel BV: Gabapentin for postherpetic neuralgia. JAMA 282(2):134–135, 1999 10411191

Conesa ML, Rojo LM, Plumed J, et al: Pregabalin in the treatment of refractory bipolar disorders. CNS Neurosci Ther 18(3):269–270, 2012 22449111

Coryell W, Solomon D, Leon AC, et al: Lithium discontinuation and subsequent effectiveness. Am J Psychiatry 155(7):895–898, 1998 9659853

Cowdry RW, Gardner DL: Pharmacotherapy of borderline personality disorder: alprazolam, carbamazepine, trifluoperazine, and tranylcypromine. Arch Gen Psychiatry 45(2):111–119, 1988 3276280

D'Andrea G, Granella F, Cadaldini M, et al: Effectiveness of lamotrigine in the prophylaxis of migraine with aura: an open pilot study. Cephalalgia 19(1):64–66, 1999 10099862

Dauphinais D, Knable M, Rosenthal J, et al: Zonisamide for bipolar disorder, mania or mixed states: a randomized, double blind, placebo-controlled adjunctive trial. Psychopharmacol Bull 44(1):5–17, 2011 22506436

DeBattista C, Solomon A, Arnow B, et al: The efficacy of divalproex sodium in the treatment of agitation associated with major depression. J Clin Psychopharmacol 25(5):476–479, 2005 16160625

De Berardis D, Serroni N, Moschetta FS, et al: Reversal of aripiprazole-induced tardive akathisia by addition of pregabalin. J Neuropsychiatry Clin Neurosci 25(2):E9–E10, 2013 23686043

Del Matto L, Muscas M, Murru A, et al: Lithium and suicide prevention in mood disorders and in the general population: a systematic review. Neurosci Biobehav Rev 116:142–153, 2020 32561344

Diav-Citrin O, Shechtman S, Tahover E, et al: Pregnancy outcome following in utero exposure to lithium: a prospective, comparative, observational study. Am J Psychiatry 171(7):785–794, 2014 24781368

Do A, Keramatian K, Schaffer A, et al: Cariprazine in the treatment of bipolar disorder: within and beyond clinical trials. Front Psychiatry 12:769897, 2021 34970166

Donovan SJ, Susser ES, Nunes EV, et al: Divalproex treatment of disruptive adolescents: a report of 10 cases. J Clin Psychiatry 58(1):12–15, 1997 9055831

Dubovsky SL, Franks RD, Lifschitz M, et al: Effectiveness of verapamil in the treatment of a manic patient. Am J Psychiatry 139(4):502–504, 1982 7065298

Durgam S, Earley W, Lipschitz A, et al: An 8-week randomized, double-blind, placebo-controlled evaluation of the safety and efficacy of cariprazine in patients with bipolar I depression. Am J Psychiatry 173(3):271–281, 2016 26541814

Eberle AJ: Valproate and polycystic ovaries. J Am Acad Child Adolesc Psychiatry 37(10):1009, 1998 9785710

Emrich HM: Studies with oxcarbazepine (Trileptal) in acute mania. Int Clin Psychopharmacol 5(suppl):83–88, 1990

Erfurth A, Kammerer C, Grunze H, et al: An open label study of gabapentin in the treatment of acute mania. J Psychiatr Res 32(5):261–264, 1998a 9789203

Erfurth A, Walden J, Grunze H: Lamotrigine in the treatment of schizoaffective disorder. Neuropsychobiology 38(3):204–205, 1998b 9778612

Faedda GL, Tondo L, Baldessarini RJ, et al: Outcome after rapid vs gradual discontinuation of lithium treatment in bipolar disorders. Arch Gen Psychiatry 50(6):448–455, 1993 8498879

Fatemi SH, Rapport DJ, Calabrese JR, et al: Lamotrigine in rapid-cycling bipolar disorder. J Clin Psychiatry 58(12):522–527, 1997 9448654

Filaković P, Erić AP: Pharmacotherapy of suicidal behaviour in major depression, schizophrenia and bipolar disorder. Coll Antropol 37(3):1039–1044, 2013 24308257

Fogelson DL, Sternbach H: Lamotrigine treatment of refractory bipolar disorder. J Clin Psychiatry 58(6):271–273, 1997 9228895

Fountoulakis KN, Kontis D, Gonda X, et al: A systematic review of the evidence on the treatment of rapid cycling bipolar disorder. Bipolar Disord 15(2):115–137, 2013 23437958

Frampton JE, Foster RH: Pregabalin: in the treatment of generalised anxiety disorder. CNS Drugs 20(8):685–693, 2006 16863276

Frangou S, Lewis M, McCrone P: Efficacy of ethyl-eicosapentaenoic acid in bipolar depression: randomised double-blind placebo-controlled study. Br J Psychiatry 188:46–50, 2006 16388069

Freeman MP, Hibbeln JR, Wisner KL, et al: Randomized dose-ranging pilot trial of omega-3 fatty acids for postpartum depression. Acta Psychiatr Scand 113(1):31–35, 2006 16390366

Freeman TW, Clothier JL, Pazzaglia P, et al: A double-blind comparison of valproate and lithium in the treatment of acute mania. Am J Psychiatry 149(1):108–111, 1992 1728157

Frye MA, Ketter TA, Kimbrell TA, et al: A placebo-controlled study of lamotrigine and gabapentin monotherapy in refractory mood disorders. J Clin Psychopharmacol 20(6):607–614, 2000 11106131

Geddes JR, Burgess S, Hawton K, et al: Long-term lithium therapy for bipolar disorder: systematic review and meta-analysis of randomized controlled trials. Am J Psychiatry 161(2):217–222, 2004 14754766

Gentile S: Lithium in pregnancy: the need to treat, the duty to ensure safety. Expert Opin Drug Saf 11(3):425–437, 2012 22400907

Geracioti TD, Jr: Valproic acid treatment of episodic explosiveness related to brain injury. J Clin Psychiatry 55(9):416–417, 1994 7929025

Ghaemi SN, Zablotsky B, Filkowski MM, et al: An open prospective study of zonisamide in acute bipolar depression. J Clin Psychopharmacol 26(4):385–388, 2006 16855456

Ghaemi SN, Shirzadi AA, Klugman J, et al: Is adjunctive open-label zonisamide effective for bipolar disorder? J Affect Disord 105(1–3):311–314, 2008 17586053

Giles JJ, Bannigan JG: Teratogenic and developmental effects of lithium. Curr Pharm Des 12(12):1531–1541, 2006 16611133

Gitlin MJ: Lithium-induced renal insufficiency. J Clin Psychopharmacol 13(4):276–279, 1993 8376615

Gitlin M: Lithium and the kidney: an updated review. Drug Saf 20(3):231–243, 1999 10221853

Goedhard LE, Stolker JJ, Heerdink ER, et al: Pharmacotherapy for the treatment of aggressive behavior in general adult psychiatry: a systematic review. J Clin Psychiatry 67(7):1013–1024, 2006 16889443

Goodwin FK, Jamison KR: Manic-Depressive Illness. New York, Oxford University Press, 1990

Goodwin GM, Bowden CL, Calabrese JR, et al: A pooled analysis of 2 placebo-controlled 18-month trials of lamotrigine and lithium maintenance in bipolar I disorder. J Clin Psychiatry 65(3):432–441, 2004 15096085

Gordon A, Price LH: Mood stabilization and weight loss with topiramate. Am J Psychiatry 156(6):968–969, 1999 10360144

Gorson KC, Schott C, Herman R, et al: Gabapentin in the treatment of painful diabetic neuropathy: a placebo controlled, double blind, crossover trial. J Neurol Neurosurg Psychiatry 66(2):251–252, 1999 10071116

Green AI, Tohen M, Patel JK, et al: Clozapine in the treatment of refractory psychotic mania. Am J Psychiatry 157(6):982–986, 2000 10831480

Greil W, Kleindienst N, Erazo N, et al: Differential response to lithium and carbamazepine in the prophylaxis of bipolar disorder. J Clin Psychopharmacol 18(6):455–460, 1998 9864077

Grunze H, Erfurth A, Amann B, et al: Intravenous valproate loading in acutely manic and depressed bipolar I patients. J Clin Psychopharmacol 19(4):303–309, 1999a 10440456

Grunze H, Erfurth A, Marcuse A, et al: Tiagabine appears not to be efficacious in the treatment of acute mania. J Clin Psychiatry 60(11):759–762, 1999b 10584764

Grunze H, Kotlik E, Costa R, et al: Assessment of the efficacy and safety of eslicarbazepine acetate in acute mania and prevention of recurrence: experience from multicentre, double-blind, randomised phase II clinical studies in patients with bipolar disorder I. J Affect Disord 174:70–82, 2015 25484179

Guzzetta F, Tondo L, Centorrino F, et al: Lithium treatment reduces suicide risk in recurrent major depressive disorder. J Clin Psychiatry 68(3):380–383, 2007 17388706

Hardoy MC, Hardoy MJ, Carta MG, et al: Gabapentin as a promising treatment for antipsychotic-induced movement disorders in schizoaffective and bipolar patients. J Affect Disord 54(3):315–317, 1999 10467977

Häuser W, Bernardy K, Uçeyler N, et al: Treatment of fibromyalgia syndrome with gabapentin and pregabalin—a meta-analysis of randomized controlled trials. Pain 145(1–2):69–81, 2009 19539427

Herrmann N: Valproic acid treatment of agitation in dementia. Can J Psychiatry 43(1):69–72, 1998 9494750

Hilty DM, Rodriguez GD, Hales RE: Intravenous valproate for rapid stabilization of agitation in neuropsychiatric disorders. J Neuropsychiatry Clin Neurosci 10(3):365–366, 1998 9706547

Hirschman S, Dolberg OT, Stern L, et al: The use of valproic acid in the treatment of borderline personality disorder [in Hebrew]. Harefuah 133(5–6):205–208, 1997 9461692

Hollander E, Swann AC, Coccaro EF, et al: Impact of trait impulsivity and state aggression on divalproex versus placebo response in borderline personality disorder. Am J Psychiatry 162(3):621–624, 2005 15741486

Horton S, Tuerk A, Cook D, et al: Maximum recommended dosage of lithium for pregnant women based on a PBPK model for lithium absorption. Adv Bioinforma 2012:352729, 2012 22693500

Hsiao YT, Wei IH, Huang CC: Oxcarbazepine-related neutropenia: a case report. J Clin Psychopharmacol 30(1):94–95, 2010 20075666

Huband N, Ferriter M, Nathan R, et al: Antiepileptics for aggression and associated impulsivity. Cochrane Database Syst Rev 2010(2):CD003499, 2010 20166067

Isojärvi JI, Laatikainen TJ, Pakarinen AJ, et al: Polycystic ovaries and hyperandrogenism in women taking valproate for epilepsy. N Engl J Med 329(19):1383–1388, 1993 8413434

Jacobsen FM: Low-dose valproate: a new treatment for cyclothymia, mild rapid cycling disorders, and premenstrual syndrome. J Clin Psychiatry 54(6):229–234, 1993 8331092

Jefferson JW, Greist JH, Ackerman DL, et al: Lithium Encyclopedia for Clinical Practice, 2nd Edition. Washington, DC, American Psychiatric Press, 1987

Joffe H, Cohen LS: Presentation at the 157th Annual Meeting of the American Psychiatric Association, New York City, May 1–6, 2004

Joffe H, Cohen LS, Suppes T, et al: Longitudinal follow-up of reproductive and metabolic features of valproate-associated polycystic ovarian syndrome features: a preliminary report. Biol Psychiatry 60(12):1378–1381, 2006 16950230

Jope RS: Anti-bipolar therapy: mechanism of action of lithium. Mol Psychiatry 4(2):117–128, 1999 10208444

Judd LL, Schettler PJ, Akiskal HS, et al: Long-term symptomatic status of bipolar I vs. bipolar II disorders. Int J Neuropsychopharmacol 6(2):127–137, 2003 12890306

Juruena MF, Ottoni GL, Machado-Vieira R, et al: Bipolar I and II disorder residual symptoms: oxcarbazepine and carbamazepine as add-on treatment to lithium in a double-blind, randomized trial. Prog Neuropsychopharmacol Biol Psychiatry 33(1):94–99, 2009 19007842

Kamali M, Krishnamurthy VB, Baweja R, et al: Lithium, in The American Psychiatric Association Publishing Textbook of Psychopharmacology, 5th Edition. Edited by Schatzberg AF, Nemeroff CB. Washington, DC, American Psychiatric Association Publishing, 2017, pp 889–921

Katz IR, Rogers MP, Lew R, et al: Lithium treatment in the prevention of repeat suicide-related outcomes in veterans with major depression or bipolar disorder: a randomized clinical trial. JAMA Psychiatry 79(1):24–32, 2022 34787653

Kaufman KR, Gerner R: Lamotrigine toxicity secondary to sertraline. Seizure 7(2):163–165, 1998 9627209

Keck PE Jr, McElroy SL, Tugrul KC, et al: Valproate oral loading in the treatment of acute mania. J Clin Psychiatry 54(8):305–308, 1993a 8253698

Keck PE Jr, Taylor VE, Tugrul KC, et al: Valproate treatment of panic disorder and lactate-induced panic attacks. Biol Psychiatry 33(7):542–546, 1993b 8513040

Keck PE Jr, Marcus R, Tourkodimitris S, et al: A placebo-controlled, double-blind study of the efficacy and safety of aripiprazole in patients with acute bipolar mania. Am J Psychiatry 160(9):1651–1658, 2003a 12944341

Keck PE Jr, Versiani M, Potkin S, et al: Ziprasidone in the treatment of acute bipolar mania: a three-week, placebo-controlled, double-blind, randomized trial. Am J Psychiatry 160(4):741–748, 2003b 12668364

Keck PE Jr, Mintz J, McElroy SL, et al: Double-blind, randomized, placebo-controlled trials of ethyl-eicosapentanoate in the treatment of bipolar depression and rapid cycling bipolar disorder. Biol Psychiatry 60(9):1020–1022, 2006 16814257

Kemp DE, Gao K, Fein EB, et al: Lamotrigine as add-on treatment to lithium and divalproex: lessons learned from a double-blind, placebo-controlled trial in rapid-cycling bipolar disorder. Bipolar Disord 14(7):780–789, 2012 23107222

Kessel JB, Verghese C, Simpson GM: Neurotoxicity related to lithium and neuroleptic combinations? A retrospective review. J Psychiatry Neurosci 17(1):28–30, 1992 1349826

Ketter TA: Monotherapy versus combined treatment with second-generation antipsychotics in bipolar disorder. J Clin Psychiatry 69(Suppl 5):9–15, 2008 19265635

Ketter TA, Winsberg ME, DeGolia SG, et al: Rapid efficacy of olanzapine augmentation in nonpsychotic bipolar mixed states. J Clin Psychiatry 59(2):83–85, 1998 9501894

Kimmel SE, Calabrese JR, Woyshville MJ, et al: Clozapine in treatment-refractory mood disorders. J Clin Psychiatry 55(Suppl B):91–93, 1994 7961583

Kishimoto A, Ogura C, Hazama H, et al: Long-term prophylactic effects of carbamazepine in affective disorder. Br J Psychiatry 143:327–331, 1983 6626851

Kocsis JH, Shaw ED, Stokes PE, et al: Neuropsychologic effects of lithium discontinuation. J Clin Psychopharmacol 13(4):268–275, 1993 8376614

Koek RJ, Yerevanian BI: Is lamotrigine effective for treatment-refractory mania? Pharmacopsychiatry 31(1):35, 1998 9524984

Kotler M, Matar MA: Lamotrigine in the treatment of resistant bipolar disorder. Clin Neuropharmacol 21(1):65–67, 1998 9579289

Kotwal R, Guerdjikova A, McElroy SL, et al: Lithium augmentation of topiramate for bipolar disorder with comorbid binge eating disorder and obesity. Hum Psychopharmacol 21(7):425–431, 2006 16941522

Krüger S, Trevor Young L, Bräunig P: Pharmacotherapy of bipolar mixed states. Bipolar Disord 7(3):205–215, 2005 15898959

Kunik ME, Puryear L, Orengo CA, et al: The efficacy and tolerability of divalproex sodium in elderly demented patients with behavioral disturbances. Int J Geriatr Psychiatry 13(1):29–34, 1998 9489578

Kushner SF, Khan A, Lane R, et al: Topiramate monotherapy in the management of acute mania: results of four double-blind placebo-controlled trials. Bipolar Disord 8(1):15–27, 2006 16411977

Kusumakar V, Yatham LN: Lamotrigine treatment of rapid cycling bipolar disorder. Am J Psychiatry 154(8):1171–1172, 1997a 9247416

Kusumakar V, Yatham LN: An open study of lamotrigine in refractory bipolar depression. Psychiatry Res 72(2):145–148, 1997b 9335206

Lambert PA, Venaud G: A comparative study of valpromide versus lithium in the treatment of affective disorders. Nervure 5(2):57–65, 1992

Lampl C, Buzath A, Klinger D, et al: Lamotrigine in the prophylactic treatment of migraine aura—a pilot study. Cephalalgia 19(1):58–63, 1999 10099861

Lenox RH, Newhouse PA, Creelman WL, et al: Adjunctive treatment of manic agitation with lorazepam versus haloperidol: a double-blind study. J Clin Psychiatry 53(2):47–52, 1992 1541605

Letterman L, Markowitz JS: Gabapentin: a review of published experience in the treatment of bipolar disorder and other psychiatric conditions. Pharmacotherapy 19(5):565–572, 1999 10331819

Lindenmayer JP, Klebanov R: Olanzapine-induced manic-like syndrome. J Clin Psychiatry 59(6):318–319, 1998 9671347

Loebel A, Cucchiaro J, Silva R, et al: Lurasidone as adjunctive therapy with lithium or valproate for the treatment of bipolar I depression: a randomized, double-blind, placebo-controlled study. Am J Psychiatry 171(2):169–177, 2014 24170221

Lonergan ET, Cameron M, Luxenberg J: Valproic acid for agitation in dementia. Cochrane Database Syst Rev 2(2):CD003945, 2004 15106227

Lott AD, McElroy SL, Keys MA: Valproate in the treatment of behavioral agitation in elderly patients with dementia. J Neuropsychiatry Clin Neurosci 7(3):314–319, 1995 7580190

MacMillan CM, Korndörfer SR, Rao S, et al: A comparison of divalproex and oxcarbazepine in aggressive youth with bipolar disorder. J Psychiatr Pract 12(4):214–222, 2006 16883146

Mahmoudi-Gharaei J, Shahrivar Z, Faghihi T, et al: Topiramate versus valproate sodium as adjunctive therapies to a combination of lithium and risperidone for adolescents with bipolar I disorder: effects on weight and serum lipid profiles. Iran J Psychiatry 7(1):1–10, 2012 23056111

Marangell LB, Martinez JM, Zboyan HA, et al: A double-blind, placebo-controlled study of the omega-3 fatty acid docosahexaenoic acid in the treatment of major depression. Am J Psychiatry 160(5):996–998, 2003 12727707

Mason BJ, Crean R, Goodell V, et al: A proof-of-concept randomized controlled study of gabapentin: effects on cannabis use, withdrawal and executive function deficits in cannabis-dependent adults. Neuropsychopharmacology 37(7):1689–1698, 2012 22373942

Mason BJ, Quello S, Goodell V, et al: Gabapentin treatment for alcohol dependence: a randomized clinical trial. JAMA Intern Med 174(1):70–77, 2014 24190578

Massot O, Rousselle JC, Fillion MP, et al: 5-HT1B receptors: a novel target for lithium: possible involvement in mood disorders. Neuropsychopharmacology 21(4):530–541, 1999 10481837

McElroy SL, Keck PE Jr, Tugrul KC, et al: Valproate as a loading treatment in acute mania. Neuropsychobiology 27(3):146–149, 1993 8232829

McElroy SL, Suppes T, Keck PE Jr, et al: Open-label adjunctive zonisamide in the treatment of bipolar disorders: a prospective trial. J Clin Psychiatry 66(5):617–624, 2005 15889949

McElroy SL, Winstanley E, Mori N, et al: A randomized, placebo-controlled study of zonisamide to prevent olanzapine-associated weight gain. J Clin Psychopharmacol 32(2):165–172, 2012 22367654

McIntyre RS, Alsuwaidan M, Goldstein BI, et al: The Canadian Network for Mood and Anxiety Treatments (CANMAT) task force recommendations for the management of patients with mood disorders and comorbid metabolic disorders. Ann Clin Psychiatry 24(1):69–81, 2012 22303523

Meador KJ, Baker GA, Browning N, et al: Cognitive function at 3 years of age after fetal exposure to antiepileptic drugs. N Engl J Med 360(16):1597–1605, 2009 19369666

Meador KJ, Baker GA, Browning N, et al: Fetal antiepileptic drug exposure and cognitive outcomes at age 6 years (NEAD study): a prospective observational study. Lancet Neurol 12(3):244–252, 2013 23352199

Mishory A, Yaroslavsky Y, Bersudsky Y, et al: Phenytoin as an antimanic anticonvulsant: a controlled study. Am J Psychiatry 157(3):463–465, 2000 10698828

Morello CM, Leckband SG, Stoner CP, et al: Randomized double-blind study comparing the efficacy of gabapentin with amitriptyline on diabetic peripheral neuropathy pain. Arch Intern Med 159(16):1931–1937, 1999 10493324

Morrell MJ, Hayes FJ, Sluss PM, et al: Hyperandrogenism, ovulatory dysfunction, and polycystic ovary syndrome with valproate versus lamotrigine. Ann Neurol 64(2):200–211, 2008 18756476

Muzina DJ, Gao K, Kemp DE, et al: Acute efficacy of divalproex sodium versus placebo in mood stabilizer-naive bipolar I or II depression: a double-blind, randomized, placebo-controlled trial. J Clin Psychiatry 72(6):813–819, 2011 20816041

Mylonakis E, Vittorio CC, Hollik DA, et al: Lamotrigine overdose presenting as anticonvulsant hypersensitivity syndrome. Ann Pharmacother 33(5):557–559, 1999 10369617

Myrick H, Malcolm R, Brady KT: Gabapentin treatment of alcohol withdrawal. Am J Psychiatry 155(11):1632, 1998 9812141

Nath K, Bhattacharya A, Praharaj SK: Eslicarbazepine acetate in the management of refractory bipolar disorder. Clin Neuropharmacol 35(6):295, 2012 23151469

Nemets H, Nemets B, Apter A, et al: Omega-3 treatment of childhood depression: a controlled, double-blind pilot study. Am J Psychiatry 163(6):1098–1100, 2006 16741212

Nierenberg AA, Fava M, Trivedi MH, et al: A comparison of lithium and T(3) augmentation following two failed medication treatments for depression: a STAR*D report. Am J Psychiatry 163(9):1519–1530, quiz 1665, 2006a 16946176

Nierenberg AA, Ostacher MJ, Calabrese JR, et al: Treatment-resistant bipolar depression: a STEP-BD equipoise randomized effectiveness trial of antidepressant augmentation with lamotrigine, inositol, or risperidone. Am J Psychiatry 163(2):210–216, 2006b 16449473

Nierenberg AA, Friedman ES, Bowden CL, et al: Lithium treatment moderate-dose use study (LiTMUS) for bipolar disorder: a randomized comparative effectiveness trial of optimized personalized treatment with and without lithium. Am J Psychiatry 170(1):102–110, 2013 23288387

Nierenberg AA, McElroy SF, Friedman ES, et al: Bipolar CHOICE: a pragmatic 6-month trial of lithium versus quetiapine for bipolar disorder. J Clin Psychiatry 77:90–99, 2016 26845264

Okuma T: Effects of carbamazepine and lithium on affective disorders. Neuropsychobiology 27(3):138–145, 1993 8232828

Ontiveros A, Fontaine R: Sodium valproate and clonazepam for treatment-resistant panic disorder. J Psychiatry Neurosci 17(2):78–80, 1992 1637803

Owen RT: Extended-release carbamazepine for acute bipolar mania: a review. Drugs Today (Barc) 42(5):283–289, 2006 16801991

Padhy R, Saxena K, Remsing L, et al: Symptomatic response to divalproex in subtypes of conduct disorder. Child Psychiatry Hum Dev 42(5):584–593, 2011 21706221

Pande AC, Davidson JR, Jefferson JW, et al: Treatment of social phobia with gabapentin: a placebo-controlled study. J Clin Psychopharmacol 19(4):341–348, 1999 10440462

Patkar A, Gilmer W, Pae CU, et al: A 6 week randomized double-blind placebo-controlled trial of ziprasidone for the acute depressive mixed state. PLoS One 7(4):e34757, 2012 22545088

Patorno E, Huybrechts KF, Bateman BT, et al: Lithium use in pregnancy and the risk of cardiac malformations. N Engl J Med 376(23):2245–2254, 2017 28591541

Perlis RH, Baker RW, Zarate CA Jr, et al: Olanzapine versus risperidone in the treatment of manic or mixed states in bipolar I disorder: a randomized, double-blind trial. J Clin Psychiatry 67(11):1747–1753, 2006 17196055

Pinto OC, Akiskal HS: Lamotrigine as a promising approach to borderline personality: an open case series without concurrent DSM-IV major mood disorder. J Affect Disord 51(3):333–343, 1998 10333987

Pope HGJr, McElroy SL, Keck PE Jr, et al: Valproate in the treatment of acute mania: a placebo-controlled study. Arch Gen Psychiatry 48(1):62–68, 1991 1984763

Post RM, Weiss SR, Chuang DM: Mechanisms of action of anticonvulsants in affective disorders: comparisons with lithium. J Clin Psychopharmacol 12(1)(suppl):23S–35S, 1992 1541715

Post RM, Leverich GS, Altshuler LL, et al: An overview of recent findings of the Stanley Foundation Bipolar Network (part I). Bipolar Disord 5(5):310–319, 2003 14525551

Post RM, Altshuler LL, Frye MA, et al: Preliminary observations on the effectiveness of levetiracetam in the open adjunctive treatment of refractory bipolar disorder. J Clin Psychiatry 66(3):370–374, 2005 15766304

Pratoomsri W, Yatham LN, Sohn CH, et al: Oxcarbazepine add-on in the treatment of refractory bipolar disorder. Bipolar Disord 7(Suppl 5):37–42, 2005 16225559

Preskorn SH, Zeller S, Citrome L, et al: Effect of sublingual dexmedetomidine vs placebo on acute agitation associated with bipolar disorder: a randomized clinical trial. JAMA 327(8):727–736, 2022 35191924

Prien RF, Kupfer DJ, Mansky PA, et al: Drug therapy in the prevention of recurrences in unipolar and bipolar affective disorders. Report of the NIMH Collaborative Study Group comparing lithium carbonate, imipramine, and a lithium carbonate-imipramine combination. Arch Gen Psychiatry 41(11):1096–1104, 1984 6437366

Rasgon N: The relationship between polycystic ovary syndrome and antiepileptic drugs: a review of the evidence. J Clin Psychopharmacol 24(3):322–334, 2004 15118487

Rasgon NL, Altshuler LL, Fairbanks L, et al: Reproductive function and risk for PCOS in women treated for bipolar disorder. Bipolar Disord 7(3):246–259, 2005 15898962

Ravindran AV, Jones BW, al-Zaid K, et al: Effective treatment of mania with olanzapine: 2 case reports. J Psychiatry Neurosci 22(5):345–346, 1997 9401315

Reeves RR, McBride WA, Brannon GE: Olanzapine-induced mania. J Am Osteopath Assoc 98(10):549–550, 1998 9821737

Rowbotham M, Harden N, Stacey B, et al: Gabapentin for the treatment of postherpetic neuralgia: a randomized controlled trial. JAMA 280(21):1837–1842, 1998 9846778

Ruedrich S, Swales TP, Fossaceca C, et al: Effect of divalproex sodium on aggression and self-injurious behaviour in adults with intellectual disability: a retrospective review. J Intellect Disabil Res 43(Pt 2):105–111, 1999 10221790

Sachs G, Bowden C, Calabrese JR, et al: Effects of lamotrigine and lithium on body weight during maintenance treatment of bipolar I disorder. Bipolar Disord 8(2):175–181, 2006 16542188

Sachs GS, Nierenberg AA, Calabrese JR, et al: Effectiveness of adjunctive antidepressant treatment for bipolar depression. N Engl J Med 356(17):1711–1722, 2007 17392295

Sachs GS, Greenberg WM, Starace A, et al: Cariprazine in the treatment of acute mania in bipolar I disorder: a double-blind, placebo-controlled, Phase III trial. J Affect Disord 174:296–302, 2015 25532076

Salzman C, Solomon D, Miyawaki E, et al: Parenteral lorazepam versus parenteral haloperidol for the control of psychotic disruptive behavior. J Clin Psychiatry 52(4):177–180, 1991 1673123

Saricicek A, Maloney K, Muralidharan A, et al: Levetiracetam in the management of bipolar depression: a randomized, double-blind, placebo-controlled trial. J Clin Psychiatry 72(6):744–750, 2011 21034692

Saxena K, Howe M, Simeonova D, et al: Divalproex sodium reduces overall aggression in youth at high risk for bipolar disorder. J Child Adolesc Psychopharmacol 16(3):252–259, 2006 16768633

Schaffer LC, Schaffer CB, Miller AR, et al: An open trial of pregabalin as an acute and maintenance adjunctive treatment for outpatients with treatment resistant bipolar disorder. J Affect Disord 147(1–3):407–410, 2013 23040739

Scherk H, Pajonk FG, Leucht S: Second-generation antipsychotic agents in the treatment of acute mania: a systematic review and meta-analysis of randomized controlled trials. Arch Gen Psychiatry 64(4):442–455, 2007 17404121

Schou M: The range of clinical uses of lithium, in Lithium in Medical Practice. Edited by Johnson FN, Johnson S. Baltimore, MD, University Park Press, 1978, pp 21–39

Schou M: Artistic productivity and lithium prophylaxis in manic-depressive illness. Br J Psychiatry 135:97–103, 1979 497639

Sobotka JL, Alexander B, Cook BL: A review of carbamazepine's hematologic reactions and monitoring recommendations. DICP 24(12):1214–1219, 1990 2089834

Solmi M, Veronese N, Zaninotto L, et al: Lamotrigine compared to placebo and other agents with antidepressant activity in patients with unipolar and bipolar depression: a comprehensive meta-analysis of efficacy and safety outcomes in short-term trials. CNS Spectr 21(5):403–418, 2016 27686028

Song J, Sjölander A, Joas E, et al: Suicidal behavior during lithium and valproate treatment: a within-individual 8-year prospective study of 50,000 patients with bipolar disorder. Am J Psychiatry 174(8):795–802, 2017 28595491

Stein DJ, Simeon D, Frenkel M, et al: An open trial of valproate in borderline personality disorder. J Clin Psychiatry 56(11):506–510, 1995 7592502

Steiner H, Petersen ML, Saxena K, et al: Divalproex sodium for the treatment of conduct disorder: a randomized controlled clinical trial. J Clin Psychiatry 64(10):1183–1191, 2003 14658966

Stephen LJ, Sills GJ, Brodie MJ: Lamotrigine and topiramate may be a useful combination. Lancet 351(9107):958–959, 1998 9734949

Stoll AL, Severus WE, Freeman MP, et al: Omega 3 fatty acids in bipolar disorder: a preliminary double-blind, placebo-controlled trial. Arch Gen Psychiatry 56(5):407–412, 1999 10232294

Suppes T, Baldessarini RJ, Faedda GL, et al: Discontinuation of maintenance treatment in bipolar disorder: risks and implications. Harv Rev Psychiatry 1(3):131–144, 1993 9384841

Suppes T, Phillips KA, Judd CR: Clozapine treatment of nonpsychotic rapid cycling bipolar disorder: a report of three cases. Biol Psychiatry 36(5):338–340, 1994 7993960

Suppes T, Chisholm KA, Dhavale D, et al: Tiagabine in treatment refractory bipolar disorder: a clinical case series. Bipolar Disord 4(5):283–289, 2002 12479659

Suppes T, Kelly DI, Hynan LS, et al: Comparison of two anticonvulsants in a randomized, single-blind treatment of hypomanic symptoms in patients with bipolar disorder. Aust N Z J Psychiatry 41(5):397–402, 2007 17464731

Suppes T, Silva R, Cucchiaro J, et al: Lurasidone for the treatment of major depressive disorder with mixed features: a randomized, double-blind, placebo-controlled study. Am J Psychiatry 173(4):400–407, 2016 26552942

Szczepankiewicz A: Evidence for single nucleotide polymorphisms and their association with bipolar disorder. Neuropsychiatr Dis Treat 9:1573–1582, 2013 24143106

Tariot PN, Schneider LS, Cummings J, et al: Chronic divalproex sodium to attenuate agitation and clinical progression of Alzheimer disease. Arch Gen Psychiatry 68(8):853–861, 2011 21810649

Tohen M, Sanger TM, McElroy SL, et al: Olanzapine versus placebo in the treatment of acute mania. Am J Psychiatry 156(5):702–709, 1999 10327902

Tohen M, Ketter TA, Zarate CA, et al: Olanzapine versus divalproex sodium for the treatment of acute mania and maintenance of remission: a 47-week study. Am J Psychiatry 160(7):1263–1271, 2003a 12832240

Tohen M, Vieta E, Calabrese J, et al: Efficacy of olanzapine and olanzapine-fluoxetine combination in the treatment of bipolar I depression. Arch Gen Psychiatry 60(11):1079–1088, 2003b 14609883

Tondo L, Hennen J, Baldessarini RJ: Lower suicide risk with long-term lithium treatment in major affective illness: a meta-analysis. Acta Psychiatr Scand 104(3):163–172, 2001 11531653

Tupin J: Management of violent patients, in Manual of Psychiatric Therapeutics. Edited by Shader RI. Boston, MA, Little, Brown, 1975, pp 125–133 van der Loos ML, Mulder PG, Hartong EG, et al: Efficacy and safety of lamotrigine as add-on treatment to lithium in bipolar depression: a multicenter, double-blind, placebo-controlled trial. J Clin Psychiatry 70(2):223–231, 2009 19200421

Vasudev A, Macritchie K, Watson S, et al: Oxcarbazepine in the maintenance treatment of bipolar disorder. Cochrane Database Syst Rev 2008(1):CD005171, 2008 18254071

Vasudev A, Macritchie K, Rao SN, et al: Tiagabine in the maintenance treatment of bipolar disorder. Cochrane Database Syst Rev 2011(12):CD005173, 2011a 22161389

Vasudev A, Macritchie K, Vasudev K, et al: Oxcarbazepine for acute affective episodes in bipolar disorder. Cochrane Database Syst Rev 2011(12):CD004857, 2011b 22161387

Vasudev A, Macritchie K, Rao SK, et al: Tiagabine for acute affective episodes in bipolar disorder. Cochrane Database Syst Rev 2012(12):CD004694, 2012 23235614

Vieta E, Sánchez-Moreno J, Goikolea JM, et al: Effects on weight and outcome of long-term olanzapine-topiramate combination treatment in bipolar disorder. J Clin Psychopharmacol 24(4):374–378, 2004 15232327

Vieta E, Cruz N, García-Campayo J, et al: A double-blind, randomized, placebo-controlled prophylaxis trial of oxcarbazepine as adjunctive treatment to lithium in the long-term treatment of bipolar I and II disorder. Int J Neuropsychopharmacol 11(4):445–452, 2008 18346292

Vinten J, Adab N, Kini U, et al: Neuropsychological effects of exposure to anticonvulsant medication in utero. Neurology 64(6):949–954, 2005 15781806

Wagner KD, Kowatch RA, Emslie GJ, et al: A double-blind, randomized, placebo-controlled trial of oxcarbazepine in the treatment of bipolar disorder in children and adolescents (erratum: Am J Psychiatry 163:1843, 2006). Am J Psychiatry 163(7):1179–1186, 2006 16816222

Wang PW, Yang YS, Chandler RA, et al: Adjunctive zonisamide for weight loss in euthymic bipolar disorder patients: a pilot study. J Psychiatr Res 42(6):451–457, 2008 17628595

Weisler RH, Ahearn EP, Davidson JR, et al: Adjunctive use of olanzapine in mood disorders: five case reports. Ann Clin Psychiatry 9(4):259–262, 1997 9511951

Weisler RH, Hirschfeld R, Cutler AJ, et al: Extended-release carbamazepine capsules as monotherapy in bipolar disorder: pooled results from two randomised, double-blind, placebo-controlled trials. CNS Drugs 20(3):219–231, 2006 16529527

Wensel TM, Powe KW, Cates ME: Pregabalin for the treatment of generalized anxiety disorder. Ann Pharmacother 46(3):424–429, 2012 22395254

Wilcox JA: Divalproex sodium as a treatment for borderline personality disorder. Ann Clin Psychiatry 7(1):33–37, 1995 8541935

Woodman CL, Noyes R Jr: Panic disorder: treatment with valproate. J Clin Psychiatry 55(4):134–136, 1994 8071256

Wroblewski BA, Joseph AB, Kupfer J, et al: Effectiveness of valproic acid on destructive and aggressive behaviours in patients with acquired brain injury. Brain Inj 11(1):37–47, 1997 9012550

Xie X, Hagan RM: Cellular and molecular actions of lamotrigine: possible mechanisms of efficacy in bipolar disorder. Neuropsychobiology 38(3):119–130, 1998 9778599

Yip VL, Marson AG, Jorgensen AL, et al: HLA genotype and carbamazepine-induced cutaneous adverse drug reactions: a systematic review. Clin Pharmacol Ther 92(6):757–765, 2012 23132554

Young AH, Geddes JR, Macritchie K, et al: Tiagabine in the maintenance treatment of bipolar disorders. Cochrane Database Syst Rev 3(3):CD005173, 2006a 16856081

Young AH, Geddes JR, Macritchie K, et al: Tiagabine in the treatment of acute affective episodes in bipolar disorder: efficacy and acceptability. Cochrane Database Syst Rev 3(3):CD004694, 2006b 16856056

Zajecka JM, Weisler R, Sachs G, et al: A comparison of the efficacy, safety, and tolerability of divalproex sodium and olanzapine in the treatment of bipolar disorder. J Clin Psychiatry 63(12):1148–1155, 2002 12523875

Zarghami M, Sheikhmoonesi F, Ala S, et al: A comparative study of beneficial effects of olanzapine and sodium valproate on aggressive behavior of patients who are on methadone maintenance therapy: a randomized triple blind clinical trial. Eur Rev Med Pharmacol Sci 17(8):1073–1081, 2013 23661521

Zullino D, Baumann P: Olanzapine for mixed episodes of bipolar disorder (letter). J Psychopharmacol 13(2):198, 1999 10475728

6

Antianxiety Agents

Anxiolytic agents—usually defined in the past as chiefly the benzodiazepines—are among the most commonly used psychotropic drugs. The vast majority of prescriptions for these medications are written by primary care physicians. Psychiatrists write less than 20% of the prescriptions for anxiolytics in this country, reflecting, in part, the fact that most anxious patients never see psychiatrists. Moreover, anxiolytics are prescribed for a wide variety of patients who do not have a primary anxiety disorder—namely, patients who present to primary care physicians with somatic complaints or true somatic disease.

Antianxiety agents may be divided into many subclasses, of which the benzodiazepines are the most frequently prescribed. Several of the subclasses of anxiolytics (e.g., benzodiazepines) include agents that were originally marketed primarily as hypnotics (e.g., flurazepam). In this manual, we have separated the pharmacological treatments of anxiety from those of insomnia. The distinction, however, is rather artificial because most antianxiety drugs can be used at a low dose in the daytime for anxiety and at a similar or higher dose for difficulty in sleeping. Some hypnotics, such as eszopiclone, have somewhat more selective properties for sedation rather than anxiety, but even eszopiclone has some anxiolytic properties. This reflects common pharmacological effects on GABA$_A$ receptors. The Z-drugs, however, have less preferential or even little binding at benzodiazepine sites as compared with the benzodiazepines. On the other hand, it is clear that the sleep agent ramelteon (Rozerem), a melatonin agonist, does not appear to be a useful anxiolytic, and buspirone, an anxiolytic that is a partial agonist of the serotonin$_{1A}$ (5-HT$_{1A}$) receptor, does not appear to be a useful hypnotic. Likewise, dual orexin receptor antagonists—such as suvorexant—have not shown consistent anxiolytic properties.

The first major anxiolytic group, the *barbiturates*, were developed as sedative-hypnotic and antiepileptic agents and were first introduced in the early 1900s. These drugs are also discussed in Chapter 7 ("Hypnotics"). Meprobamate, a *carbamate* derivative, was introduced almost 60 years later as a sedative-anxiolytic agent. Although use of the two classes—barbiturates and carbamates—has waned dramatically in recent decades, they are still used on occasion.

Benzodiazepines, introduced in the early 1960s, dramatically changed the pharmacological approach to anxiety. Although they were first developed as muscle relaxants, their anxiolytic-hypnotic properties, wider safety margin in overdose, and potential to elicit physical dependence quickly became apparent. Buspirone, a 5-HT$_{1A}$ agonist with some mixed dopaminergic effects, was released in the United States in 1987 for use in anxiety. Its use by psychiatrists in the treatment of anxiety and related conditions was less than its use in primary care and nursing home settings (see "Buspirone" section in this chapter) (Cole and Yonkers 1995).

Increasingly, anticonvulsants are being used in the treatment of anxiety states. Agents such as gabapentin and pregabalin may be alternatives or adjuncts to the more commonly used antidepressants and benzodiazepines in treating some anxiety disorders.

Less widely used pharmacological approaches to anxiety include antihistamines and autonomic agents (e.g., β-blockers). The former have primarily a general sedative action; the latter are more commonly used than antihistamines and act by blocking peripheral or central noradrenergic activity and many of the manifestations of anxiety (e.g., tremor, palpitations, sweating). Several of the antipsychotics also have indications in anxiety, although in the United States they have become less widely used in recent years for this purpose. There is strong evidence, for example, that quetiapine is efficacious in the treatment of generalized anxiety disorder (GAD), but the FDA chose not to allow an indication for GAD because of the wide availability of anxiolytics that did not have the metabolic side effects of quetiapine. Thus, the safety concerns about the second-generation antipsychotics (SGAs) render them second- or third-line agents in the management of anxiety disorders.

Many antidepressants (mainly selective serotonin reuptake inhibitors [SSRIs] and serotonin-norepinephrine reuptake inhibitors [SNRIs] such as venlafaxine) have taken center stage in the treatment of the whole range of anxiety disorders but not in the treatment of insomnia. On the other hand, mirtazapine and trazodone are commonly used as hypnotic agents. Clomipramine is the only tricyclic antidepressant (TCA) shown to be consistently effective in the treatment of OCD. However, all the SSRIs are also presumably effective treatments for OCD (see "Obsessive-Compulsive Disorder" section later in this chapter). The SSRIs and related or unrelated drugs (e.g., gabapentin, venlafaxine) may already have become the primary drugs used by psychiatrists for the treatment of specific anxiety disorders, whereas benzodiazepines may still be the first drugs prescribed by primary care physicians.

In addition to this major shift in the patterns of treatment of anxiety disorders, there has been a major upsurge of interest in cognitive-behavioral therapy (CBT), whose efficacy has been shown in well-designed studies. Specific or semispecific programs have been designed to address the symptoms and treatment requirements of individual anxiety disorders. Almost all these programs, however, have elements of desensitization, exposure, and cognitive restructuring and include having the patient demonstrate new learning in real-life situations.

As a very general overview: benzodiazepines often work fastest in relieving symptoms, antidepressants (SSRIs and newer agents) take several weeks, and CBT may take 2 months or longer. There is some evidence that patients who show improvement while participating in CBT programs maintain the improvement longer after treatment is stopped than do patients who show improvement while receiving drug therapies (Barlow et al. 2000; DiMauro et al. 2013). Some older studies suggested that pharmacotherapy may enhance the effects of CBT in the treatment of anxiety disorders. For example, D-cycloserine, a glutamatergic agent, was shown to augment the effects of behavior therapy in several types of anxiety disorders (Hofmann et al. 2006; Norberg et al. 2008; Ressler et al. 2004). However, more recent evidence suggests that D-cycloserine probably does not add much to CBT (Ori et al. 2015). On the other hand, it may augment transcranial magnetic stimulation response (Cole et al. 2021).

We begin this chapter by discussing the use of benzodiazepines in treating general and panic anxiety. We then address the use of antidepressants in treating anxiety disorders, such as social phobia; trauma- and stressor-related disorders, such as PTSD; and obsessive-compulsive and related disorders, such as OCD and body dysmorphic disorder. Finally, we discuss the use of other classes of medication for anxiety and other conditions, such as catatonia, a syndrome uniquely responsive to sedative drugs and electroconvulsive therapy.

Because the SSRIs have already been considered in some detail in Chapter 3 ("Antidepressants"), we give them less detailed attention here. Several of the SSRIs and SNRIs have been approved by the FDA for one or more specific anxiety diagnoses, including paroxetine for GAD, PTSD, OCD, panic disorder, premenstrual dysphoric disorder (PMDD) (controlled-release form only), and social phobia; fluoxetine for OCD, bulimia, panic disorder, and PMDD; sertraline for OCD, panic disorder, PMDD, social anxiety disorder, and PTSD; escitalopram for GAD; venlafaxine (extended-release form) for GAD and social anxiety disorder; duloxetine for GAD; and fluvoxamine for social anxiety disorder and OCD. It is our position that until studies clearly show differences in efficacy between these drugs in the treatment of specific anxiety disorders, all SSRIs and at least some SNRIs are probably reasonably effective across most anxiety disorders. Their use in such conditions may require adjustments, but these apply to the specific disorder and the whole class of SSRIs. For example, use very low dosages (particularly initially) in patients with panic disorder with agoraphobia; use higher dosages and wait even longer for clinical response in patients with OCD.

Benzodiazepines

Clinical Indications

In addition to anxiety, benzodiazepines are indicated for muscle tension, insomnia, status epilepticus (diazepam), myoclonic epilepsy (clonazepam), preoperative anesthesia, and alcohol withdrawal. One benzodiazepine, the triazolo-benzodiazepine alprazolam, is also indicated for anxiety associated with depression (as is lorazepam), and some studies have shown that alprazolam also parallels many antidepressants in having both antipanic and antidepressant properties (see Chapter 3). Clonazepam is also approved in the

Benzodiazepines (e.g., diazepam, clonazepam, alprazolam): overview	
Efficacy	Generalized anxiety (FDA approved)
	Panic disorder (FDA approved for alprazolam, clonazepam)
	Insomnia (FDA approved)
	Seizure disorder (FDA approved for clonazepam)
	Muscle relaxation
	Anesthesia
	Alcohol withdrawal
Side effects	Sedation
	Lethargy
	Dependence/withdrawal
Safety in overdose	Safe in overdose up to 30 times the normal daily dose. Usual symptoms of overdose include sedation, drowsiness, ataxia, and slurred speech. May result in respiratory depression in combination with other CNS depressants. Management includes gastric lavage, forced emesis, and assisted ventilation.
Dosage and administration	Varies by benzodiazepine and indication (see Table 6–1)
Discontinuation	Taper by no more than 25% of total dose per week after long-term administration. Withdrawal includes insomnia, agitation, anxiety, and, rarely, seizures.
Drug interactions	Additive CNS depression with ethanol, barbiturates, and other CNS depressants
	Drugs that ↑ triazolo-benzodiazepine levels include CYP3A4 inhibitors, ketoconazole, fluconazole, nefazodone
	Drugs that ↓ triazolo-benzodiazepine levels include carbamazepine

Note. CYP = cytochrome P450.

treatment of panic disorder, and it is likely that all benzodiazepines are effective in the treatment of panic if given at high enough doses.

Likewise, all currently available benzodiazepines are useful in treating both chronic anxiety and anxiety secondary to life stresses or medical conditions. The definition of GAD in DSM-5-TR (American Psychiatric Association 2022) is probably too restrictive to cover all the forms of anxiety for which benzodiazepines can be helpful. It is even likely that there are "double anxiety" disorders, analogous to the concept of double depression; some patients have lifelong mild to moderate anxiety symptoms with episodic periods of worsening during which they seek therapy.

Panic disorder with or without agoraphobia is a chronic, fluctuating condition; some patients experience episodes of illness (like depressive episodes), whereas other patients have mild, infrequent attacks during some life phases and incapacitating symptoms at other times. Alprazolam is the only benzodiazepine officially deemed effective and well studied in the treatment of panic disorder with or without agoraphobia, although other benzodiazepines are also likely to be effective.

Both panic and GAD are conditions often accompanying other disorders, such as major depression, PTSD, and borderline personality disorder, as well as other specific anxiety disorders (e.g., social phobia). However, benzodiazepines are often counterproductive in the treatment of PTSD and Cluster B personality disorders.

It is likely that patients seen in primary care settings may show even more complex mixtures of milder anxiety and depressive symptoms than do patients seen by psychiatrists. The old-fashioned wastebasket diagnosis of mixed anxiety and depression may still deserve recognition because of the prevalence of such a presentation, even though recent diagnostic systems (e.g., DSM-5-TR) have not fully endorsed the condition. Such disorders could explain why antidepressants and antianxiety agents often work in the same types of patients (Rickels and Schweizer 1995).

Clonazepam has been reported to speed response in patients with major depression treated with fluoxetine (Smith et al. 1998) and in panic disorder patients treated with sertraline (Goddard et al. 2001). The drug appeared to have a calming effect and to offset any anxiogenic effect associated with initiation of the SSRI. The benzodiazepine was used for brief periods (approximately 3 weeks) at doses of 0.5–1.5 mg hs and was then discontinued. Such uses are discussed in Chapter 9 ("Augmentation Strategies for Treatment-Resistant Disorders").

Pharmacological Effects

In recent years, considerable attention has been paid to the mode of action of benzodiazepines, spurred on by the identification of specific benzodiazepine sites on the $GABA_A$ receptor. This receptor complex appears to mediate the anxiolytic, sedative, and anticonvulsant actions of the benzodiazepines. The location of specific receptors may be related to the relative anticonvulsant, anxiolytic, or sedative properties of the various benzodiazepines.

It has been hypothesized that it may be possible to develop increasingly specific agents that act as site-specific agonists or partial agonists to produce anxiolysis without sedation or sedation without much muscle relaxation. These approaches are being explored. Thus far, drugs more specifically binding to the benzodiazepine α_1 site (e.g., the nonbenzodiazepine zolpidem) do not seem particularly unique but appear to have more potent sedative than muscle-relaxing properties. Partial agonists or drugs with more specific binding could substantially reduce the risk for tolerance, dependence, and withdrawal effects. Unfortunately, so far, neither partial agonists nor more uniquely binding drugs appear to be different from available benzodiazepines.

The triazolo-benzodiazepine alprazolam appears to also have effects on noradrenergic systems, causing downregulation of postsynaptic β-adrenergic receptors in reserpine-treated mice and increasing the activity of the N protein in humans (the protein that couples the postsynaptic receptor to the intraneuronal energy system). These effects may help to explain the drug's antipanic and moderate antidepressant effects beyond the effects mediated by the benzodiazepine-GABA receptor complex.

Subclasses

The anxiolytic benzodiazepines are commonly divided into three subclasses on the basis of structure: 2-keto (chlordiazepoxide, clonazepam, clorazepate, diazepam, and the hypnotic flurazepam); 3-hydroxy (lorazepam, oxazepam, and the hypnotic temazepam); and triazolo (alprazolam, adinazolam, estazolam, and the hypnotic triazolam) (Figure 6–1 and Table 6–1).

The pharmacokinetic properties (e.g., half-lives) vary among these classes, in part reflecting differences in their modes of drug metabolism, as summarized in Table 6–2. The 2-keto drugs and their active metabolites are oxidized in the liver, and because this process is relatively slow, these compounds have relatively long half-lives. For example, the half-life of diazepam is approximately 40 hours. One active metabolite (desmethyldiazepam) has an even longer half-life (about 60 hours). Moreover, because desmethyldiazepam is further metabolized to oxazepam, which is also active as an anxiolytic (see Table 6–1), diazepam imparts long-range sedative and anxiolytic effects. The half-life of clonazepam is approximately 40 hours. Many of the marketed 2-keto drugs are

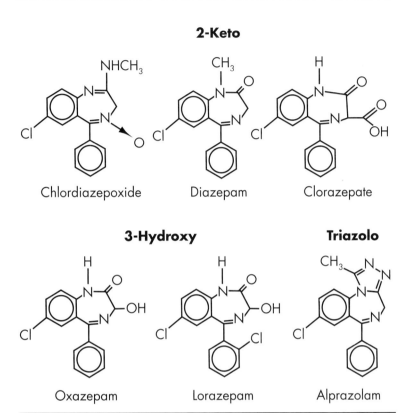

Figure 6–1.   Chemical structures of anxiolytic benzodiazepines.

prodrugs—they are themselves inactive but eventually form active metabolites. Thus, clorazepate is a mere precursor to desmethyldiazepam, as is diazepam. Differences among these specific 2-keto compounds revolve around the rates of absorption and the specific active metabolites formed.

In contrast, the 3-hydroxy compounds are metabolized via direct conjugation with a glucuronide radical, a process that is more rapid than oxidation and does not involve the formation of active metabolites. The two major examples of this subclass are oxazepam and lorazepam, which have considerably shorter half-lives (9 and 14 hours, respectively) than do their 2-keto counter-

Table 6–1.   Anxiolytic benzodiazepines: names, formulations and strengths, and anxiolytic dosage range

Generic name	Brand name[a]	Formulations and strengths	Anxiolytic dosage range[b] (mg/day)
2-Keto			
Chlordiazepoxide hydrochloride	Librium	Capsules: 5, 10, 25 mg	15–40
Clobazam	Clobazam	Tablets: 5, 10, 20 mg	NA
	Onfi	Suspension: 2.5 mg/mL	NA
		Tablets: 10, 20 mg	NA
	Sympazan	Film: 5, 10, 20 mg	NA
Clonazepam	Clonazepam	Orally disintegrating tablets: 0.125, 0.25, 0.5, 1, 2 mg	
	Klonopin	Tablets: 0.5, 1, 2 mg	0.5–1
Clorazepate dipotassium	Clorazepate dipotassium	Tablets: 3.75, 7.5, 15 mg	0.5–1
		Tablets: 7.5 mg	0.5–1
Diazepam	Diastat	Rectal gel: 2.5 mg/0.5 mL (5 mg/mL)	5–40
	Diastat AcuDial	Rectal gel: 10 mg/2 mL (5 mg/mL)	5–20
		Rectal gel: 20 mg/4 mL (5 mg/mL)	5–20
	Diazepam	Injection: 10 mg/2 mL (5 mg/mL)	5–40
		Injection: 50 mg/10 mL (5 mg/mL)	5–40
		Solution: 5 mg/5 mL	5–40

Table 6–1.   Anxiolytic benzodiazepines: names, formulations and strengths, and anxiolytic dosage range *(continued)*

Generic name	Brand name[a]	Formulations and strengths	Anxiolytic dosage range[b] (mg/day)
2-Keto *(continued)*			
Diazepam *(continued)*	Diazepam Intensol	Concentrate: 5 mg/mL	5–40
	Valium	Tablets: 2, 5, 10 mg	
	Valtoco	Spray: 5 mg/spray Spray: 7.5 mg/spray Spray: 10 mg/spray	
3-Hydroxy			
Lorazepam	Ativan	Injection: 2 mg/mL Injection: 4 mg/mL Tablets: 0.5, 1, 2 mg	
	Lorazepam Intensol	Concentrate: 2 mg/mL	
	Loreev XR	Capsules: 1, 1.5, 2, 3 mg	1–6
Oxazepam	Oxazepam	Capsules: 10, 15, 30 mg	15–120
Triazolo			
Alprazolam	Alprazolam	Concentrate: 1 mg/mL	0.5–10

Table 6–1. Anxiolytic benzodiazepines: names, formulations and strengths, and anxiolytic dosage range (*continued*)

Generic name	Brand name[a]	Formulations and strengths	Anxiolytic dosage range[b] (mg/day)
	Xanax	Orally disintegrating tablets: 0.25, 0.5, 1, 2 mg Tablets: 0.25, 0.5, 1, 2 mg	1–4
	Xanax XR	Tablets: 0.5, 1, 2, 3 mg	
Midazolam	Midazolam in 0.9% sodium chloride	Solution (intravenous): 50 mg/50 mL (1 mg/mL) Solution (intravenous): 100 mg/100 mL (1 mg/1 mL)	
	Nayzilam	Spray: 5 mg/spray	
Midazolam hydrochloride	Midazolam hydrochloride	Injection: 1 mg/mL Injection: 5 mg/mL Syrup: 2 mg/mL	NA
	Seizalam	Solution (intramuscular): 50 mg/10 mL (5 mg/mL)	
Remimazolam besylate	Byfavo	Powder: 20 mg/vial	NA

Note. NA=not indicated for treatment of anxiety; XR=extended release.
[a]Where the brand name is the same as the generic name, the brand-name products may no longer be available.
[b]Approximate dosage ranges. Some patients will require higher dosages; others may respond to dosages below the range. Range is dosage-form specific.

Table 6–2. Benzodiazepines: absorption and pharmacokinetics

Generic name	Oral absorption	Major active components	Approximate half-life[a] (hours)
2-Keto			
Chlordiazepoxide	Intermediate	Chlordiazepoxide	20
		Desmethylchlordiazepoxide	30
		Demoxepam	Unknown
		Desmethyldiazepam	60
Clorazepate	Fast	Desmethyldiazepam	60
Diazepam	Fast	Diazepam	40
		Desmethyldiazepam	60
		Methyloxazepam	10
3-Hydroxy			
Lorazepam	Intermediate	Lorazepam	14
Oxazepam	Slow to intermediate	Oxazepam	9
Triazolo			
Alprazolam	Intermediate	Alprazolam	14
Alprazolam XR			

Note. XR = extended release.

[a]Based on ranges of half-lives reported in young, psychiatrically and physically healthy volunteers.

parts. Similarly, the hypnotic temazepam has a half-life (8 hours) that is much shorter than that of flurazepam.

The triazolo compounds are also oxidized; however, they appear to have more limited active metabolites and thus relatively shorter half-lives. The half-life of alprazolam is about 14 hours; adinazolam, 2 hours; and *N*-desmethyladinazolam (adinazolam's active metabolite), 4 hours; the half-life of the hypnotic triazolam is 3–4 hours.

The pharmacokinetic properties of benzodiazepines that are oxidized in the liver may be affected by other medications. Of particular note, nefazodone, fluoxetine, fluvoxamine, sertraline, cimetidine, and contraceptive pills inhibit the liver oxidative enzyme cytochrome P450 3A3/4 and thus slow the degradation of the 2-keto and triazolo compounds. Clinicians should keep this in mind when treating anxious patients who are also taking these drugs. Fluoxetine's effects on alprazolam metabolism have not appeared to be clinically meaningful.

Other differences among benzodiazepines revolve around their rates of absorption and distribution. These agents may differ in terms of the metabolic processes required for absorption and, thus, in the rates at which they appear in blood (see Table 6–2). The lipophilic and hydrophilic properties of these drugs also vary, resulting in pronounced differences in how quickly they work and for how long. Drugs that are more lipophilic (e.g., diazepam) enter the brain more quickly, "turning on" the effect promptly, but "turning off" the effect more quickly as well as they disappear into body fat. Less lipophilic compounds (e.g., lorazepam) produce clinical effects more slowly but may provide more sustained relief. These properties are largely independent of pharmacokinetics. Some drugs with long half-lives (e.g., diazepam) can also be highly lipophilic, providing rapid relief but for shorter periods than might be predicted from half-life data alone. In contrast, lorazepam is less lipophilic and turns on and off more slowly, potentially providing more sustained effects despite its shorter half-life compared with diazepam. In short, traditional half-life pharmacokinetics can be misleading and tell only part of the story of how drugs work.

In addition, investigators have begun to pay more attention to relative receptor affinity, a property that may play a more important role than was previously thought in determining the duration of action. High-potency benzodiazepines, such as alprazolam, may have such high receptor affinity that withdrawal symptoms may be far more intense than might be expected from inspecting other variables such as half-lives. Interestingly, oxazepam, which is similar in lipid solubility and half-life to lorazepam, appears to produce fewer withdrawal symptoms. This position was stated most eloquently by Lader (1982) in the United Kingdom. Unfortunately, there are few data in the past 40 years to confirm or refute this assertion.

Although several of the benzodiazepines are available for parenteral use (see Table 6–1), there is wide variability in the absorption properties of these compounds when given intramuscularly. For example, lorazepam is relatively rapidly absorbed when given intramuscularly. In contrast, diazepam is slowly absorbed. Lorazepam is popular as an adjunctive treatment for agitation in acutely psychotic patients and also often relieves catatonic and depressive stupor. Oral concentrate forms of some benzodiazepines, such as diazepam, lorazepam, and alprazolam, are available in the United States. In addition, lorazepam and clonazepam tablets are given sublingually in some emergency department situations to promote rapid absorption of the drug from the oral mucosa. Clonazepam is available as a rapidly disintegrating tablet, and some anxious patients or patients with panic find the sublingual wafer quite helpful. In some studies, alprazolam given by nasal spray at the onset of panic attacks proved effective in aborting the attack. An American pharmaceutical company acquired the rights to intranasal alprazolam (Panistat) in 2001. However, drug development of intranasal alprazolam was discontinued in 2005. Among the concerns was the abuse potential of an intranasal benzodiazepine. Another inhaled oral form of alprazolam (Staccato alprazolam) is currently under development as a rescue medication in epilepsy (Reissig et al. 2015). A rectal form of diazepam (Diastat) is also available for use in seizure disorders. Attempts to develop alternative delivery through nasal or buccal administration have failed to demonstrate efficacy.

Dosage and Administration

The efficacy of benzodiazepines in treating patients with symptomatic anxiety or diagnosable anxiety disorders has been established in many double-blind, random-assignment comparisons with placebo. When treating a patient with GAD, the clinician might begin with a benzodiazepine (e.g., diazepam at approximately 2 mg tid, with increases as needed to a maximum regular daily dosage of 40 mg). A modal dosage of diazepam for GAD is 15–20 mg/day.

Chlordiazepoxide has a much wider dosage range: the recommended starting dosage is 5–10 mg PO tid, with a maximum of 60 mg/day for anxiety. The dosage of chlordiazepoxide for acute alcohol withdrawal is much higher: 50–200 mg/day. Generally, clinicians prescribe chlordiazepoxide 25 mg every 1–2 hours until symptomatic relief or sedation occurs, up to a maximum dosage of 200 mg/day. For lorazepam, the starting dosage is 0.5 mg tid, with titration upward as needed to 6 mg/day. Higher daily dosages are approved but are frequently associated with intense sedation. Dosage ranges for the anxiolytic benzodiazepines are listed in Table 6–1.

Clonazepam is generally started at 0.5–1 mg/day. Dosages up to 4 mg/day are sometimes needed to control panic attacks, but most patients do well with 1–2 mg/day. Clonazepam, like other benzodiazepines, works much faster than antidepressants. We often treat a panic disorder for the first 4–6 weeks with a benzodiazepine such as clonazepam while simultaneously starting an antidepressant. Studies have suggested that the addition of clonazepam to an SSRI speeds up treatment effects in panic disorder (Pollack et al. 2003).

The use of alprazolam in patients with panic disorder often requires higher dosages than those used in GAD. Currently, alprazolam is approved in dosages up to 10 mg/day, but generally, 4–5 mg/day or less are used. In our early studies on depression, we used the much higher dosage regimen, but we have been impressed that patients generally do not require more than 4 mg/day for a response, and some are even oversedated at 2–3 mg/day. Because of concern about dependence, this drug should be used at the lowest effective dose possible. There is evidence from controlled, fixed-dose studies that blood levels of alprazolam in the range of 20–40 ng/mL are optimal for improvement in patients with panic disorder. At higher plasma levels (40–60 ng/mL), some additional patients may improve, but sedative-type side effects and ataxia increase (Greenblatt et al. 1993). Alprazolam is available in an extended-release formulation (XR) for once-a-day or twice-a-day dosing (Glue et al. 2006). The XR form generally allows for once-a-day dosing and may mitigate some of the withdrawal associated with missed doses. There is some evidence that alprazolam XR may have a lower abuse potential (Mumford et al. 1995). However, alprazolam XR can still be abused, and cessation of the drug can result in withdrawal symptoms. Several biotechnology start-up companies are attempting to develop more rapidly absorbed or longer-acting formulations.

The starting dosage of alprazolam in both GAD and panic disorder should be 1.5 mg/day or less, given in divided doses, with a gradual increase in dosage as tolerated by the patient. In treating patients with panic disorder, alprazolam dosage may be increased, to block not only panic attacks but anticipatory anxiety as well. This often requires higher dosages (4–5 mg/day) in the first 6 or more weeks. Over time, however, as patients overcome their anticipatory anxiety, the dosage can be reduced to 2–3 mg/day for continued blocking of panic attacks. Although alprazolam was thought to have unique antipanic properties, subsequent reports have indicated that lorazepam, clonazepam, and diazepam may all be effective in ameliorating or preventing panic symptoms. Clonazepam is used at dosages of 1–3 mg/day.

Although TCAs, monoamine oxidase inhibitors (MAOIs), and SSRIs are all probably as effective as alprazolam or clonazepam in treating patients with panic disorder with agoraphobia, only the benzodiazepines provide rapid relief; the other drug groups take at least 4–6 weeks, compared with 1 week or less for alprazolam. With the more conventional antidepressants, more patients drop out early in treatment because of side effects, and there is a general belief that some panic patients are even more sensitive to antidepressant drug side effects than are depressed patients. In patients who have occasional bouts of moderate anxiety occurring only every few days or weeks, benzodiazepines may be preferable to maintenance antidepressants because they work as an as-needed medication. Diazepam's ability to act rapidly without prolonged sedation makes it particularly useful in such situations with patients not prone to drug abuse. Other benzodiazepines can also be used in this manner, of course. Oxazepam's slow absorption rate raises concern about its utility as an as-needed medication. However, patient acceptance of oxazepam is fairly good, and its relatively low abuse liability makes it a reasonable choice for some patients.

In patients with long histories of panic disorder with agoraphobia, 6-month and 18-month courses of alprazolam therapy were studied in terms of relapse or recurrence rates after the alprazolam was tapered and stopped; longer period was found to be associated with symptomatic relief (Ballenger et al. 1993).

One major area of debate revolves around how long to use these drugs for patients with significant anxiety. For patients whose anxiety is very acute and related to specific stressors, use of these agents should be directed at reduction of acute symptoms; thus, prolonged use beyond 1–2 weeks is generally not required or advised. In patients whose anxiety symptoms are of several months' or greater duration, we recommend treatment for 4–6 weeks at doses that provide relief, then reduction of the dosage to the minimum needed for maintenance for the next few months, followed by discontinuation when possible. Patients who meet DSM-5-TR criteria for GAD have, by definition, an even more chronic condition and require even longer treatment (e.g., 4–6 months or longer) before discontinuation is attempted. For these patients, SSRIs may be the preferred agent to use first. Unfortunately, psychiatrists often first see patients with histories compatible with GAD only after they have received benzodiazepines for years from other physicians; there are many such patients who obtain relief from these drugs but relapse when the drugs are stopped. Further, because many patients seem to do well with reasonable dosages over longer periods, the clinician may be faced with the difficult decision of how long to maintain use of the benzodiazepine. This dilemma is intensified by the observation that tolerance can develop to some effects of benzodiazepines (e.g., hypnosis), suggesting that the apparent relief experienced by patients could reflect a nonspecific psychological effect.

Although tolerance can occur, it is our belief that most patients do not develop tolerance but are still responding. We base this observation on the number of patients we have seen over the years who have functioned well on a given daily dose of benzodiazepine and have not found themselves escalating their total daily intake. Longer-term data from alprazolam studies indicate that panic patients do not escalate their daily dosages but, rather, frequently lower them over time. There does not appear to be a loss of efficacy of alprazolam in patients followed for up to 1 year. It is our impression that animal and human models of tolerance may not be totally applicable to chronic anxiety per se. Rather, such models emphasize self-administration of a drug or drug-induced ataxia produced in "normal" specimens but do not fully take into account the biological and clinical status of the anxious patient.

If possible, the clinician should attempt to taper benzodiazepines gradually, using psychotherapy, behavior therapy, or other drug therapies to help patients deal with their anxiety (see "Withdrawal" subsection later in this chapter). Some patients, however, may require continued benzodiazepine therapy. Overlapping an SSRI with the benzodiazepine for several weeks, in the hope that the patient will feel still further relief of symptoms, before tapering the benzodiazepine appears to be a useful strategy. For example, Goddard and colleagues (2001) found that the coadministration of sertraline and clonazepam in patients with panic disorder facilitated early improvement of symptoms when compared with sertraline alone.

Although the clear trend has been to use antidepressants as the preferred treatment for the long-term management of GAD and panic disorder, the evidence suggests that benzodiazepines are clearly faster acting, better tolerated, and probably more effective than antidepressants in the management of anxiety disorders (Offidani et al. 2013). That being said, there is a defined subset of patients who are at greater risk for developing dependence on benzodiazepines, such as those with a personal or family history of alcohol use disorders, and the benzodiazepines are best avoided in these patients.

True longer-term harmful effects of benzodiazepines have not been convincingly described. For example, Lader (1982) reported CT scan abnormalities in a series of patients who had taken benzodiazepines for a long time. Although these observations could be interpreted as indicating that these drugs produce organic or structural changes in brain tissue (as chronic alcohol use does), an equally acceptable explanation is that some anxious patients who require chronic treatment with benzodiazepines may have neuropsychiatric disorders, as evidenced by CT scan abnormalities. A study by Lucki et al. (1986) of patients receiving chronic long-term benzodiazepine treatment failed to show significant cognitive impairment on psychometric tests. The data on the cognitive effects of long-term benzodiazepine use have been mixed, with some studies suggesting no significant effects (Gladsjo et al. 2001) but other analyses suggesting residual cognitive deficit with long-term benzodiazepine use even after stopping the drug (Crowe and Stranks 2018; Stewart 2005). An elevated risk of cognitive decline associated with chronic benzodiazepine use has not been consistently demonstrated in studies. However, the risk may be greater in females and with the chronic use of high doses of short-half-life benzodiazepines (Torres-Bondia et al. 2022). It is not likely that benzodiazepines contribute to dementia, but long-term exposure to high doses of benzodiazepines at least weakly is associated with longer-term cognitive problems. In addition, the elderly may be particularly vulnerable to the short-term cognitive side effects of benzodiazepines. Certainly, elderly medical patients taking long-acting benzodiazepines (or antidepressants) are at increased risk for falls leading to hip fractures.

How addictive are benzodiazepines? How long does one have to take a benzodiazepine before withdrawal is seen with discontinuation? Studies in animals have indicated that benzodiazepines can reinforce use and can produce physical dependence and tolerance. Available survey and treatment facility data suggest that benzodiazepines are rarely sought after or craved in the sense that heroin and cocaine are. Rather, they are used as part of a polysubstance abuse pattern to modulate the effects of primary drugs of abuse (e.g., cocaine) or as backup drugs when more euphoriant drugs are not available.

Risk factors for benzodiazepine abuse include a history of alcohol or other substance abuse and the presence of a personality disorder. In patients with a history of substance abuse, benzodiazepines generally should not be prescribed routinely. However, they can be used in some recreational drug users with anxiety, particularly if trials of other agents have failed. In patients with a major psychiatric disorder, benzodiazepines should be administered only if necessary and for brief periods at low doses. Benzodiazepine dependence is mainly, or at least partially, an iatrogenic problem in that patients receive the medication from physicians originally for legitimate reasons but may then take it for too long or at too large a dosage. Possible length of treatment with these drugs should be thought out in advance of their prescription, and longer-term trials should be monitored carefully.

Withdrawal

Should one attempt to gradually discontinue benzodiazepines from patients who have taken them regularly over longer periods? As a rule, this approach is sensible; reduction should be made at a maximum rate of approximately 25% per week. Many patients, however, will require much slower tapering. In their classic study of benzodiazepine withdrawal, Rickels et al. (1983) noted that when benzodiazepines were abruptly discontinued under double-blind conditions, withdrawal symptoms were demonstrated more in patients who had been taking benzodiazepines for more than 8 months (43%) than patients who had been taking them for shorter periods (5%). In a subsequent study, this group reported similar rates of withdrawal symptoms in patients who had been receiving maintenance therapy with clorazepate for 6 months (Rickels et al. 1988). Pecknold et al. (1988) reported that sudden discontinuation after an 8-week trial of alprazolam resulted in symptoms of anxiety in about 35% of patients with panic disorder. Some of these patients may have experienced re-emergence of their panic symptoms rather than withdrawal.

Common symptoms of benzodiazepine withdrawal include jitteriness, anxiety, palpitations, clamminess, sweating, nausea, confusion, and heightened sensitivity to light and sound. Seizures represent the most worrisome of withdrawal reactions, but fortunately, they are generally rare. No patients in the study by Rickels et al. (1983) experienced seizures. Seizures with abrupt diazepam withdrawal occur about 5–7 days after the drug is stopped and not within 24 hours, reflecting the long half-lives of both diazepam and desmethyldiazepam. With shorter-acting drugs (e.g., lorazepam, alprazolam), withdrawal symptoms emerge more rapidly—within 2–3 days. Thus, with diazepam, physicians cannot be confident that seizures will not occur unless the patient has stopped taking the drug for at least 1 week. Any signs of withdrawal (even at day 5) should be reviewed carefully, and consideration should be given to reinstituting the drug and then withdrawing it more gradually. A few days after discontinuation of benzodiazepines, some patients reexperience their original anxiety symptoms but in a more severe form (so-called rebound anxiety). (In the case of hypnotics, this takes the form of rebound insomnia.) This syndrome is generally transient, usually lasting 48–72 hours.

As Rickels and Schweizer (1995) suggested, withdrawal symptoms usually occur during benzodiazepine tapering and in approximately the week following cessation and pass after the patient has been without benzodiazepines for 3 weeks. Symptoms of the preexisting anxiety disorder usually reemerge more rapidly.

It is becoming increasingly clear that many patients stop adhering to withdrawal regimens for benzodiazepines early in the process, well before appreciable withdrawal symptoms could occur (for more details, see Rickels et al. 1999 and the entire supplement of the journal in which their article appears). This strongly suggests a psychological belief that the medications are necessary and a strong overreaction to somatic symptoms related to anxiety. Not surprisingly, CBT of the kind used in treating panic disorder with agoraphobia and instituted well before tapering of the benzodiazepines can be very effective in facilitating tapering and allowing the patient to become free of these drugs (Spiegel 1999). In a follow-up of patients who had been in benzodiazepine tapering trials 2–3 years earlier, Rickels et al. (1999) found patients who were still free of benzodiazepines to be less symptomatic than patients who did not complete the taper or had returned to benzodiazepine use. These data unfortunately do not unscramble cause and effect.

Generally, the first half of the benzodiazepine dose can be tapered over a 4-week period, but tapering the remaining half of the dose can be a prolonged process. Patients may need to be kept at the 50% dose for several months before further tapering is attempted. However, mainly for personality reasons, many patients drop out of tapering attempts very early before any significant withdrawal symptoms occur.

Factors that make benzodiazepine withdrawal more difficult include higher daily dosage, shorter half-life of the drug, longer duration of prior benzodiazepine therapy, and more rapid taper. At the patient level, a diagnosis of panic disorder, higher pretaper levels of anxiety or depression, the presence of a significant personality disorder, and concomitant alcohol or substance abuse make tapering more difficult. Successful tapering of benzodiazepines is often demanding of the clinician's time and energy (Rickels et al. 1999). The clinician needs to be available at all hours to provide counseling, support, and reassurance. If a patient is to undertake benzodiazepine withdrawal with any real prospect of success, prewithdrawal symptoms of anxiety and depression need to be actively treated with either pharmacological or psychological therapies.

So far, adjunctive therapy with other nonbenzodiazepine drugs—carbamazepine, trazodone, valproate, buspirone, and imipramine—has not been shown to be of help in decreasing withdrawal symptoms. However, use of imipramine and valproate may enable some patients to remain free of benzodiazepines for a few weeks.

Panic control treatment (PCT), a type of CBT, is an educational-experiential approach aimed at having patients learn to tolerate somatic symptoms of panic without undue anxiety. A controlled study has shown that use of PCT in combination with a very slow and cautious benzodiazepine taper (0.125 mg of alprazolam every 2 days for patients taking more than 1 mg/day initially, or 0.25 mg every 8 days once the dosage has been reduced to 1 mg/day) is effective. In another study, the taper was even slower. In both studies, PCT plus very slow taper was substantially better than medical management plus slow taper, although the sample sizes were small. Most of the patients whose benzodiazepine use had been successfully tapered with PCT were still free of benzodiazepines 3 years later (Spiegel 1999). Some informal clinical experience suggests that for better long-term success, CBT should be continued for at least a few weeks after benzodiazepine taper is completed. As noted later in this chapter, other forms of CBT are now being successfully used in treating most of the anxiety disorders and may well prove useful in the primary treatment of drug-free patients as well as in assisting benzodiazepine withdrawal.

Side Effects

Compared with many other classes of psychotropic agents, benzodiazepines have relatively favorable side-effect profiles. The most common side effect is sedation, which is in part related to dose and can be managed by reducing the dose. Other effects include dizziness, weakness, ataxia, anterograde amnesia (particularly with the short-acting benzodiazepines [e.g., triazolam]), decreased motoric performance (e.g., driving), nausea, and slight hypotension. Falls in elderly patients have been reported to be related to the use of longer-acting benzodiazepines as well as to the use of antidepressants (see Chapter 12, "Pharmacotherapy of Specific Populations"). In the popular press, there have been reports of severe dyscontrol syndromes in patients taking certain benzodiazepines, particularly triazolam. We personally have not encountered any such syndrome in our clinical practice.

Overdose

Fortunately, benzodiazepines have a relatively wide safety margin, and deaths due to benzodiazepine ingestion alone are rare. Most deaths that have involved these drugs have been associated with concomitant ingestion of other agents (e.g., alcohol, TCAs). In 2016, the FDA issued a class warning about the combination of opioids and benzodiazepines. Patients can, and have, accidentally died from a respiratory depression when opioids and benzodiazepines were combined. In addition, there have been intentional lethal overdoses of the combination of benzodiazepines and opioids. As a result, benzodiazepines and opioids (including cough preparations that contain opioids) now include black box warnings about the risk of combining the drugs. The combination remains fairly common, and there may be legitimate reasons for the combination in some patients. We have some chronic back pain patients, for example, who have been taking the combination of an opioid and a benzodiazepine for years and are resistant to going off or lowering the benzodiazepine because it has been more helpful than other medications in relieving chronic muscle spasm. Patients should nonetheless be advised of the risk, and an alternative to a benzodiazepine should be considered if one exists.

Antidepressants

Because the antidepressants are considered in some detail in Chapter 3, we give them less detailed attention here. Although several of the SSRIs have been FDA approved for one or more specific anxiety diagnoses (e.g., paroxetine for social anxiety, GAD, OCD, panic disorder, PMDD, and PTSD; sertraline for panic disorder, OCD, PMDD, social anxiety disorder, and PTSD), it is our position, as noted earlier, that until studies clearly show differences between these drugs in treating specific anxiety disorders, all SSRIs are probably reasonably effective across the whole range of anxiety disorders. Their use for such conditions may require adjustments, but these apply to the specific disorder and the whole class of SSRIs. For example, in treating patients with panic with agoraphobia, begin with very low dosages; in treating patients with OCD, use higher dosages and wait even longer for clinical response. Likewise, the SNRIs are probably useful for a range of anxiety disorders. Venlafaxine is approved in the treatment of panic disorder, GAD, and social anxiety disorder; the manufacturer of duloxetine has sought and received approval only for GAD.

Agoraphobia and Panic

Several antidepressants exert major antianxiety effects. Imipramine was first reported by Klein and various colleagues in the 1960s (Klein 1967) to have potent anxiolytic effects in agoraphobic patients with panic. Clinically, it appears that most, if not all, TCAs and SSRIs exert similar antipanic effects. In addition, the MAOI phenelzine is a potent antipanic agent, as probably are the other MAOIs and trazodone. However, not all antidepressants are as effective in treating panic. Most notably, bupropion does not appear to exert antipanic effects and may be anxiogenic in some patients. The noradrenergic effects of various antidepressants (particularly the TCAs and MAOIs) on the locus coeruleus generally have been invoked to explain their antipanic activity. Whether such a mode of action explains the possible antipanic effects of trazodone is unclear.

The SSRIs appear to prevent or lessen panic attacks. Indeed, paroxetine and sertraline have FDA approval for use in panic disorder. Generally speaking, doses for paroxetine are higher in treating panic than in treating major depression. The starting dosage is 10 mg/day, and the therapeutic dosage range is 40–60 mg/day.

Early on, the general rule of thumb was that patients with panic disorder required only low dosages of TCAs (e.g., 50 mg/day of imipramine) for a response to occur. Over the years, it became more evident that, as in depression, many patients with panic disorder require relatively higher doses of TCAs or MAOIs, although a small proportion are very sensitive to TCAs, tolerating only 10–25 mg/day of imipramine. We recommend, when indicated, using the general dosage regimens of TCAs that are used for depression (see Chapter 3).

Klein (1993) proposed that TCAs are effective in panic disorder by affecting a supersensitive threshold for feeling smothered. In a second international collaborative study comparing imipramine with alprazolam and placebo in patients with panic disorder, patients with prominent respiratory panic symptoms (e.g., shortness of breath, choking feelings) showed more improvement with imipramine, whereas patients who did not have these symptoms during panic attacks did better with alprazolam. We know of no similar data on SSRIs.

Given the utility of TCAs in the treatment of panic disorder, it is not surprising that the SNRIs also appear effective. In 2005, venlafaxine received FDA approval for the treatment of panic disorder. Two controlled registration trials of 12 weeks' duration indicated that venlafaxine XR reduces the frequency of panic attacks at dosages ranging from 75 to 225 mg/day. It would be expected that the other SNRIs are also useful in the treatment of panic disorder, although no others have been approved for this purpose as of this writing. In addition, because all the other SNRIs are more noradrenergic than is venlafaxine, tolerability in patients with panic disorder may vary among this class of drugs.

Generalized Anxiety Disorder

Studies have pointed out that TCAs also exert effects in GAD. In one major study, imipramine was as effective at 4–6 weeks as the benzodiazepine chlordiazepoxide in patients with this disorder. However, in the first 2 weeks, the benzodiazepine was more effective. More recent studies have led to FDA approvals for venlafaxine, duloxetine, and escitalopram in the treatment of GAD.

Given the current DSM-5-TR criteria for GAD as a chronic disorder—one that probably requires long-term treatment—the role of benzodiazepines has been reduced to the short-term relief of symptoms, if clinically necessary, while a longer-term non-dependence-inducing therapeutic program is implemented. Currently, venlafaxine, escitalopram, and paroxetine are FDA approved for use in GAD, but probably all SSRIs are effective, and all the newer drugs are probably more benign than the older TCAs, although we know of no direct comparisons between newer and older antidepressants in treating this condition. CBT approaches are available for the symptoms of GAD. Again, we know of no direct comparisons of specific drugs and specific CBT approaches for GAD, but the use of multimodal approaches is a function of the cost, the patient's response to the initial treatment trial, and the availability of skilled CBT therapists in the geographic area.

Social Anxiety Disorder

Seriously symptomatic patients with social anxiety disorder experience marked anxiety in a range of social situations, such as eating in public, signing checks, public speaking, and even being in large groups. The condition, as defined in DSM-5-TR, may also include more limited fears of performing or speaking in public, often called *performance anxiety.* Performance anxiety is less incapacitating than generalized social phobia but may affect an area vital to a patient's career or interests. There is reasonable evidence that milder degrees of performance anxiety studied in volunteers (e.g., music students) respond to β-blockers given a couple of hours before the performance. Several β-blockers, including propranolol, oxprenolol, alprenolol, and atenolol, have been a bit more effective than placebo in individual controlled studies (see subsection "Noradrenergic Agents" later in this chapter). Likewise, the β-blockers appear to be helpful in managing test anxiety without the cognitive impairing effects of benzodiazepines. A number of open studies have suggested that a single dose of propranolol 10–40 mg before an exam reduces the peripheral symptoms of anxiety and appears to enhance test performance in individuals who may be incapacitated by severe anxiety. Atenolol is cardioselective and does not cross the blood-brain barrier easily, suggesting that β-blockers may act, at least in part, by suppressing tachycardia and tremor. Side effects may include hypotension and bradycardia. Thus, some caution is required in using the β-blockers for test or performance anxiety.

Social anxiety disorder has been increasingly well studied over the past 20 years. This disorder is often comorbid with a variety of other disorders, such as panic disorder, major depressive disorder, body dysmorphic disorder, and substance abuse. Because social anxiety disorder appears to begin in childhood or adolescence, early identification and treatment may be of special value in preventing the onset of other complicating disorders.

At present, there is good evidence that a variety of drug therapies are more effective than placebo. Paroxetine has been very well studied and has an FDA-approved indication for the treatment of social phobia. Dosages from 20 to 60 mg/day appeared equally effective in one multisite study (Davidson et al. 2004; Westenberg et al. 2004). Other SSRIs are presumably also effective, and several have shown efficacy in smaller double-blind or open studies. For example, several multicenter trials have demonstrated that fluvoxamine is effective in the treatment of social anxiety. Fluvoxamine at an average dosage of about 200 mg/day was effective in reducing social anxiety compared with a placebo. Venlafaxine is also approved for the treatment of social anxiety disorder and appears to be at least as effective as the SSRIs. β-Blockers (or at least atenolol) were not much better than placebo in controlled studies in the treatment of generalized social phobia, despite their efficacy in ameliorating performance anxiety.

MAOIs also are effective in social anxiety disorder, with the conventional MAOI phenelzine being the most effective and best studied of this class of antidepressants. Moclobemide, a short-acting, reversible MAOI available in Canada and Europe, appears to be somewhat less effective. Brofaromine, another reversible MAOI, was reported to not separate from placebo in social phobia. Clonazepam has been well studied by Davidson's group (Davidson 2000) and is substantially more effective than placebo. Alprazolam, in other studies, has had a weaker effect.

Only a few small studies compared CBT with pharmacotherapy, and these studies showed equivalent efficacy. Interesting reasons have been suggested as to why the exposure socially phobic patients receive to anxiety-producing situations in the course of their lives does not extinguish the anxiety; CBT programs have been developed that get around this problem and are quite successful. In double-blind studies, significant effects were seen for D-cycloserine versus placebo in patients with social anxiety receiving behavior therapy (Hofmann et al. 2006; Rodebaugh and Lenze 2013).

One tentative algorithm for treating new patients with generalized social phobia is to begin with a benzodiazepine to reduce initial apprehension. An SSRI is added, and the benzodiazepine is stopped after the SSRI has begun to work. Finally, CBT is added before phasing out the SSRI.

Duration of treatment for patients with generalized social anxiety has not been well studied. Because the condition is generally chronic, pharmacotherapy of at least a year's duration with evidence that the patient can handle previously feared situations seems reasonable before attempts are made to taper medication. Some patients may require medication indefinitely.

It should be noted that gabapentin—an α_2-δ calcium channel blocker—at dosages averaging about 3,000 mg/day has been shown to be more effective than placebo in treating social anxiety disorder. The reason for its presumed efficacy is unclear. However, an analog, pregabalin, has been reported in multiple studies of GAD to be effective (see below). For patients who have not responded to SSRIs and CBT, an MAOI trial is obviously the next step. Clomipramine may also be effective in treating social phobia. On the basis of the available evidence, mild social and/or performance anxiety could be treated first with a β-blocker, and patients with more severe impairment could be given an SSRI before a trial of phenelzine. Clomipramine could be tried in patients averse to trying MAOIs who have not had a response to SSRIs either because of discontinuation due to side effects or because of lack of improvement. If both clonazepam and alprazolam are effective in treating social phobia, clonazepam should be tried first because of its longer half-life. Benzodiazepines probably rapidly exert an effect on social anxiety; SSRIs or MAOIs may take weeks to obtain a full effect.

Posttraumatic Stress Disorder

Prior to DSM-5 (American Psychiatric Association 2013), PTSD was listed as an anxiety disorder with a presumed cause: exposure to a markedly traumatic event or series of events. In DSM-5, PTSD became part of the new category *trauma- and stressor-related disorders*. In general, studies show that about 20% of persons exposed to a severe stress develop the disorder. Probably a variety of factors predispose individuals to developing the full syndrome and needing treatment, including preexisting exposure to other stresses, prior psychiatric disorders, and the severity and prolongation of the traumatic experience(s). Group cohesion during major stresses may offer some protection. Most patients with PTSD have one or more comorbid psychiatric disorders; depression, various other anxiety disorders, dissociative disorders, and substance abuse are all relatively common and both increase morbidity and complicate treatment. Further, PTSD syndromes occurring after a single adverse event (e.g., rape, fire, motor vehicle accident, volcanic eruption) may be different from PTSD seen in combat veterans or in patients who were sexually or physically abused as children.

Although one might assume that PTSD is a close chronological sequela of the bad event (and it sometimes is), some patients may be fine or at least may function well for months or years until some factor—known, hypothetical, or unknown—causes a sudden emergence or reemergence of the typical patterns of symptoms. An episode of PTSD has been estimated to last about 7 years; however, some patients adapt to the memories and symptoms and recover early, whereas others have symptoms that vary in intensity but seem to persist for decades. PTSD was reported in some World War I veterans in studies published as late as the 1980s.

It is generally presumed that patients with PTSD have overactive autonomic nervous systems and that their cortisol responses to stress or dexamethasone are blunted—the opposite of the status in severe depression. There are reports that at the point of trauma the administration of cortisol can prevent PTSD (Zohar et al. 2011). Some patients with PTSD feel much better after being given a single dose of an opioid antagonist (nalmefene), whereas others feel much worse (Glover 1993). In one study of PTSD patients, a serotonin agonist, *m*-chlorophenylpiperazine, induced an exacerbation of PTSD symptoms, whereas yohimbine, an adrenergic agonist, induced panic and flashback symptoms (Southwick et al. 1997). In a similar small study, the pure benzodiazepine antagonist flumazenil relieved symptoms in patients with PTSD (Coupland et al. 1997).

Further, most published clinical trials of treatments for PTSD have involved outpatients who were not taking any medications and whose illness was presumably less severe than that of patients in their seventh inpatient psychiatric hospital admission whose condition had worsened despite having received prolonged trials of a variety of concomitant medications and, often, psychosocial therapies. In these days of limited hospital stays, it is no longer an option to withdraw a patient's numerous drug therapies to see whether any are helping or hurting. In many cases, such readmissions for severe PTSD usually involve women with histories of childhood sexual abuse who meet the criteria for a number of other psychiatric disorders in addition to PTSD. These patients often dissociate a lot; have severe insomnia, severe depression, and recurrent substance abuse; and exhibit self-injurious behavior. They are likely to be taking clonazepam, valproic acid, gabapentin, olanzapine, SSRIs, bupropion, clonidine, or lamotrigine, as well as butabital plus acetaminophen for headaches, and despite their medications they still feel terrible. It may be that severe symptoms and self-destructive behavior elicit overprescribing in psychiatrists and that the presence of such patients on psychiatric wards encourages other, more naive patients to emulate an expanding repertoire of symptoms. Although some reported trauma histories sound rather incredible, most seem valid and are likely true.

Given all the above factors, the most widely studied drugs for the treatment of PTSD are the SSRIs. They are often more effective than placebo, although only 40%–50% of patients taking SSRIs for PTSD show major improvement. The older MAOIs and brofaromine, a short-acting reversible MAOI no longer in development, may be effective more often than SSRIs, but these drugs' serious adverse effects in unstable, self-destructive outpatients make it hard to risk prescribing them. Nefazodone was found to be helpful in several small open studies, and lamotrigine was helpful in one small placebo-controlled study. Uncontrolled studies of moclobemide, fluvoxamine, paroxetine, mirtazapine, venlafaxine, valproate, and carbamazepine have all shown some benefit. Both paroxetine and sertraline were significantly more effective than placebo in patients with PTSD, and both now have FDA approval for the disorder. It may be that anticonvulsants are better for rage and instability, whereas antidepressants are better for depression and anxiety. Clonidine and guanfacine appear to suppress nightmares but have not been well studied (Kerbage and Richa 2015; Pearlstein 2000). Prazosin, an α_1 antagonist, appeared to reduce nightmares in patients with PTSD at dosages of 1–16 mg/day (Kung et al. 2012; Miller 2008; Thompson et al. 2008). As described below, dramatic effects were observed in men at dosages up to 25 mg/day and in women at dosages up to 12 mg/day in a multicenter Department of Veterans Affairs study (Raskind et al. 2013). Unfortunately, a rigorous follow-up study of prazosin by Raskind and colleagues (2018) in 304 combat veterans failed to show any benefit of prazosin for helping with either nightmares or sleep quality.

Patients with PTSD who experience intrusive sounds and images (flashbacks) of traumatic events and "paranoid" ideas (e.g., fear of being attacked when exposed in public places) have found the first-generation antipsychotics (e.g., perphenazine 16 mg/day) helpful, although the psychotic-like symptoms do not completely abate. The SGAs have been investigated in PTSD. At least 10 controlled trials have been completed to date on the use of risperidone, olanzapine, and quetiapine in the treatment of PTSD (Ahearn et al. 2011). In general, the effect size of the antipsychotics in the treatment of PTSD is small, but the greatest effects are seen in the reduction of intrusive traumatic ideation and hypervigilance. The combination of antidepressants with SGAs in the treatment of PTSD has been useful clinically in some patients but is not well studied. The side effects, including weight gain and metabolic issues, limit the SGAs to adjunctive use or use as second-line agents. The U.S. Department of Veterans Affairs and Department of Defense (2017) guidelines for the treatment of PTSD concluded that antipsychotics, particularly risperidone, do not appear to have much utility and should be avoided.

Propranolol has been suggested for treating PTSD symptoms, although there is no clear evidence of efficacy. Propranolol appeared to block the development of PTSD symptoms when administered to patients seen acutely in the emergency department (Pitman and Delahanty 2005), although its efficacy in later studies has been less impressive (McGhee et al. 2009). Its use was based on observations in rodents that surges of epinephrine in the brain were needed for memory consolidation of specific events.

One study showed that among recent trauma survivors, acute use of a benzodiazepine for several weeks after the traumatic experience tended to increase the likelihood that PTSD would develop. After PTSD is well established, patients often have severe initial insomnia and severe anxiety and thus almost invariably are prescribed benzodiazepines. There is even suggestive evidence that using alcohol regularly may delay onset of PTSD and that concurrent use of benzodiazepines may limit the benefits of exposure therapy (Pollack et al. 2011). Because of the risks of substance abuse in PTSD patients and the potential for disinhibition in some PTSD patients who have trouble modulating anger, benzodiazepines should generally be avoided.

In short, for milder or less intractable PTSD, SSRIs are the current treatment of choice. In one study of PTSD patients, longer-term treatment with fluvoxamine led to a better outcome, with more improvement in PTSD symptoms after 1 year than had been seen at 6 weeks. Because PTSD in the majority of patients seems to have a prolonged, chronic course, long-term use of any substantially helpful medication seems sensible.

Among investigational approaches, 3,4-methylenedioxymethamphetamine (MDMA)-assisted psychotherapy has shown substantial promise in randomized trials of PTSD to date. MDMA, commonly known by its street namem Ecstasy, is thought to act on all three monoamines via reuptake blockade as well as bind to vesicular monoamine transporter type 2 and monoamine oxidase A. MDMA has both stimulant and psychedelic properties. MDMA was first synthesized in 1912 by Merck, and its utility as a possible aid to psychotherapy was first recognized in the San Francisco Bay Area by Alexander Shulgin, who published a paper in 1976 describing its associated altered state of consciousness and its potential to strip away habits and help the individual see the world more clearly. Shulgin supplied the drug as a relaxant to friends and associates, including a Bay Area psychotherapist who had worked with psychedelics, and he recognized the therapeutic potential of MDMA for a variety of conditions. The drug eventually became popular as a recreational drug at dances and raves and was banned under the Controlled Substances Act in 1985 as a Schedule I drug.

MDMA has been studied in several conditions, including alcohol use disorder, depression, and PTSD. On the basis of preliminary studies, MDMA-assisted psychotherapy for PTSD received a breakthrough designation in 2018, which could lead to subsequent approval if those initial results confirm MDMA's efficacy and safety. Among its actions, MDMA is thought to increase plasticity in a way that helps patients with PTSD process their traumas without becoming overwhelmed by them.

A number of Phase II studies have suggested that MDMA-assisted psychotherapy may be effective in the treatment of PTSD. One of the early studies of MDMA involved 20 participants with chronic PTSD who received either MDMA-assisted psychotherapy or placebo-assisted psychotherapy in a randomized, double-blind, crossover study design (Mithoefer et al. 2019). The study found that 83% of participants who received MDMA-assisted psychotherapy experienced significant reductions in PTSD symptoms, including flashbacks, nightmares, and hyperarousal, versus only 25% of patients who received placebo-assisted psychotherapy. The study also found that the treatment was well tolerated and safe. The positive effects of the treatment were sustained at a 12-month follow-up, suggesting that the treatment may have long-lasting benefits.

In a widely cited analysis of six pooled MDMA-assisted Phase II trials, Mithoefer et al. (2019) found that 54% of participants no longer met criteria for PTSD after two sessions with MDMA-assisted psychotherapy involving doses of 75–125 mg per session. A more recent Phase III clinical trial by Mitchell and colleagues (2021) involved 90 participants with severe PTSD. This study found that two sessions of MDMA-assisted psychotherapy led to significant reductions in PTSD symptoms compared with placebo-assisted psychotherapy, with 67% of participants no longer meeting criteria for PTSD at the end of the study. No increases in suicidality, abuse potential, or QT prolongation were associated with MDMA-assisted therapy. As with previous studies, MDMA appeared to be well tolerated at the doses employed.

Overall, the clinical trials conducted so far suggest that MDMA-assisted psychotherapy has the potential to be an effective treatment for PTSD. In fact, the MDMA studies suggest a much greater efficacy than has been seen with previous treatments such as the SSRIs. In addition, the effects appear to be sustained. However, MDMA is not a completely benign agent. MDMA does have known abuse potential. Even at recreational doses, it can have prominent autonomic and sympathomimetic effects. In addition, MDMA has been associated with neurotoxic effects when abused at high doses. More research is needed to further establish the efficacy and safety of this treatment. That being said, MDMA is a potentially approvable drug for the treatment of PTSD (in conjunction with a specific therapy) and could change the paradigm on how PTSD might be most effectively treated.

Expert opinion on psychosocial therapies (Bisson et al. 2013; Hembree and Foa 2000) favors exposure therapies (although frequent experiencing of flashbacks is clearly not helpful), CBT, and eye movement desensitization and reprocessing therapy (EMDR). Certainly, PTSD patients often have "bad" cognitions: typically, that the world is much more dangerous than it really is and that they are much more helpless and inadequate than they really are. EMDR therapy—having the patient reexperience traumatic memories while the therapist's fingers are waved back and forth before the patient's eyes and the patient moves their eyes from side to side—has been assessed in controlled trials and seems to be a form of exposure therapy.

All in all, the treatment of PTSD is now in the state that treatment of OCD was before the advent of clomipramine. There is no very effective or definitive pharmacotherapy. SSRIs are probably the best studied, relatively effective medications, and here the resemblance to OCD occurs: both PTSD and OCD are long-term conditions, and prolonged drug therapy, at least with the SSRIs, is likely to yield better results over time. A wide variety of other agents are said to be helpful sometimes but are not well studied. In PTSD, memory consolidation and stress arousal systems are probably malfunctioning. There is little evidence that the anticonvulsants are effective in PTSD, although some patients with concurrent traumatic brain injury or those patients with impulsive aggression may benefit. Benzodiazepines, ketamine (with its tendency to exacerbate dissociation), and D-cycloserine (lack of evidence) are best avoided in the treatment of PTSD.

Obsessive-Compulsive Disorder

Like PTSD, OCD was moved out of the anxiety disorders category in DSM-5, meriting its own category (obsessive-compulsive and related disorders). When the second edition of this manual was published in 1991, only one drug, clomipramine, had been approved by the FDA for use in treating OCD. By 1996, fluoxetine and paroxetine were approved for use in treating both OCD and depression, and fluvoxamine was approved for use only in OCD. Over the past 30 years, the evidence is that essentially all SSRIs are effective for both major depression and OCD.

Despite this overlap in indications, the evidence is strong that the way all the SSRIs work in OCD is different from the way they work in depression. Depression tends to respond relatively rapidly—in 2–6 weeks—and most patients improve; there is a substantial placebo response. In OCD, improvement is delayed and may take 6–12 weeks, only half the patients improve, and the placebo response is smaller. The presence of coexisting or comorbid depression in patients with OCD does not affect the response of their OCD to serotonergic antidepressants. Generally, patients with OCD do better with higher doses of SSRIs (e.g., 40–80 mg of fluoxetine), whereas patients with depression often respond to 20 mg. Noradrenergic drugs (desipramine, nortriptyline, and bupropion), which are quite effective in depression, are ineffective in OCD. However, SNRIs such as venlafaxine appear to be helpful, perhaps because of the higher serotonin to norepinephrine reuptake inhibition relative to the other SNRIs.

If one accepts that all currently prescribed SSRIs are effective in OCD, it is hard to make choices among them. All cause a fair amount of sexual dysfunction, although paroxetine seems the worst among the SSRIs. Some differences in their degrees of binding to various receptors and their interactions with drug metabolism exist. It is hard to compare efficacies of these drugs, even in meta-analyses, because the kinds of patients being recruited have likely changed over time. In early clomipramine studies, most patients had never had an adequate trial of an effective drug, and drug response rates and placebo rates were around 50% and 5%, respectively. Since then, placebo rates have risen, and drug improvement rates have dropped.

The principles of treating patients with any of the SSRIs remain clear: begin with a standard antidepressant dose and increase gradually to three to four times that dose if improvement does not clearly occur. Prepare the patient for at least an 8- to 12-week trial before changing drugs or adding other drugs to the SSRI.

Over the years a variety of drugs have been tried alone or added to clomipramine or one of the SSRIs to elicit or increase a therapeutic effect: lithium, buspirone, L-tryptophan, fenfluramine, antipsychotics, opiates, clonazepam. So far, none has had any consistently demonstrated success, although case reports suggest that an occasional patient may improve when one of these drugs is added. Buspirone appeared very effective as an augmenter in open trials but did not separate from placebo in a double-blind study. It should be noted that buspirone *could* elicit a serotonin syndrome when added to an SSRI (although this was not commonly seen) and that L-tryptophan and fenfluramine are no longer available in the United States. In the last few years, as evidence has increased on the overlap of OCD with Tourette's disorder, the SGAs have been added to SSRIs in patients with OCD, with impressive improvements in symptoms seen in occasional patients. Such a response is perhaps more likely if the patient also has schizotypal features or has a history or family history of tics. At this point, risperidone at dosages up to 3 mg/day seems safest in terms of weight gain and oversedation, but orthostatic hypotension has occurred in older depressed patients when risperidone and an SSRI were combined. Conversely, consider, as an illustration that almost any drug or drug class stretches across DSM-defined boundaries, a controlled study showing that fluvoxamine was substantially more effective than placebo in about half of a group of male autistic adults, improving sociability as well as autistic compulsions (McDougle 1997). The bottom line is that about half of patients with OCD are a good deal better while taking an SSRI or clomipramine and about 15%–20% drop out of drug therapy because of side effects. Not an ideal situation.

Rodriguez et al. (2013) reported that intravenous ketamine appeared to be more effective than placebo in improving symptoms in patients with refractory OCD, with the effects lasting at least a week. Some years ago, Larry Koran's group reported in a double-blind study that oral morphine produced significantly greater relief than did placebo one day after taking it and that the effects lasted for about 5 days (Koran et al. 2005).

CBT is about as effective as pharmacotherapy if adequately done (Baer and Greist 1997); relaxation therapy does not help, but therapies involving in vivo exposure and ritual prevention are typically quite effective. Patients with OCD who have cleanliness or counting rituals do much better than patients with pure mental obsessions and no compulsive behaviors, hoarders, or patients with compulsive slowness. Perhaps all patients with OCD should receive both CBT and medication. However, therapists capable of doing CBT are mainly at major university centers with specialized OCD programs, so availability of CBT is a major problem (as is cost, sometimes). Early efforts that incorporated computerized programs and books that patients can use to carry out their own CBT with backup from a live professional seem to be effective (Baer and Greist 1997).

With or without CBT, patients with OCD should receive, in adequate dose and duration, separate trials of at least two of the SSRIs and of clomipramine before going on to more elaborate or complex therapies. For extremely treatment-resistant OCD, either intravenous clomipramine therapy (not available in the United States) or stereotactic psychosurgery (Baer et al. 1995; Mindus and Jenike 1992), both of which have some reported benefit, could be tried. The FDA approved deep brain stimulation (DBS) in 2009 for resistant OCD. Although the approval of DBS was based on minimal data (26 subjects with resistant OCD), DBS was given a "humanitarian device exemption," given the limited options available to patients with resistant OCD and the debilitating nature of the illness. The limited data available suggest that patients who have undergone a DBS implant appear to have improvement in both OCD symptom relief and general quality of life (Ooms et al. 2014). However, more rigorous data on the efficacy and safety of DBS for OCD is forthcoming.

If a patient has long-standing OCD symptoms and improves on a drug regimen, long-term maintenance therapy on that regimen seems advisable. Patients who are taken off medications tend to relapse fairly rapidly. With CBT, it is more likely that a series of treatments—say, 12 sessions—with marked behavioral improvement will lead to maintained improvement after CBT is stopped, although occasional "booster" sessions may be useful.

Anticonvulsants

A number of anticonvulsants have been used for the treatment of anxiety disorders. Many of these drugs were thought to act primarily on the GABAergic system and would be expected to have anxiolytic properties. They also tend to have utility in the treatment of neuropathic pain. Among these anticonvulsants are gabapentin, tiagabine, and pregabalin. The anticonvulsants probably work slower than benzodiazepines and faster than antidepressants in the treatment of anxiety. Among the advantages of the anticonvulsants relative to benzodiazepines is a lower risk of dependence and withdrawal.

Gabapentin (Neurontin) has been used as a less habit-forming alternative to benzodiazepines in the treatment of anxiety states. Although gabapentin was once thought to be primarily GABAergic, it appears now that it binds to an α_2-δ subunit of calcium channels found in brain, and this is the more relevant mechanism of action. On the other hand, there is more evidence that gabapentin is at least modestly effective in the treatment of social anxiety, including public speaking, generalized anxiety, and panic disorder. Our experience is that gabapentin is much less effective than either benzodiazepines or antidepressants in the treatment of anxiety. However, gabapentin has relatively few side effects or drug interactions and has only a limited risk for dependence. There have been a few cases of gabapentin dependence and withdrawal in individuals with a history of substance abuse, but the risks appear small (Bonnet and Scherbaum 2017). Doses as low as 300–400 mg may be helpful in the treatment of social anxiety, but most patients seem to need between 900 and 2,700 mg/day (in divided doses) for the treatment of panic or more serious anxiety. The primary side effects are somnolence and fatigue.

Pregabalin (Lyrica), an analog of GABA that is related to gabapentin, has been extensively studied in the treatment of GAD, fibromyalgia, neuropathic pain, and partial complex seizures. It appears to act even more selectively on the α_2-δ subunit of calcium channels found in brain than does gabapentin. Pregabalin received FDA approval in late 2004 for use in treating neuropathic pain and epilepsy. In 2008, it became the first drug approved for the treatment of fibromyalgia. Even though pregabalin received approval for the treatment of GAD in the European Union in 2006, the FDA has not approved pregabalin for GAD in the United States as of this writing. With the consistent efficacy in clinical trials and the known safety of pregabalin in clinical experience, it is not completely clear what has held up approval of pregabalin for GAD. There was reported concern about the risk-benefit ratio for the drug, given the hepatotoxicity seen in mice, but this has not proven to be a problem postrelease in humans. The drug is currently under re-review by the FDA.

At least seven placebo-controlled trials suggest that pregabalin is at least as effective as alprazolam and venlafaxine and more effective than placebo in the treatment of GAD. Pregabalin was more rapidly acting than venlafaxine and controlled somatic symptoms as well as did alprazolam (Montgomery 2006). In addition, pregabalin looks about as effective as venlafaxine in treating GAD but is better tolerated and probably more rapidly acting (Montgomery et al. 2006). The starting dosage of pregabalin in the treatment of anxiety is expected to be 150 mg/day, with the dosage increasing to 300 mg/day. Most patients should do fine at 300–400 mg/day, but the dosage can be increased by 150 mg every few days to the maximum of 600 mg/day. Arnold et al. (2015) reported that pregabalin was effective in reducing anxiety and depressive symptoms in patients with fibromyalgia and comorbid depression who were taking antidepressants. Although the studies suggest pregabalin should be a good first-line agent for the treatment of GAD, other promising anxiolytics, such as buspirone, did not live up to expectations. Still, we expect pregabalin will fill an important niche. We have seen some patients who have either not tolerated or not responded to SSRIs who have done well with pregabalin. Patients requiring immediate relief of anxiety in an emergency setting will still receive benzodiazepines. However, pregabalin is a more rapidly acting and probably better alternative to the SSRIs for some patients. The most common side effects of pregabalin have been dizziness, somnolence, and weight gain. In the adult trials in epilepsy, 9% gained 7% or more of their body weight as compared to 2% of subjects receiving placebo. This drug, like gabapentin, lacks the sexual side effects of most antidepressants.

Tiagabine (Gabitril) is a more potent drug than gabapentin and selectively inhibits GABA reuptake and the GAT1 GABA transporter. Tiagabine has been studied primarily in GAD either as a monotherapy or in combination with SSRIs. In one study, tiagabine was as effective as paroxetine and more effective than placebo in the treatment of GAD. There are anecdotal reports of tiagabine's efficacy as an adjunctive agent in treating PTSD and in treating panic disorder. However, at least two Phase III studies of tiagabine in the treatment of GAD failed to meet their primary endpoint. Thus, development of tiagabine for GAD was discontinued. The other difficulty with tiagabine has been tolerability. Tiagabine's risks for seizures, cognitive problems, and sedation have limited its application in treating psychiatric disorders. That being said, we have seen a few patients do well with tiagabine at small dosages (2–4 mg/day) when other strategies were less successful.

Antipsychotics

Antipsychotics have long been used as adjunctive agents in the treatment of anxiety associated with disorders such as schizophrenia and bipolar disorder (Hirschfeld et al. 2006; Kung et al. 2012). In addition, early work with agents such as trifluoperazine suggested that antipsychotics might be as effective as benzodiazepines in the treatment of GAD. The SGAs, with their 5-HT_2 and 5-HT_{1A} effects, would be expected to have some benefits in anxiety disorders. Indeed, quetiapine does appear to be effective in controlled trials in the treatment of GAD (see Chapter 4, "Antipsychotic Drugs"). Additional controlled studies of antipsychotics in anxiety states have involved the adjunctive use of SGAs to augment antidepressant effects in OCD and PTSD. Although the data are somewhat conflicting, most of the studies suggest that the SGAs, especially risperidone (Dold et al. 2013), may be useful adjunctive agents in the treatment of refractory OCD. In addition, the SGAs have sometimes been said to be effective in the adjunctive treatment of panic disorder and OCD.

We have seen many instances when the SGAs have been well tolerated and effective as monotherapy of anxiety states when other conventional agents were not. Of the SGAs, quetiapine XR has the best data supporting its use in moderate to severe GAD (Montgomery et al. 2014). Dosages of quetiapine in the 150–300 mg/day range appear to be effective in the treatment of GAD. Even dosages as low as 25 mg twice daily may be helpful in some patients. However, given the metabolic risks, the use of an SGA such as quetiapine should generally be considered for the treatment of GAD only after other conventional treatments, such as an SSRI, have been tried. Although newer agents such as lumateperone have not been studied in the treatment of GAD, the high 5-HT-to-dopamine$_2$ ratio of the drug along with a relatively good metabolic and extrapyramidal symptoms profile might make it another reasonable candidate for the treatment of GAD.

Noradrenergic Agents

A number of studies have pointed to the potential use of β-blockers (e.g., propranolol) and primarily presynaptic but also postsynaptic α_2 receptor agonists (e.g., clonidine) to ameliorate symptoms of anxiety. Use of these agents stems from the observation that certain symptoms of anxiety (e.g., palpitations, sweating) suggest involvement of the sympathetic nervous system. Investigations were first directed toward the use of β-blockers in anxious musical performers. Many years ago, clonidine was shown by Gold et al. (1978) to be effective in blocking physiological symptoms associated with opioid withdrawal, resulting in its eventual study in patients with anxiety disorders and possibly nicotine withdrawal. This drug exerts α_2 (presynaptic) receptor agonist effects; however, because it is also a postsynaptic α_2 agonist, its pharmacological actions are complex.

Clinical Indications

β-Blockers (e.g., propranolol) are indicated for hypertension and for prophylaxis against angina, arrhythmias, migraine headaches, and hypertrophic subaortic stenosis. They are often quite useful in relieving akathisia in patients taking antipsychotics, although they are not approved by the FDA for this use (see Chapter 4). They are also not approved by the FDA for use in anxiety, although several studies have suggested that propranolol may be useful. These studies, originally conducted in Great Britain, pointed to β-blockers' having particularly potent effects on the somatic manifestations of anxiety (e.g., palpitations, tremors) and little or no effects on the psychic component of anxiety. The antitremor properties of these drugs have resulted in their being commonly used in treating patients whose hand tremors developed secondary to lithium carbonate use (see Chapter 5, "Mood Stabilizers").

A number of reports suggested that although β-blockers had some use in generalized anxiety, they were not particularly effective in blocking panic attacks. Indeed, Gorman et al. (1983) reported that propranolol failed to block lactate-induced panic attacks. However, some investigators noted that propranolol might block panic anxiety resulting from isoproterenol (an adrenergic agonist) infusions and thus could still be effective in treating some patients with panic attacks. Pindolol, a mixed β-adrenergic receptor agonist and antagonist with serotonergic properties, has been reported to augment antidepressant response to SSRIs (see Chapter 9).

As reported earlier in this chapter, β-blockers are widely believed to be useful in allaying anxiety during speaking or performing in public. Such use means that either the several weakly positive controlled studies of the efficacy of β-blockers in such situations are somehow flawed or placebos that have convincing rationales for efficacy can have a powerful effect. Again, open-label data also support the use of β-blockers for treating test anxiety.

Clonidine has an FDA-approved indication for the treatment of hypertension. As noted earlier, clonidine has been widely studied as a means of blocking physiological symptoms of opioid withdrawal (e.g., palpitations, sweating). The drug has also been studied in anxiety and in panic disorder and has been shown to be effective in both, although tolerance to the antianxiety effects frequently develops. Clonidine may be useful for treating the nightmares and hyperarousal associated with PTSD (Alao et al. 2012). It is conceivable that the drug's mixed, partial presynaptic and postsynaptic receptor agonist properties may enter into the development of tolerance. Clonidine has also been used to test various aspects of the catecholamine hypotheses of affective and anxiety disorders. Studies on nicotine withdrawal have yielded mixed results (Franks et al. 1989; Glassman et al. 1988). Clonidine has also been used to block the tachycardia and excessive salivation seen with clozapine use (see Chapter 4).

As reported earlier in this chapter, prazosin has been used, with mixed results, in the treatment of PTSD-associated nightmares. Dosages of prazosin for the treatment of PTSD have traditionally ranged from 1 to 16 mg/day (Kung et al. 2012), but there are case reports of much higher dosages being well tolerated and effective in treating the nightmares associated with PTSD (Koola et al. 2014). Even though the most definitive study to date (Raskind et al. 2018) did not show a clear benefit of prazosin treatment, the risks are relatively small, particularly with lower doses, and prazosin may still be worth a try if other strategies prove unsuccessful.

Dosage and Administration

Using propranolol as a model, clinicians should begin patients with peripheral symptoms of anxiety or patients with lithium-induced tremor or familial tremor at 10 mg bid and increase the dosage incrementally to approximately 30–120 mg/day. Although the usual maintenance dosage of the drug in patients with hypertension is as high as 240 mg/day, such a dosage is rarely needed for anxious or tremulous patients. Generally, the use of these agents in patients with anxiety disorders should parallel that of the benzodiazepines; trials should be made of having patients stop the drug after a few weeks of treatment.

Many patients with tremors secondary to lithium carbonate treated with a β-blocker show a reemergence of their tremors after discontinuation of the β-blocker, resulting in their continuing to take a β-blocker for a prolonged period. We know of no major untoward effects; however, some patients may become lethargic and even depressed while taking β-blockers, so clinicians need to keep this in mind when treating patients with a major affective disorder (see "Side Effects" subsection below). This potential effect is a matter of some debate. We have also used propranolol for TCA-induced tremor without affecting depression in most patients.

If propranolol or another β-blocker is to be used as an as-needed medication to decrease the physiological and, perhaps, psychological effects of performance anxiety or other circumscribed, predictable situations that induce social phobia, the patient should try the proposed dose (usually 10 or 20 mg) once or twice before using it before a performance to block stage fright to make sure they can tolerate the drug comfortably at that dose (Jefferson 1995). Clonidine should be started at a dosage of 0.1 mg bid, and the dosage should be increased by 0.1 mg every 1–2 days to a total daily dosage of 0.4–0.6 mg. Because some studies have indicated that tolerance to this drug develops, clinicians should attempt to limit the duration of exposure whenever possible.

Side Effects

Side effects of the β-blockers include bradycardia, hypotension, weakness, fatigue, clouded sensorium, impotence, gastrointestinal upset, and bronchospasm. For the psychiatrist, a few caveats appear warranted. Clinicians need to remember that these drugs are contraindicated in asthmatic patients because they may produce bronchospasm and in patients with Raynaud's disease because of the risk of increased peripheral vasoconstriction. Pindolol, which acts as a mixed β-adrenergic receptor agonist and antagonist, has less effect on receptors that control bronchial constriction and has been argued to be potentially safe in patients with asthma. However, its marked agonist effects can result in unpleasant stimulation, and we have not found it particularly useful in treating anxious patients. As for the capacity of β-blockers to cause depression, we have not seen patients who have developed true depressive disorders. Rather, we have noted that some patients may feel "washed out" or lethargic. However, clinicians at other institutions have reported cases of propranolol-induced depression with endogenous features that remitted on discontinuation of the drug.

One strategy is to switch to a β-blocker that is less lipophilic and that exerts fewer CNS effects (e.g., atenolol). This strategy may be particularly useful in men who have experienced decreased sexual potency while taking propranolol. When stopping β-blockers, it is wisest to taper the dose to avoid any rebound phenomena that could result in untoward cardiac or blood pressure effects.

Clonidine has a mixed side-effect profile. Its major side effects include dry mouth, sedation or fatigue, and hypotension. These effects are often found unacceptable by anxious patients. In hypertensive patients, scheduling twice-daily dosing (with two-thirds of the dose given at bedtime) has been advocated to deal with its sedating effects. Discontinuation should be gradual to avoid rebound autonomic symptoms or the hypertensive crises that have been reported in hypertensive patients who were suddenly withdrawn from the drug.

Prazosin's primary side effects are dizziness, headaches, sedation, and fatigue. Most patients are able to tolerate the 1–8 mg/day of prazosin that has been used to help sleep disturbance and anxiety in patients with PTSD. However, there are case reports of patients benefiting from dosages as high as 30 mg/day or more. Monitoring of blood pressure is important as prazosin doses are increased because orthostatic hypotension can be a substantial problem in some patients.

Antihistamines

The antihistamine hydroxyzine has an old indication for the treatment of anxiety and tension associated with "psychoneurotic conditions" or physical disease states. It is also indicated in the treatment of pruritus due to allergic conditions and for preoperative and postoperative sedation. In psychiatric practice, antihistamines are less commonly used in treating anxious patients, reflecting their less potent anxiolytic effect. Hydroxyzine's major side effects are drowsiness and dry mouth. It does not produce physical dependence; it may produce CNS depression when added to alcohol, narcotic analgesics, CNS depressants, or TCAs. Another antihistamine, diphenhydramine, is commonly used in medicine and psychiatry as a sedative-hypnotic (see Chapter 7).

Buspirone

The development of buspirone—a nonbenzodiazepine, generally nonsedating anxiolytic—stirred considerable excitement in psychopharmacological circles in the 1980s. It represented the first prominent anxiolytic to be intro-

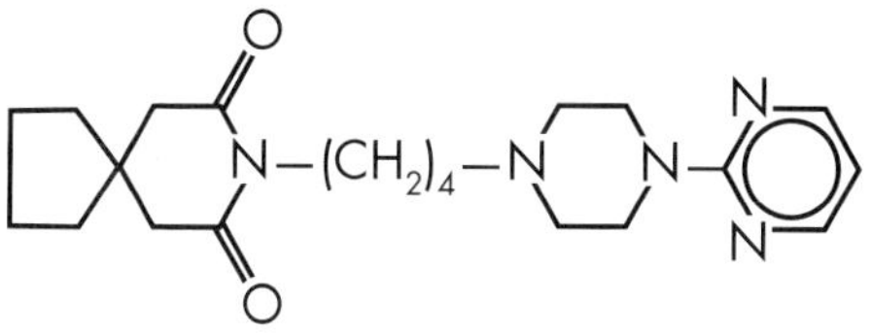

Figure 6–2. Chemical structure of buspirone.

duced since the benzodiazepines. The drug was originally developed as a potential antipsychotic agent. Although found in early clinical trials to have little antipsychotic potency, buspirone was eventually shown to have antiaggression effects in primates and antianxiety effects in humans. The structure of buspirone is shown in Figure 6–2. Buspirone went off patent in 2001 and is now available generically in the United States.

Buspirone does not bind with high affinity to benzodiazepine and GABA receptors, although it may have an effect on the chloride channel coupled to the benzodiazepine-GABA receptor complex. Buspirone has little antiseizure effect. Its anxiolytic effects were originally postulated to occur via dopaminergic properties, although the drug's central dopaminergic effects were not entirely clear. Later, buspirone was shown to exert its antianxiety effects by acting as a partial agonist of the 5-HT_{1A} receptor. This action is shared by gepirone and ipsapirone, related antianxiety drugs that do not have effects on the dopaminergic system.

Buspirone is an interesting, frustrating drug (Cole and Yonkers 1995) with properties that should make it the drug of choice in treating GAD and related anxiety disorders (e.g., social anxiety disorder, mixed anxiety and depression, anxiety in patients with a history of substance abuse). Buspirone was as effective as diazepam and superior to placebo in double-blind trials involving anxious outpatients. The available data from such studies do not show diazepam to be faster acting than buspirone, although most physicians assume that benzodiazepines are faster acting. One small subanalysis showed that patients with a history of benzodiazepine treatment did less well while taking buspirone than did patients who had never taken a benzodiazepine. Although the difference was statistically significant, half of the patients with a history of benzodiazepine use did improve while taking buspirone.

Most psychiatrists and many physicians assume that buspirone is weaker and slower in onset than are benzodiazepines, and many believe it is never effective in patients who have had a benzodiazepine in the past. These assumptions are not true. Buspirone is lacking in benzodiazepine-like effects and will not relieve benzodiazepine withdrawal symptoms. If patients like the sedation they feel after a single dose of a benzodiazepine (most do not like it), they will not get that "pause that refreshes" from buspirone. Unfortunately, both buspirone and benzodiazepines take 2–4 weeks to cause a full antianxiety effect. Psychiatrists rarely see patients with anxiety who have never taken a benzodiazepine and therefore may never see buspirone-appropriate patients and do not believe that buspirone is effective. Primary care physicians tend to learn from psychiatrists about drugs with complex dosage requirements that take weeks to act. Buspirone therefore is rarely used in adequate dosages—up to 30 mg/day or higher for 4–6 weeks—and is consequently widely believed not to work. Some, but not all, more recent studies show that buspirone is more effective than placebo in patients with depression, with social anxiety disorder, and with combined anxiety and alcoholism, at dosages of 30–60 mg/day, which patients do not tolerate as initial dosages. The best part of the buspirone story is therefore seldom reached.

Patients receiving drug therapy for anxiety disorders often do not need years of maintenance medication. Benzodiazepines can pose problems when they are tapered (particularly abruptly) and stopped. Anxious patients find that benzodiazepine withdrawal symptoms resemble the anxiety symptoms that first brought them to the doctor, become upset, and often end up taking diazepam or alprazolam again. If the patient had been taking buspirone instead, no withdrawal symptoms would have occurred; in fact, patients tend to improve a bit more in the first 2 weeks after buspirone is stopped. Buspirone is therefore a much more flexible drug to use in treating anxious patients: it can be tapered and withdrawn easily, and it enables the treating doctor to know readily whether it is still needed—without the patient's having to struggle with physical symptoms of drug withdrawal.

Buspirone should be initiated at a dosage of 5 mg bid, and the dosage should be increased gradually to 30–60 mg/day. Buspirone is not helpful in patients who are just stopping a benzodiazepine. However, if buspirone is added to the benzodiazepine for 2–6 weeks, the patient may feel "more better" because the two antianxiety drugs work by different mechanisms. Even if this effect does not occur, the benzodiazepine can be slowly tapered, often quite smoothly (Udelman and Udelman 1990), and the patient can be stabilized while taking buspirone.

Buspirone is well tolerated by medically ill elderly patients, does not depress respiration in patients with lung disease, and has some utility in patients with organic impulse disorders and in AIDS patients with anxiety. It does not adversely affect coordination or cognition. In short, it ought to be a major improvement over the benzodiazepines. However, its use in psychiatry has been limited to mainly adjunctive treatment.

Side effects of buspirone include headache, nausea, dizziness, and tension, which generally are not major problems. Indeed, the drug appears to have a more desirable side-effect profile than do the benzodiazepines. It does not appear to impair motor coordination, and it shows little untoward interaction with alcohol. It is also not sedating. According to an early report, the drug may exacerbate psychosis in patients with schizoaffective disorder, an effect that reflects complex prodopaminergic properties. This has not been a problem in clinical usage in the United States. High doses have, on the other hand, been reported to improve dyskinesia in patients with severe tardive dyskinesia. As noted in Chapter 11 ("Pharmacotherapy for Substance Use Disorders"), buspirone use also can result in reduced drinking in alcoholic outpatients.

The relative merits and side effects of buspirone versus the antidepressants in treating GAD have not been well studied. Davidson and colleagues (1999) found that venlafaxine XR appeared somewhat more effective in the treatment of GAD than did buspirone. It seems safe to say that buspirone has even fewer discontinuation effects than does venlafaxine or any of the antidepressants.

Novel Anxiolytic Agents

Although clinicians have a number of effective antianxiety agents to choose from, there are still significant limitations to the available agents. The benzodiazepines, although rapidly acting and effective, carry the risk of dependence and cognitive side effects. Likewise, the antidepressants, although effective in the long run, are slow to act and are poorly tolerated by a subset of patients. The antipsychotics have well-known limitations and are considered third-line agents. Many clinicians regard buspirone as a weak anxiolytic at best.

The search for safer, more effective, and rapidly acting agents has been ongoing since the 1960s (Griebel and Holmes 2013). The vast majority of truly novel compounds have proven ineffective or toxic in clinical trials. For example, agents targeting subunits of the $GABA_A$ receptor appeared to have anxiolytic properties but proved too sedating or amnestic to be pursued further. A variety of neuropeptides, including cholecystokinin type 2 receptor antagonists, corticotropin-releasing factor type 1 receptor antagonists, and neurokinin-2 agents, all proved either unreliable as anxiolytics or toxic.

Partial agonists of the $5-HT_{1A}$ receptor, such as buspirone, have moved far along in the clinical trial process, but most have failed to demonstrate enough efficacy to be approved. For example, gepirone made it to Phase III trials but was not effective enough to be released to the U.S. market. Tandospirone, another partial $5-HT_{1A}$ receptor agonist, has now been released in China and Japan but not elsewhere.

Among the more actively studied agents for the treatment of anxiety are agents that act on the glutamate receptor. Glutamate, the primary excitatory neurotransmitter, has long been investigated as a potential target for anxiolytic agents. Metabotropic glutamate receptors mGluR1, mGluR2, mGluR3, and mGluR5 are known to mediate anxiety behavior in animal models. Several mGluR2-mGluR3 receptor modulators have shown promise in clinical trials in GAD but not in panic disorder. One caution about these agents is that have been shown to lower seizure threshold in animal models. D-cycloserine, which potentiates glutamate N-methyl-D-aspartate receptor signaling, has shown some benefit in the adjunctive treatment of some disorders such as PTSD (Rodebaugh and Lenze 2013). A related compound, bitopertin, has shown promise in the treatment of OCD and schizophrenia (Hashimoto et al. 2013).

As discussed in Chapter 3, the serotonergic psychedelics, including psilocybin and N-dimethyltryptamine, have shown potential to mitigate anxiety in some patient populations and will no doubt be studied further for indications such as GAD. MDMA may also have applications in treating anxiety states other than PTSD.

It is unclear whether any of the novel agents discussed in this section will prove to be useful in the treatment of anxiety disorders. However, the quest for better anxiolytic agents will continue well into the future.

Suggested Readings

American Psychiatric Association: Diagnostic and Statistical Manual of Mental Disorders, 3rd Edition, Revised. Washington, DC, American Psychiatric Association, 1987

American Psychiatric Association: Diagnostic and Statistical Manual of Mental Disorders, 4th Edition. Washington, DC, American Psychiatric Association, 1994

American Psychiatric Association: Diagnostic and Statistical Manual of Mental Disorders, 4th Edition, Text Revision. Washington, DC, American Psychiatric Association, 2000

Ballenger JC, Burrows GD, DuPont RL Jr, et al: Alprazolam in panic disorder and agoraphobia: results from a multicenter trial I: efficacy in short-term treatment. Arch Gen Psychiatry 45(5):413–422, 1988 3282478

Baxter LR Jr, Thompson JM, Schwartz JM, et al: Trazodone treatment response in obsessive-compulsive disorder—correlated with shifts in glucose metabolism in the caudate nuclei. Psychopathology 20(Suppl 1):114–122, 1987 3501130

Benzodiazepine seizures: an update. Int Drug Ther Newsl 24:5–7, 1989

Bloch MH, Landeros-Weisenberger A, Kelmendi B, et al: A systematic review: antipsychotic augmentation with treatment refractory obsessive-compulsive disorder (erratum: Mol Psychiatry 11:795, 2006). Mol Psychiatry 11(7):622–632, 2006 16585942

Bogan AM, Koran LM, Chuong HW, et al: Quetiapine augmentation in obsessive-compulsive disorder resistant to serotonin reuptake inhibitors: an open-label study. J Clin Psychiatry 66(1):73–79, 2005 15669891

Braestrup C, Squires RF: Brain specific benzodiazepine receptors. Br J Psychiatry 133:249–260, 1978 698493

Bystritsky A, Ackerman DL, Rosen RM, et al: Augmentation of serotonin reuptake inhibitors in refractory obsessive-compulsive disorder using adjunctive olanzapine: a placebo-controlled trial. J Clin Psychiatry 65(4):565–568, 2004 15119922

Chao I: Olanzapine augmentation in panic disorder: a case report. Pharmacopsychiatry 37(5):239–240, 2004 15470803

de Beurs E, van Balkom AJ, Lange A, et al: Treatment of panic disorder with agoraphobia: comparison of fluvoxamine, placebo, and psychological panic management combined with exposure and of exposure in vivo alone. Am J Psychiatry 152(5):683–691, 1995 7726307

DeVeaugh-Geiss J, Landau P, Katz R: Preliminary results from a multicenter trial of clomipramine in obsessive-compulsive disorder. Psychopharmacol Bull 25(1):36–40, 1989 2672070

Fink M: Catatonia: syndrome or schizophrenia subtype? Recognition and treatment. J Neural Transm (Vienna) 108(6):637–644, 2001 11478416

Fink M: Treating neuroleptic malignant syndrome as catatonia. J Clin Psychopharmacol 21(1):121–122, 2001 11199941

Fluvoxamine for obsessive-compulsive disorder. Med Lett Drugs Ther 37(942):13–14, 1995 7845314

Foa EB: Psychosocial treatment of posttraumatic stress disorder. J Clin Psychiatry 61(5)(Suppl 5):43–48, discussion 49–51, 2000 10761678

Frank JB, Kosten TR, Giller EL Jr, et al: A randomized clinical trial of phenelzine and imipramine for posttraumatic stress disorder. Am J Psychiatry 145(10):1289–1291, 1988 3048121

Freeman CP, Trimble MR, Deakin JF, et al: Fluvoxamine versus clomipramine in the treatment of obsessive compulsive disorder: a multicenter, randomized, double-blind, parallel group comparison. J Clin Psychiatry 55(7):301–305, 1994 8071291

Friedman MJ: Toward rational pharmacotherapy for posttraumatic stress disorder: an interim report. Am J Psychiatry 145(3):281–285, 1988 2894174

Friedman MJ: What might the psychobiology of posttraumatic stress disorder teach us about future approaches to pharmacotherapy? J Clin Psychiatry 61(7)(Suppl 7):44–51, 2000 10795609

Fyer AJ, Liebowitz MR, Gorman JM, et al: Discontinuation of alprazolam treatment in panic patients. Am J Psychiatry 144(3):303–308, 1987 3826428

Gao K, Muzina D, Gajwani P, et al: Efficacy of typical and atypical antipsychotics for primary and comorbid anxiety symptoms or disorders: a review. J Clin Psychiatry 67(9):1327–1340, 2006 17017818

Gelpin E, Bonne O, Peri T, et al: Treatment of recent trauma survivors with benzodiazepines: a prospective study. J Clin Psychiatry 57(9):390–394, 1996 9746445

Goldberg HL: Buspirone hydrochloride: a unique new anxiolytic agent. Pharmacokinetics, clinical pharmacology, abuse potential and clinical efficacy. Pharmacotherapy 4(6):315–324, 1984 6151170

Granville-Grossman KL, Turner P: The effect of propranolol on anxiety. Lancet 1(7441):788–790, 1966 4159809

Greenblatt DJ, Shader RI, Abernethy DR: Drug therapy: current status of benzodiazepines. N Engl J Med 309(6):354–358, 1983 6135156

Greenblatt DJ, Shader RI, Abernethy DR: Drug therapy: current status of benzodiazepines. N Engl J Med 309(7):410–416, 1983 6135990

Hale WE, May FE, Moore MT, et al: Meprobamate use in the elderly: a report from the Dunedin program. J Am Geriatr Soc 36(11):1003–1005, 1988 2902115

Heimberg RG: Current status of psychotherapeutic interventions for social phobia. J Clin Psychiatry 62(1)(Suppl 1):36–42, 2001 11206032

Henry M, Fishman JR, Youngner SJ: Propranolol and the prevention of post-traumatic stress disorder: is it wrong to erase the "sting" of bad memories? Am J Bioeth 7(9):12–20, 2007 17849331

Herman JB, Rosenbaum JF, Brotman AW: The alprazolam to clonazepam switch for the treatment of panic disorder. J Clin Psychopharmacol 7(3):175–178, 1987 3597803

Insel TR (ed): New Findings in Obsessive-Compulsive Disorder. Washington, DC, American Psychiatric Press, 1984

Insel TR, Murphy DL, Cohen RM, et al: Obsessive-compulsive disorder: a double-blind trial of clomipramine and clorgyline. Arch Gen Psychiatry 40(6):605–612, 1983 6342562

Isbell H, Altschul S, Kornetsky CH, et al: Chronic barbiturate intoxication: an experimental study. Arch Neurol Psychiatry 64(1):1–28, 1950 15426447

Jerome L, Feduccia AA, Wang JB, et al: Long-term follow-up outcomes of MDMA-assisted psychotherapy for treatment of PTSD: a longitudinal pooled analysis of six phase 2 trials. Psychopharmacology (Berl) 237(8):2485–2497, 2020 32500209

Kahn R, McNair D, Covi L, et al: Effects of psychotropic agents in high anxiety subjects. Psychopharmacol Bull 17:97–100, 1981

Kavirajan H: The amobarbital interview revisited: a review of the literature since 1966. Harv Rev Psychiatry 7(3):153–165, 1999 10483934

Keck PE Jr, Strawn JR, McElroy SL: Pharmacologic treatment considerations in co-occurring bipolar and anxiety disorders. J Clin Psychiatry 67(Suppl 1):8–15, 2006 16426111

Liebowitz MR, Gorman JM, Fyer AJ, et al: Social phobia: review of a neglected anxiety disorder. Arch Gen Psychiatry 42(7):729–736, 1985 2861796

Liebowitz MR, Fyer AJ, Gorman JM, et al: Phenelzine in social phobia. J Clin Psychopharmacol 6(2):93–98, 1986 3700704

Lydiard RB, Falsetti SA: Treatment options for social phobia. Psychiatr Ann 17:409–423, 1994

Marazziti D, Pfanner C, Dell'Osso B, et al: Augmentation strategy with olanzapine in resistant obsessive compulsive disorder: an Italian long-term open-label study. J Psychopharmacol 19(4):392–394, 2005 15982994

McDougle CJ, Naylor ST, Cohen DJ, et al: A double-blind, placebo-controlled study of fluvoxamine in adults with autistic disorder. Arch Gen Psychiatry 53(11):1001–1008, 1996 8911223

Meltzer HY, Flemming R, Robertson A: The effect of buspirone on prolactin and growth hormone secretion in man. Arch Gen Psychiatry 40(10):1099–1102, 1983 6138009

Menza MA, Harris D: Benzodiazepines and catatonia: an overview. Biol Psychiatry 26(8):842–846, 1989 2574056

Mithoefer MC, Mithoefer AT, Feduccia AA, et al: 3,4-methylenedioxymethamphetamine (MDMA)-assisted psychotherapy for post-traumatic stress disorder in military veterans, firefighters, and police officers: a randomised, double-blind, dose-response, Phase 2 clinical trial. Lancet Psychiatry 5(6):486–497, 2018 29728331

Mooney JJ, Schatzberg AF, Cole JO, et al: Enhanced signal transduction by adenylate cyclase in platelet membranes of patients showing antidepressant responses to alprazolam: preliminary data. J Psychiatr Res 19(1):65–75, 1985 2985777

Nemeroff CB: Use of atypical antipsychotics in refractory depression and anxiety. J Clin Psychiatry 66(Suppl 8):13–21, 2005 16336032

Noyes R Jr, Anderson DJ, Clancy J, et al: Diazepam and propranolol in panic disorder and agoraphobia. Arch Gen Psychiatry 41(3):287–292, 1984 6367691

Noyes R Jr, DuPont RL Jr, Pecknold JC, et al: Alprazolam in panic disorder and agoraphobia: results from a multicenter trial II: patient acceptance, side effects, and safety. Arch Gen Psychiatry 45(5):423–428, 1988 3358644

Nutt DJ: The psychobiology of posttraumatic stress disorder. J Clin Psychiatry 61(5)(Suppl 5):24–29, discussion 30–32, 2000 10761676

Pande AC, Davidson JR, Jefferson JW, et al: Treatment of social phobia with gabapentin: a placebo-controlled study. J Clin Psychopharmacol 19(4):341–348, 1999 10440462

Petrides G, Fink M: Choosing a dosing strategy for electrical stimulation in ECT. J Clin Psychiatry 57(10):487–488, 1996 8909337

Petrides G, Fink M, Husain MM, et al: ECT remission rates in psychotic versus nonpsychotic depressed patients: a report from CORE. J ECT 17(4):244–253, 2001 11731725

Pivac N, Kozaric-Kovacic D, Muck-Seler D: Olanzapine versus fluphenazine in an open trial in patients with psychotic combat-related post-traumatic stress disorder. Psychopharmacology (Berl) 175(4):451–456, 2004 15064916

Pollack MH, Tesar GE, Rosenbaum JF, et al: Clonazepam in the treatment of panic disorder and agoraphobia: a one-year follow-up. J Clin Psychopharmacol 6(5):302–304, 1986 3771814

Pollack MH, Simon NM, Zalta AK, et al: Olanzapine augmentation of fluoxetine for refractory generalized anxiety disorder: a placebo controlled study. Biol Psychiatry 59(3):211–215, 2006 16139813

Problems associated with alprazolam therapy. Int Drug Ther Newsl 23:29–31, 1988

Riba J, Rodríguez-Fornells A, Strassman RJ, et al: Psychometric assessment of the Hallucinogen Rating Scale. Drug Alcohol Depend 62(3):215–223, 2001 11295326

Rickels K: Alprazolam extended-release in panic disorder. Expert Opin Pharmacother 5(7):1599–1611, 2004 15212610

Ries RK, Roy-Byrne PP, Ward NG, et al: Carbamazepine treatment for benzodiazepine withdrawal. Am J Psychiatry 146(4):536–537, 1989 2929759

Sathananthan GL, Sanghvi I, Phillips N, et al: MJ 9022: correlation between neuroleptic potential and stereotypy. Curr Ther Res Clin Exp 18(5):701–705, 1975 1208

Schneier FR: Treatment of social phobia with antidepressants. J Clin Psychiatry 62(1)(Suppl 1):43–48, discussion 49, 2001 11206033

Schweizer E, Rickels K, Lucki I: Resistance to the anti-anxiety effect of buspirone in patients with a history of benzodiazepine use. N Engl J Med 314(11):719–720, 1986 2869408

Sheehan DV, Ballenger J, Jacobsen G: Treatment of endogenous anxiety with phobic, hysterical, and hypochondriacal symptoms. Arch Gen Psychiatry 37(1):51–59, 1980 7352840

Solomon SD, Gerrity ET, Muff AM: Efficacy of treatments for posttraumatic stress disorder: an empirical review. JAMA 268(5):633–638, 1992 1629993

Strassman RJ: Hallucinogenic drugs in psychiatric research and treatment: perspectives and prospects. J Nerv Ment Dis 183(3):127–138, 1995 7891058

Sutherland SM, Davidson JRT: Pharmacotherapy for post-traumatic stress disorder. Psychiatr Clin North Am 17(2):409–423, 1994 7937367

Swedo SE, Leonard HL, Rapoport JL, et al: A double-blind comparison of clomipramine and desipramine in the treatment of trichotillomania (hair pulling). N Engl J Med 321(8):497–501, 1989 2761586

Tesar GE, Rosenbaum JF: Successful use of clonazepam in patients with treatment-resistant panic disorder. J Nerv Ment Dis 174(8):477–482, 1986 3734770

Tyrer PJ, Lader MH: Response to propranolol and diazepam in somatic and psychic anxiety. BMJ 2(5909):14–16, 1974 4595181

Tyrer P, Shawcross C: Monoamine oxidase inhibitors in anxiety disorders. J Psychiatr Res 22(Suppl 1):87–98, 1988 3050061

Uhlenhuth EH (ed): Benzodiazepine dependence and withdrawal: myths and management. J Clin Psychopharmacol 19(Suppl 2):1S–29S, 1999 10587277

van der Kolk BA: The drug treatment of post-traumatic stress disorder. J Affect Disord 13(2):203–213, 1987 2960712

van der Kolk BA, Dreyfuss D, Michaels M, et al: Fluoxetine in posttraumatic stress disorder. J Clin Psychiatry 55(12):517–522, 1994 7814344

Zitrin CM, Klein DF, Woerner MG, et al: Treatment of phobias I: comparison of imipramine hydrochloride and placebo. Arch Gen Psychiatry 40(2):125–138, 1983 6337578

References

Ahearn EP, Juergens T, Cordes T, et al: A review of atypical antipsychotic medications for posttraumatic stress disorder. Int Clin Psychopharmacol 26(4):193–200, 2011 21597381

Alao A, Selvarajah J, Razi S: The use of clonidine in the treatment of nightmares among patients with co-morbid PTSD and traumatic brain injury. Int J Psychiatry Med 44(2):165–169, 2012 23413663

American Psychiatric Association: Diagnostic and Statistical Manual of Mental Disorders, 5th Edition. Arlington, VA, American Psychiatric Association, 2013

American Psychiatric Association: Diagnostic and Statistical Manual of Mental Disorders, 5th Edition, Text Revision. Washington, DC, American Psychiatric Association, 2022

Arnold LM, Sarzi-Puttini P, Arsenault P, et al: Efficacy and safety of pregabalin in patients with fibromyalgia and comorbid depression taking concurrent antidepressant medication: a randomized placebo-controlled study. J Rheumatol 42(7):1237–1244, 2015 26034150

Baer L, Greist JH: An interactive computer-administered self-assessment and self-help program for behavior therapy. J Clin Psychiatry 58(12)(Suppl 12):23–28, 1997 9393393

Baer L, Rauch SL, Ballantine HT Jr, et al: Cingulotomy for intractable obsessive-compulsive disorder: prospective long-term follow-up of 18 patients. Arch Gen Psychiatry 52(5):384–392, 1995 7726719

Ballenger JC, Pecknold J, Rickels K, et al: Medication discontinuation in panic disorder. J Clin Psychiatry 54(10)(suppl):15–21, discussion 22–24, 1993 8262887

Barlow DH, Gorman JM, Shear MK, et al: Cognitive-behavioral therapy, imipramine, or their combination for panic disorder: a randomized controlled trial. JAMA 283(19):2529–2536, 2000 10815116

Bisson JI, Roberts NP, Andrew M, et al: Psychological therapies for chronic post-traumatic stress disorder (PTSD) in adults. Cochrane Database Syst Rev 2013(12):CD003388, 2013 24338345

Bonnet U, Scherbaum N: How addictive are gabapentin and pregabalin? A systematic review. Eur Neuropsychopharmacol 27(12):1185–1215, 2017 28988943

Cole JO, Yonkers KA: Non-benzodiazepine anxiolytics, in American Psychiatric Press Textbook of Psychopharmacology. Edited by Schatzberg AF, Nemeroff CB. Washington, DC, American Psychiatric Press, 1995, pp 231–244

Cole J, Selby B, Ismail Z, et al: D-cycloserine normalizes long-term motor plasticity after transcranial magnetic intermittent theta-burst stimulation in major depressive disorder. Clin Neurophysiol 132(8):1770–1776, 2021 34130243

Coupland NJ, Lillywhite A, Bell CE, et al: A pilot controlled study of the effects of flumazenil in posttraumatic stress disorder. Biol Psychiatry 41(9):988–990, 1997 9110106

Crowe SF, Stranks EK: The residual medium and long-term cognitive effects of benzodiazepine use: an updated meta-analysis. Arch Clin Neuropsychol 33(9):901–911, 2018 29244060

Davidson JRT: Pharmacotherapy of posttraumatic stress disorder: treatment options, long-term follow-up, and predictors of outcome. J Clin Psychiatry 61(5)(Suppl 5):52–56, discussion 57–59, 2000 10761679

Davidson JR, DuPont RL, Hedges D, et al: Efficacy, safety, and tolerability of venlafaxine extended release and buspirone in outpatients with generalized anxiety disorder. J Clin Psychiatry 60(8):528–535, 1999 10485635

Davidson J, Yaryura-Tobias J, DuPont R, et al: Fluvoxamine-controlled release formulation for the treatment of generalized social anxiety disorder. J Clin Psychopharmacol 24(2):118–125, 2004 15206657

DiMauro J, Domingues J, Fernandez G, et al: Long-term effectiveness of CBT for anxiety disorders in an adult outpatient clinic sample: a follow-up study. Behav Res Ther 51(2):82–86, 2013 23262115

Dold M, Aigner M, Lanzenberger R, et al: Antipsychotic augmentation of serotonin reuptake inhibitors in treatment-resistant obsessive-compulsive disorder: a meta-analysis of double-blind, randomized, placebo-controlled trials. Int J Neuropsychopharmacol 16(3):557–574, 2013 22932229

Franks P, Harp J, Bell B: Randomized, controlled trial of clonidine for smoking cessation in a primary care setting. JAMA 262(21):3011–3013, 1989 2681856

Gladsjo JA, Rapaport MH, McKinney R, et al: Absence of neuropsychologic deficits in patients receiving long-term treatment with alprazolam-XR for panic disorder. J Clin Psychopharmacol 21(2):131–138, 2001 11270908

Glassman AH, Stetner F, Walsh BT, et al: Heavy smokers, smoking cessation, and clonidine: results of a double-blind, randomized trial. JAMA 259(19):2863–2866, 1988 3367452

Glover H: A preliminary trial of nalmefene for the treatment of emotional numbing in combat veterans with post-traumatic stress disorder. Isr J Psychiatry Relat Sci 30(4):255–263, 1993 8163362

Glue P, Fang A, Gandelman K, et al: Pharmacokinetics of an extended release formulation of alprazolam (Xanax XR) in healthy normal adolescent and adult volunteers. Am J Ther 13(5):418–422, 2006 16988537

Goddard AW, Brouette T, Almai A, et al: Early coadministration of clonazepam with sertraline for panic disorder. Arch Gen Psychiatry 58(7):681–686, 2001 11448376

Gold MS, Redmond DE Jr, Kleber HD: Clonidine in opiate withdrawal. Lancet 1(8070):929–930, 1978 76860

Gorman JM, Levy GF, Liebowitz MR, et al: Effect of acute beta-adrenergic blockade on lactate-induced panic. Arch Gen Psychiatry 40(10):1079–1082, 1983 6312917

Greenblatt DJ, von Moltke LL, Harmatz JS, et al: Alprazolam pharmacokinetics, metabolism, and plasma levels: clinical implications. J Clin Psychiatry 54(10)(suppl):4–11, discussion 12–14, 1993 8262889

Griebel G, Holmes A: 50 years of hurdles and hope in anxiolytic drug discovery. Nat Rev Drug Discov 12(9):667–687, 2013 23989795

Hashimoto K, Malchow B, Falkai P, et al: Glutamate modulators as potential therapeutic drugs in schizophrenia and affective disorders. Eur Arch Psychiatry Clin Neurosci 263(5):367–377, 2013 23455590

Hembree EA, Foa EB: Posttraumatic stress disorder: psychological factors and psychosocial interventions. J Clin Psychiatry 61(7)(Suppl 7):33–39, 2000 10795607

Hirschfeld RM, Weisler RH, Raines SR, et al: Quetiapine in the treatment of anxiety in patients with bipolar I or II depression: a secondary analysis from a randomized, double-blind, placebo-controlled study. J Clin Psychiatry 67(3):355–362, 2006 16649820

Hofmann SG, Pollack MH, Otto MW: Augmentation treatment of psychotherapy for anxiety disorders with D-cycloserine. CNS Drug Rev 12(3–4):208–217, 2006 17227287

Jefferson JW: Social phobia: a pharmacologic treatment overview. J Clin Psychiatry 56(5)(Suppl 5):18–24, 1995 7782272

Kerbage H, Richa S: Non-antidepressant long-term treatment in post-traumatic stress disorder (PTSD). Curr Clin Pharmacol 10(2):116–125, 2015 23438728

Klein DF: Importance of psychiatric diagnosis in prediction of clinical drug effects. Arch Gen Psychiatry 16(1):118–126, 1967 5333776

Klein DF: False suffocation alarms, spontaneous panics, and related conditions: an integrative hypothesis. Arch Gen Psychiatry 50(4):306–317, 1993 8466392

Koola MM, Varghese SP, Fawcett JA: High-dose prazosin for the treatment of posttraumatic stress disorder. Ther Adv Psychopharmacol 4(1):43–47, 2014 24490030

Koran LM, Aboujaoude E, Bullock KD, et al: Double-blind treatment with oral morphine in treatment-resistant obsessive-compulsive disorder. J Clin Psychiatry 66(3):353–359, 2005 15766302

Kung S, Espinel Z, Lapid MI: Treatment of nightmares with prazosin: a systematic review. Mayo Clin Proc 87(9):890–900, 2012 22883741

Lader M: Summary and commentary, in Pharmacology of Benzodiazepines. Edited by Usdin E, Skolnick P, Tallman JF, et al. New York, Macmillan, 1982, pp 53–60

Lucki I, Rickels K, Geller AM: Chronic use of benzodiazepines and psychomotor and cognitive test performance. Psychopharmacology (Berl) 88(4):426–433, 1986 2871579

McDougle CJ: Update on pharmacologic management of OCD: agents and augmentation. J Clin Psychiatry 58(Suppl 12):11–17, 1997 9393391

McGhee LL, Maani CV, Garza TH, et al: The effect of propranolol on posttraumatic stress disorder in burned service members. J Burn Care Res 30(1):92–97, 2009 19060728

Miller LJ: Prazosin for the treatment of posttraumatic stress disorder sleep disturbances. Pharmacotherapy 28(5):656–666, 2008 18447662

Mindus P, Jenike MA: Neurosurgical treatment of malignant obsessive compulsive disorder. Psychiatr Clin North Am 15(4):921–938, 1992 1461805

Mitchell JM, Bogenschutz M, Lilienstein A, et al: MDMA-assisted therapy for severe PTSD: a randomized, double-blind, placebo-controlled phase 3 study. Nat Med 27(6):1025–1033, 2021 33972795

Mithoefer MC, Feduccia AA, Jerome L, et al: MDMA-assisted psychotherapy for treatment of PTSD: study design and rationale for phase 3 trials based on pooled analysis of six Phase 2 randomized controlled trials. Psychopharmacology (Berl) 236(9):2735–2745, 2019 31065731

Montgomery SA: Pregabalin for the treatment of generalised anxiety disorder. Expert Opin Pharmacother 7(15):2139–2154, 2006 17020438

Montgomery SA, Tobias K, Zornberg GL, et al: Efficacy and safety of pregabalin in the treatment of generalized anxiety disorder: a 6-week, multicenter, randomized, double-blind, placebo-controlled comparison of pregabalin and venlafaxine. J Clin Psychiatry 67(5):771–782, 2006 16841627

Montgomery SA, Locklear JC, Svedsäter H, et al: Efficacy of once-daily extended release quetiapine fumarate in patients with different levels of severity of generalized anxiety disorder. Int Clin Psychopharmacol 29(5):252–262, 2014 24394383

Mumford GK, Evans SM, Fleishaker JC, et al: Alprazolam absorption kinetics affects abuse liability. Clin Pharmacol Ther 57(3):356–365, 1995 7697954

Norberg MM, Krystal JH, Tolin DF: A meta-analysis of D-cycloserine and the facilitation of fear extinction and exposure therapy. Biol Psychiatry 63(12):1118–1126, 2008 18313643

Offidani E, Guidi J, Tomba E, et al: Efficacy and tolerability of benzodiazepines versus antidepressants in anxiety disorders: a systematic review and meta-analysis. Psychother Psychosom 82(6):355–362, 2013 24061211

Ooms P, Mantione M, Figee M, et al: Deep brain stimulation for obsessive-compulsive disorders: long-term analysis of quality of life. J Neurol Neurosurg Psychiatry 85(2):153–158, 2014 23715912

Ori R, Amos T, Bergman H, et al: Augmentation of cognitive and behavioural therapies (CBT) with d-cycloserine for anxiety and related disorders. Cochrane Database Syst Rev 2015(5):CD007803, 2015 25957940

Pearlstein T: Antidepressant treatment of posttraumatic stress disorder. J Clin Psychiatry 61(7)(Suppl 7):40–43, 2000 10795608

Pecknold JC, Swinson RP, Kuch K, et al: Alprazolam in panic disorder and agoraphobia: results from a multicenter trial. III. Discontinuation effects. Arch Gen Psychiatry 45(5):429–436, 1988 3282479

Pitman RK, Delahanty DL: Conceptually driven pharmacologic approaches to acute trauma. CNS Spectr 10(2):99–106, 2005 15685120

Pollack MH, Simon NM, Worthington JJ, et al: Combined paroxetine and clonazepam treatment strategies compared to paroxetine monotherapy for panic disorder. J Psychopharmacol 17(3):276–282, 2003 14513919

Pollack MH, Hoge EA, Worthington JJ, et al: Eszopiclone for the treatment of posttraumatic stress disorder and associated insomnia: a randomized, double-blind, placebo-controlled trial. J Clin Psychiatry 72(7):892–897, 2011 21367352

Raskind MA, Peterson K, Williams T, et al: A trial of prazosin for combat trauma PTSD with nightmares in active-duty soldiers returned from Iraq and Afghanistan. Am J Psychiatry 170(9):1003–1010, 2013 23846759

Raskind MA, Peskind ER, Chow B, et al: Trial of prazosin for posttraumatic stress disorder in military veterans. N Engl J Med 378(6):507–517, 2018 29414272

Reissig CJ, Harrison JA, Carter LP, et al: Inhaled vs. oral alprazolam: subjective, behavioral and cognitive effects, and modestly increased abuse potential. Psychopharmacology (Berl) 232(5):871–883, 2015 25199955

Ressler KJ, Rothbaum BO, Tannenbaum L, et al: Cognitive enhancers as adjuncts to psychotherapy: use of D-cycloserine in phobic individuals to facilitate extinction of fear. Arch Gen Psychiatry 61(11):1136–1144, 2004 15520361

Rickels K, Schweizer E: Maintenance treatment studies in anxiety disorders: some methodological notes. Psychopharmacol Bull 31(1):115–123, 1995 7675975

Rickels K, Case WG, Downing RW, et al: Long-term diazepam therapy and clinical outcome. JAMA 250(6):767–771, 1983 6348314

Rickels K, Schweizer E, Csanalosi I, et al: Long-term treatment of anxiety and risk of withdrawal. Prospective comparison of clorazepate and buspirone. Arch Gen Psychiatry 45(5):444–450, 1988 2895993

Rickels K, DeMartinis N, Rynn M, et al: Pharmacologic strategies for discontinuing benzodiazepine treatment. J Clin Psychopharmacol 19(6)(Suppl 2):12S–16S, 1999 10587279

Rodebaugh TL, Lenze EJ: Lessons learned from D-cycloserine: the promise and limits of drug facilitation of exposure therapy. J Clin Psychiatry 74(4):415–416, 2013 23656850

Rodriguez CI, Kegeles LS, Levinson A, et al: Randomized controlled crossover trial of ketamine in obsessive-compulsive disorder: proof-of-concept. Neuropsychopharmacology 38(12):2475–2483, 2013 23783065

Smith WT, Londborg PD, Glaudin V, et al: Short-term augmentation of fluoxetine with clonazepam in the treatment of depression: a double-blind study. Am J Psychiatry 155(10):1339–1345, 1998 9766764

Southwick SM, Krystal JH, Bremner JD, et al: Noradrenergic and serotonergic function in posttraumatic stress disorder. Arch Gen Psychiatry 54(8):749–758, 1997 9283511

Spiegel DA: Psychological strategies for discontinuing benzodiazepine treatment. J Clin Psychopharmacol 19(6)(Suppl 2):17S–22S, 1999 10587280

Stewart SA: The effects of benzodiazepines on cognition. J Clin Psychiatry 66(Suppl 2):9–13, 2005 15762814

Thompson CE, Taylor FB, McFall ME, et al: Nonnightmare distressed awakenings in veterans with posttraumatic stress disorder: response to prazosin. J Trauma Stress 21(4):417–420, 2008 18720392

Torres-Bondia F, Dakterzada F, Galván L, et al: Benzodiazepine and Z-drug use and the risk of developing dementia. Int J Neuropsychopharmacol 25(4):261–268, 2022 34727174

Udelman HD, Udelman DL: Concurrent use of buspirone in anxious patients during withdrawal from alprazolam therapy. J Clin Psychiatry 51(9)(suppl):46–50, 1990 2211568

U.S. Department of Veterans Affairs; Department of Defense: VA/DoD Clinical Practice Guideline for the Management of Posttraumatic Stress Disorder and Acute Stress Disorder, Version 3.0. Washington, DC, U.S Department of Veterans Affairs, June 2017. Available at: www.healthquality.va.gov/guidelines/MH/ptsd/VADoDPTSDCPGFinal012418.pdf. Accessed January 15, 2022.

Westenberg HG, Stein DJ, Yang H, et al: A double-blind placebo-controlled study of controlled release fluvoxamine for the treatment of generalized social anxiety disorder. J Clin Psychopharmacol 24(1):49–55, 2004 14709947

Zohar J, Juven-Wetzler A, Sonnino R, et al: New insights into secondary prevention in post-traumatic stress disorder. Dialogues Clin Neurosci 13(3):301–309, 2011 22033784

7

Hypnotics

Insomnia

Insomnia is generally defined as a difficulty initiating or maintaining sleep or a poor quality of sleep. Insomnia may be primary or secondary to other conditions such as depression, anxiety, mania, or substance abuse. Previously, insomnia was divided into primary and secondary types, but that classification has now been abandoned. Various population surveys have found self-reported symptoms of insomnia in about a third of adults. About 10% of the U.S. population report having experienced symptoms of chronic insomnia that may have lasted for many years. However, a smaller percentage of patients have insomnia with significant daytime impairment. According to the "NIH State of the Science Conference Statement on Manifestations and Management of Chronic Insomnia in Adults Statement" (2005), perhaps 10% of the population has clinically significant insomnia if the criterion of daytime impairment is included in the criteria. According to a 2014 survey by the Sleep Foundation, about 17% of the population use a hypnotic at least once a week, and 10% of the population use some kind of sleeping aid on a daily basis (National

Sleep Foundation 2014). Women and older adults appear to be the demographic groups at greatest risk for significant insomnia (Zhang et al. 2006), but of course transient insomnia can affect anyone.

The chronic use of hypnotics is typically discouraged in the medical literature, and it is assumed that the sleepless public will go to physicians or sleep clinics, where staff will find types of insomnia that respond to behavioral or other nonsedative medical therapies. However, for some patients, chronic use of a hypnotic is beneficial and not subject to abuse. Certainly, conditions such as sleep apnea, narcolepsy, and restless legs syndrome do occur, and they can be treated in a variety of ways. Sleep apnea can be life-threatening. Some insomnia may respond to treatment of the underlying illness (e.g., hyperthyroidism, depression, mania). One U.S. National Institutes of Health (NIH) Consensus Conference spent a great deal of time worrying about the possible adverse effects of hypnotics and suggested that, at most, hypnotics be prescribed for brief periods or be used only every third night. Grandner and Pack (2011), in an editorial in *JAMA*, noted that insomnia and sleep deprivation are associated with a significant increase in all-cause mortality as well as associated leading causes of mortality, including motor vehicle accidents and cardiovascular disorders. Thus, the risk associated with the use of hypnotics must be counterbalanced by the very real public health risk of inadequate sleep. About 3% of the population regularly takes over-the-counter hypnotics containing sedative antihistamines or sedative antihistamines plus mild analgesics. Sales of both types of sleep aids have been escalating, essentially unstudied, for many years.

We therefore have a situation in which a growing number of hypnotics are available for prescription use but are rather unpopular with some polysomnographers and sleep experts in particular and with physicians in general. One gets the odd impression that many individuals with chronic insomnia make do with diphenhydramine or with wakefulness while more effective hypnotics are withheld from them. Although eszopiclone, zolpidem, and ramelteon are now approved for chronic use, the perceived risk of dependence tends to limit their extended use as hypnotics even when better alternatives may be lacking.

The availability of ramelteon has altered the discourse on hypnotics somewhat. Ramelteon, a melatonin agonist, does not have the habit-forming potential of traditional hypnotics and is not sedating. On the other hand, ramelteon may not be as effective in addressing the spectrum of sleep difficulties as benzodiazepine and nonbenzodiazepine hypnotics.

When insomnia does lead patients to seek help from a psychiatrist or a sleep disorder specialist, the patients complain, often despairingly, of very poor sleep or total insomnia, but they nevertheless appear, on all-night sleep recordings or from nurses' or relatives' observations, to be sleeping most of the night. Attempts to objectify insomnia in terms of the time it takes for the person to fall asleep or the length of time actually slept have often not proved useful. Further, the psychiatrist is not uncommonly faced with patients who are actually awake all night, particularly those with marked depression and anxiety, whose sleep is so disturbed that they feel exhausted the next day and claim that they "can't function" or, in reality, cannot function.

Primary care physicians often see patients with untreated and undiagnosed insomnia. The physician can guess at presence of two of the treatable sleep disorders by asking questions of the patient and their bed partner. Sleep apnea is likely present when the partner notes the patient stops breathing in the night then snorts and gasps; snoring is also likely. The patient may note daytime sleepiness instead of wakefulness at night. Restless legs syndrome is subjectively obvious to the patient as a discomfort in his or her limbs that is relieved by movement, much like akathisia. The restlessness is worse later in the day and can disturb sleep or can disturb the bed partner because jerky leg movements at night feel like kicks. Periodic leg movement disorder is diagnosed when the leg movements occur mainly during sleep and may cause awakenings.

Falling asleep during the day can be a symptom of narcolepsy and responds well to older stimulants and to modafinil (Provigil) or armodafinil (Nuvigil).

However, most patients coming to psychiatrists or psychiatric clinics with insomnia will already be taking medication. In these cases, the clinical problems are as follows:

1. Is a diagnosable, specific sleep disorder being missed? Is referral to a sleep clinic indicated?
2. Are any of the patient's prescribed or self-administered medications (selective serotonin reuptake inhibitors [SSRIs], bronchodilators, caffeine, cocaine) causing the problem, or is the problem due to a medical condition (e.g., chronic pain, urinary frequency)?

3. Is the insomnia due to an undertreated or recurrent psychiatric condition or medical disorder?
4. If the patient is already taking a hypnotic and it is (or is not) working, should the medication be continued or stopped? If the medication is stopped, should a new medication be started?

Among psychiatric patients, troublesome insomnia is often one feature of a wider symptom complex, which may also include diurnal rhythm disturbances of activity, mood, and so forth. Insomnia related to depression and anxiety disorders is far more common than is primary insomnia that is not related to a psychiatric disorder. Depressed patients classically experience early morning awakening and diurnal variation. Many, however, have marked difficulty falling asleep and staying asleep as well. Patients with pronounced initial insomnia may be separated into those who sleep fitfully and poorly even after falling asleep and those who sleep well even after several hours of initial insomnia. Such patients can sleep from 4:00 A.M. until noon. A few patients with very severe depression complain of almost complete insomnia, reporting that they lie in bed all night without sleeping, often experiencing dysphoric, miserable ruminations.

Other psychiatric conditions are also manifested by sleep disturbances. Patients with anxiety disorders are more likely to have trouble falling asleep. Patients with mania or hypomania may stay up all night, either happily overactive or dysphorically agitated, as may patients with schizophrenia or schizophreniform psychoses. Classically, manic patients do not necessarily complain of experiencing sleeplessness; rather, they may claim that they are not sleeping much and do not seem to miss the usual sleep they get. Patients with dementia may become more confused and agitated toward evening (sundowning) and may also be agitated at night after sleeping all day. Fatigue is often a factor in sundowning. Patients who are very upset by major stressors—for example, bereavement, rejections, or physical trauma—may have insomnia as part of an acute stress response. Patients with PTSD may be afraid of falling asleep and thus have initial insomnia.

Insomnia in all the relatively acute psychiatric conditions mentioned above may be fairly straightforward to treat. Protriptyline was once reported to be a good treatment for sleep apnea. Insomnia as part of a depressive disorder often responds to a standard antidepressant; in fact, some of the more sedating antidepressants (mirtazapine, amitriptyline, doxepin, trazodone) may be useful hypnotics even in the absence of depression (see the section "Sedative Antihistamines and Other Nonbenzodiazepine Psychoactive Drugs With Hypnotic Properties" later in this chapter). For depression with poor sleep, it is sensible to begin with a sedative antidepressant (see Chapter 3, "Antidepressants"), but antidepressants with more stimulant effects, such as bupropion and fluoxetine, usually improve sleep as the depressive syndrome improves. In a study at McLean Hospital of more than 100 depressed patients taking fluoxetine, we found that insomnia at intake was not associated with a poorer clinical response to fluoxetine, even though fluoxetine can cause insomnia and negatively impact sleep architecture as a side effect. In cases of manic and schizophrenic excitement and in some cases of agitation, the insomnia often responds well to antipsychotic drugs of any class, although one of the sedating second-generation antipsychotics such as quetiapine may initially be more effective as a hypnotic before the general syndrome is ameliorated.

Thus, the best general approach is to treat the psychiatric condition that underlies the insomnia with drugs that are appropriate to that condition rather than first prescribing a benzodiazepine or other hypnotic drug for the insomnia and then treating the depression or psychosis. If a patient should be taking a drug that turns out to aggravate or cause insomnia, short-term use of a hypnotic or a drug such as trazodone or mirtazapine may be useful. A recent survey found that 100% of sleep specialists, versus 40% of non-sleep clinicians, believed that insomnia needed to be addressed directly in patients who had insomnia with a comorbid disorder (Morin et al. 2023). This gap may reflect the nature of the patients that each group sees rather than a lack of appreciation for the negative consequences of insomnia.

In principle, a psychiatrist can run an inpatient ward or treat outpatients without ever prescribing a hypnotic. In practice, however, life often is (or appears to be) more complicated. Other patients, families, and nursing staff members become very upset if patients do not retire to bed and sleep without disturbing them. Often, hypnotics end up being prescribed to reduce the patient's distress and distress in their milieu. Such prescribing is often justifiable but can pose problems. First, the hypnotic may not put the patient to sleep, but instead may leave the patient (unpredictably) groggy, confused, and even more agitated. Second, a long-acting hypnotic, such as flurazepam, may leave the patient groggy the next day. Third, once the patient is used to getting a hypnotic (and the doctor is used to prescribing it), the practice may continue for weeks or even months, long after the initial phase of the illness or the stress of hospitalization has passed. When the sleeping pill is finally stopped, rebound insomnia is likely to occur, and hypnotic use is likely to be resumed to control it. (*Rebound insomnia* is a transient worsening of sleep disturbance occurring soon after discontinuation of the hypnotic.) In fact, with short-acting hypnotics such as triazolam (or alcohol), rebound insomnia can occur even 4 hours after the medication is taken. Such an effect can precipitate overuse of the compound: some patients will take additional doses to help them fall back to sleep.

Another problematic situation involves the new patient being admitted to the hospital (or visiting a new psychiatrist) who is thoroughly accustomed to taking 10 mg of zolpidem, 3 mg of eszopiclone, or 30 mg of temazepam at bedtime (having taken the medication for months or years) but still complains of poor sleep. As might be expected, the quality of sleep is reportedly much worse if the hypnotic is stopped. Here, two obvious options are available: taper the hypnotic gradually while treating the major psychiatric disorder or continue it while dealing with the disorder. The difficulty with the second, interpersonally easier, option is that the hypnotic may never be discontinued. A more complicated version of this scenario is when the patient, at the time they come to the psychiatrist for treatment, is taking several psychoactive drugs of different classes, all of which need to be withdrawn or changed. In this situation, it is common to leave the hypnotic at a stable dose and taper and stop the other drugs first. This method avoids combining, and thus confusing, the effects of stopping the hypnotic with the already potentially complex effects of discontinuing an antidepressant or an antipsychotic.

At present, the most widely approved indications for hypnotics in treating insomnia are 1) brief (3- to 7-day) use and 2) occasional use for transitory insomnia caused by either acute life stressors or major shifts in diurnal rhythm (as in jet lag or in changing from one work shift to another).

Although it is wise to avoid prolonged hypnotic use, prolonged use of a benzodiazepine hypnotic may be less harmful than is often said and may, in fact, provide some benefit. In addition to contributing to a variety of health issues and an increase in accidents, sleep loss is widely believed to sometimes precipitate manic or depressive episodes. The available evidence from sleep laboratories suggests that hypnotics improve sleep measurably for only a few weeks, although placebo-controlled studies have shown no diminution in the efficacy of hypnotics for up to 24 weeks, and single-blind studies show efficacy up to a year. So far, no studies have clearly established a treatment duration after which benzodiazepine hypnotics fail to "work." Many confirmed users of hypnotics swear that the hypnotics are always helpful and even vitally necessary for years. Perhaps the initial sedation at peak blood levels provides a familiar, conditioned cue conducive to falling asleep. There is also evidence that benzodiazepines cause the patient to forget episodes of wakefulness; when the patient is no longer taking benzodiazepines, sleep may objectively be no worse, but they perceive (recall) it as being worse. Certainly, some patients who have taken a hypnotic every night for several years continue to complain of poor sleep and daytime fatigue and dysphoria for months after the hypnotic is stopped.

The current evidence is that zolpidem, zaleplon, and eszopiclone continued to be effective (i.e., improve sleep as measured by polysomnographic criteria) for 4–5 weeks in placebo-controlled studies and for as long as 6 months in single-blind studies. Studies using other, less formal criteria (subject or observer ratings of sleep) have shown benefit for up to a year. Data are not available beyond that point. Since publication of earlier editions of this manual, sleep experts appear to have become more permissive about the possible benefits of longer-term use of benzodiazepine-like hypnotics (Buysse and Dorsey 2002). However, package inserts still limit the use of such hypnotics to durations of use validated by placebo-controlled studies. Patients sometimes interpret such restrictions to mean that serious toxicity has been shown to occur if the hypnotic is taken for longer than specified in the *Physicians' Desk Reference*. Such an interpretation does not seem to be accurate. Oversedation, poor coordination, and memory problems are more likely to occur very early in treatment. The evidence for serious behavioral or other toxicity (e.g., impaired psychomotor performance early in treatment, auto accidents, falls in the elderly) is mixed and inconclusive (Buysse and Dorsey 2002).

Behavioral Approaches

Sleep hygiene recommendations are often useful to patients with both primary and secondary insomnia. However, insomnia secondary to another condition is not likely to resolve with improved sleep hygiene alone. Thus, it is important to first identify and then treat the underlying condition.

Sleep Hygiene Recommendations

- Sleep only when sleepy.
- If you can't fall asleep within 20 minutes, get up and do something until you feel sleepy.
- Don't take naps.
- Get up and go to bed the same time every day.
- Refrain from exercise at least 4 hours before bedtime.
- Develop a sleep routine.
- Use your bed only for sleeping or sex.
- Stay away from caffeine, nicotine, and alcohol at least 4 hours before bedtime.
- Do not eat heavy, spicy, or rich foods 4 hours before bedtime.
- Make sure your bed and bedroom are quiet and comfortable.
- Use sunlight to set your biological clock.

Cognitive-behavioral therapy for insomnia (CBT-I) is one of the most consistently effective approaches to the long-term management of primary insomnia (Edinger and Means 2005). The more clinically and scientifically validated (non-pharmacological) approaches to insomnia are as follows:

1. *Stimulus control therapy (sleep hygiene).* The patient learns to associate being in bed only with sleep (or sex) by getting out of bed when they do not fall asleep rapidly in order to avoid linking bed and bedroom with miserable sleepless nights.
2. *Sleep restriction therapy.* The patient reduces time in bed progressively (with daytime naps forbidden) until they are asleep for 80%–90% of the time they are allowed to be in bed.
3. *Continuous positive airway pressure* (for patients with sleep apnea). The patient learns to wear a mask that delivers light, constant positive air pressure to the pharynx and thereby prevents the choking spells from occurring.
4. *Bright light therapy.* A patient who sleeps an adequate amount but at the wrong time of the night or day can have their sleep-wake rhythm reset through exposure to a light box.

Obviously, behavioral approaches require patient involvement and cooperation and are best managed by experts in sleep problems.

Pharmacological Approaches

For much of the past 30 years, the major efforts to develop better hypnotics have focused entirely on chemicals that bind to at least some form of benzodiazepine receptor. It was hoped that these agents would turn out to be better than, say, temazepam by being faster acting, being less likely to cause a morning hangover, not being abusable or addictive, and not causing any change in polysomnographic sleep records (or, perhaps, causing only an increase in stage 3 and rapid eye movement [REM] sleep).

So far, this semisystematic approach has yielded a plethora of benzodiazepines, one of which, quazepam, may be selective for benzodiazepine$_1$ receptors, and three agents (zolpidem, zaleplon, and eszopiclone) that are active at benzodiazepine receptors but are not chemically benzodiazepines and may bind to fewer types of GABA-A receptors (Krystal, in press). So far, none of these drugs has been shown to be remarkably different in effect from the older benzodiazepine hypnotics, though zolpidem, eszopiclone, and zaleplon may have some advantages in that they are less likely to cause rebound insomnia, are less likely to exacerbate obstructive airway problems through muscle relaxation, and may show continued efficacy, when given nightly, for much longer. Eszopiclone has approval for long-term use.

In the interim, in fact for decades, drugs developed for other purposes end up being used for insomnia, at least by psychiatrists. Trazodone in doses of 50–200 mg at night is used more frequently for insomnia than for its original FDA-approved indication, depression. Unfortunately, trazodone's use for insomnia began only as the company's patent was expiring, so no systematic or extensive studies of its effects on sleep and insomnia have been done. Still, smaller studies have suggested that trazodone is effective and well tolerated as a hypnotic, with modest negative effects in most patients (Camargos et al. 2014; Tanimukai et al. 2013). Most clinicians agree that it works. Its problems are morning drowsiness and, conceivably (although very rarely), priapism. If tolerance to its hypnotic effect occurs, it develops only after months or years. The drug has no known abuse liability and has no clear withdrawal symptoms. Trazodone is a potent antagonist for 5-HT$_2$ receptors, an effect shared with other agents such as the antidepressant mirtazapine and second-generation antipsychotics such as olanzapine and quetiapine. Indeed, quetiapine at low dosages of 25–100 mg/day has become a commonly used hypnotic for patients with mood and personality disorders. The American Academy of Sleep Medicine (AASM; Sateia et al. 2017) does not recommend its use in chronic insomnia because of limited positive data. However, a recent national survey of practitioners did indicate that more than half thought the drug effective (Pelayo et al. 2023).

A new generation of $5\text{-}HT_2$ antagonists or inverse agonists were at one time in development as hypnotics. Among these, eplivanserin was perhaps farthest along. Eplivanserin, given in a 1-mg or 5-mg dose at bedtime, appeared to reduce sleep latency and the number of nocturnal awakenings. Its primary side effect at these doses was dry mouth. Its development was stopped in 2009 by the manufacturer.

Among the older tricyclic antidepressants (TCAs), amitriptyline, imipramine, doxepin, and trimipramine, and probably nortriptyline, are good hypnotics, although other than doxepin, they are rarely studied as such. Katz et al. (1991), in a report from the National Institute of Mental Health Collaborative Depression Study, noted that sleep ratings improved strikingly in the first 2 weeks with amitriptyline but that this hypnotic effect did not predict an overall improvement in the depressions being treated. Trimipramine appears to be the only TCA to facilitate sleep but not to affect REM latency or nocturnal penile tumescence. If it did not sometimes cause morning drowsiness, dry mouth, constipation, and weight gain, trimipramine might be the ideal hypnotic at doses of 25–100 mg at bedtime. It is not safe for use by suicidal patients. Doxepin (Silenor) is the best studied of the TCAs for the treatment of insomnia and the only one to receive an FDA indication for sleep maintenance in the treatment of insomnia. It is also approved for chronic use. The efficacy of doxepin 3–6 mg/day in the treatment of insomnia was established in several large multicenter controlled trials in adults, including elderly individuals. Doxepin, more than other TCAs, is a potent histamine H_1 receptor antagonist and has prominent antimuscarinic effects. However, in a 4-week trial of 265 elderly patients with chronic insomnia, doxepin 6 mg/day was effective in sleep maintenance and did not produce memory problems or anticholinergic effects (Lankford et al. 2012). The AASM notes that doxepin has no clear side effects at the doses approved for insomnia (Sateia et al. 2017). Because it is prescribed at such low doses, even an overdose of a month's supply would not be lethal. As with other TCAs, doxepin does not carry a risk of dependence with chronic use, and withdrawal effects were not seen with suddenly stopping the 6-mg dose.

Since gabapentin was released for use in seizures, its use has widely spread into treating pain, anxiety, and insomnia. It seems quite safe in doses from 100 to 900 mg at bedtime and maybe higher. It is not metabolized by the body and seems quite safe in overdose because the intestine appears not to be able to absorb more than about 900 mg at any one time. It appears to have limited abuse liability, but there are rare cases of recreational abuse of both gabapentin and pregabalin (Schifano 2014). Given the low abuse potential, gabapentin is sometimes used in patients with alcohol dependence as an alternative to benzodiazepines. One open study found that in alcoholic patients with sleep disturbance, gabapentin appeared more effective than trazodone as a hypnotic (Karam-Hage and Brower 2003). In one of the few controlled studies to date, gabapentin in doses of 250 mg taken at night was found to increase total sleep duration without residual daytime somnolence (Furey et al. 2014). Again, although commonly prescribed by neurologists and psychiatrists in treating insomnia, gabapentin is not approved by the FDA for this indication.

All these nonbenzodiazepines (as well as diphenhydramine and maybe melatonin and valerian) may be nonabusable, relatively safe and effective ways to treat insomnia, but prescribing clinicians would sleep better if someone— perhaps the NIH or, in the case of gabapentin, the drug company—would undertake the studies necessary to document their potential safety and efficacy.

After review of the data, the AASM guidelines (Sateia et al. 2017) recommend the following for use in chronic insomnia: benzodiazepines (triazolam and temazepam), Z-drugs (eszopiclone and zolpidem), ramelteon, doxepin, and the orexin antagonists (specifically suvorexant as an example) on the basis of their all having positive clinical data. The guidelines recommend against using trazodone, melatonin, antihistamines, valerian, and tryptophan, generally on the basis of inadequate data supporting efficacy. However, a recent meta-analysis was more negative about ramelteon but less negative about the antihistamines and trazodone (De Crescenzo et al. 2022).

The various classes of drugs (e.g., benzodiazepines), over-the-counter preparations (e.g., melatonin, antihistamines), and health foods or herbals (valerian) are discussed in the following sections.

Benzodiazepine Hypnotics

The benzodiazepines are still among the most widely prescribed sedative-hypnotics in the United States today. Although most benzodiazepines have hypnotic properties, as of this writing, only five benzodiazepines have an FDA-approved indication as a hypnotic: flurazepam, temazepam, estazolam, quazepam, and triazolam. Five nonbenzodiazepines—zolpidem, zaleplon, eszopiclone, doxepin, and ramelteon—are also FDA approved as hypnotics.

The principles for discriminating among these drugs are similar to those described in Chapter 6 ("Antianxiety Agents") for the anxiolytic benzodiazepines: structure, pharmacokinetics, absorption, and distribution (Table 7–1). For example, most of the benzodiazepine hypnotics belong to separate structural subclasses: 2-keto (flurazepam), 3-hydroxy (temazepam), and triazolo (triazolam and estazolam) (Figure 7–1).

The metabolism and half-lives of these subclass members parallel those of their anxiolytic counterparts. Flurazepam is oxidized in the liver and, like diazepam, has a relatively long half-life (40 hours). It also forms a long-acting (100 hours) metabolite, desalkylflurazepam, a metabolite shared with quazepam. Temazepam is conjugated with a glucuronide radical in the liver and has a much shorter half-life (8 hours) and no active metabolites. Triazolam and estazolam are oxidized but with no clearly active metabolites; triazolam has an extremely short half-life (3–6 hours) (see Table 7–1), whereas estazolam is more like temazepam. Flurazepam and triazolam have more rapid absorption (peak blood levels at 30 and 20 minutes, respectively) than temazepam, which may not be absorbed for 45–60 minutes. The slower absorption accounts for patients' not falling asleep rapidly after taking this medication. Clinicians should advise patients to take temazepam approximately 1 hour before bedtime to avoid anticipatory discomfort and their resorting to premature repeat dosing.

A benzodiazepine hypnotic, quazepam, was released in the early 1990s. Chemically, it does not fall into any of the three classes described in Chapter 6. However, the drug's pharmacokinetics are in the same range as those of flurazepam, and it is metabolized to desalkylflurazepam in the body; the drug and its metabolite have half-lives of about 40 hours. Metabolism and elimination are slowed in elderly patients. This pattern suggests that sedation the next morning should be more of a problem than early rebound insomnia. Quazepam's only special feature is that it binds selectively to type 1 benzodi-

Table 7–1. Benzodiazepine hypnotics

Generic name	Brand name	Formulation and strengths	Anxiolytic dosage range[a] (mg/day)	Absorption	Major active metabolites	Approximate half-life (hours)
Estazolam		Tablets: 1, 2 mg	1–4	Intermediate	None	10–24
Flurazepam hydrochloride		Capsules: 15, 30 mg	15–30	Intermediate	Hydroxyethylflurazepam, desalkylflurazepam	Flurazepam 2.3; desalkylflurazepam 47–100
Quazepam	Doral	Tablets:15 mg	7.5–15	Intermediate	Oxoquazepam, desalkyloxoquazepam	Quazepam and oxoquazepam about 39; desalkyl-2-oxoquazepam about 73
Temazepam	Restoril	Capsules: 7.5, 15, 22.5, 30 mg	15–30	Intermediate	None	Biphasic, a short half-life ranging from 0.4 to 0.6 and a terminal half-life from 3.5 to 18.4
Triazolam	Halcion	Tablets: 0.125, 0.25 mg	0.125–0.5	Intermediate	None	1.5–5.5

[a]Approximate dosage ranges. Some patients will require higher dosages; others may respond to dosages below the range. Range is dosage -orm specific.

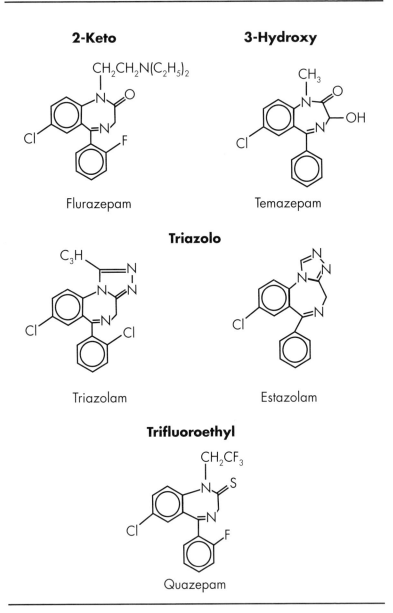

Figure 7–1.   Chemical structures of benzodiazepine hypnotics.

azepine receptors, whereas flurazepam and other older benzodiazepines bind equally to both type 1 and type 2 sites in the brain. There is no evidence that this special binding property is of particular clinical value. Quazepam's active metabolite does bind to both receptor types. Quazepam is a long-acting hypnotic, probably similar to flurazepam in its clinical utility. It is available in 7.5-mg and 15-mg tablets.

The distribution of the sedative benzodiazepines is relatively rapid. Indeed, the acute formation of high peak blood levels is thought to account for patients' falling asleep relatively quickly with these drugs. The decline from peak levels may account for why patients can awaken often, even when significant drug plasma levels are still apparent. Moreover, the decline from peak levels and the need for peak levels to induce sleep also explain why patients treated with longer-acting benzodiazepines such as flurazepam require nightly doses.

Some investigators and clinicians have argued that a non-long-acting compound (e.g., temazepam, zolpidem) offers great advantages over longer-acting agents because it is largely excreted before the next morning. Although at least one study has pointed to the safe use of triazolam for inducing sleep on transatlantic flights and preventing jet lag, there may be disadvantages associated with very-short-acting hypnotics, particularly rebound insomnia and anterograde amnesia. With some short-acting hypnotics, rebound insomnia occurs within the first 2 nights after discontinuation and can be troublesome for patients. Although acutely apparent with shorter-acting compounds, it may occur 5–7 days after discontinuation of benzodiazepines with longer half-lives and may be misinterpreted as a reemergence of the underlying insomnia rather than as a rebound phenomenon. It seems less likely to occur with zolpidem and zaleplon. When rebound insomnia occurs, clinicians should avoid resumption of the drug. Rather, reassurance and the prescription of antihistamine sedatives (e.g., 50 mg of diphenhydramine), sedating antidepressants (e.g., 50–100 mg of trazodone), or gabapentin (100 or 300 mg hs) for a few days may prove beneficial. When this does not work, reinstituting the benzodiazepine and gradually tapering the dose is an alternative strategy.

The side effects of the sedative-hypnotic benzodiazepines are similar to those of their anxiolytic counterparts. They include sedation, ataxia, anterograde amnesia, slurred speech, and nausea. These side effects are not particularly dangerous, although sedation can be a problem if the individual attempts to drive, to operate heavy machinery, or similar actions. There is weak evidence to suggest that the longer-half-life compounds cause clinically important cognitive problems the following day; however, this area has not been well studied. Refined and detailed psychological testing can usually detect impairment of cognitive or psychomotor function the morning after a benzodiazepine hypnotic has been used to induce sleep. The real question is whether this impairment is clinically important; the vast majority of users of hypnotics do not note behavioral impairment the next day unless they note persistent sedation as well. However, as noted earlier, there have been reports of pronounced anterograde amnesia ("blackouts") in patients treated with triazolam. Indeed, some healthy individuals who have used triazolam to induce sleep during a transatlantic flight have described not remembering arriving in Europe or what they did the next day. In the few personal accounts from patients and their friends and colleagues of blackouts after taking a benzodiazepine, the individuals appear to have done their usual activities during the period they cannot recall. Similar reactions have been observed with other benzodiazepines and with zolpidem and zaleplon. By far, the greater number of published or FDA reports of anterograde amnesia concern triazolam, but it is difficult to tell whether this difference is real or due to the extensive media publicity about triazolam (Bunney et al. 1999).

One possible problem with longer-acting benzodiazepines is illustrated by the case of a patient who had been treated with flurazepam nightly for years and then was shifted to an equivalent dose of temazepam. He developed a clear benzodiazepine withdrawal syndrome; the shorter-acting drug could not adequately replace the longer-acting one for the full 24 hours between doses.

In addition to pharmacologically explainable differences in shifting from one hypnotic to another, some patients claim (vigorously) that, say, lorazepam works beautifully, whereas temazepam in its new formulation does nothing. Beyond this, zolpidem, eszopiclone, and zaleplon are often rejected or criticized by patients who are used to triazolam or flurazepam; in these cases, these agents may be just different enough in their subjective effects from benzodiazepines to leave the patient worried that the hypnotic "isn't working," even though these same agents do fine as hypnotics in patients with insomnia who have never taken a benzodiazepine. The newer drugs affect mainly sleep latency; they may get the patient to sleep but may not keep them sleeping for long enough. Zolpidem, zaleplon, and eszopiclone appear to be different enough from benzodiazepines to be relatively free of rebound insomnia but may not have less danger of abuse than older benzodiazepines (Rush and Griffiths 1996; Rush et al. 1999; Victorri-Vigneau et al. 2007).

Time (and further studies) will tell, but these newer, not-quite-a-benzodiazepine hypnotics seem effective and relatively well tolerated by both young and old. They deserve the benefit of the doubt as being safer than chloral hydrate or pentobarbital, probably better than the benzodiazepine hypnotics, and probably more effective than the over-the-counter types of antihistamine preparations such as diphenhydramine (Benadryl).

The American Geriatrics Society (AGS) warns that benzodiazepines for chronic insomnia in the elderly verge on inappropriate because of potential side effects (American Geriatrics Society Beers Criteria Update Expert Panel 2019). There are no data on the long-term efficacy of benzodiazepines for sleep.

Nonbenzodiazepine Hypnotics

Drugs such as zolpidem, zaleplon, and eszopiclone lack the chemical structure of the benzodiazepines (Figure 7–2). However, these drugs still act on α_1 benzodiazepine sites on the GABA-A receptor. The nonbenzodiazepine hypnotics lack activity at α_2 and peripheral α_3 benzodiazepine sites. Thus, the nonbenzodiazepine hypnotics are not as potent muscle-relaxing and anticonvulsant agents as the benzodiazepines. The specific hypnotic effects of these drugs have distinct advantages in some patients. For example, the muscle-relaxing properties of benzodiazepines may further compromise the airways of patients with sleep apnea. The nonbenzodiazepine hypnotics appear to be less of a problem for obstructive sleep apnea patients. Likewise, we prefer that patients undergoing electroconvulsive therapy (ECT) use a nonbenzodiazepine hypnotic rather than a benzodiazepine hypnotic in the evening prior to ECT because a nonbenzodiazepine is somewhat less likely to raise the seizure threshold.

The nonbenzodiazepines have a reputation of being somewhat less addictive than benzodiazepines. It is unclear whether this reputation is deserved. High doses of the nonbenzodiazepines may induce euphoria (Gelenberg 2000), and a growing number of cases of dependence and abuse have been described in the world literature. In a survey of the scientific literature, only 36 cases of zolpidem dependence and 22 cases of zopiclone (related to eszopiclone) dependence had been described by 2003 (Hajak et al. 2003). More recent surveys suggested that reports of dependence and abuse of these agents may be

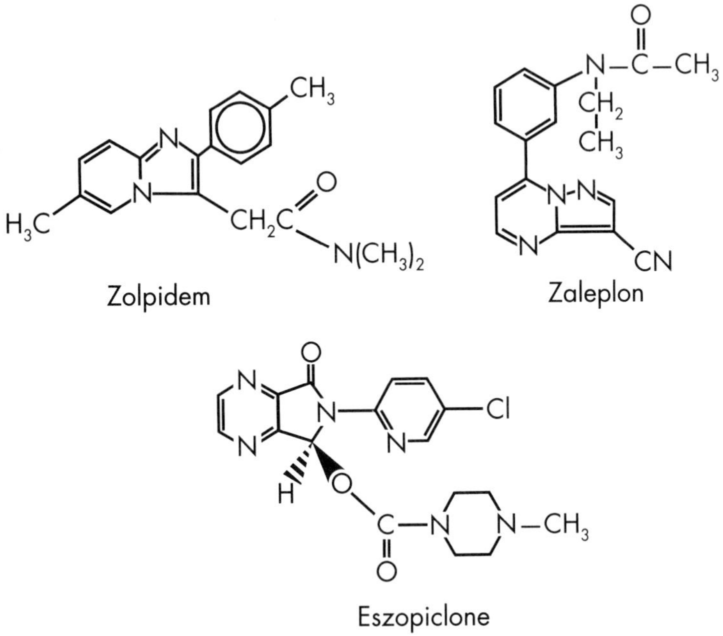

Figure 7–2.   Chemical structures of the nonbenzodiazepine hypnotics zolpidem, zaleplon, and eszopiclone.

rising (Shukla et al. 2017; Victorri-Vigneau et al. 2007). More than half of the patients who end up abusing drugs such as zolpidem have a previous history of abuse, but about 40% were prescribed the drug for sleep, developed a tolerance, and then started taking more and more of the drug. In the literature, dosages of 300 mg/day or more of zolpidem have been reported in some insomnia patients who have become dependent on the drug. Although these cases appear to be the exception, it is not clear that the abuse potential of the nonbenzodiazepine hypnotics is substantially lower than that of the benzodiazepines.

At the time of this writing, zolpidem still is among the most common of the hypnotics prescribed in the United States. There are probably more prescriptions written for benzodiazepine hypnotics, but these are available in generic form and are less expensive. Although all nonbenzodiazepines have short half-lives in healthy subjects (zaleplon, about 1–2 hours; zolpidem, 2–4 hours;

eszopiclone, 4–5 hours), many patients who are taking these medications, particularly zolpidem and eszopiclone, are able to sleep through the night. The extended-release form of zolpidem (Ambien CR) has the same half-life as the immediate-release form but is absorbed more slowly and so may allow patients to sleep longer. Zaleplon is somewhat lighter, and some patients complain of not being able to fall or stay asleep as well as they do with zolpidem. However, zaleplon is the only hypnotic that one could effectively take in the middle of the night and not feel too groggy in the morning. It has an indication for return to sleep.

Eszopiclone has been studied extensively in the treatment of insomnia associated with depression. At least two large multicenter trials have indicated that 1–3 mg of eszopiclone does help with insomnia associated with depression and may help with some aspects of mood (Fava et al. 2006; Joffe et al. 2010). It is likely that the treatment of insomnia is driving improvement in mood in these patients.

The most common side effects of the nonbenzodiazepines are drowsiness and dizziness. Other benzodiazepine side effects, such as ataxia, slurred speech, and amnestic symptoms, are less common with the nonbenzodiazepine hypnotics. However, withdrawal symptoms, including insomnia, muscle cramps, and even seizures, have been (rarely) reported.

The nonbenzodiazepine hypnotics should be taken on an empty stomach to induce more rapid onset of sleep. Zolpidem is usually dosed at 5–10 mg at night. Some patients seem to need 20 mg, although there is little evidence that this dose is much more effective than 10 mg. But there is little evidence it presents more of a problem than smaller doses. Zaleplon can be taken in doses of 10–20 mg at night. If the patient wakes up in the middle of the night, a 10-mg dose may be taken. Eszopiclone has usually been initiated at a dose of 1–2 mg to facilitate falling asleep and 3 mg to sustain sleep if 2 mg is inadequate. In the elderly, the recommended dosage is 1–2 mg/day. Unlike most hypnotics, eszopiclone has been studied in the management of insomnia for periods of 12 months with no substantial evidence of tolerance.

As with the benzodiazepines, the American Geriatric Society warns that the Z-drugs in the elderly verge on inappropriate use for chronic insomnia (American Geriatrics Society Beers Criteria Update Expert Panel 2019) because of potential side effects. Of the available Z-drugs, only eszopiclone has data supporting its FDA approval for long-term use.

Melatonin Receptor Agonists: Ramelteon and Tasimelteon

Although melatonin has been available over the counter for many years as a potential treatment of insomnia and phase shift disorders, melatonin supplements are not subject to careful and consistent manufacturing. In addition, the efficacy of most melatonin supplements appears to range from modest to minimal. In 2005, the FDA approved ramelteon (Rozerem), a specific melatonin MT_1/MT_2 receptor agonist, as the first hypnotic that is not a controlled substance. In 2014, a second MT_1/MT_2 agonist, tasimelteon, was approved for the treatment of non-24-hour sleep-wake disorder in totally blind individuals. Although not approved for other forms of insomnia, tasimelteon has a clinical profile like that of ramelteon. Both drugs appear to act on melatonin receptors in the suprachiasmatic nucleus responsible for sleep-wake cycles. Because they have no effects on the benzodiazepine receptor, they are not associated with abuse potential, rebound insomnia, motor deficits, or exacerbation of problems such as chronic obstructive pulmonary disease or obstructive sleep apnea. In addition, they are not likely to contribute to confusion or memory deficits in geriatric patients in the way that benzodiazepine or nonbenzodiazepine agents can. On the other hand, the primary utility of both agents is in reducing sleep latency, or the time it takes to fall asleep, and regulating sleep cycles; they may be of less utility than standard hypnotics in keeping patients asleep. Studies with both drugs demonstrate that they decrease the time to persistent sleep relative to placebo and have more modest effects on sleep maintenance (Erman et al. 2006; Rajaratnam et al. 2009). Both drugs appear to be useful in shifting disorders associated with phase delay of the sleep cycle, such as in jet lag, insomnia in the elderly, and insomnia associated with other neuropsychiatric disorders (Hardeland 2009; McGechan and Wellington 2005).

The primary side effects of the melatonin agonists have included headache, somnolence, fatigue, and a modest increase in hepatic alanine transaminase levels, but these have generally been mild and may improve after several weeks of treatment. High-fat meals can reduce absorption, and thus patients should be informed not to take either drug shortly after a rich meal. Both ramelteon and tasimelteon are metabolized via cytochrome P450 (CYP) 3A4 and 1A2, and serum levels may be substantially increased by fluvoxamine or ketoconazole and decreased by carbamazepine.

It is not an unreasonable question to ask what the benefits of prescription melatonin agonists are over less expensive melatonin supplements. Certainly, the consistency of the manufacturing of both ramelteon and tasimelteon is substantially greater than the much more variable manufacturing of over-the-counter supplements such as melatonin. The potency of the prescribed agents might be expected to be greater than that of over-the-counter melatonin, but this has not been established, and no direct comparisons of ramelteon or tasimelteon and over-the-counter melatonin have been reported. Nonetheless, the melatonin receptor agonists have a unique niche among currently available hypnotics as well-tolerated agents with no abuse potential. In patients with a history of substance abuse, geriatric patients, and patients with initial insomnia, the melatonin receptor agonists might be worth trying before other benzodiazepine and related hypnotics. Our general sense is that the melatonin agonists may not be as consistently effective as more traditional hypnotics but are less likely to cause mischief as well.

Ramelteon and tasimelteon are best taken at the same time every evening, about 30 minutes before bedtime. In the treatment of jet lag, the drugs should be taken 30–60 minutes before the desired sleep time for the first several days in the new time zone to adapt to the new circadian cycle. The recommended dosage of ramelteon is 8–16 mg/day, whereas tasimelteon is typically dosed at 20 mg/day. The AGS has no warning about using ramelteon in the elderly. Ramelteon is approved for long-term use.

Dual Orexin Receptor Antagonists: Suvorexant, Lemborexant, and Daridorexant

Orexin (also sometimes called hypocretin) is a naturally occurring neuropeptide found in the hypothalamus that appears to be important in the regulation of sleep-wake cycles, arousal, and appetite. The orexin receptors (OxR1 and OxR2) were discovered in the late 1990s, and an orexin receptor mutation appears to be responsible for a form of canine narcolepsy. Although there are only about 10,000–20,000 orexin-secreting neurons in the hypothalamus, these neurons project to many areas of the brain and spinal cord. Thus, orexin pathways may have broad effects not only on sleep but also on mood and appetite. Low levels of orexin are associated with depression, whereas higher levels are associated with improved mood. Thus, an orexin receptor antagonist could have negative effects on mood.

Three dual orexin receptor antagonists (DORAs) are approved for use as hypnotics (Table 7–2). The first approved DORA was suvorexant, which received an FDA-approved indication in 2014 for use in adults with insomnia who have difficulty falling or staying asleep. Suvorexant appears to be useful in increasing sleep efficiency and in reducing sleep latency from the first dose, on the basis of the results of several multicenter controlled trials (Herring et al. 2012; Michelson et al. 2014). Suvorexant is metabolized primarily via CYP3A and interacts with CYP3A inhibitors such as fluconazole and fluvoxamine in ways that increase serum levels and side effects. Similarly, inducers of CYP3A, such as rifampin, lower suvorexant levels.

A number of dose-related side effects have been seen with suvorexant. The most prominent among these is impaired driving the day after use with higher dosages. Although dosages up to 100 mg/day were studied, use at these higher dosages was problematic. The recommended dosage is 10–20 mg at night approximately 30–60 minutes before bedtime and with at least 7 hours before awakening. Suvorexant is not an agent that should be taken in the middle of the night because of residual daytime somnolence. Patients should be cautioned that driving may be impaired the day after taking the medication. Another dose-related side effect is an increase in suicidal ideation and depressive symptoms. These effects are predicted from the effects of orexin antagonism. Other side effects reported with suvorexant include headaches, dizziness, memory problems, unusual dreams, and somnambulism. Suvorexant is a Drug Enforcement Administration Schedule IV drug, indicating some potential for abuse as with benzodiazepine sleepers. In addition, withdrawal may occur if the drug is stopped abruptly.

Lemborexant is a more selective OxR2 antagonist than is suvorexant. It was approved for the treatment of insomnia in 2019. In the Study of the Efficacy and Safety of Lemborexant in Subjects 55 Years and Older With Insomnia Disorder (SUNRISE 1, SUNRISE 2, and SUNRISE 2 extension) involving more than 2,000 patients with insomnia, lemborexant significantly improved sleep onset latency and total sleep time compared with placebo. The drug has a dosage range of 5–10 mg given immediately before bedtime. Like suvorexant, lemborexant is a CYP3A4 substrate and requires a lower dose when given with a CYP3A4 inhibitor.

Table 7–2.   Dual orexin receptor antagonists (DORAs)

DORA	Trade name	Dose (mg)	Half-life	Onset
Suvorexant	Belsomra	5–20	12 hours	30 min
Lemborexant	Dayvigo	5–10	17–19 hours	<30 min
Daridorexant	Quviviq	25–50	8 hours	<30 min

Daridorexant was approved in 2022. It was evaluated in two pivotal Phase III studies (NAT-105 and NAT-201) involving more than 1,500 patients with insomnia. In these studies, daridorexant significantly improved sleep onset latency and total sleep time compared with placebo. In NAT-105, patients receiving daridorexant had a 28-minute reduction in sleep onset latency and a 54-minute increase in total sleep time compared with placebo. In NAT-201, patients receiving daridorexant had a 24-minute reduction in sleep onset latency and a 48-minute increase in total sleep time compared with placebo. The standard dose of daridorexant is 25–50 mg taken nightly about 30 minutes before bedtime. It has a more ideal half-life of 8 hours, which may translate to less daytime somnolence than with the other DORAs. Like suvorexant and lemborexant, daridorexant is a CYP3A4 substrate.

The place of DORAs among the other available hypnotics is not completely clear. The novel mechanism of the DORAs may allow them to be effective when other hypnotics are not. However, given the cost and side-effect profile, there are few cases in which DORAs would be a first-line hypnotic. In addition, there are cases in which suvorexant should probably be avoided or used with caution, including in the treatment of depressed, suicidal patients and patients with narcolepsy. Time will tell what the best application of the DORAs is in clinical practice. Lemborexant is approved for long-term use.

Sedative Antihistamines and Other Nonbenzodiazepine Psychoactive Drugs With Hypnotic Properties

Hydroxyzine compounds are the only antihistamines with some documented efficacy in the treatment of anxiety disorders. They also have an indication for preoperative and postanesthesia sedation. These drugs are available in capsules or tablets ranging from 10 to 100 mg each. However, our clinical experience with psychiatric patients suggests that the drugs are neither much appreciated by patients nor particularly effective on the few occasions when we have tried them. They are reasonably free of side effects, although hydroxyzine and the other antihistamines exert anticholinergic effects. When taken with other anticholinergic agents, hydroxyzine and related compounds can pose problems, particularly at high doses. Because they do not produce either physical or psychological dependence, the main value of these drugs may be as a delaying action for patients who are inclined to abuse sedative-hypnotic or benzodiazepine drugs.

Diphenhydramine (Benadryl) is another antihistamine sometimes used for its sedative or alleged hypnotic effects. It has not been well studied in either capacity but has some sedative properties and is judged by many patients to be acceptable. There is a well-controlled study showing some efficacy for diphenhydramine in treating insomnia (Rickels et al. 1983). The dose for sleep is 50–100 mg. Diphenhydramine has long been available over the counter in 25-mg formulations. The drug is anticholinergic and can be used for acute dystonic reactions to antipsychotics (see Chapter 4, "Antipsychotic Drugs"). Promethazine (Phenergan) is a phenothiazine without antipsychotic properties that is marketed as an antihistamine with sedative properties. Again, it is occasionally found useful as a mild sedative at doses of 25–100 mg, but it is not a major psychiatric drug. Doxylamine, another antihistamine, is the ingredient used in most over-the-counter preparations (e.g., Unisom) that are used for either tranquilization or hypnosis. It also has positive data in support of its use (De Crescenzo et al. 2022). However, the AASM does not recommend its use, and the AGS recommends against its use in the elderly.

Several TCAs exert marked antihistaminergic effects and from our perspective are excellent hypnotics (see discussion of doxepin earlier in this chapter). So is trazodone, a heterocyclic antidepressant. Amitriptyline and trimipramine can be used in doses of 25–75 mg at bedtime, and doxepin is approved as a hypnotic at modest dosages (3–6 mg/day). As a hypnotic, trazodone is best begun at a dose of 25–50 mg hs, with 50-mg increments up to 200 mg hs. At some dose in that range, improved sleep should occur, perhaps with undesirable sedation on the following morning. Some patients lose this side effect if the dose is held steady for 3–5 days; others require a lower dose that, it is hoped, will be effective without inducing a hangover. Sometimes, adult patients taking trazodone as a hypnotic on an empty stomach faint from postural hypotension if they do not go to bed soon after taking it. Occasionally, elderly patients develop orthostatic hypotension the day after taking this agent at bedtime. Some studies of trazodone's effects on sleep and of its utility have emerged in other, unexpected areas, such as agitation in the elderly, if given in 25-mg doses, and PTSD (Bajor et al. 2011). So far, it retains its record with us of mixing relatively innocuously with all other psychiatric drugs, including SSRIs and monoamine oxidase inhibitors. There is even a study showing that vis-à-vis triazolam or zolpidem, trazodone has no euphoriant effects in individuals with a history of substance abuse (Rush et al. 1999). The AASM recommends clinicians not use it for sleep onset or maintenance (Sateia et al. 2017). A recent survey (Pelayo et al. 2023) polled sleep specialists and other clinicians on the following statement: "Trazodone should never be used as a first-line medication for insomnia." All the sleep specialists agreed with the statement, largely on the basis of limited positive data for trazodone on sleep and sleep architecture. In contrast, about 50% of the other clinicians did not agree with the statement. The gap is puzzling, but understandable, in part on the basis of the specific question posed. For our patients, we have often found trazodone helpful. Mirtazapine can also be an effective hypnotic at dosages of 7.5–15 mg/day. The drug is a potent serotonin$_2$ (5-HT$_2$) receptor antagonist and has antihistaminic properties as well.

Gabapentin and pregabalin are probably also as safe and useful as trazodone in treating insomnia. They have the added potential benefit of having both analgesic and hypnotic effects, as shown in large placebo-controlled studies involving patients with postherpetic or diabetic neuralgia, and are reported to be potentially useful in the treatment of other painful conditions that interfere with sleep. The dose to be used is more of a problem, with dosages ranging between 300 mg and 1,200 mg taken at bedtime for gabapentin and between 150 and 600 mg/day for pregabalin. GABA analogs such as gabapentin and pregabalin appear to be more useful for insomnia or anxiety symptoms in psychiatric patients than as a primary mood stabilizer, although occasional patients with bipolar disorder appear to do uniquely well while taking gabapentin (see Chapter 5, "Mood Stabilizers") (Ketter et al. 1999). There is one disturbing report describing withdrawal symptoms (i.e., anxiety, agitation, and dysphoria) that were worse than those occurring at baseline (Corá-Locatelli et al. 1998), but no one we know of locally has observed or heard of such a phenomenon. Again, gabapentin has been mixed with a wide variety of other psychoactive drugs, mainly in treating bipolar patients, without evidence of adverse interactions (Chouinard et al. 1998).

It is hard to make clear recommendations about the use of benzodiazepine or related hypnotics versus trazodone, mirtazapine, gabapentin, or pregabalin. A recent large meta-analysis favored the benzodiazepines and Z-drugs as hypnotics over placebo, melatonin, and ramelteon on the basis of efficacy but found less convincing evidence for these other psychotropics that are not themselves approved for treating insomnia (De Crescenzo et al. 2022). Clearly, patients with an abuse potential may be at greater risk for dependence while taking benzodiazepines and related agents. However, those patients with significant anxiety or depression might do better when an agent such as trazodone, pregabalin, or mirtazapine is used to also help sleep. The TCAs are less safe in overdose than other potential hypnotics and generally should be avoided for hypnotic use.

Other Hypnotics

In the late 1940s and the 1950s, several hypnotic drugs were developed in the hope that they would be safer and better than the barbiturates (Figure 7–3). Unfortunately, this hope was not realized. The drugs generally proved to have as many limitations as the barbiturates, and none of them are currently available for use; chloral hydrate was discontinued in 2013. Chloral hydrate was a somewhat effective and reasonably safe sleeping medication in doses between 500 and 1,500 mg at bedtime (Table 7–3). Early prescription levels of 500 mg at bedtime often proved inadequate to produce sedation, and most prescribers came to favor 1,000 mg, particularly in younger adult patients. The drug was often used in double-blind trials of other psychiatric medications as an adjunct medication because of its presumed safety and "cleanliness." This reputation was not fully deserved. Chloral hydrate has a very low margin of safety, with the lethal dose being about 10 times the hypnotic dose, and it is irritating to the stomach. Chloral hydrate had once been widely abused in England in the early 1900s. It was also used with alcohol as a "Mickey Finn" to knock out victims who were being shanghaied. Trichloroethanol, the metabolite and active principal of chloral hydrate, is presumed to interact with alcohol, increasing the potency of the drug. Trichloroethanol slows the metabolism of ethanol, while ethanol speeds the conversion of chloral hydrate to trichlo-

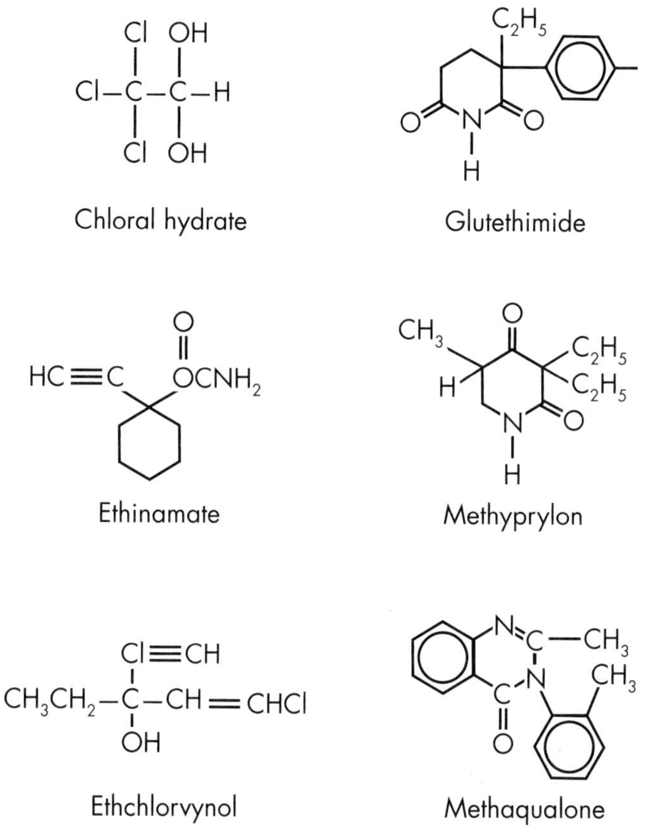

Figure 7–3.   Chemical structures of nonbarbiturate hypnotics.

roethanol (Rall 1993). As a result of safety concerns and better alternatives, chloral hydrate is no longer available.

Barbiturates were used for many years in the treatment of insomnia but were replaced in the 1960s by the benzodiazepines. The barbiturates, although effective, have a much lower therapeutic index than do the benzodiazepines and related hypnotics and a much greater risk of abuse. Other nonbarbiturate hypnotics, including glutethimide, ethinamate, methyprylon, and ethchlorvynol, were developed because of the known dangers of addiction

Table 7–3.   Other nighttime hypnotic agents[a]

Generic name	Brand name	Formulations and strengths	Dosage[b] (mg/day)
Zolpidem	Ambien[c,d]	Tablets: 5, 10 mg	5–10
	Ambien-CR[c]	Tablets (extended release): 6.25, 12.5 mg	
	Edular	Sublingual tablets: 5, 10 mg	
	Intermezzo[c]	Sublingual tablets: 1.75, 3.5 mg	
	Zolpimist	Oral spray solution: 5 mg/ spray (60 mL)	
Zaleplon	Sonata[c,d]	Capsules: 5, 10 mg	5–10
Eszopiclone	Lunesta[c,d]	Tablets: 1, 2, 3 mg	1–3
Ramelteon	Rozerem	Tablet: 8 mg	8
Tasimelteon	Hetlioz	Capsule: 20 mg	20

[a]Chloral hydrate and ethchlorvynol are no longer available.
[b]Adult dosages. Patients may require slightly higher dosages of chloral hydrate or ethchlorvynol. For child dosages, consult the latest edition of Goodman and Gilman's.
[c]Available in generic form.
[d]Lower doses may be indicated when combined with potent cytochrome P450 3A4 inhibitors (e.g., fluoxetine).

and lethality on suicidal ingestion of barbiturates. Unfortunately, none of these drugs proved to be either safer or less capable of producing physical or psychological dependence than the drugs that they were supposed to replace. Likewise, paraldehyde was introduced in the 1880s and was used for many years as a hypnotic. Today, paraldehyde is used only rarely as a rescue medication for seizure disorders. There are currently no logical reasons for using any of these older agents in preference to the safer newer hypnotics.

Conclusion

For the physician seeing a patient with recent-onset insomnia without evident primary medical, psychiatric, or sleep diagnoses (e.g., restless legs, sleep apnea) that would account for it, good sleep hygiene practices are the first intervention before any prescription. However, if sleep hygiene practices fail, prescribing a small amount of a shorter-acting hypnotic (zolpidem, temazepam, lorazepam) in the lowest dose taken every 3 days for up to 4 weeks seems reasonable, assuming the patient has no history of substance abuse.

For short-term relief of insomnia, zolpidem 5–10 mg hs has been generally satisfactory, although it would be hard to prove that it is the best of the available benzodiazepine-like drugs. Zaleplon probably produces a briefer hypnotic effect than zolpidem, and it has not been as well adopted as has zolpidem. Eszopiclone may turn out to be a major addition—effective acutely as well as over extended periods. Patients who awaken too early after taking zolpidem may do better taking temazepam as a longer-acting sedative. However, any of the benzodiazepines may be effective when the right dose for the patient is determined, although flurazepam, quazepam, and possibly clonazepam may have long enough half-lives to cause morning sedation and, perhaps, psychomotor impairment.

For patients with long-standing insomnia who are already accustomed to a nightly hypnotic of the benzodiazepine class, physical dependence probably exists, and a slow but purposeful taper of dosage over months, not days or weeks, may be needed. If shifting to a nonbenzodiazepine hypnotic (e.g., trazodone), it would seem sensible to first add the new hypnotic and make sure it improves sleep for at least 2 weeks before beginning to taper the benzodiazepine.

Trazodone 25–50 mg hs, mirtazapine 7.5–15 mg hs, doxepin 3–6 mg hs, or gabapentin 100–600 mg hs may do as well as a benzodiazepine and can be taken nightly with little concern about physical dependence. However, except for doxepin, because these are off-label (non-FDA-approved) uses, written justification for their use should be made in the medical record. Likewise, sedating second-generation antipsychotics such as quetiapine at doses of 25–100 mg may benefit some patients with insomnia, including those with depression or anxiety. Since quetiapine became available generically, its use as a hypnotic at low doses appears to be more common. However, the side effects and dangers of medications such as doxepin or quetiapine may outweigh the advantages for some patients. Two 25-mg capsules of over-the-counter diphenhydramine may be almost as effective. The rare occurrence of priapism with trazodone deserves mention to male patients, with a warning to seek emergency department help if an erection persists beyond 4 hours (Thompson et al. 1990).

All the above except the benzodiazepine-like drugs could be used in patients with a history of substance abuse problems, although such patients can sometimes escalate the dose of any drug rapidly and unwisely. In very unstable, impulsive individuals, gabapentin or trazodone is probably safest. On the other hand, if an alcoholic individual in prolonged remission comes to a physician's office with either a credible history of intractable, severe, untreated insomnia or a history of safe, cautious, appropriate use of a hypnotic such as clonazepam for months or years, continuing or starting a benzodiazepine-like hypnotic with careful monitoring is probably safe.

For patients with long-term insomnia being treated with hypnotics and without diagnosable sleep problems that require treatment with nonhypnotics, having the patient continue to take the hypnotic while evaluating and treating any concurrent major psychiatric disorder is sensible. Once the patient's condition and the patient-physician relationship are stable, alternatives can be considered. These include shifting to nonbenzodiazepine sleep-inducing drugs, tapering the original hypnotic very slowly, referring the patient to a sleep program for more specialized diagnosis and possible behavioral or other nonsedative treatments, or making and documenting a conscious, responsible treatment plan in which the patient continues to take a stable benzodiazepine dose for a defined period, say, a year, for sensible reasons (e.g., waiting for a divorce to become final, finishing a major job, recovering fully from a manic episode).

At the other extreme, clinicians see patients with a desperate, frantic need for a full night's sleep who have been taking large doses of several drugs (e.g., temazepam 90 mg plus trazodone 200 mg plus gabapentin 600 mg per night) with little benefit. In our experience, such patients need to be referred to a sleep clinic. Referral to a psychologist for CBT-I appears at least as effective as prescribing the long-term use of a hypnotic and without the cognitive, abuse, or fall risks of many hypnotics. CBT-I is recommended as the first-line treatment for insomnia by the American College of Physicians, but it may not be easily available for many patients. If the program is not successful or a program is unavailable, patients need to be told that hypnotic medications are not the answer, that even 90 mg of temazepam either will not work or will harm them, and that they need to have their bedtime medications gradually but firmly tapered while they engage in psychotherapy and a search is made for other, more appropriate treatments.

Suggested Readings

Backonja M, Beydoun A, Edwards KR, et al: Gabapentin for the symptomatic treatment of painful neuropathy in patients with diabetes mellitus: a randomized controlled trial. JAMA 280(21):1831–1836, 1998 9846777

Dement W, Seidel W, Carskadon M, et al: Changes in daytime sleepiness/alertness with nighttime benzodiazepines, in Pharmacology of Benzodiazepines. Edited by Usdin E, Skolnick P, Tallman JF, et al. New York, Macmillan, 1982, pp 219–228

Earley CJ, Allen RP: Pergolide and carbidopa/levodopa treatment of the restless legs syndrome and periodic leg movements in sleep in a consecutive series of patients. Sleep 19(10):801–810, 1996 9085489

Ehrenberg BL, Eisensehr I, Corbett KE, et al: Valproate for sleep consolidation in periodic limb movement disorder. J Clin Psychopharmacol 20(5):574–578, 2000 11001243

Elie R, Rüther E, Farr I, et al: Sleep latency is shortened during 4 weeks of treatment with zaleplon, a novel nonbenzodiazepine hypnotic. J Clin Psychiatry 60(8):536–544, 1999 10485636

Falco M: Methaqualone misuse: foreign experience and United States drug control policy. Int J Addict 11(4):597–610, 1976 992915

Garfinkel D, Laudon M, Nof D, et al: Improvement of sleep quality in elderly people by controlled-release melatonin. Lancet 346(8974):541–544, 1995 7658780

Gillin JC, Byerley WF: Drug therapy: the diagnosis and management of insomnia. N Engl J Med 322(4):239–248, 1990 2242104

Gillin JC, Reynolds CF, Shipley JE: Sleep studies in selected adult neuropsychiatric disorders, in Psychiatry Update: American Psychiatric Association Annual Review, Vol 4. Edited by Hales RE, Frances AJ. Washington, DC, American Psychiatric Press, 1985, pp 352–360

Greenblatt DJ, Shader RI, Abernethy DR: Drug therapy: current status of benzodiazepines. N Engl J Med 309(6):354–358, 1983 6135156

Greenblatt DJ, Shader RI, Abernethy DR: Drug therapy: current status of benzodiazepines. N Engl J Med 309(7):410–416, 1983 6135990

Hauri PJ, Sateia MJ: Nonpharmacological treatment of sleep disorders, in Psychiatry Update: American Psychiatric Association Annual Review, Vol 4. Edited by Hales RE, Frances AJ. Washington, DC, American Psychiatric Press, 1985, pp 361–378

Hertzman PA, Blevins WL, Mayer J, et al: Association of the eosinophilia-myalgia syndrome with the ingestion of tryptophan. N Engl J Med 322(13):869–873, 1990 2314421

Houghton PJ: The scientific basis for the reputed activity of valerian. J Pharm Pharmacol 51(5):505–512, 1999 10411208

Hughes RJ, Sack RL, Lewy AJ: The role of melatonin and circadian phase in age-related sleep-maintenance insomnia: assessment in a clinical trial of melatonin replacement. Sleep 21(1):52–68, 1998 9485533

Johnsa JD, Neville MW: Tasimelteon: a melatonin receptor agonist for non-24-hour sleep-wake disorder. Ann Pharmacother 48(12):1636–1641, 2014 25204464

Johnson MW, Suess PE, Griffiths RR: Ramelteon: a novel hypnotic lacking abuse liability and sedative adverse effects. Arch Gen Psychiatry 63(10):1149–1157, 2006 17015817

Kales A: Benzodiazepines in the treatment of insomnia, in Pharmacology of Benzodiazepines. Edited by Usdin E, Skolnick P, Tallman JF, et al. New York, Macmillan, 1982, pp 199–217

Kales A: Quazepam: hypnotic efficacy and side effects. Pharmacotherapy 10(1):1–10, discussion 10–12, 1990 1969151

Katz MM, Koslow SH, Maas JW, et al: The timing, specificity and clinical prediction of tricyclic drug effects in depression. Psychol Med 17(2):297–309, 1987 3299439

Krystal AD, Lankford A, Durrence HH, et al: Efficacy and safety of doxepin 3 and 6 mg in a 35-day sleep laboratory trial in adults with chronic primary insomnia. Sleep 34(10):1433–1442, 2011 21966075

Lasagna L: Update to "Over-the-counter hypnotics and chronic insomnia in the elderly" (guest editorial, J Clin Psychopharmacol 1995;15:383–6). J Clin Psychopharmacol 16(2):191, 1996 8690837

Melatonin. Med Lett Drugs Ther 37(962):111–112, 1995 7476672

Mendelson WB (ed): Current strategies in the treatment of insomnia. J Clin Psychiatry 53(12)(suppl):1–45, 1992

Mignot E, Mayleben D, Fietze I, et al: Safety and efficacy of daridorexant in patients with insomnia disorder: results from two multicentre, randomised, double-blind, placebo-controlled, phase 3 trials. Lancet Neurol 21(2):125–139, 2022 35065036

National Center on Sleep Disorders Research: Insomnia: Assessment and Management in Primary Care (NIH Publ No 98-4088). Washington, DC, National Center on Sleep Disorders Research, 1998

Nishino S, Okuro M: Armodafinil for excessive daytime sleepiness. Drugs Today (Barc) 44(6):395–414, 2008 18596995

Regestein QR: Specific effects of sedative/hypnotic drugs in the treatment of incapacitating chronic insomnia. Am J Med 83(5):909–916, 1987 2445202

Reiter RJ, Melchiorri D, Sewerynek E, et al: A review of the evidence supporting melatonin's role as an antioxidant. J Pineal Res 18(1):1–11, 1995 7776173

Reynolds CF, Buysse DJ, Kupfer DJ: Disordered sleep: developmental and biopsychosocial perspectives on the diagnosis and treatment of persistent insomnia, in Psychopharmacology: The Fourth Generation of Progress. Edited by Bloom FE, Kupfer DJ. New York, Raven, 1995, pp 1617–1629

Rickels K, Ginsberg J, Morris RJ, et al: Doxylamine succinate in insomniac family practice patients: a double-blind study. Curr Ther Res Clin Exp 35:532–540, 1984

Roffwarg H, Erman M: Evaluation and diagnosis of the sleep disorders: implications for psychiatry and other clinical specialties, in Psychiatry Update: American Psychiatric Association Annual Review, Vol 4. Edited by Hales RE, Frances AJ. Washington, DC, American Psychiatric Press, 1985, pp 294–328

Rosenberg R, Murphy P, Zammit G, et al: Comparison of lemborexant with placebo and zolpidem tartrate extended release for the treatment of older adults with insomnia disorder: a phase 3 randomized clinical trial. JAMA Netw Open 2(12):e1918254, 2019 31880796

Roth T, Seiden D, Sainati S, et al: Effects of ramelteon on patient-reported sleep latency in older adults with chronic insomnia. Sleep Med 7(4):312–318, 2006 16709464

Rowbotham M, Harden N, Stacey B, et al: Gabapentin for the treatment of postherpetic neuralgia: a randomized controlled trial. JAMA 280(21):1837–1842, 1998 9846778

Scharf MB, Mayleben DW, Kaffeman M, et al: Dose response effects of zolpidem in normal geriatric subjects. J Clin Psychiatry 52(2):77–83, 1991 1993640

Schneider-Helmert D: Why low-dose benzodiazepine-dependent insomniacs can't escape their sleeping pills. Acta Psychiatr Scand 78(6):706–711, 1988 2906215

Seidel WF, Roth T, Roehrs T, et al: Treatment of a 12-hour shift of sleep schedule with benzodiazepines. Science 224(4654):1262–1264, 1984 6729454

Shamir E, Laudon M, Barak Y, et al: Melatonin improves sleep quality of patients with chronic schizophrenia. J Clin Psychiatry 61(5):373–377, 2000 10847313

Sun H, Kennedy WP, Wilbraham D, et al: Effects of suvorexant, an orexin receptor antagonist, on sleep parameters as measured by polysomnography in healthy men. Sleep 36(2):259–267, 2013 23372274

Wang MY, Wang SY, Tsai PS: Cognitive behavioural therapy for primary insomnia: a systematic review. J Adv Nurs 50(5):553–564, 2005 15882372

Wong AH, Smith M, Boon HS: Herbal remedies in psychiatric practice. Arch Gen Psychiatry 55(11):1033–1044, 1998 9819073

Yardley J, Kärppä M, Inoue Y, et al: Long-term effectiveness and safety of lemborexant in adults with insomnia disorder: results from a Phase 3 randomized clinical trial. Sleep Med 80:333–342, 2021 33636648

Zhdanova IV, Lynch HJ, Wurtman RJ: Melatonin: a sleep-promoting hormone. Sleep 20(10):899–907, 1997 9415953

References

American Geriatrics Society Beers Criteria Update Expert Panel: American Geriatrics Society 2019 Updated AGS Beers Criteria for Potentially Inappropriate Medication Use in Older Adults. J Am Geriatr Soc 67(4):674–694, 2019 30693946

Bajor LA, Ticlea AN, Osser DN: The Psychopharmacology Algorithm Project at the Harvard South Shore Program: an update on posttraumatic stress disorder. Harv Rev Psychiatry 19(5):240–258, 2011 21916826

Bunney WE Jr, Azarnoff DL, Brown BW Jr, et al: Report of the Institute of Medicine Committee on the Efficacy and Safety of Halcion. Arch Gen Psychiatry 56(4):349–352, 1999 10197830

Buysse DJ, Dorsey CM: Current and experimental therapeutics of insomnia, in American College of Neuro-Psychopharmacology: A Fifth Generation of Progress. Edited by Davis JM, Charney D, Coyle J, et al. Philadelphia, PA, Lippincott Williams & Wilkins, 2002, pp 1931–1943

Camargos EF, Louzada LL, Quintas JL, et al: Trazodone improves sleep parameters in Alzheimer disease patients: a randomized, double-blind, and placebo-controlled study. Am J Geriatr Psychiatry 22(12):1565–1574, 2014 24495406

Chouinard G, Beauclair L, Bélanger MC: Gabapentin: long-term antianxiety and hypnotic effects in psychiatric patients with comorbid anxiety-related disorders. Can J Psychiatry 43(3):305, 1998 9561320

Corá-Locatelli G, Greenberg BD, Martin JD, et al: Rebound psychiatric and physical symptoms after gabapentin discontinuation (letter). J Clin Psychiatry 59(3):131, 1998 9541157

De Crescenzo F, D'Alò GL, Ostinelli EG, et al: Comparative effects of pharmacological interventions for the acute and long-term management of insomnia disorder in adults: a systematic review and network meta-analysis. Lancet 400(10347):170–184, 2022 35843245

Edinger JD, Means MK: Cognitive-behavioral therapy for primary insomnia. Clin Psychol Rev 25(5):539–558, 2005 15951083

Erman M, Seiden D, Zammit G, et al: An efficacy, safety, and dose-response study of ramelteon in patients with chronic primary insomnia. Sleep Med 7(1):17–24, 2006 16309958

Fava M, McCall WV, Krystal A, et al: Eszopiclone co-administered with fluoxetine in patients with insomnia coexisting with major depressive disorder. Biol Psychiatry 59(11):1052–1060, 2006 16581036

Furey SA, Hull SG, Leibowitz MT, et al: A randomized, double-blind, placebo-controlled, multicenter, 28-day, polysomnographic study of gabapentin in transient insomnia induced by sleep phase advance. J Clin Sleep Med 10(10):1101–1109, 2014 25317091

Gelenberg A (ed): Zaleplon: a new nonbenzodiazepine hypnotic. Biological Therapies in Psychiatry 23:5–6, 2000

Grandner MA, Pack AI: Sleep disorders, public health, and public safety. JAMA 306(23):2616–2617, 2011 22187285

Hajak G, Müller WE, Wittchen H-U, et al: Abuse and dependence potential for the non-benzodiazepine hypnotics zolpidem and zopiclone: a review of case reports and epidemiological data. Addiction 98(10):1371–1378, 2003 14519173

Hardeland R: Tasimelteon, a melatonin agonist for the treatment of insomnia and circadian rhythm sleep disorders. Curr Opin Investig Drugs 10(7):691–701, 2009 19579175

Herring WJ, Snyder E, Budd K, et al: Orexin receptor antagonism for treatment of insomnia: a randomized clinical trial of suvorexant. Neurology 79(23):2265–2274, 2012 23197752

Joffe H, Petrillo L, Viguera A, et al: Eszopiclone improves insomnia and depressive and anxious symptoms in perimenopausal and postmenopausal women with hot flashes: a randomized, double-blinded, placebo-controlled crossover trial. Am J Obstet Gynecol 202(2):171.e1–171.e11, 2010 20035910

Karam-Hage M, Brower KJ: Open pilot study of gabapentin versus trazodone to treat insomnia in alcoholic outpatients. Psychiatry Clin Neurosci 57(5):542–544, 2003 12950711

Katz MM, Koslow SH, Maas JW, et al: Identifying the specific clinical actions of amitriptyline: interrelationships of behaviour, affect and plasma levels in depression. Psychol Med 21(3):599–611, 1991 1946849

Ketter TA, Post RM, Theodore WH: Positive and negative psychiatric effects of antiepileptic drugs in patients with seizure disorders. Neurology 53(5)(Suppl 2):S53–S67, 1999 10496235

Krystal AD: Treatment of insomnia, in The American Psychiatric Association Publishing Textbook of Psychopharmacology, 6th Edition. Edited by Schatzberg AF, Nemeroff CB. Washington, DC, American Psychiatric Association Publishing (in press)

Lankford A, Rogowski R, Essink B, et al: Efficacy and safety of doxepin 6 mg in a four-week outpatient trial of elderly adults with chronic primary insomnia. Sleep Med 13(2):133–138, 2012 22197474

McGechan A, Wellington K: Ramelteon. CNS Drugs 19(12):1057–1065, 2005 16332146

Michelson D, Snyder E, Paradis E, et al: Safety and efficacy of suvorexant during 1-year treatment of insomnia with subsequent abrupt treatment discontinuation: a phase 3 randomised, double-blind, placebo-controlled trial. Lancet Neurol 13(5):461–471, 2014 24680372

Morin CM, Bertisch SM, Pelayo R, et al: What should be the focus of treatment when insomnia disorder is comorbid with depression or anxiety disorder? J Clin Med 12(5):1975, 2023 36902762

National Sleep Foundation: Sleep Health Index. National Sleep Foundation, 2014. Available at: https://www.thensf.org/sleep-health-index. Accessed October 28, 2023.

NIH State of the Science Conference statement on manifestations and management of chronic insomnia in adults statement. J Clin Sleep Med 1(4):412–421, 2005 17564412

Pelayo R, Bertisch SM, Morin CM, et al: Should trazodone be first-line therapy for insomnia? A clinical suitability appraisal. J Clin Med 12(8):2933, 2023 37109268

Rajaratnam SM, Polymeropoulos MH, Fisher DM, et al: Melatonin agonist tasimelteon (VEC-162) for transient insomnia after sleep-time shift: two randomised controlled multicentre trials. Lancet 373(9662):482–491, 2009 19054552

Rall TW: Hypnotics and sedatives, ethanol, in Goodman and Gilman's The Pharmacologic Basis of Therapeutics, 8th Edition. Edited by Gilman AG, Rall TW, Nies AS, et al. New York, McGraw-Hill, 1993, pp 345–382

Rickels K, Morris RJ, Newman H, et al: Diphenhydramine in insomnia. J Clin Psychiatry 23:235–242, 1983

Rush CR, Griffiths RR: Zolpidem, triazolam, and temazepam: behavioral and subject-rated effects in normal volunteers. J Clin Psychopharmacol 16(2):146–157, 1996 8690830

Rush CR, Baker RW, Wright K: Acute behavioral effects and abuse potential of trazodone, zolpidem and triazolam in humans. Psychopharmacology (Berl) 144(3):220–233, 1999 10435388

Sateia MJ, Buysse DJ, Krystal AD, et al: Clinical Practice Guideline for the Pharmacologic Treatment of Chronic Insomnia in Adults: an American Academy of Sleep Medicine clinical practice guideline. J Clin Sleep Med 13(2):307–349, 2017 27998379

Schifano F: Misuse and abuse of pregabalin and gabapentin: cause for concern? CNS Drugs 28(6):491–496, 2014 24760436

Shukla L, Bokka S, Shukla T, et al: Benzodiazepine and "Z-drug" dependence: data from a tertiary care center. Prim Care Companion CNS Disord 19(1)doi:10.4088/PCC.16br02025, 2017 28207998

Tanimukai H, Murai T, Okazaki N, et al: An observational study of insomnia and nightmare treated with trazodone in patients with advanced cancer. Am J Hosp Palliat Care 30(4):359–362, 2013 22777411

Thompson JW Jr, Ware MR, Blashfield RK: Psychotropic medication and priapism: a comprehensive review. J Clin Psychiatry 51(10):430–433, 1990 2211542

Victorri-Vigneau C, Dailly E, Veyrac G, et al: Evidence of zolpidem abuse and dependence: results of the French Centre for Evaluation and Information on Pharmacodependence (CEIP) network survey. Br J Clin Pharmacol 64(2):198–209, 2007 17324242

Zhang Z-J, Kang WH, Li Q, et al: Beneficial effects of ondansetron as an adjunct to haloperidol for chronic, treatment-resistant schizophrenia: a double-blind, randomized, placebo-controlled study. Schizophr Res 88(1–3):102–110, 2006 16959472

8

Stimulants and the Treatment of ADHD

Like all other drug classifications in clinical psychopharmacology, the term *stimulants* covers a range of drugs, with some overlapping actions, that may be useful in treating some disorders, syndromes, or symptoms (Table 8–1). Here, as elsewhere, we lack a tidy one-to-one correlation of drug efficacy and syndrome.

The concept of stimulants began early with caffeine and then, in 1887, with synthesis of amphetamine in Germany. However, amphetamine was a drug without an indication and was largely forgotten until the 1930s. Another stimulant, phedrine, was extracted from a Chinese herbal remedy in the 1930s. Ephedrine was known to cause euphoria, sympathetic activation, and alertness. It was used in treating asthma and has never been tested for efficacy in ADHD, obesity, or, to our knowledge, narcolepsy. From ephedrine, K.K. Chen synthesized a variant, amphetamine (Benzedrine), which was, within 10 years, separated into its two stereoisomers, D-amphetamine (Dexedrine) and L-amphetamine. The dextro isomer was much more potent and is almost the only one used clinically today. It turned out to be effective in focusing attention and/or decreasing maladaptive behaviors in children who would now be diagnosed as hav-

Table 8–1. Stimulants: names, formulations, and strengths

Generic name	Brand name	Formulations and strengths
Amphetamine[a]	Adzenys XR-ODT	Tablets: 3.1, 6.3, 9.4, 12.5, 15.7, 18.8 mg
	Adzenys XR	Suspension: 1.25 mg/mL
	Dyanavel XR	Suspension: 2.5 mg/mL
	Evekeo	Tablets (immediate release): 5, 10 mg
D-amphetamine[a]	Dexedrine Spansule	Capsules (sustained release): 5, 10, 15 mg
	Generic	Tablets (immediate release): 5, 10 mg
	Zenzedi	Tablets: 2.5, 7.5, 15, 20, 30 mg
	ProCentra	Solution: 5 mg/5 mL
Amphetamine/dextroamphetamine[a,b]	Adderall	Tablets: 5, 7.5, 10, 12.5, 15, 20, 30 mg
	Adderall XR	Capsules: 5, 10, 15, 20, 25, 30 mg
	Mydayis	Capsules (extended release): 12.5, 37.5, 50 mg
D-methamphetamine[a]	Desoxyn	Tablets: 5 mg
Methylphenidate[c]	Ritalin	Tablets: 5, 10, 20 mg
	Methylin	Tablets, chewable: 2.5, 5, 10 mg
		Oral solution: 5 mg/5 mL, 10 mg/5 mL (500 mL)
	Ritalin LA	Capsules: 10, 20, 30, 40, 60 mg
	Aptensio XR	Capsules: 10, 20, 30, 40, 50, 60 mg
	Concerta	Tablets (extended release): 18, 27, 36, 54 mg

Table 8–1.   Stimulants: names, formulations, and strengths *(continued)*

Generic name	Brand name	Formulations and strengths
Methylphenidate *(continued)*	Relexxii	Tablet (extended release): 72 mg
	Cotempla XR-ODT	Tablets: 8.6, 17.3, 25.9 mg
	QuilliChew ER	Tablets: 20, 30, 40 mg
		Suspension: 25 mg/5 mL
	Daytrana	Transdermal patch: 10, 15, 20, 30 mg/9 hours[d]
	Jornay	Tablets (extended release): 20, 40, 60, 80, 100 mg
Dexmethylphenidate[a,b]	Focalin	Tablets: 2.5, 5, 10 mg
	Focalin XR	Capsules: 5, 10, 15, 20, 25, 30, 35, 40 mg
Lisdexamfetamine	Vyvanse	Capsules: 10, 20, 30, 40, 50, 60, 70 mg
		Chewable tablets: 10, 20, 30, 40, 50, 60 mg
Modafinil[a]	Provigil	Tablets: 100, 200 mg
Armodafinil[a]	Nuvigil	Tablets: 50, 150, 200, 250 mg

[a]Available in generic form.
[b]Available in generic except the extended-release forms.
[c]Available in generic except Aptensio XR, Cotempla XR-ODT, and QuilliChew ER.
[d]Delivery rate of 1.1, 1.6, 2.2, and 3.3 mg/hour for the 10-, 15-, 20-, and 30-mg patches, respectively. In vivo delivery rate is based on a wear period of 9 hours by pediatric patients ages 6–12 years.
Note.   ER = extended release; LA = long-acting; ODT = orally disintegrating tablet; XR = extended release.

ing ADHD; in reducing sleepiness (i.e., in narcolepsy); and in reducing fatigue-induced decrements in behavior. It decreases appetite and has been widely used as an antiobesity medication. For some years, D-amphetamine was sold as a cold remedy, in an inhaler, to shrink swollen nasal membranes. It was also used in treating depression and related fatigue states, until the widespread abuse of its analog D-methamphetamine (speed) by self-injection in the 1960s led to legislation scheduling most stimulants into Drug Enforcement Agency (DEA) Schedule II along with morphine and the potent opioids. This decision was made despite the fact that almost all illicit methamphetamine was made illegally rather than being diverted from drug companies, pharmacies, or doctors.

As a result of the legislative scheduling, use of stimulants in medicine decreased sharply, and their use was sanctioned only for ADHD, narcolepsy, and obesity. Methylphenidate (Ritalin) was marketed just before the law changed and has become much more widely used than D-amphetamine for ADHD. Since the 1990s, Adderall, an "old" drug because it was effective in treating obesity when all old drugs were assessed in the early 1960s, was resurrected as a treatment for ADHD (Horrigan and Barnhill 2000). Adderall contains three different salts of D-amphetamine and one of L-amphetamine. So far, no studies are available comparing Adderall with either D-amphetamine or methylphenidate in treating ADHD, but it seems likely to be about as active as the total of its D-amphetamine salts in any of the situations in which D-amphetamine is useful. Adderall is available in tablets of various strengths (see Table 8–1); its potency is probably slightly less than the same dose of D-amphetamine, but its duration of action may be longer. By 2001, Adderall had taken over a 33% market share (Rosack 2001) and as of 2016 represented about 40% of all ADHD prescriptions, according to Express Scripts in its 2016 Drug Trends report (Managed Healthcare Executive 2017). This is almost twice the number of prescriptions than for methylphenidate or lisdexamfetamine and about eight times the number of atomoxetine prescriptions. A long-acting form of Adderall, Adderall XR, lasts as long as 10 hours and is given at a dosage of 10–30 mg/day, with the dose taken in the morning.

D-methamphetamine is still available in immediate-release form by prescription as Desoxyn from Recordati Rare Diseases. Its sustained-release form was believed by Wender (1993) to be superior in duration of action to both the current Ritalin sustained release (SR; available in a 20-mg dose) and the current Dexedrine Spansule. The last two have a reputation for discharging their main dose of stimulant in the first hour or two and may not have the prolonged effect their makers intended. Newer and better long-acting forms of methylphenidate and amphetamine are now available. One of these, Concerta, a long-acting methylphenidate formulation that lasts 12 hours, was released in July 2000 and is available in strengths of 18, 27, 36, and 54 mg. It appears to be truly long-acting.

A number of new stimulant dosing options have become available in the past 20 years (Cortese et al. 2017; Rosack 2001). Methylphenidate is available in its old, familiar immediate-release form, racemic *d,l*-methylphenidate, with effectiveness for ADHD symptoms lasting 3–4 hours, and *l*-methylphenidate sustained release (Ritalin SR), which has been available for many years and is believed to be weaker in onset of action and possibly in duration of action than immediate-release Ritalin. Novartis, manufacturer of Ritalin and Ritalin SR, has developed long-acting Ritalin (Ritalin LA), designed to release half of each dosage unit quickly and the other half slowly. However, Novartis also has obtained pure *d*-methylphenidate (Focalin), which is twice as potent as racemic Ritalin: 2.5 mg of Focalin equals 5 mg of *d,l*-methylphenidate. The *d* isomer even appears to be slightly—but statistically—more effective than twice the dose of *d,l*-methylphenidate.

To add options and perhaps confusion to the field, many once-daily formulations are now on the market. These formulations include an extended-release tablet (Relexxii), an orally disintegrating 24-hour tablet (Cotempla XR-ODT), and a chewable tablet (QuilliChew ER). Further, another company has developed a transdermal methylphenidate patch (Daytrana), which has been available for a number of years. There is even a methylphenidate formulation, approved in 2018, that is designed to be taken at night. Jornay PM is a formulation of methylphenidate with a coating that dissolves after 8 hours or so. The idea is to have a drug that is active from the time an ADHD patient is awake until the time they go to sleep but that does not interfere with sleep.

Adderall XR also releases half its dosage of mixed amphetamine metabolites rapidly and the other half slowly, both from little coated beads like those in a Dexedrine Spansule. These beads can be taken out of the capsule and sprinkled on applesauce and swallowed (but *not* chewed).

Lisdexamfetamine (Vyvanse) represents another approach: once-a-day dosing. Lisdexamfetamine is essentially a prodrug that is metabolized to dextroamphetamine. It has been studied in ADHD, and doses of 30–70 mg taken in the morning appear to be effective throughout the day. Phase III trials of lisdexamfetamine in the adjunctive treatment of major depressive disorder reported in 2014 that lisdexamfetamine failed to separate from placebo.

All these long-acting preparations cannot be smashed up without losing their prolonged action. Concerta tablets, or their residua, can sometimes be seen in the taker's feces.

The original idea behind all this ingenuity was to avoid the midday pill that may embarrass schoolchildren or complicate the lives of school nurses or that could be diverted to others. Also, some youngsters with ADHD need continued medication effect to be able to do homework or other evening activities well. These various forms allow the prescribing physician to adjust the drug formulation to the needs and side effects of individual patients. If a patient has loss of appetite for supper and insomnia, they may not need a 12-hour stimulant like Concerta.

One application of all this is to determine the twice daily or three times daily dose of *d,l*-methylphenidate or D-amphetamine and then replace these multiple doses with the appropriate longer-acting formulation. Adderall was already believed to have a 5-hour duration of action in ADHD, and Adderall XR should stretch this to possibly 10 hours.

Not all stimulants work in an identical way. Methylphenidate, D-amphetamine, and cocaine all increase release of dopamine into the postsynaptic cleft. D-Amphetamine affects presynaptic receptors as well, whereas methylphenidate does not. Clinicians have had experience with D-amphetamine, methylphenidate, and several anorexiant drugs like phentermine for many years. It is clear that occasionally, patients will do very well while taking one of these drugs but fail to respond to any of the others for no apparent reason. The use of stimulants in psychiatric practice has been reviewed extensively elsewhere (Chiarello and Cole 1987; Heal et al. 2013; Satel and Nelson 1989). It should also be noted that in hospital pharmacies, stimulants have been made into suppositories for rectal administration to patients unable to swallow pills.

Late in 1998, modafinil (Provigil) was marketed for the treatment of daytime sleepiness related to narcolepsy. Modafinil had been in use in France for several years and had not been noted to be abused. It was reported to "feel" like a stimulant in some human abuse liability trials but has slower onset of action and longer duration of action than does D-amphetamine. Further, it appears to have no observable effect on any receptor or any biogenic amine in the brain. Radioactive modafinil concentrates in the hypothalamus, whereas conventional stimulants do not. So we have yet another "stimulant" that is not conventional. Several studies have suggested that modafinil may help lessen the fatigue and sleepiness associated with a variety of conditions, such as shift work and obstructive sleep apnea. In addition, preliminary work also suggests that modafinil may be effective in the treatment of ADHD. Studies by our group and others suggest that a dosage of 100–200 mg/day of modafinil added to a selective serotonin reuptake inhibitor (SSRI) helps with fatigue and hypersomnia associated with depression.

The *R*-enantiomer of modafinil, armodafinil, was approved in 2008 for the same indications as modafinil. Armodafinil has a somewhat longer half-life than does modafinil and may have a slightly different side-effect profile. Armodafinil is being explored in the treatment of a number of conditions beyond sleep disorders, including fatigue associated with cancer and bipolar depression.

The current dilemma is that ADHD and narcolepsy (and depression when it responds) may require amphetamines as maintenance therapy for years or at least months, so the DEA Schedule II restriction that each prescription must be rewritten each month becomes a burden on both the doctor and the patient.

As can be seen, this chapter on stimulant drugs covers drugs used for the core indications of the older stimulants—ADHD, narcolepsy, and obesity—whether or not they have obvious stimulant effects in man or animals. Monoamine oxidase inhibitors (MAOIs) could be included here, but drugs whose major use is in treating depression are considered in Chapter 3 ("Antidepressants") instead.

Amphetamine Abuse

D-amphetamine and methylphenidate, but not modafinil or armodafinil, are spontaneously self-administered intravenously by laboratory animals and are well known to have abuse liability in humans. One of the most abused stimulants to date is methamphetamine. This drug was used intravenously in very high doses during the flower child period of the 1960s, resulting in some individuals, known as *speed freaks*, becoming heavily dependent. Such individuals usually took the medication in relatively large doses in runs of a few days and then withdrew from the drug for a day or two, experiencing a crash, before starting again. Patterns of oral abuse were less intense and dramatic (Grinspoon and Hedblom 1975).

Methamphetamine abuse reemerged in the 1990s. The original formulation, known as *speed*, was the hydrochloride. Crystalline methamphetamine base, known as *ice*, has been widely abused in Hawaii and California. It is chiefly smoked but is also used intravenously, the preferred route during the 1960s. When smoked, it appears to give a rush (immediate pleasurable feeling) like that of cocaine but with a longer duration of the euphoric state. This effect fits with the known relative pharmacokinetics: methamphetamine is metabolized more slowly than cocaine. In monkeys, cocaine is more abusable intravenously than is methamphetamine; monkeys will work harder and longer to get cocaine, and they will continue self-administration for days without stopping, until death occurs. In contrast, amphetamines are less reinforcing.

There is reasonable evidence that very high dosages of D-amphetamine, generally higher than 80 mg/day and sometimes as high as 1,000–2,000 mg/day, can produce an acute psychosis that generally resembles paranoid schizophrenia but can occasionally manifest with delirium and other conventional signs of toxic drug psychosis. This condition is sometimes considered a model for schizophrenia, or at least for acute paranoid psychosis. In addition, parenteral administration of methylphenidate has been used as a test to predict risk of psychotic relapse in patients with schizophrenia. These studies stirred ethical concerns and have largely been discontinued.

Although modafinil and armodafinil are Schedule IV drugs, little evidence of an abuse potential has occurred in postmarketing surveys since 1998. Because modafinil, unlike amphetamine, does not affect the dopaminergic systems that mediate reward in the cortex to the same extent, there is less physiological basis for abuse or dependence. Rapid discontinuation of the drug has generally not been associated with withdrawal symptoms. However, preclinical models in mice do suggest that repeated administration of modafinil may sensitize the nucleus accumbens in ways that promote dependence (Volkow et al. 2009; Wuo-Silva et al. 2011). Rare cases of modafinil abuse have been reported in the literature, particularly among cocaine and methamphetamine abusers, when modafinil has been used as a treatment for these disorders.

Uses of Stimulants

ADHD

ADHD is the only condition other than narcolepsy and weight reduction for which stimulants are currently approved by the FDA. In children, the syndrome is manifested by very short attention span, overactivity, irritability, poor social relations, impulsivity, occasional angry or assaultive behavior, poor school performance, and apparent inability to benefit from instruction or limit setting. Some children with the syndrome have a parent with a history or current symptoms of a similar condition. Occasionally, children with the syndrome have clear evidence of CNS damage at birth or subsequently; the majority of such patients, however, do not have "hard" neurological signs of clearly diagnosable brain injury or abnormality.

In children with ADHD, any of the stimulants is likely to be clinically better than placebo in about 70%–80% of those treated; about 30% show a clear and highly impressive degree of clinical improvement, and another 40% show some modulation of behavior that may be of some clinical importance. Occasionally, children are made more active by these drugs. In the first weeks of treatment, children often look drawn and even somewhat depressed and rarely show any euphoriant effect from the medication. It is not clear that the drugs dramatically reduce activity level. They probably act by improving attention span and organizing behavior more effectively. Some degree of growth inhibition or weight loss has been reported occasionally in children, but these are generally not major problems. (See Chapter 12, "Pharmacotherapy of Specific Populations," for further discussion of the use of stimulants in children.)

Huessey (1979), at the University of Vermont, and Wender et al. (1985), at the University of Utah, identified adults with symptoms resembling those seen in children with ADHD and showed that such adults respond to stimulant therapy. These drug responders are very likely to be remembered by their parents as having been hyperkinetic children. Some individuals who had clear clinical benefit from stimulants in childhood continue to require and to benefit from stimulant medication well into adult life. Many children with ADHD, however, seem to grow out of the major manifestations of the illness at some time in adolescence, although they are often left with residual symptoms of impaired concentration or coping ability, which may or may not be benefited by further stimulant administration. This issue is well discussed by Volkow and Swanson (2013).

The interesting and clinically useful aspect of stimulant therapy in treating either children or adults with ADHD is that clinical effects are often clear and dramatic within a day or two of reaching the appropriate dosage. Stimulant therapy, with this rapid clinical response, stands in dramatic contrast to the more conventional antidepressants and antipsychotics, which often take days or even weeks to achieve a satisfactory clinical result.

In clinical practice, adults with personality disorder, short attention span, restlessness, hyperactivity, irritability, impulsivity, and other related symptoms sometimes present with a history of illicit drug abuse. In treating such individuals, a trial of a stimulant raises an ethical problem: When it is clear that any stimulant will be abused, the drug cannot be used. Stimulants might be used in patients with a history of drug abuse under the following circumstances:

- The stimulant drug has clearly been used to improve functioning rather than to get high (produce euphoria).
- A good therapeutic alliance is available.
- The medication can be closely monitored, perhaps in an inpatient setting.
- Other approaches have failed.
- The patient's problems are seriously interfering with their life functioning.

The utility of stimulant therapy in the treatment of substance abusers with a clear history of ADHD, including individuals addicted to cocaine (Schubiner et al. 1995), has been documented in open trials, as has the lack of utility of stimulant therapy in treating cocaine users without ADHD during the early postcocaine withdrawal period; methylphenidate facilitates return to cocaine use in such patients. A smattering of studies on the use of various antidepressants (desipramine, phenelzine, bupropion, SSRIs, selegiline, and venlafaxine) in treating patients with ADHD, both childhood and adult varieties, are now available. Desipramine and bupropion are the best-documented drugs for this purpose. Most controlled studies have been positive. Some clinicians believe that, in children at least, desipramine tends to lose its effectiveness over time. With all these drugs, it is best to start with low dosages (e.g., 10 mg/day of desipramine, 75 mg/day of bupropion SR formulation) on the presumption that some patients with ADHD will be likely to respond to low dosages and show undesirable side effects at higher dosages.

The issue of the existence of ADHD (or attention-deficit disorder without hyperactivity) in adults has received more attention in the past 30 years. Ratey et al. (1994), in a clinical report, described patients with these conditions and their responses to various medications, and Spencer et al. (1995) reported positive results in a placebo-controlled trial of methylphenidate in treating adult patients with ADHD at Massachusetts General Hospital. The superior effectiveness of stimulants, compared with psychosocial treatment, for childhood ADHD received strong support from a federally sponsored multicenter study (Jensen et al. 2001). Further, the breadth of stimulant effect in conduct disorder in children was strongly supported by the results of a study by Klein et al. (1997).

Stimulants in the treatment of ADHD are generally well tolerated at the recommended dosages but can induce a number of side effects. In ADHD clinical trials, side effects led to discontinuation of the drug in 1%–7% of patients (Storebø et al. 2018). The most common side effects are decreased appetite and sleep disruption. Sleep disruption can be managed by using a stimulant preparation that allows for one-time dosing in the morning. Multiple dosing, including late afternoon doses, should be avoided if possible. The new Jornay PM evening dose may also circumvent sleep difficulties. Weight should be monitored in children who are taking stimulants. There is an association of reduced appetite and low body mass index associated with stimulant use in children, with decreases in overall height and growth (Gurbuz et al. 2016). Although the effects of stimulants on growth in children appear to be modest, they are more likely to be seen in girls and in children who start treatment before puberty (Díez-Suárez et al. 2017). In children who are not making expected weight gains or who are losing weight, nonstimulant treatments for ADHD, including atomoxetine, guanfacine, and antidepressants, might be considered. Stimulants may also increase blood pressure and heart rate. Although rarely a problem in children, cardiovascular effects may be problematic in adults with a history of coronary artery disease, arrhythmia, or uncontrolled hypertension.

Depression

The early literature on the use of amphetamines in psychiatry included a number of case reports of individuals presenting with the full syndrome of endogenous depression who responded dramatically to racemic amphetamine. A few double-blind trials completed since the early 1970s showed some evidence of clinical efficacy of stimulants in depressed outpatients. Findings from some studies were only weakly positive, and most others were clearly negative (Satel and Nelson 1989). The use of stimulants as adjunctive agents in depression is suggested by a number of uncontrolled studies and smaller controlled studies (Trivedi et al. 2013). However, the most definitive trials of a stimulant as the adjunctive agent in the treatment of major depression have involved the use of lisdexamfetamine. In these two multicenter randomized controlled trials, each with more than 300 patients, lisdexamfetamine failed to separate from placebo (Richards et al. 2017).

Given the lack of data, it not a reasonable idea to use stimulant monotherapy in the early treatment of major depressive disorder. However, in patients with a chronic treatment-resistant depression that did not respond to a range of standard antidepressants, stimulants occasionally provide excellent symptomatic relief and often enable patients to function adequately for prolonged periods without side effects or any indication that the drug is being abused or misused. Some of these patients have clear-cut vegetative symptoms; others appear to have atypical depression, and still others have major symptoms of fatigue or executive dysfunction. As it has become increasingly clear that antidepressants often do an unsatisfactory job of treating cognitive symptoms and fatigue, stimulants are being reevaluated to target those symptoms specifically.

It is not possible to tell in advance which depressed patients will benefit from stimulant therapy. Rickels et al. (1970) suggested years ago that relatively heavy intake of coffee (four cups a day or more) was a predictor of good clinical response, at least to magnesium pemoline. In contrast, patients who are intolerant of caffeine sometimes cannot tolerate stimulants. However, experience at McLean Hospital around 1990, in an informal study involving 30 patients who had done well while taking prescribed stimulants for more than 2 years, suggested that some depressed patients with excellent response to stimulants dislike or avoid caffeine-containing beverages. Only three of the patients in the study had histories suggestive of childhood ADHD, but many had a significant thought disorder (i.e., difficulty in organizing their thoughts and in functioning effectively at work or school). Almost all had significant depression, and several had bulimia. All but three had had persistent benefit from stimulants for a period ranging from 2 to 30 years.

The cases of the three patients with poor outcomes can be summarized as follows: One patient took stimulants at very high doses for 20 years, initially to lose weight. Instead, he gained a massive amount of weight, ultimately requiring a gastric bypass operation. His career was adversely affected, and a family disaster, with resulting major depression, led to his referral to McLean from another state. The second patient, a professional with clear ADHD symptoms from childhood who succeeded academically without stimulant therapy, ended up taking methylphenidate 80–120 mg/day, which, paradoxically, caused fatigue and an inability to function professionally. The third, after having had a favorable response for a decade, began to experience marital stress and developed paranoid hypomania alternating with depression. Each retrial of a stimulant to relieve her chronic depression led to hospitalization, with the patient in a paranoid excitement. The poor outcomes in these three cases must be balanced against the substantial symptom relief and improved role functioning in all the other patients seen in consultation. Many were followed for up to 15 years with continuing benefit (Cole et al. 1993).

Stimulants also have a place in the crisis management of individuals whose functioning is impaired by depression and whose life situation would deteriorate rapidly if they were not able to resume functioning within a few days. In such situations, a trial of modafinil, methylphenidate, D-amphetamine, or Adderall is worth initiating to attempt to get a patient through a crisis when failure to function might result in getting fired from a job or flunking out of college. In such situations, weaker semistimulants such as bupropion are unlikely to work rapidly enough to be useful. Modafinil or armodafinil, with favorable side-effect profiles, would seem like a good choice for many patients. However, they are still not approved for any psychiatric indication as of this writing, and insurance companies are hesitant to pay for them. For now, D-amphetamine in its generic form costs less and is a bit more likely to be effective than methylphenidate. One might begin with D-amphetamine 5 mg in the morning and increase the dosage by 5 mg every morning until the patient either feels better or feels unpleasantly stimulated. The patient should check in daily during this process. If the morning dose helps, a second, equal dose 4–6 hours later should be added. If the D-amphetamine has an unpleasant effect, it should be stopped, and methylphenidate 10 mg (5 mg in elderly or hypertensive patients) should be tried instead. Adderall, the mixture of amphetamine salts, at an initial dose of 10 mg can also be tried. Dosages up to 20 or 30 mg/

day of D-amphetamine or twice that amount of methylphenidate also can be used to see whether a response occurs.

The major problem in recommending stimulant therapy to other psychiatrists for a specific patient is the likelihood that the patient will be left taking an ineffective dosage (e.g., initial dose 5–10 mg once or twice a day) for a couple of weeks, until the drug is stopped for lack of efficacy. Using a stimulant in adult psychiatric patients requires close monitoring, at least by telephone, so that the treating psychiatrist can determine whether the drug at the dosage given had any effect. In the absence of any effect, positive or negative, the dosage should be steadily increased until something happens—up to 40 mg/day of D-amphetamine or 80 mg/day of methylphenidate. This dosing method is infrequently used, perhaps because of fear of the abuse potential of the drug (although abuse of D-amphetamine or methylphenidate is uncommon in psychiatric patients) or because psychiatrists are so accustomed to using drugs that take 7–30 days to act that they do not change their prescribing behavior when using unfamiliar but rapid-acting drugs such has D-amphetamine.

Some patients show an initial excellent response to a stimulant medication and then develop rapid tolerance, with all effect being lost, whereas others continue to benefit from the same low dose of the stimulant for months or even years. Still other patients feel anxious, agitated, and unpleasantly "wired" while taking some or all stimulants. If the drug is to be stopped, it can be either tapered or stopped abruptly. Some rebound depression may occur (see Chapter 11, "Pharmacotherapy for Substance Use Disorders"). Patients with a history of pronounced mood disturbances may require hospitalization.

D-amphetamine is available in 5-mg, 10-mg, and 15-mg Spansule (slow-release) formulations. Methamphetamine (Desoxyn) is available in a 5-mg tablet. Adderall is available in 5-mg, 7.5-mg, 10-mg, 12.5-mg, 15-mg, 20-mg, and 30-mg tablets, about equivalent in efficacy to the same dose of dextroamphetamine.

Methylphenidate is available in a 20-mg SR formulation. Better, longer-acting preparations of several stimulants have recently been marketed or are now under development. One of these, Concerta, is available in 18-mg, 27-mg, 36-mg, and 54-mg 12-hour SR tablets. A preparation of methylphenidate, Jornay PM (formerly HLD200), has a coating that allows a delayed onset of action by 8–10 hours (Childress et al. 2018). This formulation is taken at night and does not interfere with sleep but is active by the time the patient wakes up in the morning. For children with ADHD, even a 12-hour formulation of methylphenidate taken before school will take some time for the onset of action. Jornay PM ostensibly will be active even in the often difficult hours before school begins without the need for additional doses during the day. The doses used in clinical trials have ranged from 40 to 80 mg given at night.

In the late 1990s, the increasingly common use of methylphenidate was a concern to many in the community, and considerable debate occurred regarding whether it is overused. Multiple lawsuits were filed, including a class action suit against the makers of methylphenidate and the American Psychiatric Association, alleging a conspiracy to invent and promote ADHD in order to sell stimulants. These cases never progressed to trial and were all dismissed by the end of 2002.

Some depressed patients prefer taking ordinary tablets of D-amphetamine or methylphenidate and may take the entire daily dose at once on arising, even if 30–60 mg/day is being given. Such patients feel no rush or high but are relieved of depression for at least 24 hours. Others take single fast-release tablets several times a day, taking another as the effect of the previous dose wears off. Some dislike this on-off effect and prefer to use SR preparations.

After decades in which only single-dose forms of D-amphetamine and methylphenidate were available, several forms of methylphenidate with different lengths and forms of sustained release are now available. Several appear designed to avoid the necessity for a child with ADHD to take a second dose of stimulant around noon, which entails involving the school and making the child's "problem" obvious to teachers or classmates. It is too early to tell if this or other available formulations are better or worse than other established formulations. We suggest that ordinary immediate-release pills be used initially and that the dose and the formulation be adjusted to improve drug response when needed (e.g., ability to study after school) or avoid side effects (e.g., anorexia, initial insomnia).

Fatigue Associated With Chronic Viral Illness

A number of chronic viral and postviral syndromes, from AIDS and hepatitis to long COVID after infection with the virus that causes coronavirus disease 2019 (COVID-19), are associated with fatigue and cognitive deficits. Stimulants and related agents such as modafinil have a potential role to play in the treatment of these conditions.

Patients with AIDS often have a mixture of depression; fatigue; and difficulty initiating activities, perhaps a form of akinesia (see Chapter 12). Such patients may have CNS complications of AIDS, including shrinking of the basal ganglia. Standard tricyclic antidepressants (TCAs) may or may not be poorly tolerated, but they may cause increased memory problems or delirium. Methylphenidate appears to be widely used in treating such patients, with good results, although little has been written about this use. Patients can begin taking low dosages (e.g., 5 mg bid), titrated to a level that relieves symptoms without causing side effects. The dose may need to be increased gradually as the disease progresses. Local experts in Boston give us the impression that methylphenidate in treating AIDS-related depression, inertia, and confusion resembles L-dopa in treating parkinsonism—a replacement therapy needed because of changes in the brain. This idea is, of course, purely speculative. In addition, the anorexiant properties of most stimulants may be problematic in the treatment of HIV-related illness. Drug interactions with protease inhibitors and antiretroviral agents such as ritonavir are theoretically possible.

Modafinil and armodafinil have been explored as alternatives to stimulants in the treatment of HIV-related fatigue. For example, patients with HIV receiving armodafinil were significantly more likely than patients receiving placebo to report an increase in energy and mood in a double-blind, randomized controlled trial (Rabkin et al. 2010, 2011). Modafinil and armodafinil are much less likely to cause weight loss in HIV patients than are agents such as dextroamphetamine. However, because modafinil and armodafinil are substrates and mild inducers of cytochrome P450 (CYP) 3A4, the concurrent use of these agents with protease inhibitors, integrase inhibitors, and non-nucleoside reverse transcriptase inhibitors may result in lower levels of the HIV medications. Thus, monitoring of blood levels of these medications may be required if modafinil or armodafinil is used concurrently.

Many viral illnesses are associated with a chronic postviral syndrome that can persist long after the acute infection has subsided. These include illnesses caused by adenoviruses, herpesviruses, enteroviruses, paramyxoviruses, orthomyxoviruses and coronaviruses. Long COVID refers to a range of symptoms that persist for weeks or even months or years after the initial COVID-19 infection. These symptoms can include fatigue, brain fog, difficulty concentrating, insomnia, anxiety, depression, and chronic pain.

Stimulants have been used to counteract the fatigue associated with the treatment of viral illness. For example, interferon is used to treat a number of viral illnesses, including hepatitis, but is associated with depression and fatigue in a large subset of patients. Stimulants and modafinil have shown efficacy in counteracting interferon-associated fatigue (Martin et al. 2017). In addition, the use of stimulants and antidepressants has been considered as a potential treatment for some of the symptoms of long COVID. Stimulants, such as methylphenidate and modafinil, have been used to alleviate fatigue and improve cognitive function in patients with chronic fatigue syndrome and other conditions, so it makes sense that they may have a role to play in long COVID. However, to date there have been limited good studies for any treatment of long COVID.

Binge-Eating Disorder

Binge-eating disorder (BED) is a new category added in DSM-5 to differentiate repetitive bingeing without purging from bulimia. Lisdexamfetamine (Vyvanse) was reported to be significantly more effective than placebo in BED in Phase III multicenter trials. In January 2015, Vyvanse received an FDA-approved indication for treating BED in adults. It is the first drug approved for this disorder. Vyvanse for BED is started at 30 mg/day, with the dosage increased to 50 or 70 mg/day as tolerated.

Other Medical Conditions

A growing series of case reports has documented the usefulness of stimulants in treating patients on the medical wards of general hospitals. These patients have various combinations of debilitating depression and fatigue that make them unable to cooperate in necessary treatments, and they lose weight rapidly. In this situation, standard antidepressants simply do not have a fast enough onset of action. Stimulants do have a fast enough onset of effects, probably about 50% of the time. For this indication, therefore, they are being used more commonly and appear to be safe (Wallace et al. 1995).

Drug Combinations

Methylphenidate and D-amphetamine both interact with imipramine in laboratory animals to potentiate response to electrical stimulation of pleasure centers. Part of this potentiation is pharmacokinetic, in the sense that the stimulant and the TCA interfere with each other's metabolism, causing higher blood levels of each. This property was sometimes used clinically, when methylphenidate was prescribed early in TCA therapy to hasten response. However, if a patient improved with methylphenidate plus imipramine, it was impossible to know whether the clinical response was due to 1) the methylphenidate alone, 2) a longer period taking imipramine, 3) the elevation of imipramine blood level caused by methylphenidate, or 4) a true combined effect of the two drugs. Generally, we do not recommend this combination approach (see Chapter 9, "Augmentation Strategies for Treatment-Resistant Disorders"). Stimulants have been used to counteract anergia secondary to SSRI therapy in depression. Here, the plasma levels of the SSRI may be increased.

Intuitively, it should be considered clinically dangerous to combine a stimulant with an MAOI because the addition of a stimulant might precipitate a hypertensive crisis. However, we know of a few patients who have, on their own responsibility, added magnesium pemoline, methylphenidate, or D-amphetamine to reverse MAOI-induced sedation or lack of clinical response, with alleged good subjective effects and no apparent effect on blood pressure. Other such patients have been described in the literature. We have seen hypertensive crises when phenylpropanolamine or pseudoephedrine was added to an MAOI, but so far we have not encountered any such crises with stimulant-MAOI combinations. Stimulant-MAOI combinations are not recommended in general practice; however, the combination has been used cautiously to counteract MAOI-induced hypotension (see Chapter 3) and by us to reverse MAOI-induced daytime sedation, so far without adverse effects.

Psychosis

Literature from the 1930s and 1940s on the use of racemic amphetamine, D-amphetamine, and methylphenidate in treating patients with what was then called chronic schizophrenia reported mixed results: some patients improved on a stimulant given alone, some showed no change, and some worsened. However, more recent studies of single doses of intravenous methylphenidate showed that this drug increases psychosis in drug-free acutely ill patients with mania or schizophrenia but has only a mild stimulant effect when such patients are in remission. A study by Robinson et al. (1991) demonstrated that chronically ill schizophrenic outpatients who showed increased psychosis after a single dose of a stimulant were much more likely to relapse into a psychotic exacerbation than were patients who showed no worsening on stimulant administration. Other work (Lieberman et al. 1994) also supported the finding that an exacerbation of psychosis after a single dose of methylphenidate may predict higher relapse risk in stable patients whose antipsychotic dose is reduced or discontinued. This type of research became extremely controversial because of ethical concerns about worsening patients' conditions.

The most common use of stimulants in the treatment of schizophrenia is to attempt to ameliorate negative and cognitive symptoms. As reported in Chapter 4 ("Antipsychotic Drugs"), antipsychotics are best suited for treating positive symptoms. However, it is the negative and cognitive symptoms of schizophrenia that are most debilitating in vocational and interpersonal functioning (Tsang et al. 2010). Methylphenidate, amphetamine, modafinil, and armodafinil appear to have at least a modest benefit in the treatment of negative and cognitive symptoms (Lindenmayer et al. 2013; Saavedra-Velez et al. 2009). The primary risk associated with the use of these agents in schizophrenia is the exacerbation of psychosis. Although the risk appears to be small, at this time there is not enough evidence to suggest that the benefits outweigh the risks.

Stimulant Use Versus Abuse

We have occasionally seen patients who had taken prescribed stimulants for years, claiming excellent relief from depression, fatigue, or disorganized behavior, who had the drug withdrawn by a physician concerned about drug abuse. Such patients then often failed to respond to a variety of more conventional TCAs and were dysphoric and unable to function adequately for years. When the stimulant was represcribed, these patients often did quite well again for prolonged periods. It may be very hard to tell whether such individuals (who rarely have histories suggestive of ADHD) really have a uniquely stimulant-responsive disorder or whether they have somehow become dependent on stimulants. In either case, if they cope well and feel well only when taking stimulants, take low to moderate dosages as prescribed, and do not develop tolerance, the stimulant should be continued. If the physician feels uncomfortable about prescribing stimulants for such patients, consultation with a clinical psychopharmacologist may provide helpful clinical and ethical support. The risk of subsequent abuse of stimulants or other substances in children treated for ADHD appears to be quite small. In fact, some of the more rigorous studies to date suggest that childhood prescription of stimulants for ADHD might be associated with a lower risk of substance abuse in adolescence and adulthood, particularly in males (Quinn et al. 2017).

More difficult permutations of the problem exist, of course. What about a patient who recalls D-amphetamine making him feel "better," but not better enough to actually complete graduate courses or even to motivate him to pay the bill of the psychiatrist who was prescribing the pills? What about a patient for whom a host of antidepressants have failed but who refuses to try an MAOI because of the restricted diet and risks? Should she be forced to undergo a failed trial of an MAOI before a stimulant is tried or retried? What about a marginally employed, distant, mildly paranoid young man with severe ear pain of an undiagnosable nature who buys illicit stimulants to relieve the pain? The stimulants do not help him function, and they do not make him more paranoid—they only make him feel better. What about the undergraduate student or technology company manager who does not have ADHD but finds it difficult to compete without the cognitive benefits of a stimulant? We feel more comfortable prescribing stimulants when they either obviously improve functioning or, at least, relieve incapacitating distress. We would not encourage a patient to try an MAOI if they have already improved while taking a stimulant in the past, but these are personal judgments.

In summary, we suspect that the useful, rapidly acting stimulant drugs are underused in American adult psychiatric practice. They do not always work or even help, but when they do, they can be very effective. It is still unclear whether bupropion, which resembles the stimulants in some respects, or other new drugs, which do not (see Chapter 3), will prove to be safer, less abusable drugs that will help those psychiatric patients who now respond only to standard stimulants.

Nonstimulants for the Treatment of ADHD

Although the efficacy of stimulants in the treatment of ADHD is long established, not all patients respond to or tolerate stimulants. In addition, there may be a concern about abuse in some patients that may preclude the use of stimulants. Fortunately, there are a number of nonstimulants that have also

Table 8–2.   Nonstimulant medications approved for ADHD

Drug	Trade Name	Dosage range
Atomoxetine	Strattera	40–100 mg qd
Viloxazine	Qelbree	200–600 mg qd
Guanfacine	Intuniv	1–4 mg qhs
Clonidine	Kapvay	0.1–0.2 mg qhs

demonstrated efficacy without some of the side effects or liabilities of the stimulants. These medications are listed in Table 8–2.

Atomoxetine

Atomoxetine is a pure norepinephrine reuptake blocker that is FDA approved for the treatment of ADHD in children and adults. It appears to have no abuse liability potential and has been shown to be significantly more effective than placebo in children and adolescents as well as in adults with the disorder. It carries the same black box warning around suicidality as the antidepressants. In a small study in adults, Spencer et al. (1998) reported that the drug was significantly more effective than placebo. The average dosage was 76 mg/day. Subsequently, several positive trials in adults have been reported (Michelson et al. 2003). Similarly, the drug has been reported to be effective in a large study in children and adolescents (Michelson et al. 2002) (see Chapter 12). Atomoxetine appears to be more effective in improving attention than in controlling hyperactivity. Relative to the effects of stimulants, the effects of atomoxetine on ADHD are also more gradual. Stimulants tend to show more rapid benefits.

The adult daily dosage of atomoxetine is 40–100 mg; in children, the daily dosage is approximately 1.2 mg/kg and should not exceed 1.4 mg/kg, or 100 mg, whichever is less. Primary side effects appear to be loss of appetite and gastrointestinal upset in children and gastrointestinal upset, orthostatic blood pressure effects, and insomnia in adults. In contrast to the older stimulants, the dosage of atomoxetine has to be increased slowly to avoid somatic side effects.

Viloxazine

Like atomoxetine, viloxazine is a selective norepinephrine reuptake inhibitor; it has been approved for the treatment of ADHD in several countries, including a number of European countries, Canada, and Mexico. It was approved in United States in 2021 for treating children ages 6–17 and received an expanded indication for treating adults in 2022. Viloxazine is rapidly absorbed after oral administration, with peak plasma concentrations achieved within 2–4 hours. It has a half-life of approximately 6–8 hours and is metabolized primarily in the liver. The drug and its metabolites are eliminated primarily in the urine.

Several randomized controlled trials have shown that viloxazine is effective in reducing symptoms of ADHD in children and adults. In a study of 420 children with ADHD, viloxazine was shown to significantly improve inattention and hyperactivity/impulsivity compared with placebo over a 10-week treatment period (Biederman et al. 2020). Another study of 315 adults with ADHD found that viloxazine was effective in reducing ADHD symptoms and improving executive function compared with placebo over a 6-week treatment period (Wilens et al. 2021). Viloxazine is generally well tolerated, with common side effects including nausea, headache, and insomnia.

Atomoxetine has been available in a generic formulation for some time and thus is a much less expensive medication then viloxazine. However, from the efficacy and side-effect profile data, it is hard to see a clear advantage of viloxazine. One possible advantage is that viloxazine may work somewhat faster than atomoxetine, although there are no head-to-head comparisons. Viloxazine appeared to separate from placebo at about 1 week as opposed to 3 weeks for atomoxetine. Still, both drugs act much slower than do stimulants.

Guanfacine

In 2009, guanfacine, in its extended-release formulation, became the second nonstimulant, after atomoxetine, to be approved for the treatment of ADHD. Guanfacine is an old medication, used historically as an antihypertensive but rarely used for this indication currently. The drug is a selective α_{2A} antagonist whose efficacy in the treatment of ADHD in children and adolescents was established in two randomized, controlled, fixed-dose trials. Both trials included children ages 6–17. One of the trials evaluated guanfacine at dosages of 2–4 mg/day over 8 weeks (Biederman et al. 2008a, 2008b), and the other used dosages of 1–4 mg/day over 9 weeks (Sallee et al. 2009). Both studies used the ADHD Rating Scale IV (ADHD-RS-IV) to assess changes from baseline to the end of the study. Guanfacine at all dosages was reported to be superior to placebo at improving overall scores on the ADHD-RS-IV. Interestingly, there did appear to be a dose-response relationship, with higher dosages being more effective but also having more side effects than did lower dosages. No comparison studies with stimulants or atomoxetine have yet been completed, so it is unclear if there are any efficacy advantages of guanfacine over other agents.

The side effects of guanfacine can be anticipated from its α-adrenergic effects: somnolence, sedation, hypotension/dizziness, bradycardia, dry mouth, abdominal pain, and constipation. About 33% of children treated with guanfacine experienced sedation or somnolence, compared with about 12% of placebo-treated children. Sedation was the most common reason for discontinuing the drug. About 6% of children had some evidence of hypotension, and 1% had syncopal episodes. Gastrointestinal adverse events were not common reasons for discontinuing guanfacine in the acute ADHD trials.

Guanfacine extended-release is usually dosed at 1 mg/day given in the morning. Patients who experience daytime sedation may benefit from evening dosing of guanfacine. The dosage is increased by no more than 1 mg/week to a maximum of 4 mg/day. Measuring blood pressure at the start of treatment and with dosage changes is recommended. Guanfacine is metabolized via CYP3A4, and concurrent administration of inhibitors such as ketoconazole can increase plasma concentrations of the drug, whereas inducers such as carbamazepine or rifampin may lower serum levels.

Guanfacine, then, represents another nonstimulant that appears to be effective for the treatment of ADHD. We would anticipate that as a nonscheduled agent that does not have a black box warning around suicidality, guanfacine should have an important niche in the treatment of ADHD. It remains to be seen how much of an issue the cardiovascular and sedating effects of the drug will be in clinical practice.

Clonidine

Clonidine, like guanfacine, is another centrally acting α_2-adrenergic agonist that decreases sympathetic outflow from the central nervous system. Long used as an antihypertensive, it was approved in the treatment of ADHD in 2010 as a monotherapy or an adjunct to stimulants.

Clonidine undergoes significant first-pass metabolism in the liver, with only about 50% of the drug reaching systemic circulation after oral administration. The drug is extensively metabolized by the liver, with less than 1% of the dose excreted unchanged in the urine. The primary metabolite of clonidine, 4-hydroxyclonidine, is pharmacologically inactive. The elimination half-life of clonidine is approximately 12–16 hours, and the drug is eliminated primarily via the renal route. Patients with renal impairment may require dosage adjustments to avoid excessive accumulation of the drug.

Clonidine has a linear pharmacokinetic profile over the recommended dose range. The drug has a large volume of distribution, indicating that it distributes widely in the body, including into the brain. Clonidine crosses the blood-brain barrier and binds to α_2 receptors in the brain stem, resulting in a decrease in sympathetic tone, which may help in the treatment of ADHD.

Multiple clinical trials have demonstrated the efficacy of clonidine in the treatment of ADHD. A meta-analysis of randomized controlled trials found that clonidine significantly improved symptoms of hyperactivity, impulsivity, and inattention in children with ADHD (Wilens et al. 2012). Another study found that clonidine improved both subjective and objective measures of attention in adults with ADHD (Wigal et al. 2011).

Many clinicians find the α_2 drugs less effective than either the stimulants or norepinephrine-specific drugs, particularly for treating inattention. In fact, some patients complain about more brain fog with the α_2 drugs. However, some patients with ADHD seem to do well with clonidine and guanfacine, particularly as adjuncts to stimulants. Children also seem to do better with the α_2 agents than do adults.

The typical dose is 0.1 for children given at bedtime. Extended-release tablets and oral suspension are available for children who have trouble taking tablets. Clonidine is generally well tolerated, with common side effects including drowsiness, dry mouth, and constipation. Hypotension is a concern at higher doses. Clonidine should not be abruptly discontinued because that can lead to rebound hypertension, although this is less of a problem at the lower doses used by children.

Suggested Readings

Angrist B, Peselow E, Rubinstein M, et al: Amphetamine response and relapse risk after depot neuroleptic discontinuation. Psychopharmacology (Berl) 85(3):277–283, 1985 2860683

Biederman G: Fenfluramine (Pondimin) in autism. Biol Ther Psychiatry Newsl 8:25–28, 1985

Biederman J, Faraone SV: Attention-deficit hyperactivity disorder. Lancet 366(9481):237–248, 2005 16023516

Bodkin JA, Zornberg GL, Lukas SE, Cole JO: Buprenorphine treatment of refractory depression. J Clin Psychopharmacol 15(1):49–57, 1995 7714228

Cole JO (ed): The Amphetamines in Psychiatry (Seminars in Psychiatry, Vol 1, No 2). New York, Grune and Stratton, 1969, pp 128–137

Cole JO: Drug therapy of adult minimal brain dysfunction, in Psychopharmacology Update. Edited by Cole JO. Lexington, MA, Collamore, 1981, pp 69–80

Davidoff E, Reifenstein E: Treatment of schizophrenia with sympathomimetic drugs: benzedrine sulfate. Psychiatr Q 13:127–144, 1939

Drevets WC, Furey ML: Replication of scopolamine's antidepressant efficacy in major depressive disorder: a randomized, placebo-controlled clinical trial. Biol Psychiatry 67(5):432–438, 2010 20074703

Elizur A, Wintner I, Davidson S: The clinical and psychological effects of pemoline in depressed patients—a controlled study. Int Pharmacopsychiatry 14(3):127–134, 1979 391753

Ellinwood EH: Amphetamine psychosis: individuals, settings, and sequences, in Current Concepts on Amphetamine Abuse (DHEW Publ No HSM-729085). Edited by Ellinwood EH, Cohen S. Washington, DC, U.S. GPO, 1972, pp 143–158

Expert Roundtable Highlights: Stimulants and atomoxetine in the treatment of attention-deficit/hyperactivity disorder. J Clin Psychiatry Monogr 19(1):1–23, 2004

Faraone SV, Glatt SJ: Effects of extended-release guanfacine on ADHD symptoms and sedation-related adverse events in children with ADHD. J Atten Disord 13(5):532–538, 2010 19395648

Feighner JP, Herbstein J, Damlouji N: Combined MAOI, TCA, and direct stimulant therapy of treatment-resistant depression. J Clin Psychiatry 46(6):206–209, 1985 3997787

Feldman PE: Ancient psychopharmacotherapy. Bull Menninger Clin 29(5):256–263, 1965 5318413

Fernandez F, Levy JK, Galizzi H: Response of HIV-related depression to psychostimulants: case reports. Hosp Community Psychiatry 39(6):628–631, 1988 3402922

Greenhill LL, Osman BB (eds): Ritalin: Theory and Practice, 2nd Edition. Larchmont, NY, Mary Ann Liebert, 2000

Griffiths RR, Johnson MW, Carducci MA, et al: Psilocybin produces substantial and sustained decreases in depression and anxiety in patients with life-threatening cancer: a randomized double-blind trial. J Psychopharmacol 30(12):1181–1197, 2016 27909165

Hughes CH: Tranquilizer for maniacs. Alienist Neurologist 32:163–166, 1911

Jackson JG: Hazards of smokable methamphetamine. N Engl J Med 321(13):907, 1989 2770833

Kaufmann MW, Murray GB, Cassem NH: Use of psychostimulants in medically ill depressed patients. Psychosomatics 23(8):817–819, 1982 7134365

Khajavi D, Farokhnia M, Modabbernia A, et al: Oral scopolamine augmentation in moderate to severe major depressive disorder: a randomized, double-blind, placebo-controlled study. J Clin Psychiatry 73(11):1428–1433, 2012 23146150

Klein RG, Mannuzza S: Hyperactive boys almost grown up III: methylphenidate effects on ultimate height. Arch Gen Psychiatry 45(12):1131–1134, 1988 3058089

Kroft C, Cole JO: Adverse behavioral effects of psychostimulants, in Adverse Effects of Psychotropic Drugs. Edited by Kane JM, Lieberman JA. New York, Guilford, 1992, pp 153–162

Mattes JA, Boswell L, Oliver H: Methylphenidate effects on symptoms of attention deficit disorder in adults. Arch Gen Psychiatry 41(11):1059–1063, 1984 6388523

The MTA Cooperative Group: A 14-month randomized clinical trial of treatment strategies for attention deficit/hyperactivity disorder. Arch Gen Psychiatry 56:1073–1088, 1999

Myerson A: The effect of benzedrine sulfate on mood and fatigue in normal and neurotic persons. AMA Arch Neurol Psychiatry 36:816–822, 1936

Olin J, Masand P: Psychostimulants for depression in hospitalized cancer patients. Psychosomatics 37(1):57–62, 1996 8600496

Ritvo ER, Freeman BJ, Yuwiler A, et al: Study of fenfluramine in outpatients with the syndrome of autism. J Pediatr 105(5):823–828, 1984 6502317

Ross S, Bossis A, Guss J, et al: Rapid and sustained symptom reduction following psilocybin treatment for anxiety and depression in patients with life-threatening cancer: a randomized controlled trial. J Psychopharmacol 30(12):1165–1180, 2016 27909164

Savage GH: Hyoscyamine, and its uses. J Ment Sci 25:177–184, 1879

Shekim WO, Asarnow RF, Hess E, et al: A clinical and demographic profile of a sample of adults with attention deficit hyperactivity disorder, residual state. Compr Psychiatry 31(5):416–425, 1990 2225800

Spencer T, Biederman J, Wilens T, et al: A large, double-blind, randomized clinical trial of methylphenidate in the treatment of adults with attention-deficit/hyperactivity disorder. Biol Psychiatry 57(5):456–463, 2005 15737659

Stoll A, Pillay S, Diamond L, et al: Methylphenidate augmentation of SSRIs: a case series. J Clin Psychopharmacol 57:72–76, 1996

US Modafinil in Narcolepsy Multicenter Study Group: Randomized trial of modafinil for the treatment of pathological somnolence in narcolepsy. Ann Neurol 43(1):88–97, 1998 9450772

Wood DR, Reimherr FW, Wender PH, Johnson GE: Diagnosis and treatment of minimal brain dysfunction in adults: a preliminary report. Arch Gen Psychiatry 33(12):1453–1460, 1976 793563

Young CM, Findling RL: Pemoline and hepatotoxicity. Int Drug Ther Newsl 33(9):46–47, 1998

References

Biederman J, Melmed RD, Patel A, et al: Long-term, open-label extension study of guanfacine extended release in children and adolescents with ADHD. CNS Spectr 13(12):1047–1055, 2008a 19179940

Biederman J, Melmed RD, Patel A, et al; SPD503 Study Group: A randomized, double-blind, placebo-controlled study of guanfacine extended release in children and adolescents with attention-deficit/hyperactivity disorder. Pediatrics 121(1):e73–e84, 2008b

Biederman J, et al: Efficacy and safety of viloxazine for the treatment of attention-deficit/hyperactivity disorder in children and adolescents: a randomized, placebo-controlled, Phase IIb study. CNS Drugs 34(10):1057–1067, 2020

Chiarello RJ, Cole JO: The use of psychostimulants in general psychiatry: a reconsideration. Arch Gen Psychiatry 44(3):286–295, 1987 2881528

Childress A, Mehrotra S, Gobburu J, et al: Single-dose pharmacokinetics of HLD200, a delayed-release and extended-release methylphenidate formulation, in healthy adults and in adolescents and children with attention-deficit/hyperactivity disorder. J Child Adolesc Psychopharmacol 28(1):10–18, 2018 29039979

Cole JO, Boling LA, Beake BJ: Stimulant drugs: medical needs, alternative-indications and related problems, in Impact of Prescription Drug Diversion Control Systems on Medical Practice and Patient Care (NIDA Monogr No 131). Edited by Cooper JR, Czechowicz DJ, Molinari SP. Rockville, MD, National Institute on Drug Abuse, 1993, pp 89–108

Cortese S, D'Acunto G, Konofal E, et al: New formulations of methylphenidate for the treatment of attention-deficit/hyperactivity disorder: pharmacokinetics, efficacy, and tolerability. CNS Drugs 31(2):149–160, 2017 28130762

Díez-Suárez A, Vallejo-Valdivielso M, Marín-Méndez JJ, et al: Weight, height, and body mass index in patients with attention-deficit/hyperactivity disorder treated with methylphenidate. J Child Adolesc Psychopharmacol 27(8):723–730, 2017 28817309

Grinspoon L, Hedblom P: The Speed Culture: Amphetamine Use and Abuse in America. Cambridge, MA, Harvard University Press, 1975

Gurbuz F, Gurbuz BB, Celik GG, et al: Effects of methylphenidate on appetite and growth in children diagnosed with attention deficit and hyperactivity disorder. J Pediatr Endocrinol Metab 29(1):85–92, 2016 26352086

Heal DJ, Smith SL, Gosden J, Nutt DJ: Amphetamine, past and present—a pharmacological and clinical perspective. J Psychopharmacol 27(6):479–496, 2013 23539642

Horrigan JP, Barnhill LJ: Low-dose amphetamine salts and adult attention-deficit/hyperactivity disorder. J Clin Psychiatry 61(6):414–417, 2000 10901338

Huessey H: Clinical explorations in adult minimal brain dysfunction, in Psychiatric Aspects of Minimal Brain Dysfunction in Adults. Edited by Bellak L. New York, Grune and Stratton, 1979

Jensen PS, Hinshaw SP, Swanson JM, et al: Findings from the NIMH Multimodal Treatment Study of ADHD (MTA): implications and applications for primary care providers. J Dev Behav Pediatr 22(1):60–73, 2001 11265923

Klein RG, Abikoff H, Klass E, et al: Clinical efficacy of methylphenidate in conduct disorder with and without attention deficit hyperactivity disorder. Arch Gen Psychiatry 54(12):1073–1080, 1997 9400342

Lieberman JA, Alvir J, Geisler S, et al: Methylphenidate response, psychopathology and tardive dyskinesia as predictors of relapse in schizophrenia. Neuropsychopharmacology 11(2):107–118, 1994 7840862

Lindenmayer JP, Nasrallah H, Pucci M, et al: A systematic review of psychostimulant treatment of negative symptoms of schizophrenia: challenges and therapeutic opportunities. Schizophr Res 147(2–3):241–252, 2013 23619055

Managed Healthcare Executive: Express Scripts' 2016 Drug Trend Report: 7 things to know. Cranbury, NJ, Managed Healthcare Executive, February 13, 2017. Available at: www.managedhealthcareexecutive.com/view/express-scripts-2016-drug-trend-report-7-things-know. Accessed November 14, 2023.

Martin KA, Krahn LE, Balan V, Rosati MJ: Modafinil's use in combating interferon-induced fatigue. Dig Dis Sci 52(4):893–896, 2007 17318387

Michelson D, Allen AJ, Busner J, et al: Once-daily atomoxetine treatment for children and adolescents with attention deficit hyperactivity disorder: a randomized, placebo-controlled study. Am J Psychiatry 159(11):1896–1901, 2002 12411225

Michelson D, Adler L, Spencer T, et al: Atomoxetine in adults with ADHD: two randomized, placebo-controlled studies. Biol Psychiatry 53(2):112–120, 2003 12547466

Quinn PD, Chang Z, Hur K, et al: ADHD medication and substance-related problems. Am J Psychiatry 174(9):877–885, 2017 28659039

Rabkin JG, McElhiney MC, Rabkin R, McGrath PJ: Modafinil treatment for fatigue in HIV/AIDS: a randomized placebo-controlled study. J Clin Psychiatry 71(6):707–715, 2010 20492840

Rabkin JG, McElhiney MC, Rabkin R: Treatment of HIV-related fatigue with ar-modafinil: a placebo-controlled randomized trial. Psychosomatics 52(4):328–336, 2011 21777715

Ratey J, Greenberg MS, Bemporad JR, et al: Unrecognized ADHD in adults. J Child Adolesc Psychiatry 2:267–275, 1994

Richards C, Iosifescu DV, Mago R, et al: A randomized, double-blind, placebo-controlled, dose-ranging study of lisdexamfetamine dimesylate augmentation for major depressive disorder in adults with inadequate response to antidepressant therapy. J Psychopharmacol 31(9):1190–1203, 2017 28857719

Rickels K, Gordon PE, Gansman DH, et al: Pemoline and methylphenidate in midly depressed outpatients. Clin Pharmacol Ther 11(5):698–710, 1970 5455633

Robinson D, Jody D, Lieberman JA: Provocative tests with methylphenidate in schizophrenia and schizophrenia spectrum disorders, in Ritalin: Theory and Patient Management. Edited by Greenhill LL, Osman BB. New York, Mary Ann Liebert, 1991, pp 309–320

Rosack J: ADHD treatment arsenal increasing rapidly. Psychiatr News 36(24):17, 28, 2001

Saavedra-Velez C, Yusim A, Anbarasan D, Lindenmayer JP: Modafinil as an adjunctive treatment of sedation, negative symptoms, and cognition in schizophrenia: a critical review. J Clin Psychiatry 70(1):104–112, 2009 19026265

Sallee FR, Lyne A, Wigal T, McGough JJ: Long-term safety and efficacy of guanfacine extended release in children and adolescents with attention-deficit/hyperactivity disorder. J Child Adolesc Psychopharmacol 19(3):215–226, 2009 19519256

Satel SL, Nelson JC: Stimulants in the treatment of depression: a critical overview. J Clin Psychiatry 50(7):241–249, 1989 2567730

Schubiner H, Tzelepis A, Isaacson JH, et al: The dual diagnosis of attention-deficit/hyperactivity disorder and substance abuse: case reports and literature review. J Clin Psychiatry 56(4):146–150, 1995 7713853

Spencer T, Wilens T, Biederman J, et al: A double-blind, crossover comparison of methylphenidate and placebo in adults with childhood-onset attention-deficit hyperactivity disorder. Arch Gen Psychiatry 52(6):434–443, 1995 7771913

Spencer T, Biederman J, Wilens T, et al: Effectiveness and tolerability of tomoxetine in adults with attention deficit hyperactivity disorder. Am J Psychiatry 155(5):693–695, 1998 9585725

Storebø OJ, Pedersen N, Ramstad E, et al: Methylphenidate for attention deficit hyperactivity disorder (ADHD) in children and adolescents: assessment of adverse events in non-randomised studies. Cochrane Database Syst Rev May 9;5:CD012069, 2018

Trivedi MH, Cutler AJ, Richards C, et al: A randomized controlled trial of the efficacy and safety of lisdexamfetamine dimesylate as augmentation therapy in adults with residual symptoms of major depressive disorder after treatment with escitalopram. J Clin Psychiatry 74(8):802–809, 2013 24021497

Tsang HW, Leung AY, Chung RC, et al: Review on vocational predictors: a systematic review of predictors of vocational outcomes among individuals with schizophrenia: an update since 1998. Aust N Z J Psychiatry 44(6):495–504, 2010 20482409

Volkow ND, Swanson JM: Clinical practice: adult attention deficit-hyperactivity disorder. N Engl J Med 369(20):1935–1944, 2013 24224626

Volkow ND, Fowler JS, Logan J, et al: Effects of modafinil on dopamine and dopamine transporters in the male human brain: clinical implications. JAMA 301(11):1148–1154, 2009 19293415

Wallace AE, Kofoed LL, West AN: Double-blind, placebo-controlled trial of methylphenidate in older, depressed, medically ill patients. Am J Psychiatry 152(6):929–931, 1995 7755127

Wender PH: Methamphetamine in child psychiatry. J Child Adolesc Psychopharmacol 3(1):iv-vi, 1993 19630590

Wender PH, Reimherr FW, Wood D, Ward M: A controlled study of methylphenidate in the treatment of attention deficit disorder, residual type, in adults. Am J Psychiatry 142(5):547–552, 1985 3885760

Wigal SB, Kollins SH, Childress AC, et al: A 13-hour laboratory school day study of delayed-release methylphenidate and clonidine in ADHD: placebo effects and individual differences. J Atten Disord 15(5):371–384, 2011

Wilens TE, Spencer TJ, Biederman J, Girard K: A systematic review of the safety and efficacy of clonidine as adjunctive therapy for ADHD in children. J Am Acad Child Adolesc Psychiatry 51(2):155–168, 2012

Wilens TE, et al: Viloxazine extended-release capsules in adults with attention-deficit/hyperactivity disorder: a randomized, double-blind, placebo-controlled study. J Clin Psychopharmacol 41(1):13–21, 2021

Wuo-Silva R, Fukushiro DF, Borçoi AR, et al: Addictive potential of modafinil and cross-sensitization with cocaine: a pre-clinical study. Addict Biol 16(4):565–579, 2011 21790900

9

Augmentation Strategies for Treatment-Resistant Disorders

It is the general hope of all clinicians that patients will respond to a single therapeutic agent. However, such a response may be the exception rather than the rule. Although for a long time there was much warranted consternation regarding polypharmacy (patients receiving too many different types of medications), many patients do require simultaneous treatment with different classes of drugs to achieve an adequate response. There are a number of reasons for combining medications. Among the most common is to augment the effect of one agent—for example, lithium is combined with an antidepressant to enhance or bring about an antidepressant effect, or two mood stabilizers are combined to reduce breakthrough mania. A second common reason for adding one medication to another is to treat one aspect of the illness—for example, a hypnotic is added to an antidepressant to help with sleep, or a stimulant is added to combat residual fatigue. Medications are also commonly combined to reduce side effects of particular agents—for example, antiparkinsonian drugs are added to standard antipsychotics.

Unfortunately, research on combination treatments has lagged behind research on monotherapy. For many years, neither the pharmaceutical industry nor the National Institute of Mental Health (NIMH) had been particularly motivated to study the effects of medication combinations, except for adverse effects. However, around 2007, pharmaceutical companies began pursuing approval for combination strategies. The NIMH has funded several large effectiveness trials, such as Sequenced Treatment Alternatives for Resistant Depression (STAR*D) in major depression and the Systematic Treatment Enhancement Program for Bipolar Disorder (STEP-BD), that have provided some important information regarding optimal combination strategies. However, the conclusions that can be drawn from these studies are limited by the lack of placebo arms and the tendency of open-label (often nonrandomized) comparison studies to yield similar results across treatment groups. In addition, these studies tend to not employ much clinical judgment; rather, they randomly assign patients to different augmenting strategies regardless of symptom profile or other historical diagnoses. Until more is learned about the biochemistry of various disorders and the range of pharmacological effects of available and future medications, clinicians will constantly be faced with using more than one agent to effect a positive response in individual patients.

Obviously, the number of potential combinations is vast, and consideration of all of them is beyond the scope of our discussion in this chapter. Instead, we focus on combinations of agents used in augmentation (Table 9–1); medications used to counteract side effects have been discussed in previous chapters. We recommend that clinicians become familiar with a number of commonly used combination drugs or combination regimens that have been reported in recent years to be particularly effective in specific clinical situations. In addition, clinicians should become familiar with combinations that can pose difficulties because of drug-drug interactions or additive side effects.

Augmentation Strategies for Depression

Antipsychotic-Antidepressant Combinations

Currently, the second-generation antipsychotics (SGAs) cariprazine, aripiprazole, brexpiprazole, quetiapine, and olanzapine are the class of drugs that are FDA approved in the adjunctive treatment of major depression (Table 9–2). (Esketamine is also approved in the adjunctive treatment of major depression

Table 9–1. Potential augmenting agents for antidepressants

Antidepressant type	Augmenting agent
Tricyclics/tetracyclics	SGAs
	Lithium
	Thyroid supplements
	Stimulants
	Ketamine/esketamine
	Monoamine precursors
	MAOIs
SSRIs/SNRIs	SGAs
	Lithium
	Bupropion
	Thyroid supplements
	Ketamine/esketamine
	Modafinil/armodafinil
	Stimulants
	Atomoxetine
	Methylfolate
	Pramipexole/ropinirole
	Mirtazapine
	Lamotrigine
	D-cycloserine
MAOIs	Lithium
	SGAs
	Thyroid supplements
	TCAs
	Modafinil/armodafinil

Note. SGA = second-generation antipsychotic; SNRI = serotonin-norepinephrine reuptake inhibitor; SSRI = selective serotonin reuptake inhibitor; MAOI = monoamine oxidase inhibitor; TCA = tricyclic antidepressant.

Table 9–2. Second-generation antipsychotics approved in the treatment of major depressive disorder

Generic name	Brand name	Indication	Target dosage (mg/day)
Olanzapine + fluoxetine	Symbyax	Treatment-resistant depression	6/25–12/50[a]
Aripiprazole	Abilify	Adjunctive treatment of MDD	5–15
Brexpiprazole	Rexulti	Adjunctive treatment of MDD	1–3
Quetiapine	Seroquel	Adjunctive treatment of MDD	150–300
Cariprazine	Vraylar	Adjunctive treatment of MDD	1.5–4.5

Note. MDD = major depressive disorder.
[a]First value is for olanzapine; second is for fluoxetine.

but stands alone in its class of dissociative anesthetics.) However, combinations of antidepressants and antipsychotics have long been used in the treatment of both psychotic and nonpsychotic depression. Psychotic depression occurs in up to 25% of inpatients with major depression and tends to be less responsive to antidepressant therapy alone than are nondelusional depressions. The data indicate that with the exception of amoxapine, which is chemically related to the antipsychotic loxapine, an antipsychotic-antidepressant combination or electroconvulsive therapy is probably required for effective treatment of this disorder. However, some studies have suggested that monotherapy with selective serotonin reuptake inhibitors (SSRIs) and newer agents may be effective in the treatment of psychotic depression (Wijkstra et al. 2006; Zanardi et al. 2000). In addition, patients with schizophrenia or schizoaffective disorder frequently develop depressive episodes that may require the addition of an antidepressant to their antipsychotic regimen.

Most studies on psychotic depression have involved combining a tricyclic antidepressant (TCA) with a standard antipsychotic. A prepackaged amitriptyline-perphenazine combination drug is available for use in psychotic and anxious depression. This combination had appeared under two trade names

Table 9–3. Prepackaged combination antidepressants: names, formulations and strengths, and dosages

Generic name	Brand name	Formulation and strengths[a]	Dosage[b]
Chlordiazepoxide + amitriptyline	NA[c]	Tablets: 5/12.5, 10/25	3 tablets 10/25 to 6 tablets 10/25
Perphenazine + amitriptyline	NA[c]	Tablets: 2/10, 2/25, 4/10, 4/25, 4/50	2/25 tid to 4/50 qid
Olanzapine + fluoxetine	Symbyax	Capsules: 3/25, 6/25, 6/50, 12/25, 12/50	6/25 mg to 12/50 mg

[a]Formulation strengths list amount (in milligrams) of first and second ingredients, respectively.
[b]Adult dosages; some patients may require lower dosages.
[c]Available in generic form only.

(Triavil and Etrafon) that were since discontinued. Various combinations of strengths are available, coded according to the dose of each drug contained in the capsule (Table 9–3); the dose of perphenazine is given first. For example, 2/25 contains 2 mg of perphenazine and 25 mg of amitriptyline. This neuroleptic-TCA combination was widely used in the United States and was generally prescribed by primary care practitioners. However, experienced psychopharmacologists advocate prescribing each drug individually to allow for optimal flexibility in dosing.

Another antipsychotic-antidepressant combination pill is the combination of olanzapine and fluoxetine (OFC, or Symbyax). Symbyax was the first drug approved for the treatment of bipolar depression (in 2003) (see Chapter 5, "Mood Stabilizers") and also the first drug treatment approved for treatment-resistant depression (TRD) (in 2009). In a controlled trial in 853 bipolar patients treated with olanzapine alone, placebo, or OFC (6 mg/25 mg to 12 mg/50 mg), both OFC and olanzapine were better than placebo. OFC was faster and more effective than olanzapine alone (Keck 2002).

An SGA, with its serotonin$_{2C}$ (5-HT$_{2C}$) receptor antagonism, would appear to be a useful adjunctive agent with a standard antidepressant. Research in rats suggests that olanzapine in combination with an SSRI may increase release of prefrontal dopamine. Since 2003, the evidence has steadily mounted that the SGAs are effective augmenters, and currently they are the only FDA-approved drugs for the adjunctive treatment of depression. (For a more complete review of this topic, see Chapter 4, "Antipsychotic Drugs"). Aripiprazole was approved as an adjunctive treatment for unipolar depression in 2007, with target dosages of 5–15 mg/day, although we have some depressed patients who do well with just 2 mg/day. Brexpiprazole was approved as an adjunctive treatment for depression in 2015 at dosages of 1–3 mg/day. Brexpiprazole is chemically related to aripiprazole and does not seem to have many advantages over aripiprazole in side effects, drug interactions, or benefits. One disadvantage over aripiprazole is cost, so we are more likely to use generic aripiprazole over brexpiprazole. Quetiapine appears to be a useful augmenter and probably a good monotherapy for depression and for anxiety as well. In the adjunctive treatment of depression, dosages in the range of 150–300 mg/day are useful. Lurasidone has demonstrated efficacy in bipolar depression as both monotherapy and add-on. The most recent SGA to undergo comprehensive trials in the adjunctive treatment of major depressive disorder (MDD) is cariprazine. This dopamine$_{3/2}$ (D_3/D_2) partial agonist was approved in adjunctive treatment of major depression in 2023. As with brexpiprazole and aripiprazole, cariprazine has a better metabolic profile than olanzapine or quetiapine, but akathisia is more likely with cariprazine. Risperidone, ziprasidone, and lurasidone all have studies supporting their use but have somewhat less support than the other SGAs as of this writing.

Despite the clear efficacy of many SGAs in the adjunctive treatment of MDD, questions remain about how to best use these agents, including how long they should be used. Because of concerns about metabolic issues, extrapyramidal symptoms (EPS), and cost, it seems reasonable to try to taper the SGA in a patient who has responded to the combination for at least 3–6 months. Our experience is that many patients successfully treated with the combination of an antidepressant plus an SGA may be able to have the SGA discontinued after a period of stabilization. However, no studies exist to guide on whether the combination substantially diminishes the risk of relapse and whether this risk is outweighed by the risk of adverse effects. Some patients clearly do relapse readily after the SGA is discontinued. Thus, the decision to continue a successful trial of an SGA should be discussed with patients on an individual basis.

Anecdotally, we have used all of the atypical agents as augmenters in nonpsychotic depression with variable success. Anxious, agitated depressed patients or those with insomnia often seem to benefit from the addition of 5–15 mg/day of olanzapine or 100–300 mg/day of quetiapine. More lethargic patients or those in whom there is a greater concern about weight gain might benefit from augmentation with aripiprazole 5–15 mg/day or brexpiprazole 1–3 mg/day, cariprazine 1.5–4.5 mg/day, or lurasidone 20–60 mg/day. The newest antipsychotic, lumateperone, is also undergoing study as an antidepressant augmenter and should be effective. Lumateperone's potential advantages over other SGAs include favorable metabolic and EPS profiles. Akathisia seems to be a less significant problem with lumateperone than with a number of the approved SGAs. Our early experience with lumateperone has been favorable at the standard 42-mg dose. However, it is not approved as an adjunctive agent as of this writing.

Adjunctive Esketamine in Treatment-Resistant Depression

As discussed in Chapter 3 ("Antidepressants"), esketamine is the only other medication besides the SGAs to be approved in the adjunctive treatment of depression. Several clinical trials have investigated the efficacy and safety of esketamine combined with oral antidepressants for the treatment of depression. As reviewed in Chapter 3, the efficacy of esketamine in clinical trials has been mixed. In all the clinical trials, adjunctive esketamine was more effective than placebo at 4 hours, but in some studies the effect was lost at 24 hours. The TRANSFORM-2 trial showed a 4-point advantage for adjunctive esketamine compared with adjunctive placebo on the Montgomery-Åsberg Depression Rating Scale (MADRS) in patients with at least two unsuccessful medication trials. In addition, in the long-term SUSTAIN-2 study, esketamine given as a maintenance treatment every 2 weeks over 1 year demonstrated continued response and a lower rate of relapse for subjects randomly assigned to adjunctive esketamine versus adjunctive placebo.

The challenges of esketamine are many, including spotty insurance coverage; the enrollment of every patient, pharmacy, and clinical site in the Janssen Risk Evaluation and Mitigation Strategies (REMS) program; and the difficulty having the drug delivered to the clinical site. Not all pharmacies have the ability to deliver the medication on a weekly basis, and neither patients nor clinicians can pick up the drug themselves. We had some difficulty at Stanford initially finding a reliable pharmacy to deliver the drug. In addition, esketamine, as a Schedule III drug, requires careful documentation about administration, storage, and disposal. Patients cannot drive to or from visits and need to be monitored, including several blood pressure and heart rate vitals, over the course of at least 2 hours in the clinic. In our esketamine clinic, we have found that most patients do well with the 56-mg dose administered twice weekly for 4 weeks, then the standard once per week and then every 2 weeks subsequently. If the 56-mg dose has been tolerated but there is a lack of response by the fourth treatment, we tend to increase the dose to 84 mg. Although some patients are able to extend maintenance treatments to once a month, most patients require every 2 weeks indefinitely. Although late responders have been reported in the literature, we have found that if a patient has not responded by six inductions, they are probably not likely to respond. In our experience, some patients do appear to develop a tachyphylaxis as has been reported in the anesthesia literature, and the drug stops working for these patients. This occurs with a minority of patients, perhaps 20% over the course of a year.

The patients who tend to be the best candidates for ketamine or esketamine treatment are those without a significant substance abuse history or history of psychosis and those who can reliably participate in treatment. Patients with uncontrolled hypertension or advanced heart disease may be at greater risk because of the sympathomimetic effects of ketamine. As with other treatments, patients with fewer treatment failures seem to do better, and there is literature to suggest that patients with a trauma history also do better with ketamine or esketamine. We have also found that some patients with chronic suicidality may have a lysis of the suicidality without much benefit for their depression. Still, this is a good outcome.

Lithium-Antidepressant Combinations

Until the approval of SGAs and esketamine as adjunctive agents in MDD, lithium had been the best-studied augmenter to antidepressants in patients with TRD. Although there are many lithium studies in TRD, the total number of subjects in all of these trials probably does not equal the number of subjects in the registration trials of one SGA in the treatment of TRD. In addition, saying lithium is among the best-studied augmenters is different from saying lithium is the best augmenter or the strategy that should be used before others are attempted. Lithium can be cumbersome to use, requiring careful titration and serum level monitoring, and it can be lethal in overdose. An ever-growing number of augmentation strategies have been proposed, but lithium remains an important option for TRD.

Lithium has been well studied in its own right as an antidepressant. Overall, the drug is effective in some 50% of patients, with suggestions that it is best used in treating males with bipolar depression (see Chapters 3 and 5). Dé Montigny et al. (1981) reported that the addition of lithium to a TCA trial resulted in clinical improvement within 72 hours in patients who did not have a response to a TCA alone. Before 1986, studies of lithium augmentation, which were typically open-label studies, suggested that the response rate to lithium augmentation of TCAs was as high as 75%. More recent placebo-controlled studies have not typically confirmed this rapid clinical improvement or the more robust response rate. They have, however, demonstrated that the addition of lithium is more effective than addition of placebo. Although approximately one in four patients responds to lithium augmentation within 1 week, the most robust responses have typically required 3 weeks or more. Response often occurs at low dosages (600–1,200 mg/day) and at relatively low serum levels. Current data suggest that serum levels in the range of 0.5 to 0.8 mEq/L are effective in lithium augmentation of antidepressant effects (Bauer and Dopfmer 1999). The mechanism of action has been hypothesized as a potentiation of serotonergic activity via either increased biosynthesis or receptor adaptation. Our experience with the combination has generally been favorable, and we have been particularly impressed with results obtained in depressed patients with pronounced obsessionality and agitation. However, there are no controlled trial data to support thos clinical impression. Price et al. (1983) reported that lithium also elicited a response in patients with delusional depression who had not responded to the combination of amitriptyline and perphenazine.

Lithium also appears to augment responses to other antidepressants. For example, patients with bipolar depression with hypersomnia and hyperphagia (formerly termed *atypical*) may respond dramatically to the combination of lithium and the monoamine oxidase inhibitor (MAOI) tranylcypromine. In an open-label study, Price et al. (1985) found that 11 of 12 patients with TRD responded to the combination of lithium and tranylcypromine. Many of these patients had not had a response to lithium-TCA combinations. In a New Haven follow-up study, patients with unipolar depression who were treated with desipramine plus lithium remained euthymic in the community for much longer periods when not taking medication than did patients who improved while taking desipramine plus placebo (Nierenberg et al. 1990). A number of studies have confirmed the efficacy of lithium augmentation of SSRIs. In an early report, Pope et al. (1988) found that lithium appeared to augment the antidepressant effects of fluoxetine. More recent double-blind studies have confirmed this finding (Fava et al. 1994; Katona et al. 1995). Some evidence suggests that lithium may do a better job augmenting SSRIs than augmenting TCAs. In a double-blind study, lithium boosted the antidepressant actions of paroxetine more effectively than those of amitriptyline, and these effects were seen as early as 2 weeks and continued for the 6 weeks of the study (Bauer et al. 1999). In the STAR*D trial, lithium augmentation was compared with addition of L-triiodothyronine (T_3) in patients who did not respond to two previous medication trials (Nierenberg et al. 2006a). At this level (3) of the STAR*D protocol, patients received augmentation with a variety of antidepressants that could include citalopram, venlafaxine, bupropion, or sertraline. Both augmenting strategies had modest, statistically equal efficacy, but lithium was much more poorly tolerated than was T_3. About 16% of the group receiving lithium augmentation achieved a remission, versus about 25% of the group receiving T_3 augmentation. As with lithium augmentation of TCA response, the maximum potentiation of SSRI response appears to require adequate lithium serum levels and may require trials of 4 weeks or longer. (For further discussion of maintenance treatment, see Chapter 3.) Overall, we would expect about 50% of patients who did not have a response to a TCA or an SSRI to have a response after the addition of lithium.

Certain characteristics in depressed patients probably predict response to the addition of lithium to their antidepressant regimen. Depressed patients may be more likely to improve with lithium augmentation if they exhibit significant psychomotor retardation, have significant anorexia and weight loss, and have low serum cortisol levels (Alvarez et al. 1997).

If lithium is to be added, it should be initiated at 300 mg bid for 2 days, and the dosage should be increased to 900 mg/day for 3–4 days, with a further increase to 1,200 mg/day for 10–14 days. A serum level of at least 0.5 mEq/L should be achieved. If there is no response, then the dose should be gradually increased as tolerated to a serum level of 1.2 mEq/L. Given that there is probably a bimodal distribution to response, with some patients responding within the first 2 weeks and others requiring a month or more to achieve response

(Thase et al. 1998), we tend to not regard a lithium augmentation trial as failed until serum levels greater than 0.5 mEq/L are obtained for at least 6 weeks, and we would prefer a level of 0.6 mEq/L or more.

Bupropion and Mirtazapine Combinations

Among the most common augmenting agents currently used in clinical practice is bupropion. A number of studies have suggested that bupropion, as a noradrenergic-dopaminergic agent, can enhance the antidepressant effects of SSRIs and venlafaxine (Bodkin et al. 1997; Fatemi et al. 1999; Kirsch and Louie 1999). We have studied the addition of sustained-release bupropion (Wellbutrin SR) to SSRIs and believe it is a convenient and well-tolerated method of improving antidepressant response (DeBattista et al. 2003). Because all formulations of bupropion are now generic, we tend to use the extended-release formulation because of the added convenience of once-a-day dosing. We start bupropion at 150 mg and then go to 300 mg by the end of the second week of treatment. Still, no placebo-controlled studies are yet available to confirm the efficacy of this approach, and the termination of the patent life makes it less likely that such a study will ever be completed. One of the largest trials of bupropion augmentation, the open-label but randomized STAR*D trial, found that augmenting citalopram with bupropion was about as effective as augmenting with buspirone in producing a remission-level response (Trivedi et al. 2006); see also Chapter 3 in this volume. However, bupropion had an advantage over buspirone when focusing on absolute change on one of the standard depression scales used in the study (Quick Inventory of Depressive Symptomatology [QID-SR-16]). Improvement in the scale score was 25% with bupropion and only 17% with buspirone. The target dosage was 300–400 mg/day for bupropion and 45–60 mg/day for buspirone. In addition to STAR*D, the other large trial to evaluate bupropion augmentation was the Veterans Affairs Augmentation and Switching Treatments for Improving Depression Outcomes (VAST-D) trial (Mohamed et al. 2017). In that study, 1,522 Veterans Affairs patients who had not responded to at least one antidepressant were randomly assigned to one of three conditions: switching to bupropion, adding bupropion, or adding aripiprazole. In general, adding the aripiprazole was modestly better at achieving remission and response than switching to or adding bupropion. Patients in the bupropion group experienced more treatment-emergent anxiety, whereas those in the aripiprazole group had more weight gain, somnolence, and akathisia. All three regimens were equally effective at preventing relapse over a 36-week follow-up period. The use of mirtazapine to augment SSRIs in treating depression has proved very useful for some patients. Earlier evidence suggested that the combination of venlafaxine or an SSRI plus mirtazapine was efficacious and well tolerated in some patients with TRD (Carpenter et al. 1999, 2002). In the STAR*D trial, the addition of mirtazapine to venlafaxine in patients who had had three consecutive failed trials for depression was at least as effective as switching to an MAOI and was far better tolerated (McGrath et al. 2006). Unfortunately, both treatments were only modestly beneficial in patients with TRD. Only 6.9% achieved remission when a switch was made to tranylcypromine, versus 13.7% when mirtazapine was added to venlafaxine. We have found that mirtazapine 15–45 mg qhs is probably more effective than is the addition of trazodone in helping with sleep, anxiety, and depression.

Those bupropion and mirtazapine studies have been followed by two recent major trials that have explored whether combining agents can accelerate response or remission. In one—the Combining Medications to Enhance Depression Outcomes (CO-MED) study—combining bupropion with escitalopram from the start of treatment was compared with escitalopram alone and venlafaxine in combination with mirtazapine in patients with recurrent or chronic depression (Rush et al. 2011). No significant differences were found in response or remission among the three groups. In another study, mirtazapine was combined with fluoxetine, venlafaxine, or bupropion from the outset and was compared with fluoxetine alone. All three combinations were significantly more effective than fluoxetine alone (Blier et al. 2010).

Thyroid Supplement–Antidepressant Combinations

A number of years ago a debate emerged in the literature regarding whether thyroid preparations (e.g., thyroxine [T_4] and T_3) prescribed with a TCA hastened the onset of the antidepressant effect. Early studies in women suggested that they did, although subsequent studies in men, which also employed higher dosages of TCAs, failed to substantiate the earlier finding. A fallow period followed for this combination until Goodwin et al. (1982) reported that the addition of 25–50 μg/day of T_3 (Cytomel) elicited within 7 days a clinical response in patients who had previously not had a response to a seemingly adequate TCA trial. A number of subsequent clinical reports have confirmed this observation, although some clinicians have reported responses requiring 14 days or more of combined therapy. In a trial by Joffe et al. (1993), T_3 augmentation of TCAs appeared to be as effective as lithium, and both were significantly more effective than placebo. A subsequent head-to-head crossover trial also suggested that patients receiving T_3 augmentation were more likely to respond than were lithium-treated patients (Spoov and Lahdelma 1998). Statistical equivalence of T_3 augmentation to lithium augmentation was found in the STAR*D study reviewed in the previous section (Nierenberg et al. 2006a). If thyroid and lithium augmentation are both helpful in resistant depression, perhaps combining both lithium and thyroid with an antidepressant would have additive effects. Unfortunately, a study by Joffe and colleagues (2006) did not find that combining lithium with thyroid hormone had any advantages over either one alone. Thyroid augmentation of MAOIs has not been well studied.

Several case reports have suggested that thyroid augmentation of the SSRIs may also be effective. For example, Joffe (1992) found that Cytomel at 25–50 μg/mL/day when added to fluoxetine enhanced the antidepressant effects of the drug and was well tolerated. A number of other case reports suggested that thyroid supplements may potentiate SSRI antidepressant effects (Crowe et al. 1990; Gupta et al. 1991). Whether the T_3 is added at the initiation of SSRI therapy or after a patient experiences an unsuccessful trial of an SSRI may be important in the efficacy of this intervention. For example, a meta-analysis of randomized controlled trials in which the T_3 was combined with SSRIs at the beginning of treatment did not find a benefit of thyroid augmentation (Papakostas et al. 2009). However, a review of studies that examined the utility of T_3 added to an SSRI after an unsuccessful trial of SSRI monotherapy indicated that this strategy might be beneficial (Cooper-Kazaz et al. 2009).

The data suggest that thyroid supplementation may be effective in combination with a wide spectrum of antidepressants. However, good studies are still lacking, and the available studies have shown mixed results.

The mechanism of action of T_3 potentiation of antidepressants is undetermined. Generally, theories have revolved around the role of T_3 in facilitating adrenergic receptor adaptation. However, Targum et al. (1984) reported that patients who had a response to T_3 demonstrated relatively enhanced thyroid-stimulating hormone (TSH) responses to thyrotropin-releasing hormone (TRH) infusions, suggesting that a subtle form of thyroid dysfunction might play a role in these patients' condition. Targum et al. suggested that patients with refractory depression who have a normal TSH but a blunted response to the TRH stimulation test may be good candidates for thyroid augmentation. Clinicians frequently ask whether T_4 is as effective as T_3 in augmenting response to TCAs. T_4 is metabolized to T_3 in humans. One double-blind study comparing 2-week treatments of T_4 (Synthroid) and T_3 indicated that T_3 was significantly more effective. However, because T_4 has a much longer half-life, the patients may not have achieved steady state with T_4, leaving the conclusions of the study open to question (Joffe and Singer 1987). Possible explanations of the greater effectiveness of T_3 in some patients include difficulty in converting T_4 to T_3 or in transporting thyroid into the brain. Data suggest that depressed patients may demonstrate decreased cerebrospinal fluid levels of thyroid transport protein, which would limit the effect of T_4 on the brain. Clinically, we have seen a number of patients who did not respond to an antidepressant in combination with T_4 who did have a response when T_3 was substituted. In addition, an occasional patient benefits from high-dose T_4 added to their antidepressant regimen. A number of years ago, Arthur Prange's group (Bunevicius et al. 1999) reported that in patients with thyroid disease who were treated with T_4, the addition of T_3 significantly improved both mood and cognition in comparison with placebo, suggesting that individuals could have relative T_3 deficiencies in brain. An open-label trial using T_4 at an average of 482 µg/day for 8 weeks found that more than 50% of the patients with treatment-resistant depression had a robust response (Bauer et al. 1998). Although side effects were not common in this trial, the use of supraphysiological doses of T_4 for an extended time might be problematic for some patients.

Is it possible to predict which patients are the best candidates for thyroid augmentation? Clearly, those who have any evidence of thyroid abnormalities, including subclinical hypothyroidism, appear to be good candidates. There is evidence that patients with mild thyroid abnormalities (slightly elevated TSH, normal T_3 and T_4) are less likely to respond to antidepressants alone but do respond to the addition of a thyroid supplement (Sokolov et al. 1997). Women older than age 50 also appear to have high responses to thyroid augmentation, perhaps because they are most susceptible to hypothyroidism. Overall, it is our impression that Cytomel is useful in patients with pronounced psychomotor retardation. Cytomel may be experienced as energizing and may actually help with weight loss in patients with atypical features. We have on occasion found that Cytomel can also bring about a response in patients who have experienced a relapse while taking a TCA to which they had previously responded. More recently, Lerer's group has reported that responders to T_3 could be identified by their having lower T_3 levels and by being carriers for a specific allele on a single-nucleotide polymorphism for the deiodinase converting enzyme for T_4 to T_3 (Cooper-Kazaz et al. 2009). This finding is in need of replication but could explain why some patients appear to derive great benefit from thyroid augmentation. Cytomel taken from the onset in combination with antidepressants has, in a larger-scale trial, proven not more effective than adding placebo (Garlow et al. 2012).

Cytomel is typically started at 12.5–25 μg/day, with dosage increases in 1-week increments to 50 μg/day. Levothroid or Synthroid is typically initiated at 50 μg/day and increased every week or two, up to 200 μg/day. Whereas an adequate trial of T_3 may be 1–4 weeks, preparations of T_4 will probably require duration of 4–8 weeks because of its longer half-life. Thyroid preparations tend to be well tolerated, but they should be used with caution in patients who have a history of coronary artery disease, hypertension, or arrhythmia. Overdoses occasionally result in cardiac decompensation. If thyroid supplementation results in significant suppression of TSH, it is thought that bone demineralization may occur during extended treatment. However, Whybrow's group did not observe demineralization in bipolar patients with rapid cycling treated with high doses of T_4 (Whybrow 1994). If a patient responds positively, we recommend continuing the T_3 for an additional 60 days and then tapering by 12.5 μg every 3 days. Some patients will demonstrate a resumption of symptoms and will require resumption of the T_3. One of our patients required resumption of dose and maintenance for more than 1 year before T_3 could finally be tapered off. Results of thyroid function tests while the patient was taking T_3 were essentially normal. After the T_3 was tapered, the patient's T_3 uptake, TSH, and T_4 levels were all lower than normal but normalized within 2–3 weeks. This patient demonstrated none of the stigmata of decreased thyroid status immediately after discontinuation.

Estrogen, DHEA, and Testosterone Combinations With Antidepressants

For many years, estrogens have sometimes been used alone or in combination with antidepressants to treat depression in women who are postmenopausal or postpartum whose conditions are refractory to standard treatments. The results of using estrogens for depression have been uneven. Some studies found estrogens to be useful in the treatment of depression in some women, and others did not. The findings of an increased risk of breast cancer, heart attacks, and strokes in the Women's Health Initiative study in 2002 resulted in many women abandoning hormone replacement therapy. However, estrogen does have some effects on mood, and some women clearly have benefited from these effects. Coope (1981) found that estrogen had no significant antidepressant effect when used alone for perimenopausal depression. On the other hand, studies using higher dosages of conjugated estrogens (5–25 mg/day) found some partial antidepressant benefit in postmenopausal women. One published study in this area (Soares et al. 2001) found that a transdermal patch of 17-β-estradiol was significantly more effective than placebo in reducing depressive symptoms in perimenopausal women. This was a reasonably sized study (50 subjects) with a sufficient duration of treatment. On the other hand, a study by Rasgon and colleagues (2007) failed to show much benefit of adding transdermal estrogen to sertraline in depressed postmenopausal women.

The utility of estrogens in postpartum depression is also uneven. Some studies have failed to show benefit. However, one study found estrogen to be an effective prophylaxis against recurrent affective illness in the postpartum period (Sichel et al. 1995). In a Cochrane review, the administration of progesterone in the postpartum period was associated with an enhanced risk of developing depression, whereas the administration of estrogen was concluded to have modest benefit for postpartum depression (Dennis et al. 2008). Our experience with using estrogens alone in women with refractory depression has not been particularly encouraging.

The combination of estrogens with antidepressants has yielded more consistent results. Several studies before 1985 failed to show any additional benefit of combining estrogens with TCAs in depressed women. However, there have been case reports of oral contraceptives augmenting the effects of antidepressants in patients with refractory depression (Sherwin 1991). In addition, postmenopausal women may respond better to fluoxetine if they are receiving hormone replacement therapy than if they are not (Schneider et al. 1997, 2001).

Some cautions are worth considering when administering estrogens to women with mood disorders. Estrogens appear to be capable of inducing rapid cycling in some women with bipolar disorder, and progesterone may suppress rapid cycling. In addition, estrogen use carries the risk of thrombophlebitis and an increased risk of breast, cervical, and uterine cancer. Unfortunately, progesterone may induce depression in some women. Estrogens also appear to increase the bioavailability and serum levels of TCAs. Thus, lower doses of TCAs are sometimes indicated when an estrogen is added to the regimen.

At this time, the routine combination of estrogen with antidepressants is unwarranted. However, some women with refractory depression in the postpartum or perimenopausal period might benefit from such a combination. Typical dosages of estrogens in successful studies ranged from 5 to 25 mg/day of conjugated estrogens. The risks of long-term use of high-dose, unopposed estrogen, however, are probably too great to justify use of that approach for mild depression.

Dehydroepiandrosterone (DHEA), a steroid precursor of both androgens and estrogens, has become a very popular over-the-counter remedy for dysphoria (Dehydroepiandrosterone [DHEA] 1996). Some controlled reports suggested that dosages of 50–100 mg/day result in increases in physical and psychological well-being in women ages 40–70. An early study found that DHEA is more effective than placebo in augmenting a standard antidepressant at dosages up to 90 mg/day (Wolkowitz et al. 1997). Likewise, there is some evidence that DHEA is significantly more effective than placebo as a monotherapy for the treatment of dysthymia (Bloch et al. 1999). A number of studies have also found DHEA to be effective in the treatment of depressive symptoms in midlife (Schmidt et al. 2005) and in patients with HIV-related illness (Rabkin et al. 2006).

The problem with DHEA, however, is that it is not a simple food supplement; it is a prohormone of adrenal origin. Androgenic effects, including irreversible hair loss, hirsutism, and deepening of voice, have occasionally been reported. In addition, there is some concern that DHEA could accelerate tumor growth, because many malignancies, including those of the breast, endometrium, and prostate, are hormone sensitive. It will be important to collect safety data concerning long-term use of DHEA. Thus, we encourage prudence in using DHEA until further study is completed.

Testosterone gel was reported to be effective in a small double-blind, placebo-controlled trial in men with refractory depression (Pope et al. 2003). This 8-week study was undertaken in men with low or borderline low testosterone levels. In a previous trial, intramuscular testosterone had failed to separate from placebo (Seidman et al. 2001). Likewise, a later study by Seidman and colleagues (2005) in patients with SSRI-resistant depression did not show benefit to intramuscular testosterone supplementation versus the injection of a placebo. Overall, it appears that testosterone's antidepressant benefits are most consistently seen in men with hypogonadism and perhaps in elderly men and those with HIV-related depressive symptoms (Zarrouf et al. 2009). Among the more significant risks of testosterone supplementation is an increased risk of prostate cancer, although increased levels of other androgens and estrogens may play more of a role than testosterone in enhancing the risk of prostate cancer (Raynaud 2006). Regardless of the prostate risks, there may also be cardiovascular risks and altered insulin resistance with testosterone supplements. Given the unknown risks, testosterone therapy in depressed men with normal testosterone levels does not appear warranted.

As discussed in Chapter 3, a derivative of progesterone, allopregnanolone, does appear to be effective in the treatment of postpartum depression and may be useful as a monotherapy or in combination with standard antidepressants in the treatment of MDD. Allopregnanolone acts as a $GABA_A$ modulator, and there are a number of analogs that could prove useful for both men and women with MDD.

Dopamine Agonist–Antidepressant Combinations

In the early 1970s, Wharton and colleagues (1971) reported that the addition of methylphenidate increased plasma levels of TCAs through inhibition of microsomal degradation of the TCA in the liver (similar to the competitive inhibition observed with antipsychotic agents). This approach offers a possible way of increasing TCA plasma levels without increasing TCA dose. In addition to this effect, methylphenidate is a stimulant and may be useful in treating the anergia and psychomotor retardation of endogenous depression. However, as described in Chapter 8 ("Stimulants and the Treatment of ADHD"), we do not recommend adding methylphenidate to increase plasma levels because higher TCA plasma levels can be obtained by increasing the TCA doses. Rather, clinicians might want to use methylphenidate for its energizing properties, but they should keep in mind that it may increase TCA plasma levels and side effects. Fawcett et al. (1991) found that pemoline or dextroamphetamine was effective in inducing improvement when added to an MAOI in patients with severe, treatment-refractory depression. Although this combination was safe and no hypertensive crises were reported, approximately one in five patients treated developed either hypomania or mania.

The traditional stimulants do appear to still have a role in patients with TRD, those with concurrent attention-deficit disorders, and medically ill patients (see Chapter 8). Stimulants can improve energy and concentration in medically ill patients and appear to be useful adjuvants to most classes of antidepressants. Although less well studied in combination with newer antidepressants, amphetamine-type drugs have been reported in case series to augment venlafaxine and the SSRIs. In a recent trial, however, lisdexamfetamine (Vyvanse), an amphetamine preparation, failed to separate from placebo as an add-on in patients with refractory depression.

A number of other dopamine agonists have potential as augmenting agents in TRD. For example, the D_2/D_3 agonist pramipexole (Mirapex), which has an FDA-approved indication for the treatment of Parkinson's disease, has also been evaluated as a treatment for major depression. In one study, pramipexole separated from placebo to a comparable degree as fluoxetine (Corrigan et al. 2000). We have found it useful as an adjunctive agent to SSRIs in some patients with TRD at dosages up to 1 mg/day (DeBattista 1997). In addition, pramipexole appears to help with restless legs, including restless legs exacerbated by the use of SSRIs (DeBattista et al. 2000). More recently, pramipexole was found to improve depression in two small double-blind, placebo-controlled studies of bipolar depressed patients (Goldberg et al. 2004; Zarate et al. 2004). In an open-label study, we found that adjunctive ropinirole at dosages of 3–12 mg/day helped about half the 72 patients who had not had an adequate response to a standard antidepressant (DeBattista et al. 2008). These results were similar to those reported by Cassano and colleagues (2005), who used ropinirole at an average dosage of just 1 mg/day to augment standard antidepressants. Side effects of ropinirole commonly include nausea, dizziness, and headache. Rarer side effects have included compulsive behaviors such as gambling and visual hallucinations. In general, ropinirole appears to be better tolerated at lower dosages than at higher dosages, and just 1 mg/day may prove a reasonable augmentation dose if its effectiveness is confirmed by subsequent studies.

Monoamine Precursor–Antidepressant Combinations

The addition of amino acids to antidepressants is based on the rationale that supplementing the diet with precursors of monoamines may help correct a deficiency of the monoaminergic system. Phenylalanine is a precursor of dopamine and norepinephrine; tryptophan is ultimately converted into 5-HT. These amino acids have been combined with MAOIs, TCAs, and SSRIs in the treatment of refractory depression, with varying degrees of success. The "Newcastle cocktail," which has been used for treatment-refractory depression, employed a combination of clomipramine or phenelzine, lithium, and tryptophan (Montgomery 1991). This was said to be an effective combination, but one that carried some risk of serotonin syndrome. Dosages of tryptophan used for augmentation have ranged from 2 to 6 g/day. Phenylalanine has been used in dosages of 500 mg/day to 5 g/day as a supplement. We have not been particularly impressed with phenylalanine augmentation. A related strategy is the use of inositol, a precursor of an important intracellular second-messenger system: the phosphatidylinositol (Ptdlns) system. The Ptdlns system may be important in mediating the effects of lithium and various antidepressants. Levine et al. (1995) reported a small double-blind study suggesting that inositol 6 g bid was useful and was more effective than placebo in treating patients with major depression. However, in a follow-up study, no difference could be found between placebo and inositol in the augmentation of SSRIs (Levine et al. 1999). In bipolar depression, the addition of inositol 10–15 g was found to be as effective (or ineffective) as adding lamotrigine or risperidone to lithium, valproate, or carbamazepine (Nierenberg et al. 2006b). However, a small placebo-controlled trial did not demonstrate clear efficacy over placebo in the adjunctive treatment of bipolar depression (Eden Evins et al. 2006). In fact, a few subjects, especially those with high baseline irritability, appeared to get substantially worse while taking the inositol. The small size of the study ($N=17$) precluded definitive conclusions.

Other Antidepressant Augmentation Strategies

We reported on a placebo-controlled study in which atomoxetine was added to sertraline in patients who had not responded to monotherapy. Atomoxetine was not found to be superior to placebo (Michelson et al. 2006).

Modafinil is a wake-promoting agent used in the treatment of narcolepsy (Ferraro et al. 1997). It lacks the addictive potential and the hemodynamic side effects of stimulants. We have found that 100–200 mg of modafinil taken in the morning with an SSRI is well tolerated and helps with fatigue and hypersomnia in depressed patients (DeBattista et al. 2003, 2004; Fava et al.

2007). The drug appears to work quickly, within the first 2 weeks, if it is going to help. Modafinil is generally well tolerated in combination with SSRIs. Side effects of modafinil such as headache, nausea, and anxiety are usually mild and easy to manage.

In animal models, the combination of fluoxetine with desipramine produced marked and rapid downregulation of postsynaptic β-adrenergic receptors (Baron et al. 1988), suggesting that the combination should be effective. Several reports have suggested this is the case (Nelson and Price 1995; Weilburg et al. 1989). In a randomized controlled trial, Nelson and colleagues (2004) reported that depressed inpatients treated with the combination of desipramine and fluoxetine were far more likely to achieve remission than those patients treated with either agent alone. However, the TCA dosing must be done conservatively because the SSRIs slow the hepatic degradation of TCAs via competitive inhibition of cytochrome P450 (CYP) 2D6 and other CYP enzymes (see Chapter 3), resulting in potential elevation of TCA levels and increased side effects (Aranow et al. 1989; Bell and Cole 1988). If a TCA is added in patients already being treated with an SSRI, initiation of the TCA should be at low dosages: 25 mg/day of nortriptyline or 50 mg/day of imipramine, with an increase of 25 mg every 3 days as tolerated to a target dosage of 75 mg/day of nortriptyline or 150–300 mg/day of imipramine. Plasma levels of the TCA should be monitored closely, and electrocardiograms should be taken and also monitored closely. When an SSRI is added to the TCA, we recommend first gradually reducing the dosage of the TCA to 100 mg/day of nortriptyline or 150 mg/day of imipramine and monitoring plasma levels. TCA levels should be obtained before and after dosage reduction as well as after starting an SSRI.

Trazodone is often safe and useful as a hypnotic in patients who have insomnia as a result of taking fluoxetine. In the course of such use, we found patients whose depression cleared nicely after trazodone was added to the fluoxetine. One study (Nierenberg et al. 1994) found that trazodone 100 mg at night counteracted fluoxetine- or bupropion-induced insomnia in 10 of 15 patients treated. Doses of trazodone ranging from 25 to 300 mg are used for drug-induced insomnia. The literature on trazodone augmentation of fluoxetine is sparse; in one study (Nierenberg et al. 1992), trazodone seemed to potentiate the effects of fluoxetine in 3 of 8 patients treated. The combination of trazodone and the SSRIs appears to be generally well tolerated and useful but needs further study. The SSRIs have been combined with agents that act on the 5-HT$_{1A}$ receptor to augment response and reduce side effects. In addition, Nierenberg and Keck (1989) have reported on the use of trazodone to overcome insomnia associated with MAOI therapy.

Buspirone, which is a 5-HT$_{1A}$ partial agonist, has been shown to potentiate the antidepressant effects of fluoxetine in open-label studies, including the study by Joffe and Schuller (1993). Dosages of buspirone as low as 5 mg/day and as high as 50 mg/day in these studies were enough to effect a full response in the majority of patients who had not had a response or had only a partial response. On the other hand, double-blind studies have failed to show any advantage to adding buspirone to fluoxetine in the treatment of obsessive-compulsive disorder. Double-blind trials for buspirone augmentation of SSRIs for TRD have yielded mixed results; one study showed a benefit of buspirone over placebo (Bouwer and Stein 1997), and another study showed negative results (Landén et al. 1998). As reported earlier in this section, buspirone was similar in efficacy to bupropion in augmenting SSRI response in the STAR*D trial (Trivedi et al. 2006). Because buspirone is such a relatively benign agent compared with other potential augmenting agents, it is worth considering in treatment-resistant cases. A 4- to 6-week trial of dosages of buspirone from 30 to 60 mg/day is probably adequate to determine whether combination with an SSRI will be useful. In addition, buspirone may help attenuate SSRI-induced sexual dysfunction, as reported in Chapter 3. However, we have not been impressed with buspirone as an augmenting agent or in the treatment of SSRI-induced sexual dysfunction.

Another augmentation strategy is the use of pindolol, a β-blocker that also has 5-HT$_{1A}$ antagonist properties. Pindolol may enhance serotonergic tone by acting on somatodendritic autoreceptors. In two open-label studies (Artigas et al. 1994; Blier and Bergeron 1995), it was found to potentiate antidepressant response. In both studies, pindolol 2.5 mg tid seemed to speed the onset of action and lead to a response in the vast majority of patients who had not had a response. A few patients did drop out of both studies because they became more irritable. Subsequent studies of pindolol augmentation of SSRIs suggested that in addition to possibly speeding response, pindolol also resulted in more sustained response in acute treatment than monotherapy with an SSRI. In one study, 70% of patients treated with pindolol were able to sustain a response to the end of the acute trial, whereas only 40% of patients treated with fluoxetine alone had similar sustained benefits (Portella et al.

2009). Similar benefits of sustaining initial response with pindolol augmentation have also been demonstrated in studies that have included bipolar depressed patients (Geretsegger et al. 2008). However, it is not clear whether a more rapid and sustained acute response with pindolol augmentation would have any benefits in preventing later recurrence and relapse. Such studies have not been done.

Years ago we attempted to use pindolol to augment SSRI response, with at best mixed results. In a total of six controlled trials of pindolol augmentation that had been completed to date, three had positive results and three had negative results (McAskill et al. 1998). We have stopped using pindolol because we have not observed much effect in patients with refractory conditions.

D-cycloserine, a glutamatergic agent, has been used as an adjunctive agent in schizophrenia (see subsection "Other Augmentation Strategies" later in this chapter) and in anxiety disorders in combination with behavior therapy. A trial involving 26 patients indicated that D-cycloserine at a high dosage of 1,000 mg/day—much higher than was typically studied in anxiety—was significantly better than placebo as an augmenter of antidepressant response (Heresco-Levy et al. 2013). The agent can cause agitation and generally needs to be given at higher doses in combination with other drugs (e.g., SSRIs). More recently, in a large-scale clinical trial of lamotrigine augmentation up to 400 mg/day in major depression, lamotrigine failed to separate from placebo (Barbee et al. 2011).

L-methylfolate is a cofactor in the synthesis of monoamines. Depression has been associated with low serum and CNS folate levels. It thus follows that supplementation with methylfolate or folic acid may have a role to play in the treatment of depression. Research on methylfolate in the treatment of depression prior to our last edition was limited and mostly open label, with only a few controlled studies. For example, Godfrey and colleagues (1990) found that the addition of 15 mg of methylfolate to a TCA in depressed patients with low red blood cell folate levels showed greater improvement over a 6-month period than did treatment with a TCA alone. Likewise, Alpert and colleagues (2002) found that the open-label addition of folinic acid in 22 patients who had experienced no response after at least 4 weeks of SSRI therapy resulted in a modest but significant benefit. More recently, Papakostas et al. (2012) reported two controlled trials. In the larger trial, there was no difference from placebo. In the smaller trial, the agent did separate. Subsequently, this group reported that there may be biomarkers for predicting who will respond; these include genetic markers for folate metabolism (Papakostas et al. 2014). This approach is intriguing. L-methylfolate has been generally well tolerated, with side effects that do not differ in clinical trials from those seen with placebo. Methylfolate may lower the serum levels of concomitant anticonvulsants, including valproate and carbamazepine, and thus dosage adjustments may be required.

Several reports indicate that adding clonazepam to an SSRI provides more rapid responses in patients with panic disorder or major depression. In a study by Smith et al. (1998), clonazepam at a dosage of 0.5–1.0 mg hs for the first 3 weeks of fluoxetine therapy appeared to have calming effects and to accelerate overall antidepressant response. In another study (Goddard et al. 2001), clonazepam at doses of up to 1.5 mg hs accelerated response to sertraline in patients with panic disorder. More recently, a retrospective analysis of a controlled trial indicated that patients with clonazepam added to fluoxetine were significantly more likely to achieve remission than were patients taking fluoxetine alone (Papakostas et al. 2010).

Novel Augmenters Under Review

As described in Chapter 3, a number of novel antidepressants are currently under review as adjunctive treatments for treatment-resistant major depression. These include zuranolone, esmethadone, and newer SGAs. Zuranolone, discussed in Chapter 3, is an allosteric modulator of $GABA_A$ and has shown modest but significant benefit as an adjunct to standard antidepressants. Its primary advantage over available augmenters is a side-effect profile that does not include EPS or metabolic or sexual effects. In addition, because of its rapid response, it may need to be given for only 2 weeks and repeated infrequently. Zuranolone is under FDA review currently for indications including postpartum depression and MDD. Likewise, esmethadone, which is purported to act as an N-methyl-D-aspartate (NMDA) antagonist, is also being evaluated as a way to rapidly improve response to an oral antidepressant. Esmethadone also appears to have a very benign side-effect profile in studies to date. However, after a very promising Phase II study, two Phase III studies have failed. Another large multicenter adjunctive study is under way. Lamotrigine has also shown benefit as an augmenter to standard antidepressants. A meta-analysis of eight lamotrigine studies found that lamotrigine was more effective as an augmenter in patients treated with SSRIs than those treated with SNRIs and in patients with more chronic depression (Goh et al. 2019).

Given the heterogeneity of major depression, the advantage that these novel agents bring to the table is a mechanism of action that is not monoamine based. Whereas the combination of two monoamine antidepressants, such as an SSRI and bupropion, or the combination of an SNRI and an SGA, is clearly helpful to many patients, many other patients do not respond to or cannot tolerate the combination. It is conceivable—and even likely—that some patients who are nonresponsive or intolerant to a current augmenter will find relief with the newest agents. Time will tell.

Augmentation and Combination Strategies for Bipolar Disorder

Combinations of Two or More Mood Stabilizers

Monotherapy with lithium was the standard treatment for bipolar disorder in 1970, but the availability of many newer agents and the limited efficacy of lithium in a large percentage of patients have resulted in polypharmacy as the new standard of care in many, if not most, bipolar patients. Lithium may be combined with anticonvulsants in the treatment of patients with refractory mania. There are few prospective data using such combinations; however, a number of reports indicated that lithium-carbamazepine combinations are effective with patients who have not responded to these two agents given separately (see Chapter 5). In one prospective randomized study (Juruena et al. 2009), both carbamazepine and oxcarbazepine were effective in treating residual symptoms of bipolar disorder that had not responded to lithium alone. Interestingly, oxcarbazepine at an average dosage of 210 mg/day for 8 weeks was consistently more effective than carbamazepine in reducing residual manic and depressive symptoms. Retrospective reviews have also generally found the combination of lithium and carbamazepine to be useful and synergistic (Lipinski and Pope 1982; Peselow et al. 1994). However, at least one retrospective study (Fritze et al. 1994) failed to find any benefit from combining lithium and carbamazepine in bipolar patients. There is also evidence that the combination of lithium and carbamazepine may be particularly useful in rapid-cycling bipolar disorder.

The combination of lithium and carbamazepine appears to be well tolerated. There is one report of increased risk of sinus node dysfunction with this combination (Steckler 1994), but this effect appears to be rare. In addition, the combination of lithium and carbamazepine may have a cumulative antithyroid effect (Kramlinger and Post 1990). There is no evidence of increased neurotoxicity or blood dyscrasias with this combination. Dosing schedules of the lithium and carbamazepine should parallel regimens used for prescribing each drug alone. The therapeutic serum levels of both drugs should be monitored and maintained.

Lithium is commonly combined with valproate in the treatment of bipolar disorder. Patients who have breakthrough manic symptoms or depressive symptoms with lithium alone often respond to the addition of valproate. However, relatively few studies have examined the combination prospectively. Naturalistic studies have suggested that the addition of valproate to lithium is more likely to be effective in acute manic or mixed states if the lithium level is above 0.6 mEq/L (Muti et al. 2013). In addition, female sex, a recent substance abuse episode, and late onset of depressive episodes may predict poorer response to the addition of valproate to lithium (Gao et al. 2010). Valproate has been suggested to be more efficacious than lithium in the treatment of rapid-cycling bipolar disorder, but controlled studies have not necessarily supported this idea (Calabrese et al. 2005), and the addition of valproate to lithium may not be any better than lithium alone in the management of rapid-cycling bipolar disorder (Kemp et al. 2009). The largest randomized study to date on the combination of valproate and lithium in preventing relapse in bipolar I patients, the Bipolar Affective Disorder: Lithium/Anti-Convulsant Evaluation (BALANCE) trial (BALANCE Investigators and Collaborators et al. 2010), found that the combination of lithium and valproate was not more effective than lithium alone at preventing relapse but was significantly more effective than valproate monotherapy. The combination of lithium and valproate seems to be well tolerated, and the dosing should achieve adequate serum levels for both drugs.

Occasionally, valproate has been combined with carbamazepine when lithium is poorly tolerated or ineffective. There are anecdotal reports that this combination is sometimes useful. However, valproate and carbamazepine compete for hepatic metabolism, an effect that increases the risk of carbamazepine toxicity. For this reason, some investigators have suggested that the combination of valproate and carbamazepine is contraindicated. Our experience suggests that the combination may be used safely if serum levels of both drugs are closely monitored and the doses are adjusted as necessary.

As reported in Chapter 5, other anticonvulsants such as gabapentin, topiramate, and lamotrigine have sometimes been combined with lithium and divalproex sodium in patients with treatment-resistant bipolar disorder. As with most other combination treatments for bipolar disorder, combining lithium or valproate with newer anticonvulsants is poorly studied. The combination of gabapentin and lithium in the treatment of bipolar disorder has not been consistently effective. Early small studies suggested that gabapentin might help depressive symptoms when added to an existing regimen (Ghaemi et al. 1998; Perugi et al. 1999; Young et al. 1999). In addition, the only double-blind augmentation study to date (Vieta et al. 2006) found that gabapentin added to a standard mood stabilizer might have modest benefits in preventing relapse. Clearly, the combination of gabapentin with standard mood stabilizers is well tolerated and appears to be helpful with anxiety and agitation symptoms in bipolar patients even though it does not appear to be acutely effective in the treatment of either mania or depression. We typically use 900–1,200 mg/day as an adjuvant and do not recommend gabapentin as a monotherapy for bipolar disorder.

Lamotrigine is effective in the prevention of depressive episodes in bipolar patients, and the combination with other mood stabilizers may be even more effective in preventing bipolar depression. In a controlled trial, Bowden and colleagues (2012) found that the combination of lamotrigine and valproate was significantly more effective than lamotrigine alone in preventing bipolar depressive episodes. The combination of lamotrigine with valproate or carbamazepine is more difficult to manage than the combination with lithium. Valproate doubles the serum level of lamotrigine, increasing the risk of rash, whereas carbamazepine cuts the lamotrigine serum levels in half. We have found lamotrigine at dosages in the range of 50–200 mg/day particularly helpful in treating bipolar depression in combination with lithium.

Topiramate may be more useful as an adjuvant than as an augmenting agent. The addition of 50–200 mg of topiramate to a standard mood-stabilizing regimen can help mitigate weight gain. Whether topiramate also helps augment mood-stabilizing effects is less clear at this time. Controlled monotherapy trials in bipolar disorder have been disappointing.

Mood Stabilizer–Antipsychotic Combinations

The combinations of an SGA and lithium or valproate are perhaps the most common combinations used in all phases of bipolar disorder. Many of the SGAs are FDA approved as an adjunctive treatment to lithium or valproate in the treatment of acute mania or mixed states. Symbyax and the SGAs quetiapine and lurasidone are approved for the acute treatment of bipolar depression. In the maintenance phase, both ziprasidone and quetiapine are approved in combination with lithium or valproate. Lithium does have some antidopaminergic properties, and some patients may have a greater proclivity for developing EPS when lithium is combined with antipsychotics. This appears to be particularly true at higher or toxic lithium serum levels. Likewise, it has been suggested that lithium increases the risk of tardive dyskinesia in patients also treated with first-generation antipsychotics. However, whether lithium really adds to the risk of antipsychotic-induced tardive dyskinesia is still unanswered. As reported earlier, there does not appear to be evidence of an increased risk of neurotoxicity when lithium is combined with a high-potency first-generation antipsychotic.

In a pooled analysis of five of the larger controlled trials of SGAs combined with lithium or valproate in acute mania versus a mood stabilizer alone, Ketter and colleagues (2006) concluded that there was about a 20% advantage of combination treatment versus monotherapy. This is roughly equivalent to the advantage of monotherapy with a mood stabilizer or SGA over placebo in the treatment of acute mania. Thus, the authors concluded that there appeared to be a distinct advantage of combining an SGA with lithium or valproate in acute mania. On the other hand, the combination of an SGA with carbamazepine has been less successful. For example, there appeared to be no advantage to combining olanzapine with carbamazepine in the treatment of acute mania relative to carbamazepine monotherapy (Tohen et al. 2008). In addition, the combination was more poorly tolerated than was carbamazepine monotherapy.

Quetiapine was approved in 2008 in combination with valproate or lithium in the maintenance treatment of bipolar I disorder. In patients who had been stabilized on lithium or valproate, the addition of quetiapine was significantly better than the addition of placebo in preventing both depressive and manic episodes over the next 24 weeks (Suppes et al. 2009). Far fewer patients had a relapse of a mood episode while taking the combination treatment (20%) versus monotherapy with lithium or valproate (52%). As expected, the combination of quetiapine with lithium or valproate was also less well tolerated than was adjunctive placebo, with higher rates of weight gain, sedation, and discontinuation due to adverse events.

Lurasidone received FDA approval in 2013 as monotherapy and for adjunctive use with lithium or valproate in bipolar depression. The registration trial of the addition of lurasidone to either valproate or lithium at therapeutic levels found that the combination of lurasidone to a mood stabilizer at dosages of 20–120 mg/day was significantly more effective than either mood stabilizer alone in the acute treatment of bipolar depression (Loebel et al. 2014). What is not clear from this study is whether the combination treatment is any better than monotherapy with lurasidone alone.

Other SGAs, including risperidone (Geller et al. 2012; Ouyang et al. 2012), olanzapine (Katagiri et al. 2013), aripiprazole (Woo et al. 2011), and asenapine (Szegedi et al. 2012) have all been studied in the adjunctive treatment of different aspects of bipolar disorder and may have advantages over monotherapy with a mood stabilizer alone. Thus, a bipolar depression or mania that has broken through with a mood stabilizer alone should be treated with the addition of one of the approved SGAs. In addition, the combination of an SGA and a mood stabilizer is often a more effective treatment than a mood stabilizer alone in preventing relapse.

Clozapine tends to be at the bottom of the treatment algorithm for treatment-resistant bipolar disorder because of its toxicity and complexity of use. As reported in Chapter 5, patients with treatment-resistant bipolar disorder often respond to clozapine therapy. The combination of lithium and clozapine may be synergistic—an effect that is a double-edged sword. On the one hand, some patients with refractory illness have a response after addition of clozapine to their regimens. In addition, lithium may mitigate the leukopenia associated with clozapine (Adityanjee 1995). On the other hand, most of the known cases of neuroleptic malignant syndrome (NMS) associated with clozapine have been associated with concurrent lithium use. Still, for the patient with treatment-resistant bipolar disorder, the addition or substitution of clozapine in the regimen remains an important option if other mood stabilizers and antipsychotics have failed.

Mood Stabilizer–Antidepressant Combinations

It is still common practice to use an antidepressant with a mood stabilizer to treat the depressed phase of bipolar illness. However, the utility of this combination remains questionable. As reported in Chapter 4, most studies evaluating the addition of an antidepressant to a mood stabilizer for the treatment of bipolar depression have not found clear advantages over adding placebo. For example, STEP-BD found that 23% of patients with bipolar depression treated with an antidepressant in combination with a mood stabilizer achieved euthymia for at least 8 consecutive weeks, compared with 27% of patients who had placebo added to a mood stabilizer (Sachs et al. 2007). Likewise, Nemeroff and colleagues (2001) did not find an advantage for adding imipramine or paroxetine to lithium versus adding placebo in bipolar depressed patients. However, patients with lower lithium serum levels (<0.8 mEq/L) did better with the addition of an antidepressant than they did with the addition of placebo. Thus, depressed bipolar patients who cannot tolerate a higher lithium level might benefit from the addition of an antidepressant.

Because antidepressants have not fared well in combination studies, a related question is whether the addition of a second mood stabilizer is superior to the combination of an antidepressant and a mood stabilizer in the treatment of bipolar depression. A study by Young et al. (2000) attempted to answer this question. Twenty-seven depressed bipolar patients were randomly assigned to either paroxetine or an additional mood stabilizer (either lithium or valproate). Over the 6-week trial, both strategies improved the depression, but patients were more likely to benefit from the paroxetine than they were from the mood stabilizer. Because this was a short trial, it is still conceivable that the addition of an antidepressant may be more problematic than the addition of another mood stabilizer in the long run. Although many depressed bipolar patients do not appear to benefit from the addition of an antidepressant to a mood stabilizer, some patients clearly do. We have observed some bipolar patients who clearly do more poorly when an antidepressant is discontinued. In patients who are tolerating the combination and appear to be benefiting, it makes sense to continue that combination.

Among the potential drawbacks of using antidepressants in bipolar patients is the induction of rapid cycling and switching into mania (Wehr and Goodwin 1979; Wehr et al. 1988). The induction of rapid cycling has mostly been observed with TCAs and possibly SNRIs, but it may occur with MAOIs, SSRIs, and other classes of drugs.

Bupropion was initially thought to be less likely to induce rapid cycling or mixed states, but a few cases of bupropion-induced mixed states and manic episodes have been reported. On the basis of the limited data, we suggest trying bupropion or SSRIs before treating a depressed cycle of bipolar illness with a noradrenergic antidepressant, including a TCA or an SNRI. If rapid cycling is induced, the antidepressant should be discontinued if possible, and a combination of mood stabilizers, with or without thyroid supplement, should be considered.

Mood Stabilizers and Thyroid Supplements

Thyroid supplements have long been used to accelerate or augment response in bipolar depression as in unipolar depression. Most of the studies to date of adding thyroid hormone to a mood stabilizer or antidepressant in bipolar depression are small and difficult to draw definitive conclusions from. Most of the literature of thyroid supplementation in bipolar disorder consists of retrospective chart reviews and case series. However, there are a few double-blind studies in rapid-cycling and resistant bipolar depression using high-dose levothyroxine. That being said, the majority of studies suggest a benefit of adding T_3 or T_4 to the bipolar regimen (Parmentier and Sienaert 2018). The high-dose T_4 studies have shown the most benefit in bipolar patients. For example, Walshaw and colleagues (2018) randomly assigned 32 treatment-resistant rapid-cycling patients to receive adjunctive high doses of T_3 or T_4. T_3 was given at doses high enough to get patients to a T_3 serum level of 0.65–1.36, and the T_4 doses aimed at getting the free T_4 level to 4.5–7.5 or enough to suppress the TSH level to <0.1. Both T_4 and T_3 supplementation significantly improved the time spent in a euthymic condition, but the T_4 was somewhat better. In one of the few placebo-controlled studies, Stamm and colleagues (2014) randomly assigned 112 bipolar I and II depressed patients who had not responded to their current regimen to receive either add-on T_4 300 μg/day or add-on placebo. After 6 weeks of treatment, the groups did not statistically separate, but women did better than men, and there was a numerical advantage in the T_4-treated group.

Adding high-dose T_4, T_3, or the combination of the two would be a second- or third-tier option in bipolar depressed or rapid-cycling patients. In general, T_4 or the combination of T_4 and T_3 appears to have more supporting evidence than T_3 alone. The dosages of T_4 in studies have ranged from 150 to as high as 600 μg/day. Even supraphysiological doses of thyroid supplements have tended to be well tolerated, but they do carry some risks. Common side effects are weight loss, headache, nausea, and agitation. More serious side effects include the risk of atrial fibrillation, particularly in older patients. As reported earlier in this chapter, there is a risk of bone demineralization or a switch into mania, but these risks appear to be small (Ribot et al. 1990). Patients treated with high-dose thyroid augmentation should have their free T_4, T_3, and TSH levels monitored. An electrocardiogram is also prudent.

Mood Stabilizers and Omega-3 Fatty Acids

Omega-3 and omega-6 fatty acids are the building blocks of fats in the same way that amino acids are the building blocks of proteins. A number of reports since the early 1990s have suggested that affective illness may be associated with deficiencies of some omega-3 fatty acids. For example, there appears to be a higher ratio of arachidonic acid to eicosapentaenoic acid in more severely depressed patients compared with less severely depressed patients. Other studies have suggested that the red blood cell membranes of depressed patients may contain lower levels of omega-3 fatty acids compared with healthy control subjects. Furthermore, some limited evidence suggests that omega-3 fatty acids may impact signal transduction in a manner analogous to lithium.

A preliminary double-blind study reported that adding supplemental omega-3 fatty acids to the drug regimens of bipolar patients improved their outcomes (Stoll et al. 1999). In this study, 30 bipolar patients were randomly assigned to either 9.6 g/day of omega-3 supplements or olive oil (as a control) for 4 months. They continued taking standard mood stabilizers. The patients treated with omega-3 experienced longer remission and more complete resolution of symptoms than did the placebo-treated patients. More recent studies of the adjunctive use of omega-3 fatty acids in both bipolar disorder and unipolar depression have been inconclusive (see Chapter 5). A Cochrane review of five controlled trials of omega-3 fatty acids in the treatment of bipolar disorder concluded that there was little evidence that these supplements help manic symptoms, but they might help depressive symptoms in bipolar patients (Montgomery and Richardson 2008). A more recent meta-analysis of omega-3 fatty acids in MDD also suggested that the supplement might help depressive symptoms in both patients with MDD and patients who did not meet the syndromal criteria for MDD (Grosso et al. 2014).

The American Psychiatric Association (APA) has taken the position that patients with a mood disorder might benefit from the addition of omega-3 fatty acids to their diet. The APA has suggested at least two servings of fatty fish, such as salmon, per week or 1 g of eicosapentaenoic acid or docosahexaenoic acid per day. Because these fatty acids are fairly benign and may have other health benefits, we think it is not unreasonable to supplement the mood-stabilizing regimens of bipolar patients with omega-3 fatty acids. Although dramatic benefits are uncommon in our experience, the downsides are minimal. One possible downside is that omega-3 fatty acids have anticoagulant properties. Thus, they may increase the risk of bleeding in some susceptible patients, such as those taking anticoagulants, including nonsteroidal anti-inflammatory drugs. Children and pregnant women should avoid eating fish with the highest levels of mercury (and other heavy metal) concentration (i.e., shark, mackerel, swordfish). In addition, the FDA recommends eating no more than 12 oz a week of fish with lower mercury levels, such as canned light tuna, salmon, pollock, and catfish.

Augmentation Strategies for Schizophrenia

Combinations of Two Antipsychotics

Combining two or more antipsychotics (referred to as *antipsychotic polypharmacy* [APP]) is generally frowned on because the utility of this approach is not clear. Several states, including California, have made a reduction of APP an important goal in the public mental health sector. The most common reason for combining antipsychotics is the lack of adequate response to antipsychotic monotherapy in schizophrenia. Earlier onset of illness, longer duration of illness, and factors such as more frequent hospitalizations and the presence of violence as a symptom of schizophrenia are more likely to be associated with APP (Sagud et al. 2013).

The efficacy of APP versus antipsychotic monotherapy is unclear. The one meta-analysis to date of APP versus monotherapy in 19 clinical trials suggested that APP appeared superior to monotherapy in the treatment of patients with resistant schizophrenia (Correll et al. 2009). However, the various studies are difficult to interpret because they used different outcome measures and involved many different agents. Clozapine was the most common antipsychotic studied in these combination trials.

It makes intuitive sense that the combination of clozapine, which has limited D_2 antagonism, and a D_2 antagonist might be useful. Several studies have suggested that the combination of clozapine with aripiprazole or amisulpride may be more effective than clozapine monotherapy (Porcelli et al. 2012). At this time, aripiprazole probably has the most evidence supporting its use as an add-on to clozapine for the treatment of positive symptoms (Siskind et al. 2018). If a patient has not responded to the maximum tolerated dose of clozapine, these studies suggest that there may be a benefit of adding 10–15 mg of aripiprazole. Likewise, a few case reports have suggested that the addition of risperidone to clozapine might be helpful for some patients with refractory schizophrenia (see Morera et al. 1999). However, the α-adrenergic receptor–blocking properties of risperidone might be problematic in some patients being treated with clozapine, and the addition of haloperidol might work just as well and with fewer complications. The combination of other atypical antipsychotics and standard antipsychotics may also be warranted if the maximum dosage of the atypical agent has been achieved with less than satisfactory benefit. We tend to prefer the addition of high-potency agents because the weight gain and the hypotensive and sedation problems associated with the atypical antipsychotics complicate the addition of low-potency agents. Because risperidone is such a potent D_2 antagonist by itself, we push the dosage of risperidone as tolerated by the patient up to 12 mg/day rather than add another antipsychotic to it.

There may be problems with combining certain antipsychotics. For example, combining aripiprazole with other D_2 antagonists has sometimes been associated with a worsening of symptoms (Chan and Sweeting 2007; Chang et al. 2006). APP may also carry an increased risk of side effects, including parkinsonism and increased prolactin levels (Gallego et al. 2012).

Response to a given antipsychotic may occur earlier than we previously believed. In a meta-analysis of 34 studies, Samara et al. (2015) found that a lack of acute antipsychotic benefit in the first 2 weeks of treatment predicted lack of response subsequently. Thus, in the acute management of schizophrenia, it might not be unreasonable to switch or augment relatively early in an acute course of treatment. The question is what to switch to or augment with given that the data are sparse. Certainly, a switch from a first-generation drug to an SGA makes sense for many patients, as does switching to clozapine after failed antipsychotic trials of other medications. Except for tolerability reasons, switching within the class of antipsychotics does not generally seem to be associated with better outcomes. Some small studies have suggested that switching to olanzapine may benefit some patients who had an early lack of response to risperidone (Kinon et al. 2010). However, there is little evidence, in general, that switching within the class of antipsychotics improves outcome much.

Likewise, combining two first- or second-generation drugs rarely is helpful. The most common combination is a high-potency agent such as haloperidol and a low-potency agent such as chlorpromazine. The rationale for using the low-potency agent is usually to help with sleep. However, the clinician could obtain the same effect from adding higher doses of diphenhydramine (50–100 mg qhs) or, better yet, a benzodiazepine, to the antipsychotic. Combining olanzapine with risperidone in patients who experienced unsuccessful trials with one or the other medication may have small benefits but seems worth trying (Hatta and Ito 2014). However, the overall benefits of combining most antipsychotics appear small and may be outweighed by the risks, which can include compounding metabolic effects, QTc prolongation,and oversedation. There is the rare patient who clinically does better with two different standard antipsychotics, but there is rarely a time that another class of agents (antidepressants, benzodiazepines, or mood stabilizers) might not work even better.

Combinations of Antidepressants and Antipsychotics

The SSRIs and other antidepressants have been combined with antipsychotics in the treatment of negative symptoms and depression in schizophrenia, schizoaffective disorder, and psychotic depression. As of this writing, there have been more than 80 randomized controlled trials of adding antidepressants to antipsychotics in the treatment of schizophrenia, with most showing some benefit in the treatment of associated depression, negative symptoms, and quality-of-life measures without exacerbating the psychosis (Helfer et al. 2016). Open-label studies have suggested that fluoxetine and fluvoxamine may help with negative symptoms and mood problems in patients with schizophrenia (Goldman and Janecek 1990; Silver and Nassar 1992). One potential problem is that the SSRIs may raise the serum levels of standard and atypical antipsychotics. In a double-blind trial of fluoxetine added to a depot neuroleptic, negative symptoms were clearly improved with the fluoxetine treatment, but serum levels of the antipsychotic were increased an average of 65% with fluphenazine and 20% with haloperidol decanoate (Goff et al. 1995). Although EPS did not worsen in this study, some patients clearly had a worsening of akathisia and other symptoms with the addition of fluoxetine or other SSRIs to their antipsychotic regimen. Therefore, lower antipsychotic doses may be required when antipsychotics are combined with the SSRIs. As indicated previously, SSRIs, particularly fluvoxamine, can markedly elevate serum clozapine levels.

Other antidepressants may also have benefit in treating negative symptoms. Trazodone has shown modest benefits in the treatment of negative symptoms, as has moclobemide. Trazodone produces significant but modest improvements in negative symptoms compared with placebo when added to a standard antipsychotic (Decina et al. 1994). Bodkin et al. (1996) found that selegiline 5 mg bid over 6 weeks significantly improved negative symptoms and EPS in a group of 21 patients with schizophrenia or schizoaffective disorder but had no effect on positive symptoms. At these low dosages, one would not anticipate significant interactions with atypical, serotonergic antipsychotics, but caution should be exercised. Transdermal selegiline at a dosage of 6 mg/day would be expected to be at least as safe as low-dose oral selegiline. However, transdermal selegiline has not been evaluated in schizophrenia as of this writing.

Finally, low doses of standard antipsychotics may actually increase the availability of dopamine synaptically by inhibition of presynaptic dopamine autoreceptors to release more dopamine. There have been some anecdotal reports of both worsening of positive symptoms and improvement of negative symptoms with low-dose antipsychotics. In a placebo-controlled study, amisulpride, a dopamine-blocking benzamide antipsychotic, was found to significantly improve negative symptoms of schizophrenia at low doses (Boyer et al. 1995). At high doses, amisulpride and standard antipsychotics may worsen negative symptoms by dampening dopaminergic tone throughout the prefrontal cortex.

Combinations of Mood Stabilizers and Antipsychotics

As many as a third of schizophrenic patients do not respond adequately to an antipsychotic. One of the earliest augmentation strategies for treatment-resistant schizophrenia was the addition of lithium. Lithium augmentation of neuroleptics at relatively low dosages (300–900 mg/day) has been said to be helpful in the treatment of schizophrenia (Johns and Thompson 1995). However, most of the reports suggesting that lithium is a useful augmenting agent in treating schizophrenia have been anecdotal. Several randomized controlled studies have investigated the efficacy of lithium when added to an antipsychotic. None has shown any benefit of adding lithium over adding placebo in patients with well-characterized schizophrenia (Collins et al. 1991; Schulz et al. 1999; Wilson 1993). It may be that earlier reports included patients with schizoaffective disorder or psychotic mania, who may clearly benefit from lithium. Because use of lithium with antipsychotics appears to increase the risk of EPS and perhaps NMS, we suggest using lithium augmentation primarily in treating patients with suspected schizoaffective disorder. The dosage of the antipsychotic may need to be lowered in some patients treated concurrently with lithium.

Valproate has been shown to be helpful as an adjunctive treatment in combination with antipsychotics in the treatment of acute exacerbations of schizophrenia. Casey and colleagues (2003) reported that adding 15–30 mg/kg/day of valproate resulted in earlier improvement in psychotic symptoms in acutely ill schizophrenic patients. However, the effects of valproate as an augmenter tend not to be evident at the endpoint of most trials (Basan et al. 2004). Thus, valproate's primary utility might be in speeding response, or perhaps as an adjunct in treating agitation in some patients.

It has also been suggested that carbamazepine may boost antipsychotic effects. As with lithium, many anecdotal and open-label studies have suggested a role for carbamazepine in treatment-resistant schizophrenia. However, as with lithium, controlled trials have failed to show much benefit of adding carbamazepine to an antipsychotic (Llorca et al. 1993; Martín Muñoz et al. 1992). Because carbamazepine can substantially lower the serum levels of most concurrent antipsychotics, we find it difficult to use carbamazepine as an augmenting agent in treating schizophrenia.

An alternative to carbamazepine or valproate as an adjunctive agent in schizophrenia may be topiramate. The addition of topiramate to antipsychotics has been reported to be beneficial in resistant schizophrenia in a controlled trial (Tiihonen et al. 2005, 2009). Topiramate may also have the advantage of mitigating antipsychotic-induced weight gain.

There has been some evidence that adding lamotrigine to clozapine may be helpful in patients with treatment-resistant schizophrenia. At least five small open or controlled trials of adding lamotrigine to clozapine have been completed to date. In general, the addition of lamotrigine appears to modestly help both positive and negative symptoms in patients who have not responded to clozapine monotherapy (Citrome 2009). On the other hand, the addition of lamotrigine 100–400 mg/day to various other SGAs did not show much benefit (Goff et al. 2007). Lamotrigine is currently being investigated as an adjunctive agent in schizophrenia to specifically target cognitive deficits because this potential benefit has been seen in at least one of the controlled trials.

In general, mood stabilizers have been thought to have a limited role as augmenting agents in the treatment of the core symptoms of schizophrenia. We believe, on the other hand, that mood stabilizers have a role as adjuvant agents in treating aggressive outbursts and agitation in patients with schizophrenia. We have found gabapentin, at dosages up to 3,600 mg/day, and valproate, at dosages of 750–2,000 mg/day, helpful in treating agitation and aggression in some patients with schizophrenia. In addition, gabapentin may have the added benefit of helping with EPS in patients treated with standard antipsychotics (see Chapter 5).

Other Augmentation Strategies

Because cognitive and executive deficits in schizophrenia appear to be one of the major factors that limit functioning in patients with schizophrenia, the NIMH has been interested in fostering research that leads to better treatment of cognitive deficits in this population. The Measurement and Treatment Research to Improve Cognition in Schizophrenia (MATRICS) program has begun to evaluate possible treatments. Among the adjunctive medications that might have a role to play in improving cognition in schizophrenia patients are stimulants, modafinil, atomoxetine, and acetylcholinesterase inhibitors. Small studies have suggested that amphetamine can help working memory and executive dysfunction in patients with schizophrenia (Barch and Carter 2005). Although stimulants can worsen positive symptoms, they often help negative symptoms (see Chapter 4). In contrast, modafinil has not been particularly helpful for treating executive deficits in schizophrenia patients to date (Saavedra-Velez et al. 2009), although it may help on some global measures of negative symptoms. Likewise, atomoxetine and acetylcholinesterase inhibitors have also not been particularly efficacious (Kelly et al. 2009). The search continues for viable treatments for cognitive deficits in schizophrenia. A promising experimental strategy is the potential use of $\alpha 7$ nicotinic agonists (Barak et al. 2009).

Abnormalities in glutamate transmission, particularly hypofunctioning of the NMDA glutamate receptor, have been proposed in the etiology of deficit symptoms in schizophrenia. To this end, a number of studies have examined the role of glycine and D-cycloserine in augmenting the effects of antipsychotics. D-cycloserine is an agonist of the NMDA receptor, and a number of controlled trials have suggested that D-cycloserine improves negative symptoms and neuropsychological functioning in patients taking standard antipsychotics (Goff et al. 1999b; Rosse et al. 1996; Tsai et al. 1998) but not in those taking clozapine (Goff et al. 1996, 1999a; Tsai et al. 1999). The dosage of D-cycloserine that was most effective was around 50 mg/day, which tended to be well tolerated. The effects of D-cycloserine on negative symptoms and cognitive functioning, although significant, have not been particularly robust.

Glycine is an amino acid that is a co-agonist of the NMDA receptor. Early open trials suggested that glycine helps some patients with schizophrenia and worsens symptoms in others (Rosse et al. 1989). A more recent crossover trial of high-dose glycine (0.8 g/kg) added to an antipsychotic found that negative symptoms were significantly improved relative to placebo (Heresco-Levy et al. 1999). Glycine augmentation is a fairly benign strategy for improving negative symptoms. However, it is unlikely that adding glycine to a standard antipsychotic is better in improving negative symptoms than simply switching to an atypical agent. For patients who do not respond as well to an atypical antipsychotic, the addition of glycine or D-cycloserine may be an option.

Cyproheptadine (Periactin) is a general serotonin antagonist used primarily to treat migraines and allergies. Its serotonin receptor antagonist properties have made it of interest to clinicians treating negative symptoms in schizophrenia because all atypical antipsychotics are also 5-HT$_2$ antagonists. In a controlled trial, cyproheptadine at a dosage of 24 mg/day significantly improved negative symptoms and was well tolerated (Akhondzadeh et al. 1999). Cyproheptadine also has the advantage of being anticholinergic and can help with EPS. The problem with cyproheptadine is that most patients find it quite sedating, and 24 mg/day is a large dosage for many patients. It is unclear whether smaller dosages might work just as well.

The 5-HT$_3$ antagonist ondansetron has also been reported to be a useful adjunctive or augmenting agent in resistant schizophrenia. Over the past 15 years, a number of anecdotal reports have suggested that ondansetron, which is used primarily as an antinausea medication, might help the cognitive and negative symptoms of schizophrenia. The first double-blind study of ondansetron in resistant schizophrenia also seems to support the benefits of this agent (Zhang et al. 2006). Patients with schizophrenia that was unresponsive to haloperidol were more likely to see a 30% improvement in psychotic symptoms with ondansetron added to the haloperidol than were patients who had placebo added to the haloperidol. Ondansetron is well tolerated but currently quite expensive. The dosage of ondansetron used in Zhang et al.'s (2006) study was 8 mg/day administered for 12 weeks.

Oxytocin is a neuropeptide that appears to be important in social cognition, attachment, memory, and other social domains. Because schizophrenia patients are often lacking in these social domains, intranasal oxytocin at a dosage of 24-48 IU/day has sometimes been added to an antipsychotic regimen. The results of adjunctive oxytocin in schizophrenia have been inconsistent (Oya et al. 2016). Case reports have suggested benefits in social cognition, negative symptoms, and even positive symptoms, but controlled studies have been less supportive. That being said, oxytocin tends to be well tolerated and might be worth considering for negative and social interaction symptoms if strategies such as adjunctive antidepressants prove less helpful.

Another strategy for treating negative symptoms of schizophrenia has been adjunctive treatment with minocycline. Minocycline is a tetracycline antibiotic that appears to have NMDA antagonist properties similar to those of memantine. Memantine has also been shown in some studies to improve negative symptoms in schizophrenia (Di Iorio et al. 2017). There are a number of controlled trials of adjunctive treatment with minocycline that also suggest benefit in treating the negative symptoms of schizophrenia (Oya et al. 2014). The most common side effect of minocycline is gastrointestinal upset, but in rare cases anaphylactic reactions occur. The typical target dosage of minocycline is 200 mg/day. Long-term risks with minocycline are less well known. As with oxytocin, minocycline use in schizophrenia is still largely experimental and should be considered only if other strategies for treating negative symptoms have been unsuccessful.

Suggested Readings

Austin LS, Arana GW, Melvin JA: Toxicity resulting from lithium augmentation of antidepressant treatment in elderly patients. J Clin Psychiatry 51(8):344–345, 1990 2380160

Bakish D, Hooper CL, Thornton MD, et al: Fast onset: an open study of the treatment of major depressive disorder with nefazodone and pindolol combination therapy. Int Clin Psychopharmacol 12(2):91–97, 1997 9219044

Bommer M, Naber D: Subclinical hypothyroidism in recurrent mania. Biol Psychiatry 31(7):729–734, 1992 1599989

Bowden CL, Myers JE, Grossman F, et al: Risperidone in combination with mood stabilizers: a 10-week continuation phase study in bipolar I disorder. J Clin Psychiatry 65(5):707–714, 2004 15163260

Buchanan RW, Freedman R, Javitt DC, et al: Recent advances in the development of novel pharmacological agents for the treatment of cognitive impairments in schizophrenia. Schizophr Bull 33(5):1120–1130, 2007 17641146

Cattell DL, King EA: Estrogen for postnatal depression. J Fam Pract 43(1):22–23, 1996 8691173

Chambers CD, Johnson KA, Dick LM, et al: Birth outcomes in pregnant women taking fluoxetine. N Engl J Med 335(14):1010–1015, 1996 8793924

Cooke RG, Joffe RT, Levitt AJ: T3 augmentation of antidepressant treatment in T4-replaced thyroid patients. J Clin Psychiatry 53(1):16–18, 1992 1737734

DeBattista C, Schatzberg AF: Estrogen modulation of monoamines, in Gender Differences in Mood and Anxiety Disorders. Edited by Liebenluft E. Washington, DC, American Psychiatric Publishing, 1999

de Montigny C, Cournoyer G, Morissette R, et al: Lithium carbonate addition in tricyclic antidepressant–resistant unipolar depression: correlations with the neurobiologic actions of tricyclic antidepressant drugs and lithium ion on the serotonin system. Arch Gen Psychiatry 40(12):1327–1334, 1983 6418109

Eden Evins A, Demopulos C, Nierenberg A, et al: A double-blind, placebo-controlled trial of adjunctive donepezil in treatment-resistant mania. Bipolar Disord 8(1):75–80, 2006 16411983

Everett HC: The use of bethanechol chloride with tricyclic antidepressants. Am J Psychiatry 132(11):1202–1204, 1975 1166898

Feighner JP, Brauzer B, Gelenberg AJ, et al: A placebo-controlled multicenter trial of Limbitrol versus its components (amitriptyline and chlordiazepoxide) in the symptomatic treatment of depressive illness. Psychopharmacology (Berl) 61(2):217–225, 1979 108739

Flint AJ, Rifat SL: A prospective study of lithium augmentation in antidepressant-resistant geriatric depression. J Clin Psychopharmacol 14(5):353–356, 1994 7806693

Gerner RH, Stanton A: Algorithm for patient management of acute manic states: lithium, valproate, or carbamazepine? J Clin Psychopharmacol 12(1)(suppl):57S–63S, 1992 1541719

Ghaemi SN, Goodwin FK: Use of atypical antipsychotic agents in bipolar and schizoaffective disorders: review of the empirical literature. J Clin Psychopharmacol 19(4):354–361, 1999 10440464

Ghaemi SN, Sachs GS, Baldassano CF, et al: Acute treatment of bipolar disorder with adjunctive risperidone in outpatients. Can J Psychiatry 42(2):196–199, 1997 9067070

Ghaemi SN, Schrauwen E, Klugman J, et al: Long-term lamotrigine plus lithium for bipolar disorder: one year outcome. J Psychiatr Pract 12(5):300–305, 2006 16998417

Gitlin MJ, Weiner H, Fairbanks L, et al: Failure of T3 to potentiate tricyclic antidepressant response. J Affect Disord 13(3):267–272, 1987 2960719

Goh KK, Chen CH, Chiu YH, Lu ML: Lamotrigine augmentation in treatment-resistant unipolar depression: a comprehensive meta-analysis of efficacy and safety. J Psychopharmacol 33(6):700–713, 2019 31081449

Granacher RP, Baldessarini RJ: Physostigmine: its use in acute anticholinergic syndrome with antidepressant and antiparkinson drugs. Arch Gen Psychiatry 32(3):375–380, 1975 1115577

Hayes SG: Barbiturate anticonvulsants in refractory affective disorders. Ann Clin Psychiatry 5(1):35–44, 1993 8348197

Heninger GR, Charney DS, Sternberg DE: Lithium carbonate augmentation of antidepressant treatment: an effective prescription for treatment-refractory depression. Arch Gen Psychiatry 40(12):1335–1342, 1983 6418110

Hollander E, DeCaria CM, Schneier FR, et al: Fenfluramine augmentation of serotonin reuptake blockade antiobsessional treatment. J Clin Psychiatry 51(3):119–123, 1990 2106515

Holsboer F, Grasser A, Friess E, et al: Steroid effects on central neurons and implications for psychiatric and neurological disorders. Ann N Y Acad Sci 746:345–359 [discussion 359–361], 1994 2106515

Hopwood SE, Bogle S, Wildgust HJ: The combination of fluoxetine and lithium in clinical practice. Int Clin Psychopharmacol 8(4):325–327, 1993 8277157

Howland RH: Lithium augmentation of fluoxetine in the treatment of OCD and major depression: a case report. Can J Psychiatry 36(2):154–155, 1991 1904303

Howland RH: Thyroid dysfunction in refractory depression: implications for pathophysiology and treatment. J Clin Psychiatry 54(2):47–54, 1993 8444820

Hunter MD, Ganesan V, Wilkinson ID, et al: Impact of modafinil on prefrontal executive function in schizophrenia. Am J Psychiatry 163(12):2184–2186, 2006 17151173

Joffe G, Appelberg B, Rimón R: Adjunctive nefazodone in neuroleptic-treated schizophrenic patients with predominantly negative symptoms: an open prospective pilot study. Int Clin Psychopharmacol 14(4):233–238, 1999 10468316

Karunakaran K, Tungaraza TE, Harborne GC: Is clozapine-aripiprazole combination a useful regime in the management of treatment-resistant schizophrenia? J Psychopharmacol 21(4):453–456, 2007 17050662

Katona CL, Robertson MM, Abou-Saleh MT, et al: Placebo-controlled trial of lithium augmentation of fluoxetine and lofepramine. Int Clin Psychopharmacol 8(4):323–324, 1993 8277156

Keck PE Jr, McElroy SL, Vuckovic A, et al: Combined valproate and carbamazepine treatment of bipolar disorder. J Neuropsychiatry Clin Neurosci 4(3):319–322, 1992 1498585

Ketter TA, Winsberg ME, DeGolia SG, et al: Rapid efficacy of olanzapine augmentation in nonpsychotic bipolar mixed states. J Clin Psychiatry 59(2):83–85, 1998 9501894

Ketter T, Wang P, Nowakowski C: Treatment of acute mania in bipolar disorder, in Advances in Treatment of Bipolar Disorder. Edited by Ketter TA. Washington, DC, American Psychiatric Publishing, 2005, pp 11–55

Kishimoto A: The treatment of affective disorder with carbamazepine: prophylactic synergism of lithium and carbamazepine combination. Prog Neuropsychopharmacol Biol Psychiatry 16(4):483–493, 1992 1641493

Kline NS, Pare M, Hallstrom C, et al: Amitriptyline protects patients on MAOIs from tyramine reactions. J Clin Psychopharmacol 2(6):434–435, 1982 7174870

Kusalic M: Grade II and grade III hypothyroidism in rapid-cycling bipolar patients. Neuropsychobiology 25(4):177–181, 1992 1454157

Lemberger L, Rowe H, Bosomworth JC, et al: The effect of fluoxetine on the pharmacokinetics and psychomotor responses of diazepam. Clin Pharmacol Ther 43(4):412–419, 1988 3128416

McElroy SL, Pope HG Jr (eds): Use of Anticonvulsants in Psychiatry: Recent Advances. Clifton, NJ, Oxford Health Care, 1988

McGinness J, Kishimoto A, Hollister LE: Avoiding neurotoxicity with lithium-carbamazepine combinations. Psychopharmacol Bull 26(2):181–184, 1990 2236454

McIntyre A, Gendron A, McIntyre A: Quetiapine adjunct to selective serotonin reuptake inhibitors or venlafaxine in patients with major depression, comorbid anxiety, and residual depressive symptoms: a randomized, placebo-controlled pilot study. Depress Anxiety 24(7):487–494, 2007 17177199

Mitchell P, Withers K, Jacobs G, et al: Combining lithium and sodium valproate for bipolar disorder. Aust N Z J Psychiatry 28(1):141–143, 1994 8067959

Mouaffak F, Tranulis C, Gourevitch R, et al: Augmentation strategies of clozapine with antipsychotics in the treatment of ultraresistant schizophrenia. Clin Neuropharmacol 29(1):28–33, 2006 16518132

Muly EC, McDonald W, Steffens D, et al: Serotonin syndrome produced by a combination of fluoxetine and lithium. Am J Psychiatry 150(10):1565, 1993 8379573

Okuma T: Effects of carbamazepine and lithium on affective disorders. Neuropsychobiology 27(3):138–145, 1993 8232828

Ontiveros A, Fontaine R, Elie R: Refractory depression: the addition of lithium to fluoxetine or desipramine. Acta Psychiatr Scand 83(3):188–192, 1991 1903237

Palinkas LA, Barrett-Connor E: Estrogen use and depressive symptoms in postmenopausal women. Obstet Gynecol 80(1):30–36, 1992 1603493

Pare CMB, Kline N, Hallstrom C, et al: Will amitriptyline prevent the "cheese" reaction of monoamine-oxidase inhibitors? Lancet 2(8291):183–186, 1982 6123888

Rapaport MH, Gharabawi GM, Canuso CM, et al: Effects of risperidone augmentation in patients with treatment-resistant depression: results of open-label treatment followed by double-blind continuation. Neuropsychopharmacology 31(11):2505–2513, 2006 16760927

Remington G, Saha A, Chong SA, et al: Augmentation strategies in clozapine-resistant schizophrenia. CNS Drugs 19(10):843–872, 2005 16185094

Rothschild AJ, Samson JA, Bessette MP, et al: Efficacy of the combination of fluoxetine and perphenazine in the treatment of psychotic depression. J Clin Psychiatry 54(9):338–342, 1993 8104930

Rothschild AJ, Williamson DJ, Tohen MF, et al: A double-blind, randomized study of olanzapine and olanzapine/fluoxetine combination for major depression with psychotic features. J Clin Psychopharmacol 24(4):365–373, 2004 15232326

Sachs GS, Weilburg JB, Rosenbaum JF: Clonazepam vs. neuroleptics as adjuncts to lithium maintenance. Psychopharmacol Bull 26(1):137–143, 1990 1973545

Sachs GS, Grossman F, Ghaemi SN, et al: Combination of a mood stabilizer with risperidone or haloperidol for treatment of acute mania: a double-blind, placebo-controlled comparison of efficacy and safety. Am J Psychiatry 159(7):1146–1154, 2002 12091192

Schatzberg AF, DeBattista CB, DeGolia S: Valproate in the treatment of agitation associated with depression. Psychiatr Ann 26(7):S470–S473, 1996

Sharma V, Persad E: Augmentation of valproate with lithium in a case of rapid cycling affective disorder. Can J Psychiatry 37(8):584–585, 1992 1423163

Shelton RC: The combination of olanzapine and fluoxetine in mood disorders. Expert Opin Pharmacother 4(7):1175–1183, 2003 12831342

Shelton RC, Tollefson GD, Tohen M, et al: A novel augmentation strategy for treating resistant major depression. Am J Psychiatry 158(1):131–134, 2001 11136647

Shelton RC, Williamson DJ, Corya SA, et al: Olanzapine/fluoxetine combination for treatment-resistant depression: a controlled study of SSRI and nortriptyline resistance. J Clin Psychiatry 66(10):1289–1297, 2005 16259543

Simhandl C, Denk E, Thau K: The comparative efficacy of carbamazepine low and high serum level and lithium carbonate in the prophylaxis of affective disorders. J Affect Disord 28(4):221–231, 1993 8227758

Spiker DG, Weiss JC, Dealy RS, et al: The pharmacological treatment of delusional depression. Am J Psychiatry 142(4):430–436, 1985 3883815

Stein G, Bernadt M: Lithium augmentation therapy in tricyclic-resistant depression: a controlled trial using lithium in low and normal doses. Br J Psychiatry 162:634–640, 1993 8149115

Strömgren LS: The combination of lithium and carbamazepine in treatment and prevention of manic-depressive disorder: a review and a case report. Compr Psychiatry 31(3):261–265, 1990 2187656

Takahashi N, Terao T, Oga T, et al: Comparison of risperidone and mosapramine addition to neuroleptic treatment in chronic schizophrenia. Neuropsychobiology 39(2):81–85, 1999 10072664

Thase ME, Kupfer DJ, Frank E, et al: Treatment of imipramine-resistant recurrent depression II: an open clinical trial of lithium augmentation. J Clin Psychiatry 50(11):413–417, 1989 2509437

Tohen M, Chengappa KN, Suppes T, et al: Efficacy of olanzapine in combination with valproate or lithium in the treatment of mania in patients partially nonresponsive to valproate or lithium monotherapy. Arch Gen Psychiatry 59(1):62–69, 2002 11779284

Tollefson GD, Sanger TM, Anderson SW: The use of an olanzapine:fluoxetine combination in the treatment of major depression with psychotic features: results from a large, prospective double-blind trial, in Abstracts of the 40th Annual Meeting of the American College of Neuropsychopharmacology, Waikoloa, HI, 2001, p 58

The Upjohn Company: Technical Report Synopsis: A Multicenter Study to Evaluate the Pharmacokinetic and Clinical Interactions Between Alprazolam and Imipramine. Kalamazoo, MI, Upjohn, 1986

The Upjohn Company: Technical Report Synopsis: A Pharmacokinetic/Pharmacodynamic Evaluation of the Combined Administration of Alprazolam and Fluoxetine. Kalamazoo, MI, Upjohn, 1990

Vieta E, Sánchez-Moreno J, Goikolea JM, et al: Effects on weight and outcome of long-term olanzapine-topiramate combination treatment in bipolar disorder. J Clin Psychopharmacol 24(4):374–378, 2004 15232327

Vieweg V, Shutty M, Hundley P, et al: Combined treatment with lithium and carbamazepine. Am J Psychiatry 148(3):398–399, 1991 1899545

Wheatley D: Potentiation of amitriptyline by thyroid hormone. Arch Gen Psychiatry 26(3):229–233, 1972 4551047

White K, Simpson G: Combined MAOI-tricyclic antidepressant treatment: a reevaluation. J Clin Psychopharmacol 1(5):264–282, 1981 7037873

Whybrow PC, Bauer MS, Gyulai L: Thyroid axis considerations in patients with rapid cycling affective disorder. Clin Neuropharmacol 15(Suppl 1 Pt A):391A–392A, 1992 1498888

Wolkowitz OM, Reus VI, Roberts E, et al: Antidepressant and cognition-enhancing effects of DHEA in major depression. Ann NY Acad Sci 774:337–339, 1995 8597481

References

Adityanjee: Modification of clozapine-induced leukopenia and neutropenia with lithium carbonate. Am J Psychiatry 152(4):648–649, 1995 7694925

Akhondzadeh S, Mohammadi MR, Amini-Nooshabadi H, et al: Cyproheptadine in treatment of chronic schizophrenia: a double-blind, placebo-controlled study. J Clin Pharm Ther 24(1):49–52, 1999 10319907

Alpert JE, Mischoulon D, Rubenstein GE, et al: Folinic acid (Leucovorin) as an adjunctive treatment for SSRI-refractory depression. Ann Clin Psychiatry 14(1):33–38, 2002 12046638

Alvarez E, Pérez-Solá V, Pérez-Blanco J, et al: Predicting outcome of lithium added to antidepressants in resistant depression. J Affect Disord 42(2–3):179–186, 1997 9105959

Aranow AB, Hudson JI, Pope HG Jr, et al: Elevated antidepressant plasma levels after addition of fluoxetine. Am J Psychiatry 146(7):911–913, 1989 2787124

Artigas F, Perez V, Alvarez E: Pindolol induces a rapid improvement of depressed patients treated with serotonin reuptake inhibitors. Arch Gen Psychiatry 51(3):248–251, 1994 8122960

BALANCE investigators and collaborators; Geddes JR, Goodwin GM, et al: Lithium plus valproate combination therapy versus monotherapy for relapse prevention in bipolar I disorder (BALANCE): a randomised open-label trial. Lancet 375(9712):385–395, 2010 20092882

Barak S, Arad M, De Levie A, et al: Pro-cognitive and antipsychotic efficacy of the alpha7 nicotinic partial agonist SSR180711 in pharmacological and neurodevelopmental latent inhibition models of schizophrenia. Neuropsychopharmacology 34(7):1753–1763, 2009 19158670

Barbee JG, Thompson TR, Jamhour NJ, et al: A double-blind placebo-controlled trial of lamotrigine as an antidepressant augmentation agent in treatment-refractory unipolar depression. J Clin Psychiatry 72(10):1405–1412, 2011 21367355

Barch DM, Carter CS: Amphetamine improves cognitive function in medicated individuals with schizophrenia and in healthy volunteers. Schizophr Res 77(1):43–58, 2005 16005384

Baron BM, Ogden AM, Siegel BW, et al: Rapid down regulation of beta-adrenoceptors by co-administration of desipramine and fluoxetine. Eur J Pharmacol 154(2):125–134, 1988 2465908

Basan A, Kissling W, Leucht S: Valproate as an adjunct to antipsychotics for schizophrenia: a systematic review of randomized trials. Schizophr Res 70(1):33–37, 2004 15246461

Bauer M, Dopfmer S: Lithium augmentation in treatment-resistant depression: meta-analysis of placebo-controlled studies. J Clin Psychopharmacol 19(5):427–434, 1999 10505584

Bauer M, Hellweg R, Gräf KJ, et al: Treatment of refractory depression with high-dose thyroxine. Neuropsychopharmacology 18(6):444–455, 1998 9571653

Bauer M, Zaninelli R, Müller-Oerlinghausen B, et al: Paroxetine and amitriptyline augmentation of lithium in the treatment of major depression: a double-blind study. J Clin Psychopharmacol 19(2):164–171, 1999 10211918

Bell IR, Cole JO: Fluoxetine induces elevation of desipramine level and exacerbation of geriatric nonpsychotic depression (letter). J Clin Psychopharmacol 8(6):447–448, 1988 3266222

Blier P, Bergeron R: Effectiveness of pindolol with selected antidepressant drugs in the treatment of major depression. J Clin Psychopharmacol 15(3):217–222, 1995 7636000

Blier P, Ward HE, Tremblay P, et al: Combination of antidepressant medications from treatment initiation for major depressive disorder: a double-blind randomized study. Am J Psychiatry 167(3):281–288, 2010 20008946

Bloch M, Schmidt PJ, Danaceau MA, et al: Dehydroepiandrosterone treatment of midlife dysthymia. Biol Psychiatry 45(12):1533–1541, 1999 10376113

Bodkin JA, Cohen BM, Salomon MS, et al: Treatment of negative symptoms in schizophrenia and schizoaffective disorder by selegiline augmentation of antipsychotic medication: a pilot study examining the role of dopamine. J Nerv Ment Dis 184(5):295–301, 1996 8627275

Bodkin JA, Lasser RA, Wines JD Jr, et al: Combining serotonin reuptake inhibitors and bupropion in partial responders to antidepressant monotherapy. J Clin Psychiatry 58(4):137–145, 1997 9164423

Bouwer C, Stein DJ: Buspirone is an effective augmenting agent of serotonin selective reuptake inhibitors in severe treatment-refractory depression. S Afr Med J 87(4, suppl):534–537, 540, 1997 9180827

Bowden CL, Singh V, Weisler R, et al: Lamotrigine vs. lamotrigine plus divalproex in randomized, placebo-controlled maintenance treatment for bipolar depression. Acta Psychiatr Scand 126(5):342–350, 2012 22708645

Boyer P, Lecrubier Y, Puech AJ, et al: Treatment of negative symptoms in schizophrenia with amisulpride. Br J Psychiatry 166(1):68–72, 1995 7894879

Bunevicius R, Kazanavicius G, Zalinkevicius R, et al: Effects of thyroxine as compared with thyroxine plus triiodothyronine in patients with hypothyroidism. N Engl J Med 340(6):424–429, 1999 9971866

Calabrese JR, Rapport DJ, Youngstrom EA, et al: New data on the use of lithium, divalproate, and lamotrigine in rapid cycling bipolar disorder. Eur Psychiatry 20(2):92–95, 2005 15797691

Carpenter LL, Jocic Z, Hall JM, et al: Mirtazapine augmentation in the treatment of refractory depression. J Clin Psychiatry 60(1):45–49, 1999 10074878

Carpenter LL, Yasmin S, Price LH: A double-blind, placebo-controlled study of antidepressant augmentation with mirtazapine. Biol Psychiatry 51(2):183–188, 2002 11822997

Casey DE, Daniel DG, Wassef AA, et al: Effect of divalproex combined with olanzapine or risperidone in patients with an acute exacerbation of schizophrenia. Neuropsychopharmacology 28(1):182–192, 2003 12496955

Cassano P, Lattanzi L, Fava M, et al: Ropinirole in treatment-resistant depression: a 16-week pilot study. Can J Psychiatry 50(6):357–360, 2005 15999953

Chan J, Sweeting M: Review: combination therapy with non-clozapine atypical antipsychotic medication: a review of current evidence. J Psychopharmacol 21(6):657–664, 2007 17092976

Chang JS, Ha KS, Young Lee K, et al: The effects of long-term clozapine add-on therapy on the rehospitalization rate and the mood polarity patterns in bipolar disorders. J Clin Psychiatry 67(3):461–467, 2006 16649834

Citrome L: Adjunctive lithium and anticonvulsants for the treatment of schizophrenia: what is the evidence? Expert Rev Neurother 9(1):55–71, 2009 19102669

Collins PJ, Larkin EP, Shubsachs AP: Lithium carbonate in chronic schizophrenia: a brief trial of lithium carbonate added to neuroleptics for treatment of resistant schizophrenic patients. Acta Psychiatr Scand 84(2):150–154, 1991 1683094

Coope J: Is oestrogen therapy effective in the treatment of menopausal depression? J R Coll Gen Pract 31(224):134–140, 1981 6268783

Cooper-Kazaz R, van der Deure WM, Medici M, et al: Preliminary evidence that a functional polymorphism in type 1 deiodinase is associated with enhanced potentiation of the antidepressant effect of sertraline by triiodothyronine. J Affect Disord 116(1–2):113–116, 2009 19064291

Correll CU, Rummel-Kluge C, Corves C, et al: Antipsychotic combinations vs monotherapy in schizophrenia: a meta-analysis of randomized controlled trials. Schizophr Bull 35(2):443–457, 2009 18417466

Corrigan MH, Denahan AQ, Wright CE, et al: Comparison of pramipexole, fluoxetine, and placebo in patients with major depression. Depress Anxiety 11(2):58–65, 2000 10812530

Crowe D, Collins JP, Rosse RB: Thyroid hormone supplementation of fluoxetine treatment. J Clin Psychopharmacol 10(2):150–151, 1990 2341594

DeBattista C: Pramipexole in the treatment of resistant depression. Presentation at the Annual Meeting of the New Clinical Drug Evaluation Unit (NCDEU), Boca Raton, FL, June 1997

DeBattista C, Solvason HB, Breen JA, et al: Pramipexole augmentation of a selective serotonin reuptake inhibitor in the treatment of depression. J Clin Psychopharmacol 20(2):274–275, 2000 10770475

DeBattista C, Solvason HB, Poirier J, et al: A prospective trial of bupropion SR augmentation of partial and non-responders to serotonergic antidepressants. J Clin Psychopharmacol 23(1):27–30, 2003 12544372

DeBattista C, Lembke A, Solvason HB, et al: A prospective trial of modafinil as an adjunctive treatment of major depression. J Clin Psychopharmacol 24(1):87–90, 2004 14709953

DeBattista C, Patkar P, Hawkins J: Ropinirole augmentation of standard antidepressants in the treatment of resistant depression. Presented at the 48th Annual Meeting of the New Clinical Drug Evaluation Unit (NCDEU), Session 1, Phoenix, AZ, May 2008

Decina P, Mukherjee S, Bocola V, et al: Adjunctive trazodone in the treatment of negative symptoms of schizophrenia. Hosp Community Psychiatry 45(12):1220–1223, 1994 7868106

Dehydroepiandrosterone (DHEA). Med Lett Drugs Ther 38(985):91–92, 1996 8874392

Dé Montigny C, Grunberg F, Mayer A, et al: Lithium induces rapid relief of depression in tricyclic antidepressant drug non-responders. Br J Psychiatry 138:252–256, 1981 7272619

Dennis CL, Ross LE, Herxheimer A: Oestrogens and progestins for preventing and treating postpartum depression. Cochrane Database Syst Rev 2008(4):CD001690, 2008 18843619

Di Iorio G, Baroni G, Lorusso M, et al: Efficacy of memantine in schizophrenic patients: a systematic review. J Amino Acids 2017:7021071, 2017 28243470

Eden Evins A, Demopulos C, Yovel I, et al: Inositol augmentation of lithium or valproate for bipolar depression. Bipolar Disord 8(2):168–174, 2006 16542187

Fatemi SH, Emamian ES, Kist DA: Venlafaxine and bupropion combination therapy in a case of treatment-resistant depression. Ann Pharmacother 33(6):701–703, 1999 10410184

Fava M, Rosenbaum JF, McGrath PJ, et al: Lithium and tricyclic augmentation of fluoxetine treatment for resistant major depression: a double-blind, controlled study. Am J Psychiatry 151(9):1372–1374, 1994 8067495

Fava M, Thase ME, DeBattista C, et al: Modafinil augmentation of selective serotonin reuptake inhibitor therapy in MDD partial responders with persistent fatigue and sleepiness. Ann Clin Psychiatry 19(3):153–159, 2007 17729016

Fawcett J, Kravitz HM, Zajecka JM, et al: CNS stimulant potentiation of monoamine oxidase inhibitors in treatment-refractory depression. J Clin Psychopharmacol 11(2):127–132, 1991 2056139

Ferraro L, Antonelli T, O'Connor WT, et al: Modafinil: an antinarcoleptic drug with a different neurochemical profile to d-amphetamine and dopamine uptake blockers. Biol Psychiatry 42(12):1181–1183, 1997 9426889

Fritze J, Beneke M, Lanczik M, et al: Carbamazepine as adjunct or alternative to lithium in the prophylaxis of recurrent affective disorders. Pharmacopsychiatry 27(5):181–185, 1994 7838887

Gallego JA, Bonetti J, Zhang J, et al: Prevalence and correlates of antipsychotic polypharmacy: a systematic review and meta-regression of global and regional trends from the 1970s to 2009. Schizophr Res 138(1):18–28, 2012 22534420

Gao K, Kemp DE, Wang Z, et al: Predictors of non-stabilization during the combination therapy of lithium and divalproex in rapid cycling bipolar disorder: a post-hoc analysis of two studies. Psychopharmacol Bull 43(1):23–38, 2010 20581798

Garlow SJ, Dunlop BW, Ninan PT, et al: The combination of triiodothyronine (T3) and sertraline is not superior to sertraline monotherapy in the treatment of major depressive disorder. J Psychiatr Res 46(11):1406–1413, 2012 22964160

Geller B, Luby JL, Joshi P, et al: A randomized controlled trial of risperidone, lithium, or divalproex sodium for initial treatment of bipolar I disorder, manic or mixed phase, in children and adolescents. Arch Gen Psychiatry 69(5):515–528, 2012 22213771

Geretsegger C, Bitterlich W, Stelzig R, et al: Paroxetine with pindolol augmentation: a double-blind, randomized, placebo-controlled study in depressed in-patients. Eur Neuropsychopharmacol 18(2):141–146, 2008 18054209

Ghaemi SN, Katzow JJ, Desai SP, et al: Gabapentin treatment of mood disorders: a preliminary study. J Clin Psychiatry 59(8):426–429, 1998 9721823

Goddard AW, Brouette T, Almai A, et al: Early coadministration of clonazepam with sertraline for panic disorder. Arch Gen Psychiatry 58(7):681–686, 2001 11448376

Godfrey PS, Toone BK, Carney MW, et al: Enhancement of recovery from psychiatric illness by methylfolate. Lancet 336(8712):392–395, 1990 1974941

Goff DC, Midha KK, Sarid-Segal O, et al: A placebo-controlled trial of fluoxetine added to neuroleptic in patients with schizophrenia. Psychopharmacology (Berl) 117(4):417–423, 1995 7604142

Goff DC, Tsai G, Manoach DS, et al: D-cycloserine added to clozapine for patients with schizophrenia. Am J Psychiatry 153(12):1628–1630, 1996 8942463

Goff DC, Henderson DC, Evins AE, et al: A placebo-controlled crossover trial of D-cycloserine added to clozapine in patients with schizophrenia. Biol Psychiatry 45(4):512–514, 1999a 10071726

Goff DC, Tsai G, Levitt J, et al: A placebo-controlled trial of D-cycloserine added to conventional neuroleptics in patients with schizophrenia. Arch Gen Psychiatry 56(1):21–27, 1999b 9892252

Goff DC, Keefe R, Citrome L, et al: Lamotrigine as add-on therapy in schizophrenia: results of 2 placebo-controlled trials. J Clin Psychopharmacol 27(6):582–589, 2007 18004124

Goh KK, Chen CH, Chiu YH, et al: Lamotrigine augmentation in treatment-resistant unipolar depression: a comprehensive meta-analysis of efficacy and safety. J Psychopharmacol 33(6):700–713, 2019 31081449

Goldberg JF, Burdick KE, Endick CJ: Preliminary randomized, double-blind, placebo-controlled trial of pramipexole added to mood stabilizers for treatment-resistant bipolar depression. Am J Psychiatry 161(3):564–566, 2004 14992985

Goldman MB, Janecek HM: Adjunctive fluoxetine improves global function in chronic schizophrenia. J Neuropsychiatry Clin Neurosci 2(4):429–431, 1990 1983785

Goodwin FK, Prange AJ Jr, Post RM, et al: Potentiation of antidepressant effects by L-triiodothyronine in tricyclic nonresponders. Am J Psychiatry 139(1):34–38, 1982 7055275

Grosso G, Pajak A, Marventano S, et al: Role of omega-3 fatty acids in the treatment of depressive disorders: a comprehensive meta-analysis of randomized clinical trials. PLoS One 9(5):e96905, 2014 24805797

Gupta S, Masand P, Tanquary JF: Thyroid hormone supplementation of fluoxetine in the treatment of major depression. Br J Psychiatry 159:866–867, 1991 1790460

Hatta K, Ito H: Strategies for early non-response to antipsychotic drugs in the treatment of acute-phase schizophrenia. Clin Psychopharmacol Neurosci 12(1):1–7, 2014 24851115

Helfer B, Samara MT, Huhn M, et al: Efficacy and safety of antidepressants added to antipsychotics for schizophrenia: a systematic review and meta-analysis. Am J Psychiatry 173(9):876–886, 2016 27282362

Heresco-Levy U, Javitt DC, Ermilov M, et al: Efficacy of high-dose glycine in the treatment of enduring negative symptoms of schizophrenia. Arch Gen Psychiatry 56(1):29–36, 1999 9892253

Heresco-Levy U, Gelfin G, Bloch B, et al: A randomized add-on trial of high-dose D-cycloserine for treatment-resistant depression. Int J Neuropsychopharmacol 16(3):501–506, 2013 23174090

Joffe RT: Triiodothyronine potentiation of fluoxetine in depressed patients. Can J Psychiatry 37(1):48–50, 1992 1551045

Joffe RT, Schuller DR: An open study of buspirone augmentation of serotonin reuptake inhibitors in refractory depression. J Clin Psychiatry 54(7):269–271, 1993 8335654

Joffe RT, Singer W: Thyroid hormone potentiation of antidepressants. Neuroendocrinology Letters (St. Michael's Hospital) 9:172, 1987

Joffe RT, Levitt AJ, Bagby RM, et al: Predictors of response to lithium and triiodothyronine augmentation of antidepressants in tricyclic non-responders. Br J Psychiatry 163:574–578, 1993 8298824

Joffe RT, Sokolov ST, Levitt AJ: Lithium and triiodothyronine augmentation of antidepressants. Can J Psychiatry 51(12):791–793, 2006 17168254

Johns CA, Thompson JW: Adjunctive treatments in schizophrenia: pharmacotherapies and electroconvulsive therapy. Schizophr Bull 21(4):607–619, 1995 8749888

Juruena MF, Ottoni GL, Machado-Vieira R, et al: Bipolar I and II disorder residual symptoms: oxcarbazepine and carbamazepine as add-on treatment to lithium in a double-blind, randomized trial. Prog Neuropsychopharmacol Biol Psychiatry 33(1):94–99, 2009 19007842

Katagiri H, Tohen M, McDonnell DP, et al: Efficacy and safety of olanzapine for treatment of patients with bipolar depression: Japanese subpopulation analysis of a randomized, double-blind, placebo-controlled study. BMC Psychiatry 13:138, 2013 23672672

Katona CL, Abou-Saleh MT, Harrison DA, et al: Placebo-controlled trial of lithium augmentation of fluoxetine and lofepramine. Br J Psychiatry 166(1):80–86, 1995 7894881

Keck PE: A randomized, placebo-controlled trial of olanzapine and olanzapine-fluoxetine combination in the treatment of bipolar depression. Presentation at the 155th Annual Meeting of the American Psychiatric Association, Philadelphia, PA, May 2002

Kelly DL, Buchanan RW, Boggs DL, et al: A randomized double-blind trial of atomoxetine for cognitive impairments in 32 people with schizophrenia. J Clin Psychiatry 70(4):518–525, 2009 19358788

Kemp DE, Gao K, Ganocy SJ, et al: A 6-month, double-blind, maintenance trial of lithium monotherapy versus the combination of lithium and divalproex for rapid-cycling bipolar disorder and co-occurring substance abuse or dependence. J Clin Psychiatry 70(1):113–121, 2009 19192457

Ketter TA, Wang PW, Chandler RA, et al: Adjunctive aripiprazole in treatment-resistant bipolar depression. Ann Clin Psychiatry 18(3):169–172, 2006 16923655

Kinon BJ, Chen L, Ascher-Svanum H, et al: Early response to antipsychotic drug therapy as a clinical marker of subsequent response in the treatment of schizophrenia. Neuropsychopharmacology 35(2):581–590, 2010 19890258

Kirsch MA, Louie AK: Combination treatment with venlafaxine and bupropion. Am J Psychiatry 156(3):494, 1999 10080572

Kramlinger KG, Post RM: Addition of lithium carbonate to carbamazepine: hematological and thyroid effects. Am J Psychiatry 147(5):615–620, 1990 2109539

Landén M, Björling G, Agren H, et al: A randomized, double-blind, placebo-controlled trial of buspirone in combination with an SSRI in patients with treatment-refractory depression. J Clin Psychiatry 59(12):664–668, 1998 9921700

Levine J, Barak Y, Gonzalves M, et al: Double-blind, controlled trial of inositol treatment of depression. Am J Psychiatry 152(5):792–794, 1995 7726322

Levine J, Mishori A, Susnosky M, et al: Combination of inositol and serotonin reuptake inhibitors in the treatment of depression. Biol Psychiatry 45(3):270–273, 1999 10023500

Lipinski JF, Pope HG Jr: Possible synergistic action between carbamazepine and lithium carbonate in the treatment of three acutely manic patients. Am J Psychiatry 139(7):948–949, 1982 6807113

Llorca PM, Wolf MA, Lançon C, et al: Comparative efficacy of bromocriptine, carbamazepine and cyproheptadine with neuroleptics in 24 refractory chronic schizophrenic patients [in French]. Encephale 19(5):565–571, 1993 8306925

Loebel A, Cucchiaro J, Silva R, et al: Lurasidone as adjunctive therapy with lithium or valproate for the treatment of bipolar I depression: a randomized, double-blind, placebo-controlled study. Am J Psychiatry 171(2):169–177, 2014 24170221

Martín Muñoz JC, Moriñigo Domínguez AV, Mateo Martín I, et al: Carbamazepine: an efficient adjuvant treatment in schizophrenia [in Spanish]. Actas Luso Esp Neurol Psiquiatr Cienc Afines 20(1):11–16, 1992 1502960

McAskill R, Mir S, Taylor D: Pindolol augmentation of antidepressant therapy. Br J Psychiatry 173:203–208, 1998 9926094

McGrath PJ, Stewart JW, Fava M, et al: Tranylcypromine versus venlafaxine plus mirtazapine following three failed antidepressant medication trials for depression: a STAR*D report. Am J Psychiatry 163(9):1531–1541, 2006 16946177

Michelson D, Aller AA, Amsterdam JD, et al: Addition of atomoxetine for depression incompletely responsive to sertraline: a randomized, double-blind, placebo-controlled study, in Syllabus and Proceedings Summary, American Psychiatric Association Annual Meeting, Toronto, ON, Canada, May 20–25, 2006, p 74

Mohamed S, Johnson GR, Chen P, et al: Effect of antidepressant switching vs augmentation on remission among patients with major depressive disorder unresponsive to antidepressant treatment: the VAST-D randomized clinical trial. JAMA 318(2):132–145, 2017 28697253

Montgomery P, Richardson AJ: Omega-3 fatty acids for bipolar disorder. Cochrane Database Syst Rev 2008(2):CD005169, 2008 18425912

Montgomery SA: Selectivity of antidepressants and resistant depression, in Advances in Neuropsychiatry and Psychopharmacology, Vol 2: Refractory Depression. Edited by Amsterdam JD. New York, Raven, 1991, pp 93–104

Morera AL, Barreiro P, Cano-Munoz JL: Risperidone and clozapine combination for the treatment of refractory schizophrenia. Acta Psychiatr Scand 99(4):305–306 [discussion 306–307], 1999 10223435

Muti M, Del Grande C, Musetti L, et al: Prescribing patterns of lithium or lithium+valproate in manic or mixed episodes: a naturalistic study. Int Clin Psychopharmacol 28(6):305–311, 2013 23873290

Nelson JC, Price LH: Lithium or desipramine augmentation of fluoxetine treatment. Am J Psychiatry 152(10):1538–1539, 1995 7573606

Nelson JC, Mazure CM, Jatlow PI, et al: Combining norepinephrine and serotonin reuptake inhibition mechanisms for treatment of depression: a double-blind, randomized study. Biol Psychiatry 55(3):296–300, 2004 14744472

Nemeroff CB, Evans DL, Gyulai L, et al: Double-blind, placebo-controlled comparison of imipramine and paroxetine in the treatment of bipolar depression. Am J Psychiatry 158(6):906–912, 2001 11384898

Nierenberg AA, Keck PE Jr: Management of monoamine oxidase inhibitor-associated insomnia with trazodone. J Clin Psychopharmacol 9(1):42–45, 1989 2708555

Nierenberg AA, Price LH, Charney DS, et al: After lithium augmentation: a retrospective follow-up of patients with antidepressant-refractory depression. J Affect Disord 18(3):167–175, 1990 2139061

Nierenberg AA, Cole JO, Glass L: Possible trazodone potentiation of fluoxetine: a case series. J Clin Psychiatry 53(3):83–85, 1992 1548249

Nierenberg AA, Adler LA, Peselow E, et al: Trazodone for antidepressant-associated insomnia. Am J Psychiatry 151(7):1069–1072, 1994 8010365

Nierenberg AA, Fava M, Trivedi MH, et al: A comparison of lithium and T(3) augmentation following two failed medication treatments for depression: a STAR*D report. Am J Psychiatry 163(9):1519–1530, quiz 1665, 2006a 16946176

Nierenberg AA, Ostacher MJ, Calabrese JR, et al: Treatment-resistant bipolar depression: a STEP-BD equipoise randomized effectiveness trial of antidepressant augmentation with lamotrigine, inositol, or risperidone. Am J Psychiatry 163(2):210–216, 2006b 16449473

Ouyang WC, Hsu MC, Yeh IN, et al: Efficacy and safety of combination of risperidone and haloperidol with divalproate in patients with acute mania. Int J Psychiatry Clin Pract 16(3):178–188, 2012 22404731

Oya K, Kishi T, Iwata N: Efficacy and tolerability of minocycline augmentation therapy in schizophrenia: a systematic review and meta-analysis of randomized controlled trials. Hum Psychopharmacol 29(5):483–491, 2014 25087702

Oya K, Matsuda Y, Matsunaga S, et al: Efficacy and safety of oxytocin augmentation therapy for schizophrenia: an updated systematic review and meta-analysis of randomized, placebo-controlled trials. Eur Arch Psychiatry Clin Neurosci 266(5):439–450, 2016 26303414

Papakostas GI, Cooper-Kazaz R, Appelhof BC, et al: Simultaneous initiation (coinitiation) of pharmacotherapy with triiodothyronine and a selective serotonin reuptake inhibitor for major depressive disorder: a quantitative synthesis of double-blind studies. Int Clin Psychopharmacol 24(1):19–25, 2009 19092448

Papakostas GI, Clain A, Ameral VE, et al: Fluoxetine-clonazepam cotherapy for anxious depression: an exploratory, post-hoc analysis of a randomized, double blind study. Int Clin Psychopharmacol 25(1):17–21, 2010 19898245

Papakostas GI, Shelton RC, Zajecka JM, et al: L-methylfolate as adjunctive therapy for SSRI-resistant major depression: results of two randomized, double-blind, parallel-sequential trials. Am J Psychiatry 169(12):1267–1274, 2012 23212058

Papakostas GI, Shelton RC, Zajecka JM, et al: Effect of adjunctive L-methylfolate 15 mg among inadequate responders to SSRIs in depressed patients who were stratified by biomarker levels and genotype: results from a randomized clinical trial. J Clin Psychiatry 75(8):855–863, 2014 24813065

Parmentier T, Sienaert P: The use of triiodothyronine (T3) in the treatment of bipolar depression: a review of the literature. J Affect Disord 229:410–414, 2018 29331701

Perugi G, Toni C, Ruffolo G, et al: Clinical experience using adjunctive gabapentin in treatment-resistant bipolar mixed states. Pharmacopsychiatry 32(4):136–141, 1999 10505483

Peselow ED, Fieve RR, Difiglia C, et al: Lithium prophylaxis of bipolar illness: the value of combination treatment. Br J Psychiatry 164(2):208–214, 1994 7909713

Pope HG Jr, McElroy SL, Nixon RA: Possible synergism between fluoxetine and lithium in refractory depression. Am J Psychiatry 145(10):1292–1294, 1988 3262313

Pope HG Jr, Cohane GH, Kanayama G, et al: Testosterone gel supplementation for men with refractory depression: a randomized, placebo-controlled trial. Am J Psychiatry 160(1):105–111, 2003 12505808

Porcelli S, Balzarro B, Serretti A: Clozapine resistance: augmentation strategies. Eur Neuropsychopharmacol 22(3):165–182, 2012 21906915

Portella MJ, de Diego-Adeliño J, Puigdemont D, et al: Pindolol augmentation enhances response outcomes in first depressive episodes. Eur Neuropsychopharmacol 19(7):516–519, 2009 19419845

Price LH, Conwell Y, Nelson JC: Lithium augmentation of combined neuroleptic-tricyclic treatment in delusional depression. Am J Psychiatry 140(3):318–322, 1983 6131612

Price LH, Charney DS, Heninger GR: Efficacy of lithium-tranylcypromine treatment in refractory depression. Am J Psychiatry 142(5):619–623, 1985 3920923

Rabkin JG, McElhiney MC, Rabkin R, et al: Placebo-controlled trial of dehydroepiandrosterone (DHEA) for treatment of nonmajor depression in patients with HIV/AIDS. Am J Psychiatry 163(1):59–66, 2006 16390890

Rasgon NL, Dunkin J, Fairbanks L, et al: Estrogen and response to sertraline in postmenopausal women with major depressive disorder: a pilot study. J Psychiatr Res 41(3–4):338–343, 2007 16697413

Raynaud JP: Prostate cancer risk in testosterone-treated men. J Steroid Biochem Mol Biol 102(1–5):261–266, 2006 17113983

Ribot C, Tremollieres F, Pouilles JM, et al: Bone mineral density and thyroid hormone therapy. Clin Endocrinol (Oxf) 33(2):143–153, 1990 2225474

Rosse RB, Theut SK, Banay-Schwartz M, et al: Glycine adjuvant therapy to conventional neuroleptic treatment in schizophrenia: an open-label, pilot study. Clin Neuropharmacol 12(5):416–424, 1989 2611765

Rosse RB, Fay-McCarthy M, Kendrick K, et al: D-cycloserine adjuvant therapy to molindone in the treatment of schizophrenia. Clin Neuropharmacol 19(5):444–450, 1996 8889288

Rush AJ, Trivedi MH, Stewart JW, et al: Combining Medications to Enhance Depression Outcomes (CO-MED): acute and long-term outcomes of a single-blind randomized study. Am J Psychiatry 168(7):689–701, 2011 21536692

Saavedra-Velez C, Yusim A, Anbarasan D, et al: Modafinil as an adjunctive treatment of sedation, negative symptoms, and cognition in schizophrenia: a critical review. J Clin Psychiatry 70(1):104–112, 2009 19026265

Sachs GS, Nierenberg AA, Calabrese JR, et al: Effectiveness of adjunctive antidepressant treatment for bipolar depression. N Engl J Med 356(17):1711–1722, 2007 17392295

Sagud M, Vuksan-Ćusa B, Zivković M, et al: Antipsychotics: to combine or not to combine? Psychiatr Danub 25(3):306–310, 2013 24048402

Samara MT, Leucht C, Leeflang MM, et al: Early improvement as a predictor of later response to antipsychotics in schizophrenia: a diagnostic test review. Am J Psychiatry 172(7):617–629, 2015 26046338

Schmidt PJ, Daly RC, Bloch M, et al: Dehydroepiandrosterone monotherapy in midlife-onset major and minor depression. Arch Gen Psychiatry 62(2):154–162, 2005 15699292

Schneider LS, Small GW, Hamilton SH, et al: Estrogen replacement and response to fluoxetine in a multicenter geriatric depression trial. Am J Geriatr Psychiatry 5(2):97–106, 1997 9106373

Schneider LS, Small GW, Clary CM: Estrogen replacement therapy and antidepressant response to sertraline in older depressed women. Am J Geriatr Psychiatry 9(4):393–399, 2001 11739065

Schulz SC, Thompson PA, Jacobs M, et al: Lithium augmentation fails to reduce symptoms in poorly responsive schizophrenic outpatients. J Clin Psychiatry 60(6):366–372, 1999 10401914

Seidman SN, Spatz E, Rizzo C, et al: Testosterone replacement therapy for hypogonadal men with major depressive disorder: a randomized, placebo-controlled clinical trial. J Clin Psychiatry 62(6):406–412, 2001 11465516

Seidman SN, Miyazaki M, Roose SP: Intramuscular testosterone supplementation to selective serotonin reuptake inhibitor in treatment-resistant depressed men: randomized placebo-controlled clinical trial. J Clin Psychopharmacol 25(6):584–588, 2005 16282843

Sherwin BB: Estrogen in refractory depression, in Advances in Neuropsychiatry and Psychopharmacology, Vol 2: Refractory Depression. Edited by Amsterdam JD. New York, Raven, 1991, pp 209–218

Sichel DA, Cohen LS, Robertson LM, et al: Prophylactic estrogen in recurrent postpartum affective disorder. Biol Psychiatry 38(12):814–818, 1995 8750040

Silver H, Nassar A: Fluvoxamine improves negative symptoms in treated chronic schizophrenia: an add-on double-blind, placebo-controlled study. Biol Psychiatry 31(7):698–704, 1992 1599987

Siskind DJ, Lee M, Ravindran A, et al: Augmentation strategies for clozapine refractory schizophrenia: a systematic review and meta-analysis. Aust N Z J Psychiatry 52(8):751–767, 2018 29732913

Smith WT, Londborg PD, Glaudin V, et al: Short-term augmentation of fluoxetine with clonazepam in the treatment of depression: a double-blind study. Am J Psychiatry 155(10):1339–1345, 1998 9766764

Soares CN, Almeida OP, Joffe H, et al: Efficacy of estradiol for the treatment of depressive disorders in perimenopausal women: a double-blind, randomized, placebo-controlled trial. Arch Gen Psychiatry 58(6):529–534, 2001 11386980

Sokolov ST, Levitt AJ, Joffe RT: Thyroid hormone levels before unsuccessful antidepressant therapy are associated with later response to T3 augmentation. Psychiatry Res 69(2–3):203–206, 1997 9109188

Spoov J, Lahdelma L: Should thyroid augmentation precede lithium augmentation: a pilot study. J Affect Disord 49(3):235–239, 1998 9629954

Stamm TJ, Lewitzka U, Sauer C, et al: Supraphysiologic doses of levothyroxine as adjunctive therapy in bipolar depression: a randomized, double-blind, placebo-controlled study. J Clin Psychiatry 75(2):162–168, 2014 24345793

Steckler TL: Lithium- and carbamazepine-associated sinus node dysfunction: nine-year experience in a psychiatric hospital. J Clin Psychopharmacol 14(5):336–339, 1994 7806689

Stoll AL, Locke CA, Marangell LB, et al: Omega-3 fatty acids and bipolar disorder: a review. Prostaglandins Leukot Essent Fatty Acids 60(5–6):329–337, 1999 10471117

Suppes T, Vieta E, Liu S, et al: Maintenance treatment for patients with bipolar I disorder: results from a North American study of quetiapine in combination with lithium or divalproex (Trial 127). Am J Psychiatry 166(4):476–488, 2009 19289454

Szegedi A, Verweij P, van Duijnhoven W, et al: Meta-analyses of the efficacy of asenapine for acute schizophrenia: comparisons with placebo and other antipsychotics. J Clin Psychiatry 73(12):1533–1540, 2012 23290326

Targum SD, Greenberg RD, Harmon RL, et al: Thyroid hormone and the TRH stimulation test in refractory depression. J Clin Psychiatry 45(8):345–346, 1984 6746579

Thase ME, Howland RH, Friedman ES: Treating antidepressant nonresponders with augmentation strategies: an overview. J Clin Psychiatry 59(5 suppl):5–12 [discussion 13–15], 1998

Tiihonen J, Halonen P, Wahlbeck K, et al: Topiramate add-on in treatment-resistant schizophrenia: a randomized, double-blind, placebo-controlled, crossover trial. J Clin Psychiatry 66(8):1012–1015, 2005 16086616

Tiihonen J, Wahlbeck K, Kiviniemi V: The efficacy of lamotrigine in clozapine-resistant schizophrenia: a systematic review and meta-analysis. Schizophr Res 109(1–3):10–14, 2009 19186030

Tohen M, Bowden CL, Smulevich AB, et al: Olanzapine plus carbamazepine v. carbamazepine alone in treating manic episodes. Br J Psychiatry 192(2):135–143, 2008 18245032

Trivedi MH, Fava M, Wisniewski SR, et al: Medication augmentation after the failure of SSRIs for depression. N Engl J Med 354(12):1243–1252, 2006 16554526

Tsai G, Yang P, Chung LC, et al: D-serine added to antipsychotics for the treatment of schizophrenia. Biol Psychiatry 44(11):1081–1089, 1998 9836012

Tsai GE, Yang P, Chung LC, et al: D-serine added to clozapine for the treatment of schizophrenia. Am J Psychiatry 156(11):1822–1825, 1999 10553752

Vieta E, Manuel Goikolea J, Martínez-Arán A, et al: A double-blind, randomized, placebo-controlled, prophylaxis study of adjunctive gabapentin for bipolar disorder. J Clin Psychiatry 67(3):473–477, 2006 16649836

Walshaw PD, Gyulai L, Bauer M, et al: Adjunctive thyroid hormone treatment in rapid cycling bipolar disorder: a double-blind placebo-controlled trial of levothyroxine (L-T4) and triiodothyronine (T3). Bipolar Disord 20(7):594–603, 2018 29869405

Wehr TA, Goodwin FK: Rapid cycling in manic-depressives induced by tricyclic antidepressants. Arch Gen Psychiatry 36(5):555–559, 1979 435015

Wehr TA, Sack DA, Rosenthal NE, et al: Rapid cycling affective disorder: contributing factors and treatment responses in 51 patients. Am J Psychiatry 145(2):179–184, 1988 3341463

Weilburg JB, Rosenbaum JF, Biederman J, et al: Fluoxetine added to non-MAOI antidepressants converts nonresponders to responders: a preliminary report. J Clin Psychiatry 50(12):447–449, 1989 2600061

Wharton RN, Perel JM, Dayton PG, et al: A potential clinical use for methylphenidate with tricyclic antidepressants. Am J Psychiatry 127(12):1619–1625, 1971 4998422

Whybrow PC: The therapeutic use of triiodothyronine and high dose thyroxine in psychiatric disorder. Acta Med Austriaca 21(2):47–52, 1994 7998482

Wijkstra J, Lijmer J, Balk FJ, et al: Pharmacological treatment for unipolar psychotic depression: systematic review and meta-analysis. Br J Psychiatry 188:410–415, 2006 16648526

Wilson WH: Addition of lithium to haloperidol in non-affective, antipsychotic nonresponsive schizophrenia: a double blind, placebo controlled, parallel design clinical trial. Psychopharmacology (Berl) 111(3):359–366, 1993 7870975

Wolkowitz OM, Reus VI, Roberts E, et al: Dehydroepiandrosterone (DHEA) treatment of depression. Biol Psychiatry 41(3):311–318, 1997 9024954

Woo YS, Bahk WM, Chung MY, et al: Aripiprazole plus divalproex for recently manic or mixed patients with bipolar I disorder: a 6-month, randomized, placebo-controlled, double-blind maintenance trial. Hum Psychopharmacol 26(8):543–553, 2011 22134973

Young LT, Robb JC, Hasey GM, et al: Gabapentin as an adjunctive treatment in bipolar disorder. J Affect Disord 55(1):73–77, 1999 10512610

Young LT, Joffe RT, Robb JC, et al: Double-blind comparison of addition of a second mood stabilizer versus an antidepressant to an initial mood stabilizer for treatment of patients with bipolar depression. Am J Psychiatry 157(1):124–126, 2000 10618026

Zanardi R, Franchini L, Serretti A, et al: Venlafaxine versus fluvoxamine in the treatment of delusional depression: a pilot double-blind controlled study. J Clin Psychiatry 61(1):26–29, 2000 10695642

Zarate CA Jr, Payne JL, Singh J, et al: Pramipexole for bipolar II depression: a placebo-controlled proof of concept study. Biol Psychiatry 56(1):54–60, 2004 15219473

Zarrouf FA, Artz S, Griffith J, et al: Testosterone and depression: systematic review and meta-analysis. J Psychiatr Pract 15(4):289–305, 2009 19625884

Zhang ZJ, Kang WH, Li Q, et al: Beneficial effects of ondansetron as an adjunct to haloperidol for chronic, treatment-resistant schizophrenia: a double-blind, randomized, placebo-controlled study. Schizophr Res 88(1–3):102–110, 2006 16959472

10

Emergency Department Treatment

Psychiatrists see patients in crisis not only in emergency departments but also (occasionally) in their offices, during home visits, or in medical or nursing home settings. In this chapter, we address some of the more common emergencies facing the clinical psychiatrist.

In emergency situations, psychiatrists are often faced with the diagnosis and treatment of patients presenting with psychiatric symptoms of sudden or presumed recent onset. Phenomenologically, these symptoms can be crudely subdivided into the following types:

1. Agitation and violent behavior, with or without signs of alcohol or other intoxication
2. Depression with suicidal ideation, with or without a recent suicide attempt
3. Acute psychotic episodes, usually with overt thought disorder, paranoid ideation, and/or hallucinations and marked fear or anger

4. Delirium manifesting with disorientation and confusion, with or without psychotic symptoms

5. Severe anxiety without psychotic symptoms but often with physical symptoms

6. Psychogenic stupor or catatonia

In some of these situations, a history can be obtained either from the patient or from friends or relatives. Sometimes the patient may be carrying enough identification that friends or relatives can be rapidly contacted. In the worst situation, the psychiatrist has little to go on besides the patient's behavior and a brief physical examination. When the patient is severely disturbed, obtunded, or confused; can give no history; and has no diagnostic stigmata (e.g., needle tracks, obvious atropine-like toxic signs), hospitalization without specific drug treatment, or at least medical evaluation with toxic screens, electrocardiogram, and so forth in a competent medical emergency facility, is indicated.

We stress the importance of trying to ascertain which drugs the patient has been taking or may have been taking before pharmacotherapy is begun. This was particularly the case in earlier times when the various classes of agents used carried greater risks of severe reactions. For example, deaths have occurred when meperidine was given to patients who were already taking monoamine oxidase inhibitors (MAOIs). Adding sedative drugs in a patient already intoxicated on alcohol or other sedative drugs is unwise. Adding an antipsychotic in a patient with possible neuroleptic malignant syndrome (NMS) is obviously contraindicated. Similarly, drugs must be chosen carefully if a tricyclic antidepressant (TCA) overdose may have affected cardiac function. In short, when the patient may have been taking preexisting medication or may have overdosed on an unknown drug, it is better to avoid medication until the situation can be clarified.

Agitation and Violence

Few emergency department encounters are more difficult than having to contend with an agitated, violent patient. Individuals representing many diagnostic groups may present to the emergency department in an agitated, violent state. In some surveys, as many as 80% of teaching hospital emergency departments reported patient assaults of staff members, and at least 25% of these emergency departments had to restrain patients daily (Aljohani et al. 2021; Lavoie et al. 1988). Many assaults are by family members or associates of patients, rather than patients themselves. However, violence from agitated patients is extremely common. It is difficult to ascertain how frequently assaults occur by patients against medical personnel because the vast majority of these assaults are not reported (Barlow and Rizzo 1997). Violence often represents an attempt by the patient to assert control in the context of feeling frightened and helpless.

In nonpsychotic patients presenting to emergency departments with angry tantrums, as well as in similar patients with severe anxiety that seems to be based on family fights or other interpersonal crises, supportive listening, reassurance, and the elixir of time often enable the patient to gradually become calm and reasonable without specific medication. Sedative- or alcohol-related angry intoxication also often passes gradually with time, talk, and external limit setting.

From the legal perspective, use of external restraints is sometimes considered a less invasive intervention than the involuntary administration of psychotropic medications. No intervention is more effective for potentially violent patients than a sufficient show of force to restrain the patient, if necessary, along with calm reassurance. The use of restraints generally should be a last resort, when all less-restrictive options have been exhausted or are impractical. Thus, this option should be employed if the patient represents an imminent danger to themself or others. However, some patients are quite capable of exhausting or injuring themselves while in restraints. In these cases the addition of medications is frequently required.

A number of open-label studies have investigated the use of various psychotropic agents in the rapid tranquilization of agitated patients. Dr. William Dubin of Temple University used the term *rapid tranquilization* to describe the use of antipsychotics and benzodiazepines given every half-hour or hour to treat the target symptoms of agitation, motor excitement, tension, and hostility. This strategy has been studied with both psychotic and nonpsychotic patients. Although the strategy of rapid tranquilization as described by Dubin is more than 40 years old, emergency psychiatrists still tend to employ some variation of this strategy (Kim et al. 2021). There has been some movement toward using second-generation antipsychotics (SGAs) as first-line agents and a greater reliance on benzodiazepines in nonpsychotic conditions.

The typical rapid tranquilization approach employs an intramuscular route of administration for rapid absorption and increased bioavailability (Table 10–1). However, Dubin et al. (1985) suggested that oral concentrate forms of antipsychotics also provide rapid response and may decrease feelings of helplessness in an already vulnerable patient, relative to being approached with a needle. In a study of 159 agitated psychiatric patients who were randomly assigned to receive either intramuscular or oral concentrate forms of thiothixene, haloperidol, or thioridazine, there was a minimal time advantage to using the intramuscular route of administration, but fewer intramuscular doses were required to achieve a satisfactory response (Dubin et al. 1985). The SGAs also tend to be available in oral solution form, which may have similar advantages over intramuscular forms. In medical-surgical patients, the intravenous route of administration is also a common option. Möller et al. (1982) found that patients given intravenous haloperidol improved more rapidly in the first 3 hours than did patients taking oral haloperidol. However, after 3 hours there was no significant difference between the oral and intravenous haloperidol-treated groups. Several other open-label studies have confirmed the utility of intravenous haloperidol and benzodiazepines (lorazepam) in the management of agitated medical-surgical patients.

Haloperidol is still the most common first-generation antipsychotic (FGA) used for the management of acute agitation, but some emergency department doctors still regard droperidol as among the most effective agents for rapid tranquilization. In the past, shortages of droperidol have limited its availability, but it remains the drug of choice in some emergency departments for managing acute agitation. In a large study of 1,200 patients in the emergency department with acute agitation, intramuscular droperidol (average dose 5 mg) was as rapidly effective as intramuscular olanzapine, with a lower need for additional rescue medications (Cole et al. 2021). However, 6% of patients who received droperidol developed akithisia, versus 1% of olanzapine patients. In addition, droperidol may be more effective than either intramuscular ziprasidone or intramuscular lorazepam in managing acute agitation (Martel et al. 2021). Droperidol does have a black box warning about QTc prolongation, but this seems to be less of a problem with doses below 5 mg.

Intramuscular SGAs such as olanzapine, aripiprazole, and ziprasidone are being employed with increasing frequency relative to intramuscular FGAs such as haloperidol. However, there is little evidence that they are more effec-

Table 10–1. Medication options for rapid tranquilization of agitated patients (administered every 30–60 minutes)

Medication	Dose			Average total dose for tranquilization
	Intramuscular/IV	Oral	Inhalation	
Haloperidol	2.5–5 mg	5–10 mg		10–20 mg
Thiothixene	10–20 mg[a]	5–10 mg		15–30 mg
Droperidol	2.5–5 mg	Not available		5–20 mg
Loxapine	10–15 mg[a]	25 mg	10 mg/24 hr[b]	30–60 mg
				10 mg
Chlorpromazine	50 mg	100 mg		300–600 mg
Lorazepam	0.5–1 mg	1–2 mg		4–8 mg
Midazolam	0.5–1mg IV	NA		2.5 mg
Diazepam	Not applicable	5–10 mg		20–60 mg
Olanzapine	2.5–10 mg	2.5–5 mg		10–20 mg
Ziprasidone	10–20 mg	40–160 mg		10–20 mg
Aripiprazole	9.75 mg	10–30 mg		9.75–19.5 mg
Ketamine	1–5 mg/kg IM or IV	NA		5 mg/kg
Dexmedetomidine	1 μg/kg over 10 min	60–120 mg		240 mg

Note. NA=not available.
[a]No longer available in the United States.
[b]10-mg inhaler for single use; must be administered by health care provider.

tive than FGAs. Rather, the advantage of intramuscular SGAs is a reduced rate of acute extrapyramidal symptoms (EPS), especially akathisia and dystonic reactions. On the other hand, a significant disadvantage of the atypical intramuscular formulations is that they are substantially more costly than generic agents such as haloperidol. Intramuscular olanzapine has now been approved for use in treating agitation associated with psychosis. It has been studied in the acute management of schizophrenia, dementia, and bipolar disorder. In acutely agitated patients with dementia, olanzapine at 2.5 or 5 mg IM was significantly more effective than placebo in reducing agitation 2 and 24 hours postinjection; lorazepam at 1 mg was not (Meehan et al. 2002). In patients with schizophrenia, olanzapine at 5–10 mg IM was significantly more effective than placebo at 2 and 24 hours postinjection (Breier et al. 2001); similar data at 10–25 mg were observed in acutely manic patients (Meehan et al. 2001). The primary advantages of intramuscular olanzapine over intramuscular haloperidol are a faster onset of action and fewer EPS (Wright et al. 2003). The onset of action of intramuscular olanzapine is within 30 minutes, and minimal EPS have been reported. The most common side effects were somnolence and dizziness. Occasional mild hypotension and bradycardia have been reported. There is a black box warning on combined use of intramuscular lorazepam and olanzapine because of the risk of both sleepiness and cardiorespiratory depression (Garlow et al. 2017).

An injectable form of ziprasidone has been available since 2002. Ziprasidone has been evaluated in several double-blind trials in the treatment of acute agitation. Both 10 mg and 20 mg IM appear to be effective, but 2 mg IM was not effective. Like olanzapine, intramuscular ziprasidone has a low incidence of EPS. In studies of acute agitation in psychotic patients, dosages of 10–20 mg/day were as effective as haloperidol in treating agitation and more effective in treating psychosis. The most common side effects with intramuscular ziprasidone were headache, nausea, and somnolence.

Aripiprazole was the next SGA to be indicated in the treatment of acute agitation associated with bipolar disorder, schizoaffective disorder, and schizophrenia. Several studies of the acute effects of aripiprazole in the reduction of agitation have demonstrated the superiority of this agent to placebo and its equivalence to intramuscular haloperidol (see Andrezina et al. 2006a, 2006b). Intramuscular aripiprazole appears to produce EPS much less commonly than does intramuscular haloperidol, with about 2% of aripiprazole-treated patients experiencing akathisia and 1% experiencing dystonic reactions. It is likely, but untested, that repeated doses may increase the risk of EPS. Other side effects that were more commonly seen with intramuscular aripiprazole than with placebo include headache, somnolence, nausea, and dizziness.

An approved inhalant formulation of the FGA loxapine may offer some advantages for the agitated patient. Although patients may prefer an inhaler to a needle, the inhalation does require patient cooperation, which is not often possible with an agitated patient (see Chapter 4, "Antipsychotic Drugs"). The formulation (Adasuve) is prescribed in doses of 5 or 10 mg (Keating 2013).

For severely agitated or imminently violent patients, rapid tranquilization strategies employ antipsychotics every 30–60 minutes until the target symptoms of hostility, agitation, and assaultiveness are reduced. Most studies suggest that the typical dose of antipsychotics required is in the range of 300–600 mg of chlorpromazine, 10–20 mg of haloperidol, or 10–20 mg of olanzapine over a 2- to 4-hour period (see Table 10–1). The high-potency typical antipsychotics have the advantage of not producing significant adrenergic blockade in the acute setting. However, akathisia and dystonic reactions may be problematic, particularly in young males. We have found that alternating the antipsychotic with a benzodiazepine is also a sound strategy. In a common regimen, haloperidol 5 mg IM is alternated with lorazepam 1–2 mg IM every 30 minutes until tranquilization is achieved.

Lorazepam is the only benzodiazepine reliably absorbed from all routes of administration. However, for oral dosing, diazepam may offer the most rapid onset of action. The combination of benzodiazepines and antipsychotics offers several advantages. Frequently, lower doses of both classes of medications are sufficient when they are combined. The lower doses decrease the risks of side effects from either the benzodiazepines or the antipsychotics. Further, benzodiazepines may counter some antipsychotic side effects, including akathisia. Likewise, the combination with high-potency FGAs may reduce the excessive sedation associated with use of benzodiazepines alone. However, some data support the idea that benzodiazepines alone may be as effective as antipsychotics within the first 24 hours, even with floridly psychotic patients (Saklad et al. 1985).

For less severe acute agitation, especially in a nonpsychotic patient or when limited information is available, the use of benzodiazepines alone appears to be adequate. Lorazepam 1–2 mg PO every hour to a maximum of 10 mg or diazepam 5–10 mg every hour to a maximum of 60 mg is usually enough to calm the more moderately agitated patient.

A number of long-term strategies for the management of aggression in patients have been used. Mood-stabilizing agents such as lithium, carbamazepine, and valproate have proved useful in controlling aggressive, violent impulses in some patients. However, as indicated in Chapter 5 ("Mood Stabilizers"), controlled trial data on carbamazepine and valproate in both aggressive behavior and agitation have been mixed. The selective serotonin reuptake inhibitors (SSRIs) have been used with some success in studies of treating patients with aggressive personality disorders. Likewise, with long-term use, buspirone, propranolol, trazodone, and clozapine may all have a role in reducing aggression in some patients.

Ketamine for Rapid Tranquilization and Management of Acute Agitation

In some emergency situations both in the emergency department and in the field, intramuscular or intravenous ketamine has become favored over the use of antipsychotics for rapid tranquilization. The primary advantage of ketamine is the rapidity of onset. Whereas intramuscular and oral antipsychotics often take 30 minutes or more to achieve tranquilization, intramuscular or intravenous ketamine often takes as little to 2–5 minutes to achieve the same effects.

A systematic review and meta-analysis of 16 randomized controlled trials (RCTs) that evaluated the efficacy and safety of ketamine for acute agitation in the emergency department found that ketamine was more effective than placebo or other sedative agents in achieving rapid tranquilization, with no significant increase in adverse events. The study concluded that ketamine is a safe and effective option for managing acute agitation in the emergency department (Liu and Reid 2017). Similarly, a systematic review and meta-analysis of 10 RCTs that evaluated the use of ketamine for sedation in the ICU found that ketamine was effective in achieving deep sedation with minimal respiratory depression or hypotension, particularly in patients with refractory delirium or agitation (Beloucif et al. 2020). A randomized, double-blind, placebo-controlled trial of 68 patients with severe agitated behavior in the emergency department found that ketamine was more effective than placebo in achieving rapid tranquilization, with no significant increase in adverse events (Andolfatto et al. 2013).

The biggest challenge with ketamine has been respiratory depression. Although doses below 1 mg/kg are rarely a problem, anesthetic doses in the 2–5 mg/kg range have sometimes required intubation. Thus, unless experienced and qualified for moderate sedation, psychiatrists generally should not be using ketamine for the management of acute agitation.

Dexmedetomidine for the Management of Acute Agitation

Dexmedetomidine is a selective α_2-adrenergic receptor agonist that has been used in the acute management of psychiatric patients, particularly in the setting of agitated delirium, alcohol withdrawal, and sedation for procedural interventions. It was approved in 2022 for the acute management of agitation in patients with bipolar disorder and schizophrenia. It has been available as an intravenous formulation since 1999 for the management of agitation and delirium in mechanically ventilated ICU patients. Dexmedetomidine has several advantages over traditional sedatives, such as benzodiazepines and antipsychotics, including a reduced risk of respiratory depression, minimal effect on cognitive function, and shorter duration of action.

In a study of 380 patients with schizophrenia or schizoaffective disorder randomly assigned to active drug or placebo, Citrome and colleagues (2022) found that 120–180 µg of self-administered sublingual dexmedetomidine was effective at achieving control of agitation within 2 hours, with an onset of effect at 20 minutes. Similarly, in a group of 378 agitated bipolar patients randomly assigned to 120–180 µg of sublingual dexmedetomidine or placebo, dexmedetomidine showed control of the agitation starting at about 20 minutes (Preskorn et al. 2022).

The most common side effects of dexmedetomidine were somnolence, dry mouth, hypotension, and dizziness. At higher doses, oral hypoesthesia has been reported. Given the challenges of antipsychotics, having a sublingual or buccally administered drug that is rapidly active, does not cause EPS, and generally is better tolerated is a welcome addition for the management of acute agitation. However, sublingual self-administration does require a somewhat cooperative patient who is not going to swallow the medication, which would render it ineffective. Patients should not eat or drink for 15 minutes after sublingual administration or for an hour after buccal administration between the tongue and cheek.

Depression and Suicidality

Depressed suicidal patients, along with agitated patients, represent one of the most common and serious challenges confronted by the emergency department clinician. In many emergency departments, complaints of depression and suicidal ideation, with or without suicide attempts, represent the most frequent reason for psychiatric hospital admission. Predicting imminent suicide is sometimes not an easy matter, even for skilled psychiatrists. Many factors have been known to increase the risk of suicide, including advanced age, a diagnosis of major depression, male sex, concurrent alcohol use, a viable suicide plan, and a history of serious suicide attempts. The significant majority of the successful 30,000 or so suicides that occur in the United States annually involve white males older than 45. In addition, depression or alcohol is implicated in approximately 75% of all suicides (Bongar 1992). Fawcett et al. (1990) attempted to further elucidate factors that may increase the immediate risk of suicide; among these were global insomnia and severe anxiety (Table 10–2).

Suicidal depressed patients brought to an emergency department after suicide threats or nonharmful attempts present a real challenge to clinical judgment. The conservative course is to admit such patients to a secure inpatient unit. Occasionally, this may seem unwise or impractical. If the clinician can develop an alliance with and personally follow the patient, and/or if friends or relatives can reliably supervise the patient until the next appointment, the patient may be followed as an outpatient. In general, any patient with suicidal ideation or attempt and depression who is psychotic, who cannot attend to daily needs, who is acutely intoxicated, or about whose well-being the clinician has any significant doubt should be admitted and observed.

Very few somatic interventions work rapidly enough to be useful in the emergency setting. One exception is ketamine, an *N*-methyl-D-aspartate (NMDA) glutamatergic receptor antagonist that is an anesthesia agent and a potential drug of abuse. Intravenous ketamine at subanesthesia doses produces depersonalization, commonly acutely, but also produces an improvement in

Table 10–2. Short-term (6- to 12-month) risk factors for suicide in depressed patients

Obsessive-compulsive features

Severe hopelessness

Panic, severe anxiety, and agitation

Global insomnia

Severe cognitive difficulties and psychotic thinking

Lack of friends in adolescence

Acute overuse of alcohol

Recurrent depression

Source. Adapted from Fawcett et al. (1990).

mood after an hour or two that lasts up to a week. The drug has been shown to be significantly more effective than placebo (Berman et al. 2000; Zarate et al. 2006) and more recently to be better than midazolam (Murrough et al. 2013a) as an antidepressant in refractory depression. A combined analysis of improvement in suicidal symptoms in refractory depression indicated significantly greater effect for single intravenous infusions of ketamine than for placebo or midazolam, with enhanced benefit lasting for approximately 2 weeks (Wilkinson et al. 2018). These studies were not necessarily done in acutely suicidal patients. Unfortunately, it is still unclear how best to treat patients beyond a single infusion, with a variety of strategies proving ineffective. Follow-on ketamine infusions do appear to be effective over a 2-week period (Murrough et al. 2013b), but that is not a practical strategy. Other strategies with NMDA antagonists have failed to extend the effects.

It is unclear if NMDA antagonism is the putative mechanism of action for ketamine. The drug binds to μ opioid receptors as well (Bonaventura et al. 2021). Because ketamine is a drug of abuse and we do not know what to do for follow-on treatment, we had argued that clinicians should be wary about adoption of the drug for routine clinical use (Schatzberg 2014), although an argument could be made for its use in the emergency department. An Israeli study from Yovell and colleagues (2016) reported that ultra-low oral doses of the μ partial agonist buprenorphine (0.2–0.8 mg/day) was more effective than placebo in reducing suicidal symptoms, with separation being seen by 2 weeks. We are currently conducting a study in suicidal patients in which we administer ketamine intravenously and then randomly assign patients to ultra-low-dose oral buprenorphine or placebo to see if we can extend the acute antisuicidal effects.

A nasal formulation of ketamine has appeared effective (Lapidus et al. 2014). Jannsen tested an esketamine intranasal formulation and reported rapid efficacy in suicidal patients and in patients with treatment-refractory depression (Canuso et al. 2018; Daly et al. 2018). In the Canuso et al. (2018) suicide study, significant differences from placebo were observed at 4, 24, and 48 hours but not beyond, raising questions as to what the follow-up strategy should be (see Chapter 3). In 2020, intranasal esketamine was granted an expanded indication for treating depression in patients with suicidal thoughts or behaviors, although one major study showed statistically significant improvement over placebo in depression but not in suicidality (Fu et al. 2020). Although intranasal formulations of ketamine are certainly more convenient than intravenous administration, intranasal racemic ketamine has been associated with more variable absorption and can potentially result in higher peak serum levels and greater side effects. Side effects at high peak serum levels of ketamine might include hypertension, psychosis, and incoordination (Gálvez et al. 2018). Racemic ketamine has not been formulated for intranasal use and typically is created by compounding pharmacies. Esketamine, on the other hand, is formulated for the intranasal route and may be less problematic than compounded racemic ketamine.

Our group demonstrated that the rapid antidepressant effects of intravenous ketamine are blocked by pretreatment administration of the μ opioid antagonist naltrexone (Williams et al. 2018). These data suggest that opioids might be useful follow-up treatments. Indeed, Yovell et al. (2016) reported that low doses of sublingual buprenorphine reduced suicidal activity in a group of patients with depression or borderline personality disorder. Effect was noted more slowly than with esketamine (i.e., after 2 weeks) but lasted for 1 month. The starting dosage of buprenorphine in the study was 0.1 mg once or twice a day, with a mean total dosage of 0.44 mg/day.

Lithium has long been known to reduce suicidality in depressed and bipolar patients. As of this writing, no fewer than 16 RCTs and 40 years of clinical experience, as well as multiple meta-analyses, indicate that treatment with lithium significantly reduces the risk of self-harm and suicide in patients with unipolar and bipolar depression (Cipriani et al. 2013; Smith and Cipriani 2017). In a study of 50,000 bipolar patients, lithium was associated with a

14% lower rate of completed suicides and other suicide-related events relative to valproate (Song et al. 2017). There is even convincing evidence that the higher the lithium level in the drinking water, the lower the suicide rate in the general population (Helbich et al. 2015). However, lithium is a prophylaxis against suicide and is not considered an acute intervention in the suicidal patient, especially given that a lithium overdose can be quite lethal. In the inpatient setting, where administration can be monitored, lithium is underutilized in the acute treatment of suicidality.

There may also be ways of speeding up or augmenting lithium's antisuicidal properties. For example, Benedetti and colleagues (2014) combined lithium treatment with another strategy known to rapidly improve depressive symptoms in some bipolar patients: sleep deprivation. They found that when 1 week of lithium was combined concurrently with three consecutive 36-hour periods of being awake with a sleep recovery period in between, 70% of patients had a significant reduction in both depression and suicidality. Furthermore, the majority maintained benefit 1 month after treatment.

Given the types of imminent risk factors described by Fawcett et al. (1990), benzodiazepines are probably underused in the emergency and acute settings for the treatment of suicidal patients. Benzodiazepines may have an immediate effect on risk factors such as severe insomnia and anxiety. Patients' hopelessness is also attributed, in part, to the belief that they will never feel any better. When they feel better quickly with a benzodiazepine, their belief system may be altered enough to mitigate the risk of imminent suicide. We have found that lorazepam 0.5–1.0 mg qid, with the last dose given at bedtime, can make a dramatic difference even in less agitated suicidal patients. That being said, there is little empirical evidence that benzodiazepines help patients who are acutely suicidal (Youssef and Rich 2008). One also has to consider that some suicidal patients may become more depressed or disinhibited while taking benzodiazepines. Therefore, it is important that the suicidal patient be observed when starting a benzodiazepine.

A number of other somatic interventions are worth considering in the acute management of imminently suicidal patients. Among these is electroconvulsive therapy (ECT). ECT may work very rapidly in the profoundly depressed suicidal patient and may therefore be lifesaving. The average number of ECT treatments for depression in the United States is eight to nine; therefore it is not unusual to see significant benefit in the first 2 weeks of treatment.

Repetitive transcranial magnetic stimulation (r-TMS) has generally not been favored for treating acutely suicidal patients because it typically requires a course of 6 weeks of treatment to achieve efficacy. At Stanford, we are investigating Stanford Intelligent Accelerated Neuromodulation Therapy (SAINT), a protocol that employs an imaging-guided, accelerated theta burst protocol over 5 days that has shown early promise in achieving rapid response and remission in a population of patients with treatment-resistant depression (Cole et al. 2022). The FDA has cleared the device for refractory depression, but further testing is required to demonstrate the relative efficacy and safety of the device, as compared with other forms of r-TMS, in refractory depression with and without suicidal activity. However, a TMS protocol that can be demonstrated to be rapidly effective would hold promise in the treatment of acutely depressed patients.

In addition to devices, there is some evidence that the rapid titration of some antidepressants may be associated with an earlier onset of action. For example, premarketing studies (e.g., Montgomery 1993) suggested that venlafaxine may have a more rapid onset of action when the dose is titrated up to 300 mg or more in the first 7 days of treatment. Unfortunately, we have found that many patients are unable to tolerate this rapid dose titration. The combination of bupropion and dextromethorphan has been shown to be rapidly effective in some depressed patients but has not been specifically studied in suicidal patients. Other strategies that may be associated with a more rapid onset of response for depressed suicidal patients include stimulant or lithium augmentation of various antidepressants. There is perhaps more evidence of an antisuicidal property of lithium than for any other medication. Lithium appears to reduce both completed suicides and suicide attempts in patients with unipolar and bipolar depression (Cipriani et al. 2013; Kovacsics et al. 2009; Smith and Cipriani 2017), and it now has an FDA-approved indication for preventing suicide. However, lithium's low therapeutic index makes it an inappropriate drug to start in the emergency department. On the other hand, it may be a reasonable drug to consider during the acute hospitalization of a suicidal patient.

Many depressed patients have used their antidepressants in suicide attempts. TCAs are the most commonly used antidepressants in completed overdoses (Table 10–3). The usual cause of death in these cases is malignant arrhythmia. Management of TCA overdoses includes charcoal lavage (50 g slurry followed by repeat doses of 25 g via nasogastric tube), admitting the pa-

Table 10–3. Antidepressant overdoses and their management

Drug	Toxic dose	Toxicity manifestations	Management
TCAs	>1,500 mg (imipramine and most TCAs)	Anticholinergic symptoms, arrhythmia, hypotension, delirium, seizures	Gastric lavage, fluid support, cardiac monitoring
MAOIs	≥2 mg/kg	CNS excitation, hypotension or hypertension, delirium, fever, arrhythmia, seizures, rhabdomyolysis	Gastric lavage, fluids, cardiac monitoring, antihypertensives, body cooling, benzodiazepines for CNS symptoms, maintenance of MAOI diet
Bupropion	>2 g	CNS excitation, seizures	Gastric lavage, benzodiazepines, anticonvulsants
SSRIs	Unknown	CNS excitation, somnolence, GI irritation	Gastric lavage, supportive care
SNRIs (venlafaxine, duloxetine)	Unknown	Cardiotoxicity, hypertension, seizures, serotonin effects	Gastric lavage, supportive care

Note. GI=gastrointestinal; MAOI=monoamine oxidase inhibitor; SNRI=serotonin-norepinephrine reuptake inhibitor; SSRI=selective serotonin reuptake inhibitor; TCA=tricyclic antidepressant.

tient to a unit for cardiac monitoring, fluids to combat the adrenergic blockade, physostigmine 1 mg IM for severe anticholinergic symptoms, and correction of acidosis with sodium bicarbonate if necessary.

MAOI overdoses of as little as 2 mg/kg may be lethal. The cause of death in MAOI overdoses ranges from arrhythmia and cardiovascular collapse to rhabdomyolysis and renal failure. Acute management of overdose includes gastric lavage, maintenance of MAOI diet, cardiac monitoring for at least 24 hours, the use of benzodiazepines to treat central nervous system activation, and the use of sodium nitroprusside or phentolamine 5 mg IV to treat the hypertension.

MAOIs are also associated with another medical emergency: the development of a serotonin syndrome. The combination of MAOIs with serotonergic drugs such as SSRIs and clomipramine (see Chapter 3) is among the more common causes of serotonin syndrome. Symptoms of serotonin syndrome are tremor, diaphoresis, rigidity, myoclonus, and autonomic dysregulation, potentially progressing to hyperthermia, rhabdomyolysis, coma, and death. The treatment of serotonin syndrome involves discontinuing the offending drugs, monitoring vital signs, and supporting vital functions. Cooling blankets are often helpful. The drug cyproheptadine, a general serotonin (5-hydroxytryptamine [5-HT]) antagonist, has been used occasionally in oral doses up to 16 mg/day to counteract serotonin syndrome. Dantrolene in doses up to 1 mg/kg IV in divided doses has been used in severe cases to treat rigidity and prevent rhabdomyolysis. The key to treatment of the serotonin syndrome, however, is discontinuing the offending agents and providing supportive care.

Fortunately, many of the newer antidepressants present much less of a problem in overdose than do the TCAs and MAOIs. Overdoses of SSRIs and 5-HT antagonists are often asymptomatic, or patients may present with gastrointestinal distress, agitation, and somnolence. The treatment of choice is gastric lavage and supportive care. The British drug authorities warned that venlafaxine overdoses are more likely to be lethal than are SSRI overdoses. Their data suggest that risk of lethality from overdose with venlafaxine is comparable to that with TCAs. A review by the FDA indicated that venlafaxine may carry a higher risk for a fatal outcome in overdose than SSRIs but less risk than the TCAs. The risk of fatality in overdose is not just from cardiac events but is also associated with seizures, rhabdomyolysis, and other causes. Patients taking venlafaxine tend to be more ill than those taking SSRIs, and this may be associated with a greater risk of overdoses in general (Rubino et al. 2007).

One possible mechanism for the increased risk is an effect on sodium channels. Bupropion overdoses also tend to be less dangerous than overdoses of TCAs. There has, however, been at least one death related to neurotoxicity and seizures (see Chapter 3).

Acute Psychotic Episodes

Psychotic symptoms can be manifestations of drug intoxication, mania, depression, schizophrenia, dementia, delirium, or a variety of other disorders. An organic basis for the psychosis should be ruled out, whenever possible, by history, physical examination, and urine and/or blood tests for drugs of abuse.

Mixed Psychotic Features

With any psychotic episode presumptively due to toxicity from illicit or licit drugs, a variety of complicated clinical pictures can occur. Illicit drug users often take several kinds of drugs and alcohol simultaneously. When patients with schizophrenia abuse drugs and/or become intoxicated on alcohol, acute drug-induced psychosis can sometimes persist and blend into a picture indistinguishable from schizophrenia that can continue for days or weeks. The pharmacotherapeutic problem is to choose between acute doses of an antipsychotic, a benzodiazepine, and watchful waiting, while checking for illicit drugs in urine or blood, evaluating possible medical causes, and obtaining a recent history from friends or relatives. Benzodiazepines should not be used with patients who appear to be already intoxicated from alcohol or sedative drugs, but they are commonly used to manage withdrawal from CNS depressants.

Schizophrenic, Schizophreniform, and Manic Psychoses

When the likelihood of a drug-induced psychosis is low and the patient is manifestly acutely psychotic—paranoid, disorganized, hallucinated, agitated, belligerent, and so forth—the rapid tranquilization strategies described earlier are quite useful. Often, oral haloperidol is taken without objection by the patient; in that case, liquid medication is preferred because ingestion can be ensured. Likewise, asenapine (in sublingual tablets) and risperidone, olanzapine, and aripiprazole (in rapidly dissolving tablets) are fast-acting oral antipsychotics. However, swallowing a sublingual antipsychotic rather than letting it dissolve under the tongue will typically render the drug ineffective. Thus, sublingual drugs require a cooperative patient. Parenteral antipsychotics (e.g., chlorpromazine 50 mg, aripiprazole 9.75 mg, olanzapine 10–30 mg, ziprasidone 10–20 mg, haloperidol 5–10 mg) are all effective. An antiparkinsonian drug should usually be given at the same time as the typical antipsychotics to help avert dystonia.

Acute mania is managed with a combination of antipsychotics, benzodiazepines, and mood stabilizers. Although loading doses of lithium have not proved useful, loading doses of valproate may speed the onset of response. Valproate at an oral loading dosage of 20 mg/kg/day has been associated with moderate antimanic effects occurring in as little as a few days. Standard doses of mood stabilizers may take a week or longer to achieve adequate control of mania. Benzodiazepines may be as useful as antipsychotics in the acute management of nonpsychotic manic patients. However, both psychotic and nonpsychotic patients benefit equally well from an atypical agent, and these drugs are more rapidly acting than mood stabilizers in the management of acute mania. Thus, we typically prescribe an SGA for a manic patient and add a benzodiazepine or mood stabilizer as necessary.

When a psychotic patient can give some history and has a preference among available antipsychotic drugs, or when relatives or past medical records provide relevant information, the drug reported as best for the particular patient should be used.

Patients may present to the emergency department with antipsychotic complications in many forms (Table 10–4). One still fairly common form may be the development of acute EPS. The most worrisome of the acute EPS is *dystonia*. As discussed in Chapter 4, young males are most vulnerable to acute dystonic reactions, which may include oculogyric crisis, opisthotonos, torticollis, trismus, or laryngospasm. Although all dystonic reactions are very frightening to patients, laryngospasm compromises the airway and is potentially fatal. Severe dystonic reactions may occur at any time during treatment, but they usually occur in the first few days of neuroleptic use. Furthermore, high-potency typical antipsychotics may have a greater association with dystonia. The most reliable and rapid treatment for dystonia is intravenous diphenhydramine 50 mg or benztropine 2 mg every 30 minutes until the dystonia resolves. Laryngospasm may require intubation and the use of intravenous lorazepam to treat the spasm. If intravenous access cannot be secured, intramuscular injections of the drugs are necessary. Although atypical agents

Table 10–4. Emergency complications of antipsychotic use

Complication	Risk factors	Clinical findings	Management
Dystonia	Age <40, male; high-potency agents	Torticollis, opisthotonos, oculogyric crisis, trismus, laryngospasm	Diphenhydramine (IV) or benztropine (IV); lorazepam and maintenance of airway for laryngospasm
Overdose	Age <40, male, educated; schizophrenic, psychotic depression	Hypothermia/hyperthermia, EPS, hypotension, anticholinergic toxicity, seizures, arrhythmia	Gastric lavage, hydration, antiparkinsonian agents for EPS, cardiac monitoring
Neuroleptic malignant syndrome	Dehydration; lithium use; high doses	Delirium, hyperthermia, severe EPS, autonomic instability, elevated CK and LFTs	Stop antipsychotics; dantrolene (IV), bromocriptine, lorazepam (IV)

Note.   CK=creatine kinase; EPS=extrapyramidal symptoms; IV=intravenous; LFTs=liver function tests.

are less commonly associated with dystonic reactions, such reactions still sometimes occur.

An overdose of antipsychotics is rarely fatal. However, overdoses may result in hypothermia, hyperthermia, severe EPS, and occasional arrhythmias. Low-potency agents may additionally produce anticholinergic toxicity and hypotension. Hypotension is a complication of risperidone overdose as well. All antipsychotics reduce the seizure threshold, but clozapine may be particularly problematic in overdose. Psychotically depressed patients and young, educated male schizophrenic patients may be at greatest risk for antipsychotic overdoses. Antipsychotic overdoses usually respond to gastric lavage and supportive measures, including hydration, antiparkinsonian drugs for EPS, and cardiac monitoring.

NMS is a relatively rare complication of antipsychotic use (for discussion, see Chapter 4). It represents a medical emergency and is characterized by severe EPS, delirium, hyperthermia, and autonomic abnormalities. Both typical and atypical antipsychotics, including clozapine, are sometimes associated with NMS. The major risk factors for EPS appear to be dehydration, concurrent use of lithium, and rapid titration to higher doses of all standard neuroleptics. Treatment involves immediate cessation of antipsychotics, support of vital functions, and prescription of dantrolene sodium as a muscle relaxant in doses of 0.8–1 mg/kg IV every 6 hours for up to 2 weeks. Longer use may be associated with extreme respiratory suppression and muscle atrophy. Bromocriptine at a dosage of up to 5 mg tid may help relieve some of the EPS, and lorazepam 1 mg IV tid may also provide relief. In refractory cases, ECT is also reported to be of utility.

Delirium

DSM-5-TR (American Psychiatric Association 2022) criteria for delirium include a disturbance of consciousness, a change in cognition, a fluctuating course, and an organic basis for the disorder. Common causes of delirium include withdrawal syndromes, medication overdoses, endocrinopathies, metabolic abnormalities, and infections. Very old persons appear to be at greatest risk for the development of delirium, but delirium may occur at any age. The presence of delirium is a medical emergency and is associated with significant morbidity and mortality.

Clinical management of delirium centers on assessment of the underlying cause and supportive care. Physical restraints are often necessary and tend to be preferable to the administration of psychoactive agents, which may further cloud the clinical picture. When medications are required for control of an agitated, delirious patient, small doses of high-potency antipsychotics may be the treatment of choice. Drugs such as haloperidol do not cause significant anticholinergic or α-adrenergic symptoms and tend not to present problems of cardiac or respiratory depression. A typical dosage of haloperidol in the management of elderly delirious patients is 0.5 mg bid. Another pharmacological option is the use of small doses of 3-hydroxy-benzodiazepines, such as lorazepam and oxazepam, that have no active metabolites, have short half-lives, and are well metabolized even in elderly patients. Lorazepam can be administered in doses of 0.5–1 mg IV every 30 minutes, if administered slowly to avoid very high peak serum levels and subsequent respiratory depression. Oxazepam is not available in a parenteral form and has the second disadvantage of slow absorption and thus slower onset of action. If the patient is able to take medication orally, oxazepam 15 mg tid as needed for agitation is worth considering but is generally less desirable than lorazepam. Another strategy with which clinicians have had some success in the treatment of postoperative delirium is gabapentin (Leung et al. 2006). Gabapentin has also been associated with reducing perioperative pain and reducing the need for analgesics.

Severe Anxiety

Patients can present with panic, severe fear and anxiety, or multiple somatic symptoms. The symptoms of severe anxiety may be associated with a variety of medical conditions, including hypothyroidism, hypoglycemia, coronary artery disease, carcinoid syndrome, and pheochromocytoma. In addition, severe anxiety may be a feature of other psychiatric disorders, including schizophrenia, acute drug intoxication, alcohol withdrawal, and depression.

The anxiety disorders with which patients are most likely to present to the emergency department are panic disorder and PTSD. If medical illness can be rapidly ruled out or the patient has a known history of panic attacks, oral diazepam offers significant advantages because of its rapid onset of action after administration. Either 5- or 10-mg doses prn can be tried, depending on the severity of the anxiety and the patient's past responses to sedatives. If intramuscular administration is required, however, diazepam is not an ideal choice because of its erratic absorption. Lorazepam 1 mg IM repeated hourly is effective in the acute management of severe anxiety. Antidepressant drugs are indicated in the longer-term treatment of panic disorders, but they are slow in onset and of no immediate value in patients experiencing acute, severe anxiety. Thus, it may be appropriate to use a benzodiazepine with an antidepressant in the initial weeks of antipanic therapy. A month later, the benzodiazepine may be tapered off after the antidepressant has begun to work. Clonazepam is also an effective antipanic agent and can be initiated at a dosage of 0.5 mg bid. Although anticonvulsants such as gabapentin and tiagabine are occasionally useful, they do not appear to be as rapidly acting as the benzodiazepines.

Patients with PTSD may present to the emergency department with significant symptoms of autonomic arousal from flashback experiences, intrusive thoughts, and insomnia. It is important to evaluate patients for comorbid disorders such as depression and substance abuse. Violent or agitated PTSD patients should be managed by the rapid tranquilization methods described earlier. β-Blockers may also be helpful in the initial management of autonomic hyperarousal. However, long-term treatments, including the use of antidepressants and mood-stabilizing agents, are best initiated after the acute distress is reduced and long-term follow-up is secured.

Some experts prefer low-dose antipsychotic drugs in patients with borderline or other personality disorders who present in an acute crisis. If the patient has a past history of sedative abuse, olanzapine 5–10 mg, quetiapine 25–50 mg, or chlorpromazine 25–50 mg can be used. Chlorpromazine's sedation is likely to persist for many hours—at times, longer than is desired. If the patient is currently dependent on sedative drugs, consideration must be given to the problem of withdrawal reactions if the drugs are stopped abruptly. Buspirone is available for use in anxiety, but single doses are not helpful in reducing acute symptoms.

Stupor and Catatonia

Catatonia is a syndrome that may be induced by a variety of medical and psychiatric disorders. It has a separate diagnostic code in DSM-5-TR. It is characterized by cataplexy and waxy flexibility, mutism, resistance to instructions or attempts to be moved (negativism), and intermittent agitation. The causes of catatonia range from metabolic disorders such as hepatic encephalopathy and ketoacidosis to postictal states and basal ganglia lesions. Affective disorders represent the most common psychiatric cause of catatonia, although the syndrome often occurs in schizophrenia.

Nonpsychiatric etiologies account for a large percentage of catatonia cases. Therefore, a thorough history, a physical examination, and laboratory assessment are required. If medical or neurological causes for stupor can be ruled out, hospital admission to a psychiatric ward is generally indicated. If no information on the patient is available, intravenous benzodiazepines (e.g., lorazepam 1–2 mg) can sometimes facilitate obtaining a history by letting the patient talk relatively freely. Historically, intravenous amobarbital sodium was used. However, this approach required the clinician to be experienced in the technique, and, again, it was best done in an inpatient setting (see Chapter 6, "Antianxiety Agents"). Intravenous amobarbital sodium is given at a rate up to 50 mg/minute to a maximum of 700 mg. The dose is titrated to the size and age of the patient; smaller and older patients require smaller amounts. There is a significant risk of respiratory depression with larger doses, which necessitates having a crash cart available and perhaps having a second IV line in case of difficulties.

There are lethal forms of catatonia in which patients present with hyperthermia, extreme rigidity, mental status changes, rhabdomyolysis, and renal failure. This so-called lethal or malignant catatonia may be quite difficult to distinguish from NMS. The distinction is important because lethal catatonia sometimes responds to antipsychotics, whereas antipsychotics are contraindicated in treating NMS. Fortunately, both NMS and lethal catatonia may respond to ECT.

Emergency Department Referrals

Psychiatric patients are occasionally referred to a general hospital emergency department by their psychiatrist after telephone calls or office visits. Definite or possible overdose attempts, unexplained confusional states, or serious drug side effects (such as MAOI-related hypertensive crises or acute dystonia) are reasonable examples of appropriate referrals.

It is important for psychiatrists to remember that emergency department physicians may know less about the pharmacological effects of psychiatric drugs than they do, despite the natural hope that the emergency department doctor will be all-knowing and highly resourceful. Therefore, to ensure that no major gaps in knowledge exist, it is worthwhile to call the emergency department before the patient gets there and/or after the patient has been initially evaluated. At one time, many physicians had never heard that meperidine can be fatal when added to an MAOI. Some who do not know that TCAs have quinidine-like effects on cardiac conduction might give quinidine to treat an arrhythmia resulting from TCA overdose. Not uncommonly in emergency departments, a patient with a severe headache due to a hypertensive crisis may be ignored (i.e., made to wait) until the headache has passed on its own.

If a patient is sick enough to be admitted to a hospital and the psychiatrist knows of a history of benzodiazepine use, the psychiatrist should encourage the hospital staff to be concerned about withdrawal symptoms such as seizures or delirium. Also, the emergency physician may be reassured to know that overdoses of SSRIs, serotonin$_2$ antagonists, venlafaxine, and bupropion are likely to be relatively benign. In our experience, emergency department staff members seem interested and appreciative when the responsible psychiatrist calls and provides both clinical and psychopharmacological input.

Suggested Readings

Allen MH, Currier GW, Carpenter D, et al; Expert Consensus Panel for Behavioral Emergencies 2005: The expert consensus guideline series: treatment of behavioral emergencies 2005. J Psychiatr Pract 11(Suppl 1):5–108, quiz 110–112, 2005 16319571

American Psychiatric Association: Diagnostic and Statistical Manual of Mental Disorders, 4th Edition, Text Revision. Washington, DC, American Psychiatric Association, 2000

Bazire S: MAOIs and narcotic analgesics. Br J Psychiatry 151:701–710, 1987 2895679

Browne B, Linter S: Monoamine oxidase inhibitors and narcotic analgesics: a critical review of the implications for treatment. Br J Psychiatry 151:210–212, 1987 2891392

Cipriani A, Pretty H, Hawton K, Geddes JR: Lithium in the prevention of suicidal behavior and all-cause mortality in patients with mood disorders: a systematic review of randomized trials. Am J Psychiatry 162(10):1805–1819, 2005 16199826

Cole J: Drugs and seclusion and restraint. McLean Hospital Journal 10:37–53, 1985

Crome P: Antidepressant overdosage. Drugs 23(6):431–461, 1982 6213400

Dubin WR, Feld JA: Rapid tranquilization of the violent patient. Am J Emerg Med 7(3):313–320, 1989 2565724

Dubin W, Stolberg R: Emergency Psychiatry for the House Officer. New York, SP Medical and Scientific Books, 1981

Goldberg RJ, Dubin WR, Fogel BS: Behavioral emergencies: assessment and psychopharmacologic management. Clin Neuropharmacol 12(4):233–248, 1989 2680076

Hillard JR (ed): Manual of Clinical Emergency Psychiatry. Washington, DC, American Psychiatric Press, 1990

Hughes DH: Trends and treatment models in emergency psychiatry. Hosp Community Psychiatry 44(10):927–928, 1993 8225271

Hyman SE, Tesar GE: Manual of Psychiatric Emergencies, 3rd Edition. Boston, MA, Little, Brown, 1994

Müller-Oerlinghausen B, Berghöfer A, Ahrens B: The antisuicidal and mortality-reducing effect of lithium prophylaxis: consequences for guidelines in clinical psychiatry. Can J Psychiatry 48(7):433–439, 2003 12971012

Munizza C, Furlan PM, d'Elia A, et al: Emergency psychiatry: a review of the literature. Acta Psychiatr Scand Suppl 374:1–51, 1993 7905227

Prien RF, Kupfer DJ, Mansky PA, et al: Drug therapy in the prevention of recurrences in unipolar and bipolar affective disorders: report of the NIMH Collaborative Study Group comparing lithium carbonate, imipramine, and a lithium carbonate-imipramine combination. Arch Gen Psychiatry 41(11):1096–1104, 1984 6437366

Puryear DA: Proposed standards in emergency psychiatry. Hosp Community Psychiatry 43(1):14–15, 1992 1544641

Szuster RR, Schanbacher BL, McCann SC, McConnell A: Underdiagnosis of psychoactive-substance-induced organic mental disorders in emergency psychiatry. Am J Drug Alcohol Abuse 16(3–4):319–327, 1990 2288329

Weissberg MP: Emergency psychiatry: a critical educational omission. Ann Intern Med 114(3):246–247, 1991 1984751

References

Aljohani B, Burkholder J, Tran QK, et al: Workplace violence in the emergency department: a systematic review and meta-analysis. Public Health 196:186–197, 2021 34246105

American Psychiatric Association: Diagnostic and Statistical Manual of Mental Disorders, 5th Edition, Text Revision. Washington, DC, American Psychiatric Association, 2022

Andolfatto G, Willman E, Joo D, et al: Ketamine in the management of acute agitation in the emergency department. Ann Emerg Med 61(3):264–272, 2013

Andrezina R, Josiassen RC, Marcus RN, et al: Intramuscular aripiprazole for the treatment of acute agitation in patients with schizophrenia or schizoaffective disorder: a double-blind, placebo-controlled comparison with intramuscular haloperidol. Psychopharmacology (Berl) 188(3):281–292, 2006a 16953381

Andrezina R, Marcus RN, Oren DA, et al: Intramuscular aripiprazole or haloperidol and transition to oral therapy in patients with agitation associated with schizophrenia: sub-analysis of a double-blind study. Curr Med Res Opin 22(11):2209–2219, 2006b 17076982

Barlow CB, Rizzo AG: Violence against surgical residents. West J Med 167(2):74–78, 1997 9291743

Beloucif S, et al: Ketamine for sedation in the intensive care unit: a systematic review and meta-analysis. Intensive Care Med 46(7):1250–1259, 2020

Benedetti F, Riccaboni R, Locatelli C, et al: Rapid treatment response of suicidal symptoms to lithium, sleep deprivation, and light therapy (chronotherapeutics) in drug-resistant bipolar depression. J Clin Psychiatry 75(2):133–140, 2014 24345382

Berman RM, Cappiello A, Anand A, et al: Antidepressant effects of ketamine in depressed patients. Biol Psychiatry 47(4):351–354, 2000 10686270

Bonaventura J, Lam S, Carlton M, et al: Pharmacological and behavioral divergence of ketamine enantiomers: implications for abuse liability. Mol Psychiatry 26(11):6704–6722, 2021 33859356

Bongar B: Suicide Guidelines for Assessment, Management and Treatment. New York, Oxford University Press, 1992

Breier A, Wright P, Birkett M, et al: Intramuscular olanzapine: dose-related improvement in acutely agitated patients with schizophrenia. Presentation at the 154th Annual Meeting of the American Psychiatric Association, New Orleans, May 5–10, 2001

Canuso CM, Singh JB, Fedgchin M, et al: Efficacy and safety of intranasal esketamine for the rapid reduction of symptoms of depression and suicidality in patients at imminent risk for suicide: results of a double-blind, randomized, placebo-controlled study. Am J Psychiatry 175(7):620–630, 2018 29656663

Cipriani A, Hawton K, Stockton S, Geddes JR: Lithium in the prevention of suicide in mood disorders: updated systematic review and meta-analysis. BMJ 346:f3646, 2013

Citrome L, Preskorn SH, Lauriello J, et al: Sublingual dexmedetomidine for the treatment of acute agitation in adults with schizophrenia or schizoaffective disorder: a randomized placebo-controlled trial. J Clin Psychiatry 83(6):22m14447, 2022

Cole JB, Stang JL, DeVries PA, et al: A prospective study of intramuscular droperidol or olanzapine for acute agitation in the emergency department: a natural experiment owing to drug shortages. Ann Emerg Med 78(2):274–286, 2021 33846015

Cole EJ, Phillips AL, Bentzley BS, et al: Stanford neuromodulation therapy (SNT): a double-blind randomized controlled trial. Am J Psychiatry 179(2):132–141, 2022 34711062

Daly EJ, Singh JB, Fedgchin M, et al: Efficacy and safety of intranasal esketamine adjunctive to oral antidepressant therapy in treatment-resistant depression: a randomized clinical trial. JAMA Psychiatry 75(2):139–148, 2018 29282469

Dubin WR, Waxman HM, Weiss KJ, et al: Rapid tranquilization: the efficacy of oral concentrate. J Clin Psychiatry 46(11):475–478, 1985 2865251

Fawcett J, Scheftner WA, Fogg L, et al: Time-related predictors of suicide in major affective disorder. Am J Psychiatry 147(9):1189–1194, 1990 2104515

Fu DJ, Ionescu DF, Li X, et al: Esketamine nasal spray for rapid reduction of major depressive disorder symptoms in patients who have active suicidal ideation with intent: double-blind, randomized study (ASPIRE I). J Clin Psychiatry 81(3):19m13191, 2020 32412700

Gálvez V, Li A, Huggins C, et al: Repeated intranasal ketamine for treatment-resistant depression—the way to go? Results from a pilot randomised controlled trial. J Psychopharmacol 32(4):397–407, 2018 29542371

Garlow SJ, Weigel MB, D'Orio B: Treatment of psychiatric emergencies, in The American Psychiatric Association Publishing Textbook of Psychopharmacology, 5th Edition. Edited by Schatzberg AF, Nemeroff CB. Washington, DC, American Psychiatric Association Publishing, 2017, pp 1593–1621

Helbich M, Leitner M, Kapusta ND: Lithium in drinking water and suicide mortality: interplay with lithium prescriptions. Br J Psychiatry 207(1):64–71, 2015 25953888

Keating GM: Loxapine inhalation powder: a review of its use in the acute treatment of agitation in patients with bipolar disorder or schizophrenia. CNS Drugs 27(6):479–489, 2013 23740380

Kim HK, Leonard JB, Corwell BN, Connors NJ: Safety and efficacy of pharmacologic agents used for rapid tranquilization of emergency department patients with acute agitation or excited delirium. Expert Opin Drug Saf 20(2):123–138, 2021 33327811

Kovacsics CE, Gottesman II, Gould TD: Lithium's antisuicidal efficacy: elucidation of neurobiological targets using endophenotype strategies. Annu Rev Pharmacol Toxicol 49:175–198, 2009 18834309

Lapidus KA, Levitch CF, Perez AM, et al: A randomized controlled trial of intranasal ketamine in major depressive disorder. Biol Psychiatry 76(12):970–976, 2014 24821196

Lavoie FW, Carter GL, Danzl DF, Berg RL: Emergency department violence in United States teaching hospitals. Ann Emerg Med 17(11):1227–1233, 1988 3189977

Leung JM, Sands LP, Rico M, et al: Pilot clinical trial of gabapentin to decrease postoperative delirium in older patients. Neurology 67(7):1251–1253, 2006 16914695

Liu WM, Reid JJ: The effectiveness and safety of ketamine for the management of acute postoperative pain: a systematic review and meta-analysis. Can J Anaesth 64(8):880–890, 2017

Martel ML, Driver BE, Miner JR, et al: Randomized double-blind trial of intramuscular droperidol, ziprasidone, and lorazepam for acute undifferentiated agitation in the emergency department. Acad Emerg Med 28(4):421–434, 2021 32888340

Meehan K, Zhang F, David S, et al: A double-blind, randomized comparison of the efficacy and safety of intramuscular injections of olanzapine, lorazepam, or placebo in treating acutely agitated patients diagnosed with bipolar mania. J Clin Psychopharmacol 21(4):389–397, 2001 11476123

Meehan KM, Wang H, David SR, et al: Comparison of rapidly acting intramuscular olanzapine, lorazepam, and placebo: a double-blind, randomized study in acutely agitated patients with dementia. Neuropsychopharmacology 26(4):494–504, 2002 11927174

Möller HJ, Kissling W, Lang C, et al: Efficacy and side effects of haloperidol in psychotic patients: oral versus intravenous administration. Am J Psychiatry 139(12):1571–1575, 1982 7149056

Montgomery SA: Venlafaxine: a new dimension in antidepressant pharmacotherapy. J Clin Psychiatry 54(3):119–126, 1993 8468312

Murrough JW, Iosifescu DV, Chang LC, et al: Antidepressant efficacy of ketamine in treatment-resistant major depression: a two-site randomized controlled trial. Am J Psychiatry 170(10):1134–1142, 2013a 23982301

Murrough JW, Perez AM, Pillemer S, et al: Rapid and longer-term antidepressant effects of repeated ketamine infusions in treatment-resistant major depression. Biol Psychiatry 74(4):250–256, 2013b 22840761

Preskorn SH, Zeller S, Citrome L, et al: Effect of sublingual dexmedetomidine vs placebo on acute agitation associated with bipolar disorder: a randomized clinical trial. JAMA 327(8):727–736, 2022 35191924

Rubino A, Roskell N, Tennis P, et al: Risk of suicide during treatment with venlafaxine, citalopram, fluoxetine, and dothiepin: retrospective cohort study. BMJ 334(7587):242, 2007 17164297

Saklad SR, Ereshefsky L, Jann MW, et al: Usefulness of injectable and oral lorazepam in psychotic and developmentally disabled patients. Paper presented at the 138th Annual Meeting of the American Psychiatric Association, Dallas, TX, May 20–23, 1985

Schatzberg AF: A word to the wise about ketamine. Am J Psychiatry 171(3):262–264, 2014 24585328

Smith KA, Cipriani A: Lithium and suicide in mood disorders: updated meta-review of the scientific literature. Bipolar Disord 19(7):575–586, 2017 28895269

Song J, Sjölander A, Joas E, et al: Suicidal behavior during lithium and valproate treatment: a within-individual 8-year prospective study of 50,000 patients with bipolar disorder. Am J Psychiatry 174(8):795–802, 2017 28595491

Wilkinson ST, Ballard ED, Bloch MH, et al: The effect of a single dose of intravenous ketamine on suicidal ideation: a systematic review and individual participant data meta-analysis. Am J Psychiatry 175(2):150–158, 2018 28969441

Williams NR, Heifets BD, Blasey C, et al: Attenuation of antidepressant effects of ketamine by opioid receptor antagonism. Am J Psychiatry 175(12):1205–1215 2018 30153752

Wright P, Lindborg SR, Birkett M, et al: Intramuscular olanzapine and intramuscular haloperidol in acute schizophrenia: antipsychotic efficacy and extrapyramidal safety during the first 24 hours of treatment. Can J Psychiatry 48(11):716–721, 2003 14733451

Youssef NA, Rich CL: Does acute treatment with sedatives/hypnotics for anxiety in depressed patients affect suicide risk? A literature review. Ann Clin Psychiatry 20(3):157–169, 2008 18633742

Yovell Y, Bar G, Mashiah M, et al: Ultra-low-dose buprenorphine as a time-limited treatment for severe suicidal ideation: a randomized controlled trial. Am J Psychiatry 173(5):491–498, 2016 26684923

Zarate CAJr, Singh JB, Carlson PJ, et al: A randomized trial of an N-methyl-D-aspartate antagonist in treatment-resistant major depression. Arch Gen Psychiatry 63(8):856–864, 2006 16894061

11

Pharmacotherapy for Substance Use Disorders

D rug therapies for patients with substance use disorders are sometimes necessary or useful, but they are rarely sufficient to cure the disorder. If illicit drugs are overused by a patient with major depression to reduce psychic pain, by a patient with mania manifested as overactivity and uncontrolled hedonism, or by a patient with some other comorbid major mental disorder, appropriate drug therapy for the underlying major psychiatric condition can be very helpful. Unfortunately, some patients with clear syndromes (e.g., depression, bipolar disorder, schizophrenia) continue to abuse illicit drugs even when the syndromes are in full or partial remission, although others show improvement in both conditions with appropriate drug therapy.

Specific drug therapies are, however, available for some aspects of chemical dependence. Medications are useful for ameliorating withdrawal symptoms caused by physical dependence on sedative or opioid drugs. Either methadone or buprenorphine, as maintenance therapy, is a longer-acting, more manageable, less dangerous drug than heroin and can be given indefi-

663

nitely in an attempt to replace heroin. Naltrexone, an opiate antagonist, can also be given indefinitely to prevent the patient from obtaining euphoria from heroin and has been found to be useful in the maintenance therapy of alcoholism. Disulfiram (Antabuse) is sometimes used in treating chronic alcoholism to ensure that patients will become unpleasantly sick if they consume alcohol. Alternatively, a medication such as naltrexone or acamprosate can reduce the risk of relapse in an alcohol-dependent patient.

Some classes of illicit drugs, of course, do not cause any serious degree of physical dependence. These include cannabis, inhalants, and the hallucinogens (e.g., lysergic acid diethylamide [LSD], mescaline), but cannabis at the much higher concentrations currently available may convey greater risks than were found in the substance previously. Withdrawal symptoms are also seldom seen with phencyclidine (PCP) use. Such drugs can sometimes be abruptly discontinued, even in heavy and frequent users. Nevertheless, a drug therapy that would decrease or stop the use of these agents might well be clinically useful. Drug dependence syndromes for which drug therapies are sometimes or regularly useful involve stimulants, opioids, sedative-hypnotics, and alcohol.

A large variety of interesting, even promising, drug therapies for various substance use disorders have been proposed and studied, but the basic, approved, and available drug therapies have changed very little. The situation is exciting, frustrating, and sometimes even irritating. However, there is general agreement that a variety of psychosocial approaches to substance use disorders, especially opioid, cocaine, and alcohol dependence, are effective, probably more so than most available or even potential drug therapies. There is also agreement that drug therapies must be used in the context of psychosocial treatments, including 12-step and compulsory aspects of treatment.

The only new drug to be approved for the treatment of alcoholism in two decades is acamprosate (Campral). Acamprosate was approved by the FDA in 2004 but has been used in Europe since the early 1990s.

On the basis of published evidence, buprenorphine, a partial agonist (i.e., in a sense, a mixed opioid agonist-antagonist), appears to be effective both in opioid detoxification and as a maintenance treatment potentially superior to methadone, particularly if it is allowed to be used without all the legalistic complications surrounding the use of methadone and L-α-acetylmethadol (LAAM). Buprenorphine was approved for the maintenance treatment of opioid dependence in 2002. It is currently available in 2-mg and 8-mg sublingual tablets (Subutex), an injection form (Buprenex), a buccal film (Belbuca), a subcutaneous implant (Probuphine Implant Kit), a transdermal weekly patch (Butrans and generic form), and a prefilled syringe for subcutaneous injection (Sublocade). Buprenorphine is also available in combination with naloxone (Suboxone) in sublingual tablets (2 mg buprenorphine/0.5 mg naloxone and 8 mg buprenorphine/2 mg naloxone). Naloxone is used primarily to counter diversion.

A number of drug therapies (e.g., tricyclic antidepressants [TCAs]) were found to be better than placebo in the treatment of cocaine users in early controlled studies but were not effective in many other similarly controlled studies. Data supporting the use of old drugs in new bottles (e.g., disulfiram for cocaine abuse) and totally new approaches (e.g., antibodies against cocaine) still are wanting. The only other relatively solid advance in the pharmacotherapy of substance use disorders is the handful of well-controlled studies showing that patients with substance use disorders and major depression can benefit from standard antidepressants without being forced to become drug-free first. There are some reports suggesting that gabapentin can be helpful in reducing use of both alcohol and cannabis in abusers of these substances.

Drug Testing

A variety of sensitive assays are available to monitor and test for illicit drug use. The most common of these are urine drug screens that evaluate the NIDA 5, the five classes of drugs typically evaluated in federal drug testing programs run by the National Institute of Drug Abuse: cannabinoids, opioids, cocaine, amphetamine, and PCP. Many laboratories are also equipped to evaluate benzodiazepines, barbiturates, hallucinogens, and inhalants.

Urine drug screens are the least intrusive tests, and they are inexpensive and, typically, quite reliable. The cost for in-office tests ranges from about $5 to $50. Urine drug screens can be influenced by abstaining before the drug screen, which primarily detects drugs taken within 7 days of the test. However, chronic cannabis use up to 12 weeks before a urine drug screen can be detected by the screen, and a single use a few days before the test might be picked up. Saliva tests are usually processed in a laboratory and tend to be more expensive ($20–$100) than urine drug screens. Salivary tests are capable of detecting very recent use (the past hour or so) that may be missed in a urine test. Like urine tests, they primarily pick up drugs that have been used in the previous 3 days. Serum blood screens are the most sensitive assays and the most expensive. For most drugs, a serum assay is best at detecting drug use in the previous 3–7 days. Other types of tests include hair assays, which can detect most drugs that have been used in the previous 90 days, and patch or sweat tests, which are neither very accurate nor convenient. In most offices, a urine drug screen offers the best combination of convenience, cost, and reliability.

Opioids

Detoxification

Opioid abuse has become a major public health concern in the United States. Approximately 80,000 opioid overdose deaths were reported in 2022 according to the CDC (Centers for Disease Control and Prevention: 2023). Opioids are a class of drugs that include prescription painkillers, such as oxycodone, hydrocodone, and morphine, as well as illegal drugs such as heroin. Abstinence symptoms can begin as early as 6 hours after the last dose of heroin or other short-acting opioid. Withdrawal symptoms include anxiety, insomnia, yawning, sweating, and rhinorrhea, followed by dilated pupils, tremor, gooseflesh, chills, anorexia, and muscle cramps. About a day after the last dose, pulse, blood pressure, respiration, and temperature may all increase, and diarrhea, nausea, and vomiting can occur. Untreated, the syndrome peaks at 2–3 days and resolves within about 10 days, although mild variable complaints may persist for weeks.

A great deal of street heroin is so weak that some illicit heroin users may not have developed true physical dependence. In addition, both street and medical users of opioids, with or without real physical dependence, often consciously or unconsciously exaggerate their withdrawal distress in an effort to obtain more opioid medication from the physician. For these reasons, drug treatment of the withdrawal syndrome should be based on objective signs of opioid withdrawal, not on subjective complaints. These signs are listed in Table 11–1.

Unfortunately, recent years have witnessed a spike in opioid abuse and dependence, made more dangerous by the availability of extremely high-potency opioids (often available illicitly) as well as relatively inexpensive heroin as a street drug. Accidental overdoses have become all too common, and we are in the midst of an opioid crisis.

Table 11–1.   Objective opioid withdrawal signs

Pulse 10 bpm or more over baseline[a] or more than 90 bpm if no history of tachycardia and baseline unknown

Systolic blood pressure 10 mm Hg or more above baseline or blood pressure greater than 160/95 in nonhypertensive patients

Dilated pupils

Gooseflesh, sweating, rhinorrhea, or lacrimation

[a]Baseline: vital sign values 1 hour after receiving 10 mg of methadone.

Methadone, a long-acting opioid, is used to treat withdrawal because of its superior pharmacokinetics (a long half-life). A short-acting drug like morphine would have to be given every few hours to block withdrawal, whereas methadone accomplishes this when given only twice a day. The initial methadone dose should be 10 mg given orally, in liquid or crushed tablet form, so as to blind the patient to that dosage and subsequent dosages during detoxification. The patient should be evaluated every 4 hours, and an additional 10 mg of methadone should be administered if at least two of the four criteria in Table 11–1 are met. Unless the patient is being withdrawn from high-dose methadone maintenance therapy, no more than 40 mg of methadone should be required in the first 24 hours.

The total dose of methadone given in the first 24 hours should be considered the stabilization dose. This dose is then given the next day in two divided doses (e.g., 15 mg each at 8:00 A.M. and 8:00 P.M.) in crushed or liquid form. It should be consumed under the direct observation of a staff member to avoid illicit diversion. The stabilization dose should then be reduced by 5 mg/day until the patient is completely withdrawn from the drug. A patient who is physically dependent on sedative drugs and opioids should continue taking the stabilization methadone dose without tapering until they are completely withdrawn from the sedative drug.

An alternative pharmacological approach to the management of opioid withdrawal has been used for years at some centers. This approach involves the use of the non-opioid antihypertensive drug clonidine, which is mainly an α_2-adrenergic agonist. It can suppress both objective and subjective symptoms of opioid withdrawal. In beginning clonidine treatment, the method of Kleber et al. (1985) is worth following: an initial dose of 0.1 mg of clonidine should be given to assess the patient's tolerance of this approach. Hypotension, dizziness, sedation, and dry mouth are common adverse effects. If the initial dose is tolerated well by the patient, doses of 0.1–0.2 mg every 8 hours can be given during the early phases of opioid withdrawal, with increases to as high as 0.2–0.4 mg every 8 hours after 2–3 days. Blood pressure should be checked before each dose, and the dose should not be given if blood pressure is less than 85/55. Amelioration of withdrawal symptoms reaches a peak 2 or 3 hours after each dose. Muscle aches, irritability, and insomnia are not well suppressed by clonidine.

In one inpatient study of the use of clonidine in the detoxification of patients withdrawing from maintenance methadone, an average dosage of about 1 mg/day of clonidine was required for the first 8 days the patients were withdrawing from methadone. In a study using clonidine in outpatient detoxification, the medication was begun at 0.1 mg every 4–6 hours as needed, and the dose was increased to 0.2 mg every 4–6 hours, with a maximum dosage of 1.2 mg/day (average maximum total daily dose was 0.8 mg). Some variation of these dosing strategies could be used if a methadone detoxification program is to be avoided. Physicians interested in using this approach should carefully read the article by Kosten et al. (1989) or consult with a local program where this approach is being actively used.

Outpatient use of clonidine for opioid detoxification has generally met with much less success than has use in inpatient studies. Clonidine (Catapres) is available in 0.1-mg, 0.2-mg, and 0.3-mg tablets, as well as in transdermal patches that may be administered weekly.

Three interlocking developments are taking place in the area of opioid detoxification. One is the use of buprenorphine, the mixed opioid agonist-antagonist, instead of methadone to speed the detoxification process and as a maintenance treatment (Umbricht et al. 1999). Another, more experimental use of buprenorphine is to combine it with the opioid antagonist naltrexone or naloxone to precipitate rapid, severe abstinence of short duration, leaving the patient no longer physically dependent on (or having tolerance for) opioids after a day or two.

Neither buprenorphine-assisted withdrawal nor very rapid antagonist withdrawal is a procedure to be undertaken outside a specialized treatment facility. Buprenorphine certification is generally required for practitioners, and courses are available at the annual meetings organized by the American Psychiatric Association.

Maintenance

For many years, methadone maintenance has been available in major urban areas in specially licensed clinics as a replacement therapy for heroin or other illicit opioids for confirmed addicts who have failed to stay drug-free after detoxification. The dose adjustment varies from program to program; dosages as high as 80 mg/day are used in some clinics. It now has been repeatedly shown that a dosage of 60 mg/day provides much better long-term results than do lower maintenance dosages. First-line medications for treating opioid use disorder are provided in Table 11–2.

Patients usually take the drug once a day at the clinic under direct supervision and have their urine samples checked for other illicit drug use. If the patient is drug-free and doing generally well, take-home doses are often allowed so that the patient takes the methadone dose at the clinic only every other day. The drug is often dispensed in a fruit drink to avoid intravenous misuse of the alternate-day dose taken at home. Although this regimen would appear to provide a popular and useful alternative for confirmed opioid addicts, patients often drop out of methadone maintenance programs after weeks or months of participation.

Over the years it has become ever clearer that the purpose of methadone maintenance and related programs is not to gradually wean all patients off methadone entirely over weeks or months but to stabilize the patients so they can improve their psychosocial adjustment, or at least not have to resort to criminal activity to obtain heroin. Concomitantly, "dirty" urine samples showing that the patient is using other abusable drugs have become issues for counseling, not reasons to throw the patient out of the methadone program.

LAAM is even longer acting than methadone and is effective even if administered only three times a week. This feature eliminates the complications of daily clinic visits and the potential diversion of take-home doses. LAAM was approved by the FDA for the treatment of opioid dependence in 1993. However, LAAM has been associated with ventricular arrythmias and was removed from the European market in 2001. In 2003, the most common formulation of LAAM, Orlaam, was discontinued in the United States.

Table 11–2.   First-line maintenance medications for opioid use disorder

Medication	Dosing	Mechanism	DEA Schedule	Setting
Methadone	80–120 mg	Full μ agonist	II	Methadone prescription center
Buprenorphine	4–24 mg	Partial μ agonist	III	Outpatient setting

Note.   DEA = Drug Enforcement Administration.

Use of either methadone or LAAM was intended to avert withdrawal symptoms and to abolish craving for opioids in heroin-addicted individuals. Either agent was also supposed to provide so high a level of tolerance to opioids that self-administration of street heroin or other illicit morphinelike drugs will no longer cause euphoria.

Maintenance methadone is stabilizing for some opioid addicts, but it does not completely suppress drug-seeking behavior, even for heroin; patients in methadone programs often continue to get in trouble with other drugs of abuse, especially alcohol and cocaine. Maintenance therapy, even coupled with good support programs, cannot solve the multiple problems of many heroin users.

Maintenance methadone is a specialized modality in which psychiatrists cannot get involved in the ordinary course of practice. Consider the plight of the psychiatrist involved in caring for an opioid-dependent patient who is seeking, or claims to be seeking, admission to a detoxification program but has an admission date that is several days off. What can or should the physician do? It is illegal to prescribe opioids to sustain an addiction. The best procedure is to consult with the detoxification program staff as to how to proceed. It is our understanding of U.S. Drug Enforcement Administration (DEA) regulations that a physician is allowed to dispense daily doses of an opioid for up to 3 successive days to avert acute withdrawal while the patient is awaiting a planned admission for detoxification. In addition, physicians may provide maintenance treatment to an addict "who is hospitalized for medical conditions other than addiction and who requires temporary maintenance during the critical period of his [or her] hospitalization or whose enrollment in an approved program has been verified" (American Society of Health-System Pharmacists 2003, p. 2,040). Physicians should check with their local DEA office before embarking on such an enterprise. It is legal to prescribe opioids for prolonged periods outside a methadone clinic if the patient has bona fide chronic pain of substantial degree. Before getting into such a situation, the physician should certainly obtain a consultation from a pain specialist or refer the patient to a pain clinic.

Besides methadone, the other first-line maintenance treatment for an opioid use disorder is buprenorphine. It is available as sublingual tablets in generic form (the Subutex brand was discontinued in 2011), transdermal patch (Butrans), and a buprenorphine and naloxone combination (Suboxone). The combination of the partial agonist buprenorphine and the antagonist naloxone was approved by the FDA in 2002 as an alternative to methadone for maintenance treatment of opiate addiction. The approval of buprenorphine allowed the possibility of an office-based treatment outside the highly regulated methadone clinics. Buprenorphine is a Schedule III drug, whereas methadone is a Schedule II drug and requires stricter regulations for use. Studies support the contention that outpatient-based buprenorphine therapy is highly effective in reducing relapse and enhancing adherence in 12-step programs and may be safer than methadone treatment (Bell et al. 2009; Parran et al. 2010). The drug is given usually at dosages of 6–20 mg/day, with a target dosage of around 16 mg/day. Buprenorphine is taken sublingually to avoid excessive drug destruction in the liver, which occurs if the drug is taken as an ordinary pill and swallowed. This sublingual form, which is said to be the most widely used analgesic in many European countries, has been placed by the DEA in Schedule III. This area is the topic of some debate, which may reflect that high doses of buprenorphine act as comparative antagonists at μ receptors.

Buprenorphine is a good analgesic, but so are many other opioids and mixed agonist-antagonists (e.g., pentazocine). However, when buprenorphine was tested for abuse liability in humans by Jasinski et al. (1978) at the NIDA Addiction Research Center, it proved to be well tolerated and to elicit very mild dependence and withdrawal symptoms, even after prolonged high-dose administration.

Buprenorphine can substitute for other opioids and can block opioid-induced euphoria. Testing for periods of several weeks with individuals with opioid addiction has suggested that the drug is much more acceptable to patients than is naltrexone, perhaps because of the former's mild euphoriant effect. It decreases illicit drug use, as measured by urine screens, as effectively as methadone—not completely, but substantially. Studies of buprenorphine in opioid withdrawal suggest that it is equivalent in efficacy to methadone and superior to other drugs, such as clonidine (Janiri et al. 1994). A word of caution is that as a partial agonist, it can competitively antagonize other μ opioids used in close proximity and has sometimes been associated with inducing withdrawal symptoms.

Withdrawing patients from maintenance buprenorphine is easier than withdrawing them from methadone. The drug is already in pharmacies, in vials (for intramuscular administration), and, as noted above, has a less restrictive schedule status (III) than does methadone, which has Schedule II status. Clinically, we have been told that lower dosages (about 0.5 mg/day) can be harder to totally discontinue, particularly in depressed patients treated long term. Buprenorphine may become the first reasonably good maintenance therapy for chronic opioid users that could be prescribed in ordinary hospitals, clinics, and doctors' offices and dispensed in ordinary pharmacies. Such availability would avoid the bad side of methadone clinics: the massing of street users all in one clinic who can "reinfect" each other.

A second-line maintenance treatment is the opioid antagonist naltrexone (ReVia). This drug is similar to naloxone (Narcan), the opioid antagonist that has long been available for treating opioid overdose. However, naltrexone is much longer acting and is available in oral form. Either drug could, in theory, be given orally in large daily doses to create a chronic blockade of opioid receptors, which would reliably block the euphoriant effects of heroin or other morphinelike drugs. Naloxone is too weak and short acting orally to be usable as a maintenance treatment. However, naloxone is a life-saving intranasally adminsitered treatment for opioid overdose. With a growing epidemic of opioid overdoses, the FDA approved naloxone over the counter in 2022, and it is sold at all the major drug store chains around the country without a prescription.

As a maintenance treatment, naltrexone has been even less popular than methadone with patients with opioid use disorder. Thus, naltrexone requires a highly motivated patient. Naltrexone is also an option for patients for whom opioid agonist therapy is not allowed, such as some health care workers, law enforcement workers, and commercial pilots. The problem, of course, is that oral naltrexone is as easy as disulfiram to circumvent. An opioid addict needs to simply hold the dose of naltrexone for 2 or 3 days and then inject heroin to experience the full effects of the drug. For the moment, however, naltrexone is still a drug to be used mainly in special programs and not by general psychiatrists, unless they are asked to take over the care of a patient who has already been stabilized by being given naltrexone in a specialty program.

The usual dosage of naltrexone for maintenance treatment of opioid addiction is 50 mg/day. It can be given three times a week (100 mg, 100 mg, then 150 mg), but gastrointestinal side effects are more common with that regimen. A report from Australia indicated that an implantable form of naltrexone was more effective than oral naltrexone in promoting abstinence in a long-term trial (Hulse et al. 2009). In the United States, the approval and introduction of Vivitrol—a long-acting intramuscular naltrexone—has had an increasing impact on the treatment of opioid dependence. The usual dose is 380 mg once per month. The drug blocks opioid effects such that one should be careful to avoid use in patients who have recently taken an opioid for medical indications.

Another change, in process, is in our attitude toward the treatment of depression in methadone patients and other substance users. In a study by Nunes and colleagues (1998), imipramine was superior to placebo in decreasing depression in methadone-maintained patients with coexisting primary major depression. There was also some concomitant decrease in illicit drug use.

Anyone contemplating using psychiatric drugs to treat serious mental disorders in methadone clinic patients should be aware of potential drug-drug interactions. Carbamazepine, but not valproic acid or lithium, enhances hepatic metabolism and lowers methadone blood levels, perhaps justifying an increase in the daily methadone dose. Fluvoxamine, however, blocks methadone metabolism and raises the blood level (which will fall again if the fluvoxamine is discontinued).

In general, selective serotonin reuptake inhibitors (SSRIs) or other newer antidepressants that can be taken once a day and do not need much dose adjustment are easier for patients with depression and substance use disorders. With other agents, these patients are likely to be undercompliant and not experience improvement or to raise their dosages unilaterally and induce toxicity. One of us has seen such an outpatient become delirious after 5 days of taking amitriptyline; because the prescribed dosage (50 mg/day) did not give rapid relief, the patient took 500 mg/day.

Alcohol

Detoxification

Ethyl alcohol is a short-acting sedative drug that produces withdrawal syndromes similar to those caused by barbiturates. The symptoms and signs of withdrawal are the same as those described in the "Detoxification" subsection of "Sedatives and Hypnostics" in this chapter, with the caveat that alcoholic patients may be either very slightly dependent physically but in trouble with alcohol for other reasons or malnourished and/or medically quite ill. Because alcoholism programs tend to treat large numbers of patients, they usually choose a "standard" detoxification program—a program that is standard for a given institution but that may differ substantially from one facility to another. Some have used chlordiazepoxide in alcohol detoxification (see Table 11–3), which may be a good choice because it has a long half-life and may be less euphoriant than diazepam. The use of benzodiazepines for the management of acute alcohol withdrawal has become the standard of care in patients with complicated withdrawal in acute medical settings (Blondell 2005). Because of the risk of Wernicke's syndrome in alcoholic patients, thiamine 100 mg po or im must be given on admission. Thereafter, 50 mg/day is given for 1 month. Folate 1 mg/day po is also a common component of the alcohol detoxification regimen. Chlordiazepoxide is initiated at a maximum of 200 mg/day for the first 2 days, and then the dosage is reduced by approximately 25% per day to zero, with extra doses given intramuscularly or orally on an as-needed basis if the withdrawal symptoms are not adequately controlled.

An alternative and perhaps simpler approach, developed by Sellers et al. (1983), for alcoholic patients in withdrawal is to administer diazepam in 20-mg doses every 1–2 hours until withdrawal symptoms are relieved. Medication is then stopped. Detoxification was reported to proceed comfortably without further drug treatment once this loading dose of a long-acting benzodiazepine achieved symptom suppression.

Because only about 5% of alcohol-dependent patients are subject to serious withdrawal, some detoxification centers do not use pharmacological strategies at

Table 11–3. Pharmacological strategies for acute detoxification of alcohol alone

Agent	Dosage regimen	
	Fixed	Flexible
Diazepam	10–20 mg q 4–6 hours×2–3 days, then decrease by 25% per day	5–10 mg q 1–2 hours per DBP, pulse >100
Chlordiazepoxide	25–50 mg q 4–6 hours×2 days, then decrease by 25% per day	25–50 mg q 1–2 hours per DBP, pulse >100
Clonidine	0.1–0.2 mg q 4–6 hours×2 days, then decrease by 25%–33% per day	Titrate to BP and pulse

Note. BP=blood pressure; DBP=diastolic blood pressure.

all. In some hospital settings, patients without a history of complicated withdrawal are observed, and the dosing of benzodiazepines is titrated to physiological parameters. A dose of 5–10 mg of diazepam or 25–50 mg of chlordiazepoxide may be given every hour when the diastolic blood pressure or pulse is greater than 100.

Some clinicians have adopted lorazepam as the drug of choice in detoxifying alcoholic patients because it undergoes glucuronidation, has no active metabolites, and has an intermediate half-life. Therefore, patients with alcoholic liver disease might be at less risk of developing toxicity from detoxification with lorazepam than from detoxification with other benzodiazepines. On the other hand, the shorter half-life of lorazepam may be less than ideal for achieving smooth withdrawal. Unfortunately, no controlled studies have ever compared the advantages and disadvantages of various benzodiazepines in alcohol detoxification (Bird and Makela 1994), and there is no evidence for or against the routine use of lorazepam as a first-line agent in the treatment of alcohol withdrawal.

Clonidine has also become popular in some settings for decreasing the discomfort associated with alcohol withdrawal. In one study, transdermal clonidine was as well tolerated and as effective as chlordiazepoxide in the treatment of acute alcohol withdrawal (Baumgartner and Rowen 1991). Clonidine decreases the hypertension, tachycardia, and tremulousness associated with withdrawal. However, it does not prevent seizures or delirium tremens in the rarer instance of complicated withdrawal. Vital signs need to be monitored regularly with this drug. Typical oral dosages average 0.4–0.6 mg/day in two to four divided doses. Clonidine is also available in a transcutaneous patch. Each clonidine patch lasts approximately 1 week and delivers a fixed dose of 0.1–0.3 mg/ day, depending on the strength of the patch. Patches, however, do not allow for the day-to-day adjustments in dose that are often required in detoxification.

Phenytoin (Dilantin) is sometimes added in patients with a history of withdrawal seizures or in patients unable to give an adequate history. The very rare patient who develops delirium tremens despite the above regimens should be transferred to a major medical hospital for treatment.

Outpatient detoxification has been carried out in patients with adequate motivation and an adequate social support system. In the managed care era, outpatient detoxification became more common than inpatient detoxification. For outpatient detoxification, chlordiazepoxide 25 mg taken every 4 hours, or less often as needed, is probably reasonable for the first day, with tapering thereafter. For very tremulous patients who had to be handled as outpatients, chlordiazepoxide 100 mg im was used previously. The drug's slow absorption from the tissues was an asset rather than the liability it was in treating psychiatric conditions in which rapid sedation was desired. Chlordiazepoxide injectable is no longer available.

As in opioid withdrawal and maintenance treatment, the general psychiatrist will often be well advised to refer patients to specialized alcoholism programs for at least the management of detoxification and possible medical or neurological complications.

Maintenance Treatment

Most alcoholism programs rely for maintenance treatment mainly on Alcoholics Anonymous plus other educational, psychotherapeutic, and psychosocial modalities. Disulfiram (Antabuse) is sometimes prescribed (or recommended). Often, a daily dose of 125 mg is used in patients with chronic alcoholism. If the disulfiram is taken daily and alcohol is ingested, the following symptoms appear in this general order: flushing, sweating, palpitations, dyspnea, hyperventilation, tachycardia, hypotension, nausea, and vomiting. These events are usually followed by drowsiness and are usually gone after the patient has slept for a period.

Diphenhydramine 50 mg parenterally may be helpful in cases of severe disulfiram-alcohol reactions. Hypotension, shock, and arrhythmias are treated symptomatically. Oxygen is useful in respiratory distress. Hypokalemia may occur. Severe reactions require emergency treatment in a medical setting.

Obviously, willingness to take disulfiram, and thereby to commit oneself to not ingesting alcohol or suffering unpleasant effects if one drinks, is a test of motivation to remain abstinent. It is still, after all these years, not firmly established that the drug is more than a test of motivation or of compliance with therapy. Long-acting injectable or implantable disulfiram preparations have been tested abroad, but they are not available in the United States.

Patients whose motivation to remain abstinent at all costs while taking disulfiram is questionable or weak should not be prescribed disulfiram. In fact, doubts about the utility of disulfiram have probably led to the gradual decrease in its use in alcohol treatment programs over the years. Disulfiram can cause side effects such as fatigue; a metallic taste; impotence (rarely); toxic psychosis (even more rarely); and a severe, occasionally fatal toxic hepatitis (very rarely). The hepatits occurs early in treatment, usually within 2–8 weeks after disulfiram is begun, and is the basis for a labeling recommendation that liver function tests be carried out before disulfiram is begun and again after about 8 weeks of treatment. Disulfiram is a potent inhibitor of cytochrome P450 (CYP) enzymes and can substantially raise the levels of phenytoin, oral anticoagulants, and other drugs.

Naltrexone joined disulfiram as a strategy for the maintenance treatment of alcoholism in the early 1990s. Volpicelli et al. (1992) found that naltrexone 50 mg/day was twice as effective as placebo in preventing relapse in a 12-week period. In a similar study, which also incorporated either supportive therapy or coping skills and relapse prevention approaches, naltrexone was superior to placebo; it worked best when combined with supportive therapy (O'Malley et al. 1992). Naltrexone appears to modify the reinforcing effects of alcohol through its effect on endogenous opioids (Swift 1995). Further naltrexone studies have yielded mixed results; still, the drug, at dosages of approximately 50 mg/day, is an option for the maintenance treatment of alcohol dependence.

Naltrexone does not stop alcohol consumption entirely, but it appears to significantly decrease the likelihood that one drink will lead to uncontrolled binge drinking. In patients who respond well to the drug and are doing well by

3–6 months, discontinuing the drug and continuing other psychosocial treatments seems reasonable. Patients doing badly by 3 months while taking naltrexone are unlikely to improve significantly with longer treatment. However, experience with opioid users taking naltrexone suggests that prolonged treatment over 1 or more years may well be safe if the patient (or the doctor) feels more secure continuing the drug.

As a side note, a combination of naltrexone and bupropion (Contrave) has been approved for the treatment of obesity. Each combination tablet contains 8 mg of naltrexone and 90 mg of bupropion. The final recommended daily dosage is four pills per day. We have been impressed with the combination's ability to suppress appetite and promote weight loss in patients who have gained weight on psychotropics.

For alcohol abuse, naltrexone tends to be well tolerated at 50 mg/day. However, a number of side effects are common with this drug (Table 11–4). At least 10% of patients experience gastrointestinal side effects, including nausea, vomiting, anorexia, constipation, and abdominal pain. The gastrointestinal disturbance tends to attenuate with time and may be reduced by the patient's avoiding taking the drug on an empty stomach. CNS side effects such as nervousness, headache, somnolence, insomnia, and agitation are also fairly common. Lowering the dose and avoiding the drug at bedtime often help with the CNS symptoms. Joint pain and muscle pain occur in about 10% of patients, and increases in hepatic enzymes, rashes, and chills have also been reported at rates higher than those with placebo.

An alternative maintenance treatment for chronic alcoholism, acamprosate (now available only in generic after the brand Campral was discontinued), has been studied extensively in Europe and was approved in the United States in 2004. Its mechanism of action is unclear. The drug is a taurine analog that reduces alcohol intake in animal models of alcoholism, reduces symptoms of alcohol withdrawal in humans, and, as a chronic treatment, reduces relapse drinking and alcohol craving at a dosage of up to 3,000 mg/day (Sass et al. 1996; Swift 1998). In three of four multicenter U.S. trials, acamprosate was effective in maintaining abstinence in patients who were abstinent at the start of treatment. The failed trial occurred in polysubstance abusers. In contrast, the nearly 20 positive European studies had not required abstinence or detoxification, and this may account for the difference from earlier studies. The combination of acamprosate and naltrexone might be more effective than ei-

Table 11–4.   Common side effects of naltrexone therapy

Gastrointestinal effects

   Nausea and vomiting

   Abdominal pain and cramping

   Constipation

   Heartburn

   Hepatic enzyme elevation

   Anorexia

CNS effects

   Nervousness

   Agitation

   Headaches

   Insomnia

   Somnolence

Musculoskeletal effects

   Joint pain

   Muscle soreness

ther drug alone (Bouza et al. 2004). The main side effects seem to be diarrhea and headache. However, the drug is well tolerated overall. The target dosage is 666 mg given three times daily. Although the divided dosing presents a compliance challenge, many patients have been able to stick with a long-term maintenance program. There are no significant drug interactions with benzodiazepines, naltrexone, or disulfiram.

Mason and colleagues reported that gabapentin at dosages of 900 mg/day and 1,800 mg/day significantly reduced alcohol consumption in alcohol-dependent patients (Mason et al. 2014). The higher dosage appeared to be more effective than the 900 mg/day dosage. The drug was well tolerated, with no adverse side effects noted. The glucocorticoid antagonist mifepristone has been reported in a rodent model to decrease consumption of alcohol that is associated with upregulated glucocorticoid receptor activity in the amygdala (Vendruscolo et al. 2012, 2015). Mason's group has reported preliminary data in her laboratory model showing that mifepristone reduced alcohol consumption in heavy drinkers (Mason et al. 2012; Vendruscolo et al. 2015).

There was previously much interest in the potential application of serotonin (5-hydroxytryptamine [5-HT]) agonists and reuptake blockers to the management and treatment of patients with alcohol abuse or alcoholism. The rationale for their use stemmed from a number of observations in animals: in rats that are genetically bred to preferentially drink alcohol rather than water, alcohol consumption is reduced by the administration of L-tryptophan and SSRIs (e.g., fluoxetine) but not by the administration of noradrenergic TCAs (Naranjo and Sellers 1985). Abnormalities in the 5-HT receptors 5-HT$_{1B}$, 5-HT$_2$, and 5-HT$_3$ have been implicated in some cases of alcoholism (Murphy 1990). In early studies of heavy social drinkers, zimelidine, an SSRI that was once available in Europe, significantly increased the interval between bouts of consumption. However, subjects had only about 10 drinks fewer per bout, suggesting that this strategy will be only adjunctive at best. The mechanism of action may involve increasing satiety rather than acting via classical aversive or reinforcement mechanisms. The nausea-producing effects of the SSRIs also do not explain their effects on alcohol consumption. The SSRIs are not currently being pursued by pharmaceutical concerns in the United States as a treatment for alcoholism.

However, there is evidence that major depressive disorder coexisting with alcohol dependence can and probably should be treated with an antidepressant. Mason et al. (1996) and McGrath et al. (1996) showed that TCAs produce significant improvement in depression in active alcoholic patients and decrease alcohol consumption at the same time. Cornelius et al. (1997) showed similar results in a placebo-controlled study of fluoxetine. For many years, most clinicians believed that alcoholic patients should be abstinent for at least 4 weeks (and still be depressed) before receiving a drug therapy for their depression. A study by Greenfield et al. (1998) casts serious doubt on this belief. They found that *all* alcoholic patients hospitalized for detoxification who had a recent major depression diagnosis relapsed into drinking, two-thirds within a month after discharge from the hospital. None had been prescribed antidepressants, in accordance with the practice of the time. This study was completed prior to the publication of the articles showing a positive effect of antidepressants in nonsober depressed alcoholic patients. These two bodies of data combine to encourage the use of antidepressants in treating depressed alcoholic patients even if patients are or are likely to be drinking.

It has been evident for some time that pharmacotherapy and psychosocial therapies should be coordinated in treating patients with substance use disorders. The old caveat that sobriety must precede antidepressant therapy appears to be dubious. The clinician is better advised to work on the substance abuse and the non-substance-related psychiatric disorder concurrently (Weiss 2003). The SSRIs may not suppress drinking directly, but they, and other newer drugs, may be easier to use and therefore more effective (acceptable) than the TCAs in treating depressed alcoholic patients.

Obviously, if a patient has a psychiatric disorder that will respond to pharmacotherapy, such as major depression, in addition to alcoholism, the second disorder should be treated appropriately. The treatment of episodic or chronic residual anxiety symptoms after detoxification is a problem. The use of benzodiazepines is usually frowned on, probably correctly. (The case could be made, however, that chlordiazepoxide could be considered the sedative equivalent of methadone and might be able to be taken at a stable, controlled rate, whereas alcohol, if used to control anxiety, leads to uncontrolled use.) Nonabusable alternatives to sedative benzodiazepines in the treatment of anxious, abstinent alcoholic patients include propranolol, clonidine, hydroxyzine, TCAs, atypical antipsychotics, buspirone, SSRIs, and serotonin-norepinephrine reuptake inhibitors (e.g., venlafaxine).

In the past few years, a number of studies pointed to the adjunctive use of ketamine or psilocybin to treat alcohol use disorder. For example, single infusions of ketamine or multiple infusions over a few-week period have a salient effect on alcohol use disorder as measured, for example, by increasing the number of alcohol-free days (Dakwar et al. 2020; Grabski et al. 2022). Another approach has involved psilocybin, which has been reported in a 93 patient randomized controlled trial to produce significantly higher rates of alcohol-free days (Bogenschutz et al. 2022). One issue with these approaches is the difficulty in maintaining a blind. In the psilocybin study, virtually all the psilocybin subjects correctly identified that they had received the drug (Bogenschutz et al. 2022).

Sedatives and Hypnotics

Detoxification

Over the past 50 years, the problem of sedative addiction (physical and psychological dependence) shifted from being almost completely an abuse of short- or intermediate-acting barbiturates (e.g., amobarbital, pentobarbital, secobarbital) to being an abuse of newer hypnotics (glutethimide, methaqualone) and, most recently, benzodiazepines (e.g., diazepam, alprazolam). All these agents (and alcohol) produce cross-tolerance—that is, physical withdrawal symptoms in a patient who is dependent on any one of these drugs can be relieved by an adequate dose of another. The time course of withdrawal symptoms differs with the half-lives of the drugs involved, beginning within 12–16 hours after the last dose of a short-acting agent (e.g., amobarbital, alprazolam) and perhaps 2–5 days after the last dose of diazepam.

Early withdrawal symptoms include anxiety, restlessness, agitation, nausea, vomiting, and fatigue. Later, weakness develops, often with abdominal cramps, plus tachycardia, postural hypotension, hyperreflexia, and gross resting tremor. Insomnia and nightmares may occur. Peak symptoms, including grand mal seizures in some instances, occur at about 1–3 days after the last dose of short-acting drugs (amobarbital, lorazepam, alprazolam) and 5–10 days after the last dose of long-acting drugs (diazepam, clorazepate). Of patients who have seizures, about half develop delirium with disorientation, anxiety, and visual hallucinations. Even without seizures, patients in benzodiazepine withdrawal may be mildly confused, perceive lights as being too bright and sounds as too loud, become mildly paranoid, and feel depersonalized.

Sedative withdrawal, particularly from barbiturates, can be fatal once it has progressed to delirium and is not readily reversible then. For this reason, withdrawal from sedative dependence should be considered a medical emergency, and patients presenting in withdrawal should be treated as emergency patients. Withdrawal syndromes from benzodiazepines may be less severe. In contrast, opioid withdrawal symptoms are rarely life-threatening and are always reversible if an opioid is given.

Some current regimens use a long-acting sedative, such as phenobarbital, chlordiazepoxide, or diazepam, to ameliorate withdrawal from sedatives. In previous years, the most commonly recommended regimen involved using the short-acting barbiturate pentobarbital (Nembutal) to establish the degree of dependence and then converting the patient to the longer-acting phenobarbital for the real detoxification phase. This regimen, the *pentobarbital tolerance test*, is very rarely used now; the favored regimen is treatment of sedative dependence with a taper of a long-acting benzodiazepine.

Benzodiazepines

For the more common psychiatric patient who has probably become physically dependent on a prescribed benzodiazepine at moderate doses taken for more than a year, the benzodiazepine dose can be gradually decreased while the patient is followed as an outpatient, if the patient can tolerate such a program. There are reports that in patients with panic disorder who have responded to relatively higher dosages (e.g., 6 mg/day) of alprazolam, reduction in dosage at a rate of 0.5 mg every week to 2 mg/day is generally well tolerated. Further reduction below 2 mg/day at this rate of discontinuation will cause patients considerable discomfort. At or below 2 mg/day, a more gradual reduction—0.25 mg/day every week—is recommended.

A shift from short-acting benzodiazepines, such as lorazepam or alprazolam, to longer-acting ones such as clonazepam can be tried if tapering of the shorter-acting drug leads to uncomfortable symptoms. For patients with such discomfort, it is not clear whether rapid inpatient withdrawal is required, but that approach seems legitimate if outpatient withdrawal is poorly tolerated. It may be that slow withdrawal over weeks produces more discomfort than would a rapid, systematic inpatient regimen. Even with systematic inpatient withdrawal, however, there is a significant risk of relapse. A study by Joughin et al. (1991) found that most patients with long-term benzodiazepine dependence did not fare well even after successful inpatient detoxification. Only 38% of patients studied had had a "good" outcome at 6-month follow-up, and many had relapsed or encountered other difficulties, including suicide. Elderly patients and those with concurrent depressive symptoms fared particularly poorly. The authors concluded that for some patients, maintenance benzodiazepine therapy might be preferable to withdrawal.

Herman et al. (1987) reported good results in shifting patients from alprazolam to clonazepam. They substituted 1 mg of clonazepam abruptly for every 2 mg of alprazolam and allowed patients to take extra doses of alprazolam as needed during the first week they were receiving clonazepam. Patients stabilized on clonazepam could then be withdrawn more easily from the longer-acting drug. Animal studies (Galpern et al. 1991) suggested that clonazepam probably has a risk for dependence and tolerance problems similar to those of other benzodiazepines, but its long half-life may make for a smoother withdrawal. Still, we have seen patients who had difficulty in withdrawing from clonazepam.

Carbamazepine has also been used, with mixed results, to facilitate withdrawal from alprazolam and other short-acting benzodiazepines. Patients given carbamazepine at dosages of 200–800 mg/day, initiated before a benzodiazepine taper, showed longer benzodiazepine abstinence after the taper than did patients treated concurrently with placebo (Schweizer et al. 1991). Likewise, geriatric patients who did not respond to previous tapers of alprazolam were able to achieve success when the taper was initiated with concurrent carbamazepine use (Swantek et al. 1991). However, it has been difficult to demonstrate that the withdrawal is any less severe in patients using carbamazepine as an adjunct in benzodiazepine withdrawal, and not all studies have found a robust effect for this regimen. It is important to keep in mind that carbamazepine may induce CYP3A3/4 and other CYP enzymes in the liver, thus lowering alprazolam plasma levels and intensifying withdrawal symptoms. Some clinicians use valproate instead.

Another issue that warrants attention is that mild benzodiazepine withdrawal symptoms should be looked for more carefully in patients who have been admitted to psychiatric hospitals and whose prior sedative benzodiazepine medication was abruptly stopped. A few patients appear to become quite uncomfortable and to have typical withdrawal symptoms after discontinuation of dosages as low as 5 mg/day of diazepam or 30 mg/day of flurazepam if the dosages were taken regularly for many years. Withdrawal symptoms in such patients can last for weeks. Physicians may forget that sedative withdrawal may be occurring when a depressed or schizophrenic patient begins to get more agitated, and they may be painfully surprised and discomfited when the patient suddenly has a grand mal seizure.

There is a real question as to whether outpatients receiving long-term regular benzodiazepine therapy for anxiety—say, clonazepam 0.5 mg tid and 1 mg hs—need to be firmly tapered off the drug over their objections. If they have a history of a substance use disorder and have been stable while taking such a dose for months or even years, does the chronic use of prescribed medication put them at significant risk of relapse into serious substance abuse? Physicians who see "ordinary" psychiatric outpatients outside specialized drug abuse programs are sometimes not aware of their patients' history of past substance abuse. Physicians actively treating patients with serious substance use disorders are often horrified if patients are given maintenance benzodiazepines for chronic anxiety disorder.

The published literature is mixed. Expert opinion is generally against using benzodiazepines in patients with substance use disorders, but clinical reports on the adverse effects of such prescribing are lacking. On the basis of guesswork and of experience supervising residents treating such patients, we surmise that soon after alcohol, sedative, or other detoxification, patients may be at much increased risk of returning to substance abuse if they are prescribed benzodiazepines, but a bit later they may use such sedative drugs sensibly and with benefit.

Some patients with substance use disorders probably have anxiety disorders of such severity that they will relapse rapidly into taking whatever is available to relieve their discomfort; some of these patients may do better with prescribed, well-monitored sedatives than with illicit drugs (Mueller et al. 1996). Any physician regularly prescribing maintenance benzodiazepines to a large number of patients with substance use disorders needs to document the reasons for their prescribing in detail in each case and to obtain outside consultations to forestall accusations of substandard practice.

Nicotine

Nicotine dependence has been a target of drug development for many years. Initial approaches revolved around nicotine substitution using a variety of drug delivery methods (e.g., patch, gum). Two nonsubstitution agents are now approved and in common use in this country. The first is the antidepressant bupropion SR (sustained release), which was approved in 1997 under the brand Zyban. Buproprion generally reduces nicotine craving. The drug has been reported to double rates of abstinence (Hughes et al. 2014). The target dosage is 150 mg bid. The side effects are the same as those seen when it is used as an antidepressant (see Chapter 3, "Antidepressants").

A more recent approach has been to use varenicline (Chantix), an agent that was approved by the FDA in 2006. It is a specific α4-β2 nicotinic receptor partial agonist that blocks withdrawal symptoms as well as the effects of nicotine. The drug has been reported to be more effective than both bupropion and placebo (Gonzales et al. 2006; Jorenby et al. 2006). The dosage is 1 mg bid. Side effects include nausea, sleep disturbance, gastrointestinal discomfort (e.g., gas, constipation, nausea), and depression. The drug does have a black box warning for suicidal ideation, as do antidepressants. Medications used to treat nicotine use disorders are presented in Table 11–5.

Table 11–5. Medications for treating nicotine use disorders

Medication	Starting dose (mg)	Maintenance dosage (mg)	Side effects
Bupropion	150	150 bid	Dry mouth, headache, insomnia
Varenicline	0.5	1 bid	Nausea, insomnia, vivid dreams

Cannabis

Cannabis use continues to be quite prevalent in the United States and is now legal in 21 states; 18% of the population used the drug at least once in 2019. The active substance in the resin of the marijuana plant, Δ-9-tetra-hydrocannabinol (THC), results in the acute intoxication state. Symptoms of cannabis intoxication include behavioral or psychological changes such as euphoria, anxiety, impaired judgment, increased appetite, dry mouth, and increased heart rate. Motor skills and coordination are frequently affected. Rare instances of cannabis-induced delirium and psychosis have been reported (Luzi et al. 2008; Tunving 1985).

Medications are rarely required for the treatment of cannabis intoxication. The most common symptom requiring intervention is severe anxiety. This anxiety can usually be managed by modest amounts of oral benzodiazepines such as lorazepam, 1 mg every 4 hours. Often, one or two doses are sufficient to control the anxiety. Likewise, if psychotic symptoms are present, one or two doses of haloperidol 2–5 mg po will control these symptoms, which have occasionally been reported in frequent users of high-potency cannabis.

States of withdrawal from long-term cannabis dependence are quite uncommon except in chronic daily users of high-potency or high-dose cannabis. These have, however, become more common with legalization. The withdrawal state can include mild insomnia, irritability, tremor, and nausea. These symptoms usually do not require treatment. The treatment of choice for long-term dependence has been a combination of education, drug counseling, and support programs. Some 25% of substance abusers seeking treatment are dependent on cannabis. Gabapentin at 1,200 mg/day can reduce cannabis withdrawal and dependence or use (Mason et al. 2012).

Hallucinogens

The hallucinogens include LSD, mescaline, psilocybin, and related drugs whose principal effects are increased perceptual sensitivity, derealization, visual illusions, and hallucinations. Occasionally, these perceptual changes are associated with a frank panic reaction (called a "bad trip"), depression, or paranoid ideation. The symptoms of hallucinogen intoxication usually begin 1 hour after the last dose and typically last 8–12 hours. LSD use is still apparently more common in the western United States than in other parts of the country, and it is used by young males more than by other demographic groups.

Time and a calm, supportive environment enable patients who are in the midst of a hallucinogenic hallucinosis associated with panic to be talked down. Benzodiazepines such as diazepam 10–20 mg po will decrease the anxiety and commonly contribute to the patient's being able to sleep off the effects of the hallucinogen. Antipsychotics have also been used, but they are rarely necessary. Low-potency antipsychotics should probably be avoided because their anticholinergic effects can exacerbate the hallucinosis. Haloperidol 5–10 mg im or po is preferred over other antipsychotics, but there are no controlled studies to support this common clinical practice. For recurrent hallucinosis (flashbacks), benzodiazepines may be as useful as antipsychotics.

Withdrawal states for chronic hallucinogen use are very rarely reported, and no detoxification is necessary. Chronic hallucinogen use is best managed through psychosocial interventions such as drug counseling and support groups.

Stimulants

Stimulants, including cocaine, amphetamine, and their various forms, are among the most common drugs of abuse in the United States. NIDA estimates that at least 1%–2% of the population currently abuses cocaine, but rates of amphetamine abuse are lower. Stimulant overdose or abuse represents a fairly common reason for emergency department visits and hospitalization in urban settings. When a patient who is dependent on stimulants is hospitalized, stimulant administration should be stopped abruptly. No tapered withdrawal is necessary. Patients who have been taking stimulants in large amounts (e.g., more than 50 mg of D-amphetamine or several doses of cocaine a day) often have a withdrawal syndrome consisting of depression, fatigue, hyperphagia, and hypersomnia. In unstable individuals, this rebound depression can reach serious clinical proportions for a few days and may persist for weeks, usually in less severe form.

A variety of drugs, mainly dopaminergic or noradrenergic drugs (desipramine, amantadine, bromocriptine, bupropion), but even fluoxetine, have been tried in cocaine withdrawal or as possible longer-term treatments, but with no consistently demonstrated effect. Imipramine, desipramine, and venlafaxine have shown promising results in treating depressed cocaine-dependent patients, reducing both depressive symptoms and cocaine use, but the full value of these controlled, but preliminary, studies does not yet constitute a clear, valid guide for the use of such drugs in patients with major depression who use cocaine.

Carbamazepine has been used, without success, in an attempt to reduce brain stimulation caused by cocaine. Topiramate has shown preliminary success in cocaine dependence (Reis et al. 2008) and may have a role to play in alcohol and nicotine dependence. Calcium channel blockers have been tried as a way to improve brain blood flow in cocaine users.

Disulfiram (Antabuse) has been resurrected from its declining use in treating chronic alcoholism because it inhibits dopamine-β-hydroxylase, thereby raising brain cocaine and dopamine levels. One might imagine that this effect would only make the cocaine "high" better and longer, but disulfiram seems to increase anxiety, paranoia, and dysphoria when cocaine is taken concurrently. Several small studies have shown reduction in cocaine use, perhaps secondary to subjects' fear of using alcohol to modulate cocaine-induced agitation. In one study, the reduction in cocaine use in the disulfiram group occurred even in patients who disclaimed prior use of alcohol (Petrakis et al. 2000). The dosage of disulfiram used appears to be 250 mg/day. It is unclear how safe this therapy is in the long run if patients drink alcohol despite warnings and experience severe reactions.

Other investigational approaches include ecopipam, a dopamine$_1$ receptor blocker, and citicoline, previously used in treating neurological disorders to repair damaged cell membranes. Citicoline has been shown to have potential for decreasing craving for and use of cocaine as well as for treating alcohol and cannabis abuse (Wignall and Brown 2014). Even aspirin has been used to prevent platelet aggregation and improve brain blood flow and, in one study, to improve neuropsychological function (O'Leary and Weiss 2000).

As noted earlier, a cocaine "vaccine"—a large antibody that binds cocaine in body fluids—has been under development for several years. Animal experiments suggested this approach had promise. One study did suggest some potential efficacy in a human trial; however, the authors concluded that the vaccine did not produce sufficient effect and that better vaccines were required (Martell et al. 2009). A follow-up vaccine study (Kosten et al. 2014) also failed to find pronounced effects.

Any or all of the aforementioned potential therapies should be combined with appropriate addiction-focused psychotherapies (Najavits and Weiss 1994).

Amphetamine abuse, even the relatively recent advent of "crack"-style D-methamphetamine ("ice") inhalation, has not stimulated any new pharmacotherapy either conceptually or empirically. However, treatments useful for cocaine use would likely be effective for "speed" use.

The issue of abuse can be a problem with medically prescribed stimulants. If the patient has a clinical depression that responds uniquely to stimulants or clearly has adult ADHD and takes moderate doses in a stable manner to produce socially responsible functioning, stimulant use can be therapeutically helpful (see Chapter 8, "Stimulants and the Treatment of ADHD"). If the patient takes stimulants in large doses for euphoriant purposes or pushes the dosage to the point that paranoia or other serious symptoms develop, prescribing stimulants is obviously contraindicated.

Last, there are several pilot studies suggesting that repetitive transmagnetic stimulation may have potential clinical utility in patients with various substance use disorders (for a useful review, see Antonelli et al. 2021).

Phencyclidine

PCP (also called angel dust) has been used on the streets since the mid-1960s and remains relatively popular. The drug is usually smoked and is rapidly absorbed across the blood-brain barrier. PCP appears to enhance dopaminergic transmission and also to modulate N-methyl-D-aspartate and glutamate receptor activity. Acute PCP intoxication produces not only behavior that mimics paranoid schizophrenia or manic states but also even more bizarre, violent behavior than do amphetamines or LSD. Effects of the drug include muscle tension, tachycardia, hypertension, drooling, and horizontal and vertical nystagmus. Other neurological signs include analgesia, loss of proprioception, and ataxia.

Treatment of the PCP intoxication state may involve seclusion and restraints because at least one-third to two-thirds of PCP patients who come to emergency departments present in an agitated or violent state. Trying to talk down such patients is usually unsuccessful and often dangerous; isolation in a quiet area is better. These patients' agitation and violent behavior may be managed with high-potency antipsychotics alternated with benzodiazepines, as described in Chapter 10 ("Emergency Department Treatment"). Low-potency antipsychotics may compound the already significant anticholinergic effects of PCP and are sometimes associated with delirium. Acidifying the patient's urine with ammonium chloride (2.75 mEq/kg in 3 ounces saline) may facilitate excretion, as may charcoal lavage.

PCP withdrawal appears very rare in humans but is occasionally reported in animals. No detoxification is necessary other than to control the symptoms of intoxication. Unfortunately, no prospective studies on pharmacological strategies for chronic PCP abuse or dependence have been done. Maintenance treatment interventions include drug counseling, support groups (including 12-step programs such as Narcotics Anonymous), and regular drug testing to monitor progress.

Suggested Readings

Arndt IO, Dorozynsky L, Woody GE, et al: Desipramine treatment of cocaine dependence in methadone-maintained patients. Arch Gen Psychiatry 49(11):888–893, 1992 1444727

Arndt IO, McLellan AT, Dorozynsky L, et al: Desipramine treatment for cocaine dependence: role of antisocial personality disorder. J Nerv Ment Dis 182(3):151–156, 1994 8113775

Bagasra O, Forman LJ, Howeedy A, Whittle P: A potential vaccine for cocaine abuse prophylaxis. Immunopharmacology 23(3):173–179, 1992 1500284

Batki SL, Manfredi LB, Jacob P III, Jones RT: Fluoxetine for cocaine dependence in methadone maintenance: quantitative plasma and urine cocaine/benzoylecgonine concentrations. J Clin Psychopharmacol 13(4):243–250, 1993 8376611

Carroll KM, Rounsaville BJ, Nich C, et al: One-year follow-up of psychotherapy and pharmacotherapy for cocaine dependence: delayed emergence of psychotherapy effects. Arch Gen Psychiatry 51(12):989–997, 1994 7979888

Charney DS, Sternberg DE, Kleber HD, et al: The clinical use of clonidine in abrupt withdrawal from methadone: effects on blood pressure and specific signs and symptoms. Arch Gen Psychiatry 38(11):1273–1277, 1981 7305608

Cheskin LJ, Fudala PJ, Johnson RE: A controlled comparison of buprenorphine and clonidine for acute detoxification from opioids. Drug Alcohol Depend 36(2):115–121, 1994 7851278

Cole JO, Ryback RS: Pharmacological therapy, in Alcoholism: Interdisciplinary Approaches to an Enduring Problem. Edited by Tarter R, Sugarman AA. Reading, MA, Addison-Wesley, 1976, pp 687–734

Farrell M, Ward J, Mattick R, et al: Methadone maintenance treatment in opiate dependence: a review. BMJ 309(6960):997–1001, 1994 7950725

Franklin JE: Addiction medicine. JAMA 273(21):1656–1657, 1995 7752401

Galanter M: Network therapy for addiction: a model for office practice. Am J Psychiatry 150(1):28–36, 1993 8417577

Galloway GP, Newmeyer J, Knapp T, et al: Imipramine for the treatment of cocaine and methamphetamine dependence. J Addict Dis 13(4):201–216, 1994 7734470

Gawin FH, Ellinwood EH Jr: Cocaine and other stimulants: actions, abuse, and treatment. N Engl J Med 318(18):1173–1182, 1988 3283549

Gawin FH, Allen D, Humblestone B: Outpatient treatment of "crack" cocaine smoking with flupenthixol decanoate: a preliminary report. Arch Gen Psychiatry 46(4):322–325, 1989 2930329

Gawin FH, Kleber HD, Byck R, et al: Desipramine facilitation of initial cocaine abstinence. Arch Gen Psychiatry 46(2):117–121, 1989 2492422

Ginzburg HM: Naltrexone: Its Clinical Utility (DHHS Publ No ADM-84-1358). Washington, DC, U.S. Government Printing Office, 1984

Grabowski J, Rhoades H, Elk R, et al: Fluoxetine is ineffective for treatment of cocaine dependence or concurrent opiate and cocaine dependence: two placebo-controlled double-blind trials. J Clin Psychopharmacol 15(3):163–174, 1995 7635993

Higgins ST, Budney AJ, Bickel WK, et al: Incentives improve outcome in outpatient behavioral treatment of cocaine dependence. Arch Gen Psychiatry 51(7):568–576, 1994 8031230

Kampman KM, Pettinati H, Lynch KG, et al: A pilot trial of topiramate for the treatment of cocaine dependence. Drug Alcohol Depend 75(3):233–240, 2004 15283944

Kosten TR: Current pharmacotherapies for opioid dependence. Psychopharmacol Bull 26(1):69–74, 1990 2196628

Kosten TR, Kleber HD: Buprenorphine detoxification from opioid dependence: a pilot study. Life Sci 42(6):635–641, 1988 3276999

Kosten TA, Kosten TR: Pharmacological blocking agents for treating substance abuse. J Nerv Ment Dis 179(10):583–592, 1991 1919542

Kreek MJ: Rationale for maintenance pharmacotherapy of opiate dependence. Res Publ Assoc Res Nerv Ment Dis 70:205–230, 1992 1346939

Landry DW, Zhao K, Yang GX, et al: Antibody-catalyzed degradation of cocaine. Science 259(5103):1899–1901, 1993 8456315

Lejoyeux M, Solomon J, Adès J: Benzodiazepine treatment for alcohol-dependent patients. Alcohol Alcohol 33(6):563–575, 1998 9872344

Mann K: Pharmacotherapy of alcohol dependence: a review of the clinical data. CNS Drugs 18(8):485–504, 2004 15182219

Mason BJ, Crean R, Goodell V, et al: A proof-of-concept randomized controlled study of gabapentin: effects on cannabis use, withdrawal and executive function deficits in cannabis-dependent adults. Neuropsychopharmacology 37(7):1689–1698, 2012 22373942

Mason NA: Disulfiram-induced hepatitis: case report and review of the literature. DICP 23(11):872–875, 1989 2688328

Messinis L, Lyros E, Andrian V, et al: Neuropsychological functioning in buprenorphine maintained patients versus abstinent heroin abusers on naltrexone hydrochloride therapy. Hum Psychopharmacol 24(7):524–531, 2009 19650155

Miller NS: Pharmacotherapy in alcoholism. J Addict Dis 14(1):23–46, 1995 7632745

Miller NS, Sheppart LM: Addiction treatment and continuing care in forensic populations. Psychiatr Ann 30:589–596, 2000

Milne M, Crouch BI, Caravati EM: Buprenorphine for opioid dependence. J Pain Palliat Care Pharmacother 23(2):153–155, 2009 19492216

Moak DH: Assessing the efficacy of medical treatments for alcohol use disorders. Expert Opin Pharmacother 5(10):2075–2089, 2004 15461543

O'Connor PG, Kosten TR: Rapid and ultrarapid opioid detoxification techniques. JAMA 279(3):229–234, 1998 9438745

O'Connor PG, Carroll KM, Shi JM, et al: Three methods of opioid detoxification in a primary care setting: a randomized trial. Ann Intern Med 127(7):526–530, 1997 9313020

O'Malley SS: Integration of opioid antagonists and psychosocial therapy in the treatment of narcotic and alcohol dependence. J Clin Psychiatry 56(Suppl 7):30–38, 1995 7673103

O'Mara NB, Wesley LC: Naltrexone in the treatment of alcohol dependence. Ann Pharmacother 28(2):210–211, 1994 8173139

Salvato FR, Mason BJ: Changes in transaminases over the course of a 12-week, double-blind nalmefene trial in a 38-year-old female subject. Alcohol Clin Exp Res 18(5):1187–1189, 1994 7847604

Sinclair JD: Drugs to decrease alcohol drinking. Ann Med 22(5):357–362, 1990 2291844

Smith DE, Wesson DR: Phenobarbital technique for treatment of barbiturate dependence. Arch Gen Psychiatry 24(1):56–60, 1971 5538852

Stine SM, Kosten TR: Use of drug combinations in treatment of opioid withdrawal. J Clin Psychopharmacol 12(3):203–209, 1992 1629388

Stine SM, Kosten TR: Reduction of opiate withdrawal-like symptoms by cocaine abuse during methadone and buprenorphine maintenance. Am J Drug Alcohol Abuse 20(4):445–458, 1994 7832179

Teoh SK, Mello NK, Mendelson JH, et al: Buprenorphine effects on morphine- and cocaine-induced subjective responses by drug-dependent men. J Clin Psychopharmacol 14(1):15–27, 1994 8151000

U.S. Department of Justice, Drug Enforcement Administration: Controlled Substances Act as Amended to July 1, 1991. Washington, DC, West Publishing, 1991, pp 977–978

Verheul R, Lehert P, Geerlings PJ, et al: Predictors of acamprosate efficacy: results from a pooled analysis of seven European trials including 1485 alcohol-dependent patients. Psychopharmacology (Berl) 178(2–3):167–173, 2005 15322728

Washton AM, Resnick RB: Clonidine for opiate detoxification: outpatient clinical trials. Am J Psychiatry 137(9):1121–1122, 1980 7425173

References

American Society of Health-System Pharmacists: AHFS Drug Information 2003. Bethesda, MD, American Society of Health-System Pharmacists, 2003

Antonelli M, Fattore L, Sestito L, et al: Transcranial magnetic stimulation: a review about its efficacy in the treatment of alcohol, tobacco and cocaine addiction. Addict Behav 114:106760, 2021 33316590

Baumgartner GR, Rowen RC: Transdermal clonidine versus chlordiazepoxide in alcohol withdrawal: a randomized, controlled clinical trial. South Med J 84(3):312–321, 1991 2000517

Bell J, Trinh L, Butler B, et al: Comparing retention in treatment and mortality in people after initial entry to methadone and buprenorphine treatment. Addiction 104(7):1193–1200, 2009 19563562

Bird RD, Makela EH: Alcohol withdrawal: what is the benzodiazepine of choice? Ann Pharmacother 28(1):67–71, 1994 8123967

Blondell RD: Ambulatory detoxification of patients with alcohol dependence. Am Fam Physician 71(3):495–502, 2005 15712624

Bogenschutz MP, Ross S, Bhatt S, et al: Percentage of heavy drinking days following psilocybin-assisted psychotherapy vs placebo in the treatment of adult patients with alcohol use disorder: a randomized clinical trial. JAMA Psychiatry 79(10):953–962, 2022 36001306

Bouza C, Angeles M, Muñoz A, Amate JM: Efficacy and safety of naltrexone and acamprosate in the treatment of alcohol dependence: a systematic review. Addiction 99(7):811–828, 2004 15200577

Centers for Disease Control and Prevention: Vital statistics rapid release, Hyattsville, MD, National Center for Health Statistics, 2023. Available at: www.cdc.gov/nchs/products/vsrr/drug-overdose-data.htm. Accessed November 14, 2023.

Cornelius JR, Salloum IM, Ehler JG, et al: Fluoxetine in depressed alcoholics: a double-blind, placebo-controlled trial. Arch Gen Psychiatry 54(8):700–705, 1997 9283504

Dakwar E, Levin F, Hart CL, et al: A single ketamine infusion combined with motivational enhancement therapy for alcohol use disorder: a randomized midazolam-controlled pilot trial. Am J Psychiatry 177(2):125–133, 2020 31786934

Galpern WR, Lumpkin M, Greenblatt DJ, et al: Chronic benzodiazepine administration VII: behavioral tolerance and withdrawal and receptor alterations associated with clonazepam administration. Psychopharmacology (Berl) 104(2):225–230, 1991 1652144

Gonzales D, Rennard SI, Nides M, et al; Varenicline Phase 3 Study Group: Varenicline, an alpha4beta2 nicotinic acetylcholine receptor partial agonist, vs sustained-release bupropion and placebo for smoking cessation: a randomized controlled trial. JAMA 296(1):47–55, 2006 16820546

Grabski M, McAndrew A, Lawn W, et al: Adjunctive ketamine with relapse prevention-based psychological therapy in the treatment of alcohol use disorder. Am J Psychiatry 179(2):152–162, 2022 35012326

Greenfield SF, Weiss RD, Muenz LR, et al: The effect of depression on return to drinking: a prospective study. Arch Gen Psychiatry 55(3):259–265, 1998 9510220

Herman JB, Rosenbaum JF, Brotman AW: The alprazolam to clonazepam switch for the treatment of panic disorder. J Clin Psychopharmacol 7(3):175–178, 1987 3597803

Hughes JR, Stead LF, Hartmann-Boyce J, et al: Antidepressants for smoking cessation. Cochrane Database Syst Rev Jan 8(1):CD000031, 2014

Hulse GK, Morris N, Arnold-Reed D, Tait RJ: Improving clinical outcomes in treating heroin dependence: randomized, controlled trial of oral or implant naltrexone. Arch Gen Psychiatry 66(10):1108–1115, 2009 19805701

Janiri L, Mannelli P, Persico AM, et al: Opiate detoxification of methadone maintenance patients using lefetamine, clonidine and buprenorphine. Drug Alcohol Depend 36(2):139–145, 1994 7851281

Jasinski DR, Pevnick JS, Griffith JD: Human pharmacology and abuse potential of the analgesic buprenorphine: a potential agent for treating narcotic addiction. Arch Gen Psychiatry 35(4):501–516, 1978 215096

Jorenby DE, Hays JT, Rigotti NA, et al; Varenicline Phase 3 Study Group: Efficacy of varenicline, an alpha4beta2 nicotinic acetylcholine receptor partial agonist, vs placebo or sustained-release bupropion for smoking cessation: a randomized controlled trial. JAMA 296(1):56–63, 2006 16820547

Joughin N, Tata P, Collins M, et al: In-patient withdrawal from long-term benzodiazepine use. Br J Addict 86(4):449–455, 1991 1675899

Kleber HD, Riordan CE, Rounsaville B, et al: Clonidine in outpatient detoxification from methadone maintenance. Arch Gen Psychiatry 42(4):391–394, 1985 3977557

Kosten TR, Kleber HD, Morgan C: Role of opioid antagonists in treating intravenous cocaine abuse. Life Sci 44(13):887–892, 1989 2927249

Kosten TR, Domingo CB, Shorter D, et al: Vaccine for cocaine dependence: a randomized double-blind placebo-controlled efficacy trial. Drug Alcohol Depend 140:42–47, 2014 24793366

Luzi S, Morrison PD, Powell J, et al: What is the mechanism whereby cannabis use increases risk of psychosis? Neurotox Res 14(2–3):105–112, 2008 19073418

Martell BA, Orson FM, Poling J, et al: Cocaine vaccine for the treatment of cocaine dependence in methadone-maintained patients: a randomized, double-blind, placebo-controlled efficacy trial. Arch Gen Psychiatry 66(10):1116–1123, 2009 19805702

Mason BJ, Kocsis JH, Ritvo EC, Cutler RB: A double-blind, placebo-controlled trial of desipramine for primary alcohol dependence stratified on the presence or absence of major depression. JAMA 275(10):761–767, 1996 8598592

Mason BJ, Crean R, Goodell V, et al: A proof-of-concept randomized controlled study of gabapentin: effects on cannabis use, withdrawal and executive function deficits in cannabis-dependent adults. Neuropsychopharmacology 37(7):1689–1698, 2012 22373942

Mason BJ, Quello S, Goodell V, et al: Gabapentin treatment for alcohol dependence: a randomized clinical trial. JAMA Intern Med 174(1):70–77, 2014 24190578

McGrath PJ, Nunes EV, Stewart JW, et al: Imipramine treatment of alcoholics with primary depression: a placebo-controlled clinical trial. Arch Gen Psychiatry 53(3):232–240, 1996 8611060

Mueller TI, Goldenberg IM, Gordon AL, et al: Benzodiazepine use in anxiety disordered patients with and without a history of alcoholism. J Clin Psychiatry 57(2):83–89, 1996 8591974

Murphy DL: Neuropsychiatric disorders and the multiple human brain serotonin receptor subtypes and subsystems. Neuropsychopharmacology 3(5–6):457–471, 1990 2078279

Najavits LM, Weiss RD: The role of psychotherapy in the treatment of substance-use disorders. Harv Rev Psychiatry 2(2):84–96, 1994 9384886

Naranjo CA, Sellers EM: Research Advances in New Psychopharmacological Treatments for Alcoholism. New York, Excerpta Medica, 1985

Nunes EV, Quitkin FM, Donovan SJ, et al: Imipramine treatment of opiate-dependent patients with depressive disorders: a placebo-controlled trial. Arch Gen Psychiatry 55(2):153–160, 1998 9477929

O'Leary G, Weiss RD: Pharmacotherapies for cocaine dependence. Curr Psychiatry Rep 2(6):508–513, 2000 11123003

O'Malley SS, Jaffe AJ, Chang G, et al: Naltrexone and coping skills therapy for alcohol dependence: a controlled study. Arch Gen Psychiatry 49(11):881–887, 1992 1444726

Parran TV, Adelman CA, Merkin B, et al: Long-term outcomes of office-based buprenorphine/naloxone maintenance therapy. Drug Alcohol Depend 106(1):56–60, 2010 19717249

Petrakis IL, Carroll KM, Nich C, et al: Disulfiram treatment for cocaine dependence in methadone-maintained opioid addicts. Addiction 95(2):219–228, 2000 10723850

Reis AD, Castro LA, Faria R, Laranjeira R: Craving decrease with topiramate in outpatient treatment for cocaine dependence: an open label trial. Rev Bras Psiquiatr 30(2):132–135, 2008 18470406

Sass H, Soyka M, Mann K, Zieglgänsberger W: Relapse prevention by acamprosate: results from a placebo-controlled study on alcohol dependence. Arch Gen Psychiatry 53(8):673–680, 1996 8694680

Schweizer E, Rickels K, Case WG, Greenblatt DJ: Carbamazepine treatment in patients discontinuing long-term benzodiazepine therapy: effects on withdrawal severity and outcome. Arch Gen Psychiatry 48(5):448–452, 1991 2021297

Sellers EM, Naranjo CA, Harrison M, et al: Diazepam loading: simplified treatment of alcohol withdrawal. Clin Pharmacol Ther 34(6):822–826, 1983 6641099

Swantek SS, Grossberg GT, Neppe VM, et al: The use of carbamazepine to treat benzodiazepine withdrawal in a geriatric population. J Geriatr Psychiatry Neurol 4(2):106–109, 1991 1854420

Swift RM: Effect of naltrexone on human alcohol consumption. J Clin Psychiatry 56(Suppl 7):24–29, 1995 7673102

Swift RM: Pharmacological treatments for drug and alcohol dependence: experimental and standard therapies. Psychiatr Ann 28:697–702, 1998

Tunving K: Psychiatric effects of cannabis use. Acta Psychiatr Scand 72(3):209–217, 1985 3000137

Umbricht A, Montoya ID, Hoover DR, et al: Naltrexone shortened opioid detoxification with buprenorphine. Drug Alcohol Depend 56(3):181–190, 1999 10529020

Vendruscolo LF, Barbier E, Schlosburg JE, et al: Corticosteroid-dependent plasticity mediates compulsive alcohol drinking in rats. J Neurosci 32(22):7563–7571, 2012 22649234

Vendruscolo LF, Estey D, Goodell V, et al: Glucocorticoid receptor antagonism decreases alcohol seeking in alcohol-dependent individuals. J Clin Invest 125(8):3193–3197, 2015 26121746

Volpicelli JR, Alterman AI, Hayashida M, O'Brien CP: Naltrexone in the treatment of alcohol dependence. Arch Gen Psychiatry 49(11):876–880, 1992 1345133

Weiss RD: Pharmacotherapy for co-occurring mood and substance use disorders, in Integrated Treatment for Mood and Substance Disorders. Edited by Westermeyer JJ, Weiss RD, Ziedonis DM. Baltimore, MD, Johns Hopkins University Press, 2003, pp 122–139

Wignall ND, Brown ES: Citicoline in addictive disorders: a review of the literature. Am J Drug Alcohol Abuse 40(4):262–268, 2014 24950234

12

Pharmacotherapy of Specific Populations

O ne of the difficulties that clinicians face is that a typical clinic patient often does not resemble the sanitized patients selected in research studies. Most published reports evaluating the efficacy of psychoactive drugs in psychiatric patients carefully select physically healthy adult, but not geriatric, pediatric, or pregnant, patients. Unfortunately, in clinical practice, physicians frequently encounter patients with psychiatric disorders who are also pregnant, juvenile, elderly, brain injured, or medically ill but who are otherwise appropriate candidates for conventional pharmacotherapy. Over the past decade, much has been learned about treating specific populations with psychotropic agents. In this chapter, we address some of these special situations.

Pregnancy

Pregnancy, current or planned, poses a complex problem for the psychiatrist, for the psychiatric patient, and for the fetus. Folk wisdom has suggested that pregnancy is a relatively protected time in which the pregnant person may be less susceptible to psychiatric difficulties. This, unfortunately, is not the case. Pregnancy does not protect patients against the occurrence, recurrence, or exacerbation of psychiatric conditions. For example, most patients with recurrent depression who stop taking an antidepressant in anticipation of conceiving are back taking an antidepressant before delivery. At least 10% of patients meet criteria for a depressive disorder during pregnancy. Pregnancy appears to increase the risk of OCD and other anxiety disorders. Mania and schizophrenia may occur or worsen during pregnancy.

The risks of drug administration during pregnancy include teratogenesis, particularly during the first trimester, and even possible behavioral teratogenesis (Table 12–1). Until June 2015, the FDA categorized medications on the basis of known teratogenic risk from animal and human data. The categories ranged from category A, in which adequate data indicate that the drug is safe in pregnancy, to category X, which indicates that the teratogenic risks generally outweigh the benefits. For drugs released after 2015, the FDA has dropped the categories in the drug label in favor of a narrative that includes sections on pregnancy, including labor and delivery; lactation; and a new section, "Females and Males of Reproductive Potential." This new section includes information on what is known about the drug's impact on fertility, contraception recommendations, and the need for pregnancy testing. Part of the rationale for expanding the narrative and dropping the categories was to fill in gaps that clinicians and patients need in order to make decisions about a drug, but also because the FDA decided that the previous categories were overly simplistic. Many psychiatric drugs are category D, and some are category X. In some women, the benefits of even a category X drug, such as some benzodiazepines, may conceivably outweigh the risks. Also, a prescriber may mistakenly believe that because clozapine was a category B drug, it is safer to use in pregnancy than most other antipsychotics, which are category C. That would be a faulty assumption. There simply has not been enough study of clozapine in pregnancy to say anything more definitive about its risks. Given the known toxicity of clozapine, there is no reason to think it is any safer in pregnancy than other antipsychotics. On the other hand, the new narratives place more responsibility on clinicians and may result in less consistent prescribing practices among them. Rather than simply looking at the categories, a clinician must take a deeper dive into the narratives and decide whether a

Table 12–1. Teratogenic risks of psychotropic medications

Class	Drug	Previous FDA risk category[a]	Possible effects
Anxiolytics	Benzodiazepines	D	"Floppy baby," withdrawal, increased risk of cleft lip or palate
	Hypnotic benzodiazepines	X	Decreased intrauterine growth
	Buspirone	C	Unknown
Antidepressants	TCAs	D	Fetal tachycardia, fetal withdrawal, fetal anticholinergic effects, urinary retention, bowel obstruction
	Amitriptyline, imipramine, nortriptyline		
	Other TCAs	C	
	MAOIs	C	Rare fetal malformations; rarely used in pregnancy because of hypertension
	SSRIs	C	Increased perinatal complications
	Paroxetine	D	Cardiovascular malformations, increased perinatal complications
Antipsychotics	FGAs	C	Rare anomalies, fetal jaundice, fetal anticholinergic effects at birth
	SGAs		Gestational diabetes, high birth weight
	Clozapine	B	
	Aripiprazole, risperidone, olanzapine, quetiapine, ziprasidone, iloperidone, asenapine	C	

Table 12–1. Teratogenic risks of psychotropic medications *(continued)*

Class	Drug	Previous FDA risk category[a]	Possible effects
Mood stabilizers	Lithium	D	Associated with increase in birth defects, including cardiac anomalies, especially Ebstein's anomaly; behavioral effects
	Valproate	D	Neural tube defects, lowered IQ
	Carbamazepine	D	Neural tube defects, minor anomalies
	Oxcarbazepine	C	Unknown
	Lamotrigine	C	Unknown
	Gabapentin/pregabalin	C	Unknown

Note. FGA=first-generation antipsychotic; MAOI=monoamine oxidase inhibitor; SGA=second-generation antipsychotic; SSRI=selective serotonin reuptake inhibitor; TCA=tricyclic antidepressant.

[a]In December 2014, the FDA issued the final Pregnancy and Lactation Labeling Rule, which required changes to prescription drug labeling "to assist health care providers in assessing benefit versus risk and in subsequent counseling of pregnant women and nursing mothers who need to take medication" and removed pregnancy letter categories. See www.fda.gov/Drugs/DevelopmentApprovalProcess/DevelopmentResources/Labeling/ucm093307.htm for details.

given medication is suitable for a specific patient. Although, in principle, the clinician should always be as familiar as possible with the risks of a drug, in practice, many clinicians have depended on categories rather than reading detailed narratives on each medication.

There are a number of excellent reviews of the known teratogenic risks associated with psychiatric medications (Newport et al. 2009; Payne 2021; Ray-Griffith et al. 2017). All psychotropic agents cross the placenta to some degree. Gross physical malformations are easy to detect and document, and the possibility that drugs given during pregnancy may affect brain function and behavior years later exists, but there is no clear evidence that it actually occurs. Direct toxic effects on the fetus can occur later in pregnancy. Drugs can affect labor and delivery, with residual effects on the infant's behavior after delivery. All psychotropic drugs are excreted in the mother's milk during breastfeeding, to different degrees. This puts both doctor and patient in a very unpleasant bind. Ideally, every mother should be totally drug-free throughout every pregnancy. However, there are many instances in which the known risks of discontinuing psychiatric medications are greater than the unknown risks of continuing to take them.

Not treating mental illness during pregnancy has significant risks. Severely depressed pregnant patients do not take care of themselves optimally, and conflicting reports have suggested a higher risk of low birth weight and preterm delivery in untreated depressed pregnant people. When the risk of suicide is added to the equation, the risk can be overwhelming. Similarly, untreated schizophrenia has been associated with an increase in perinatal deaths. Psychosis can jeopardize both mother and fetus. There is at least a theoretical risk that elevated cortisol levels associated with severe stress during pregnancy might affect fetal brain development.

This dilemma is illustrated by the case of a markedly manic drug-free patient believed to be in the sixth week of pregnancy who was admitted to the hospital a number of years ago. She was kept drug-free in seclusion, and often in restraint, for a week because the treating psychiatrist was afraid to initiate neuroleptic treatment for fear of harming the fetus. One consultant on the case advised proceeding with haloperidol therapy, despite the presumed pregnancy, on the grounds that severe hyperactivity and distress were a risk to both patient and fetus, whereas there was no direct evidence that haloperidol or any other antipsychotic leads to any specific birth defect. The physician in charge disagreed. Finally, an ultrasound examination revealed a false pregnancy, and appropriate drug treatment was begun. This case illustrates one kind of clinical dilemma. Thalidomide, with its gross fetal deformities, still haunts all of pharmacotherapy.

As far as we can determine, the only drugs commonly used in psychiatry with proven relationships to specific birth defects are lithium, most anticonvulsants, paroxetine, and benzodiazepines. Lithium has been associated with cardiac abnormalities, especially Ebstein's anomaly, and anticonvulsants have been associated with a variety of birth defects, including facial deformity and spina bifida. However, studies in the 1990s (Cohen et al. 1994) suggested that first-trimester lithium teratogenic effects had been overestimated in the earlier studies and that the risks of stopping lithium in some patients outweighed the risks of birth defects. A recent large-scale U.S. study pointed to lower rates of Ebstein's anomaly than were previously reported, although the risk was still greater than was seen with lamotrigine (Patorno et al. 2017). The absolute risk of Ebstein's anomaly with first trimester exposure appears to be 6/1,000. However, this risk is still greater than the risk to pregnant patients without first trimester exposure to lithium.

Beyond this, there is no clear evidence that any standard psychiatric drug does (or does not) cause birth defects. Minor congenital abnormalities occur in up to 4% of infants born to drug-free mothers. However, there is a general suspicion that any drug might be bad for the fetus, and no doctor feels totally comfortable recommending drug therapy for a patient who is believed to have recently become pregnant or who intends to become pregnant. Whenever possible, drug therapy should be avoided in such instances.

Unfortunately, some patients with severe, even disabling, psychiatric disorders either want to become or actually become pregnant, and a choice must be made between treating the patient and avoiding medicating the fetus. If the situation is not a crisis, as with the patient who is taking maintenance medication but would like to become pregnant, outside consultation can be obtained from a psychiatrist experienced in working collaboratively with obstetricians or from a dysmorphologist (an expert in birth defects), a type of specialist found in major medical centers.

Telephone hotlines providing information about the effects of drugs on the fetus are also available. One of these is the MotherToBaby (MTB) organization (https://mothertobaby.org) based in California, which is part of the Organization of Teratotology Information Specialists (OTIS; https://mothertobaby.org/

about-otis). They can be reached at (866) 626-6847. Staff members are willing to accept calls and refer callers to other programs around the country when appropriate. MTB accepts calls from both patients and clinicians and provides up-to-date information on what is known about the risks of a specific medication in pregnancy. OTIS is also involved in multiple studies of teratogenic effects of drugs and offers enrollment to patients referred from physicians when appropriate. Another resource is the North American Antiepiletic Drug (AED) Pregnancy Registry for women to learn about anticonvulsant drugs in pregnancy. Women taking anticonvulsants during pregnancy are encouraged to enroll in the AED Pregnancy Registry online at www.aedpregnancyregistry.org or by calling (888) 233-2334. Major reference works in this area are listed in the Suggested Readings at the end of this chapter.

Information from a reproductive psychiatry specialist or a telephone hotline can indicate whether there is any solid evidence that a particular drug is teratogenic, but it does not solve the clinician's whole problem. The final decision must be based on the seriousness of the patient's distress and the reasonableness of the desire to have a child. Documented informed consent from the patient and family (including the patient's spouse or parents, when appropriate) for the treatment plan is necessary, whether the clinician decides to leave the patient drug-free with the risks of that course or to continue with a needed medication despite the pregnancy.

It is likely that stopping most psychotropic medication 2–3 weeks before the pregnancy is early enough to avoid malformations. If medication can be avoided for the first 3 months of pregnancy, the risk of fetal abnormality is much reduced, but other risks can occur. Babies born to individuals who are physically dependent on sedatives or opioids suffer withdrawal syndromes and need to be treated postnatally. Autonomic withdrawal symptoms presumably can occur in the newborn if the pregnant parent has been taking tricyclic antidepressants (TCAs) or short-acting antidepressants such as paroxetine and venlafaxine. One can justify withdrawing medication carefully from pregnant patients a few weeks before delivery in some circumstances. However, the risk to the fetus or newborn may be small relative to the risks posed by not treating a vulnerable patient as the postpartum period begins.

Overall, antidepressants are probably the best-studied class of agents during pregnancy relative to all other medicines. Most of the data and reviews on exposure during pregnancy (Rahimi et al. 2006; Yonkers et al. 2009) suggest that selective serotonin reuptake inhibitors (SSRIs), with the exception of paroxetine, are not associated with a higher rate of birth anomalies. Paroxetine was moved from category C to category D under the old classification because of an association with cardiac abnormalities, including atrial and septal defects. Thus, paroxetine generally should be avoided in pregnancy if possible, particularly in the first trimester. In addition, SSRI exposure during pregnancy has been associated with higher rates of spontaneous abortions (Rahimi et al. 2006); a self-limiting poor neonatal adaptation syndrome that can include a broad array of symptoms including motor effects, respiratory symptoms, feeding difficulty, irritability, and gastrointestinal upset (Moses-Kolko et al. 2005, Viguera et al. 2023); a small risk of postnatal pulmonary hypertension (absolute risk estimate 0.619/1,000) (Ng et al. 2019); and even autism (Boukhris et al. 2016). In addition, women exposed to high doses of fluoxetine in pregnancy might have a somewhat increased risk of delivering a low–birth weight infant (Hendrick et al. 2003; Simon et al. 2002). Studies on the association of SSRIs with teratogenic and perinatal complications are often contradictory. The challenge with these association studies is that they do not typically account for the confounding effect of the underlying psychiatric condition of the pregnant parent. For example, when the contribution of the maternal depression is factored in, it is difficult to show an association with low gestational birth weight with antidepressant use. Depression affects weight gain in the pregnant person and is itself associated with low gestational birth weight. Preliminary evidence suggests that citalopram and sertraline do not appear to be teratogens (Einarson et al. 2009). Given the known risk of relapse or recurrence when antidepressants are stopped, we have, along with our patients, concluded many times that patients are better off continuing their SSRIs throughout the pregnancy.

All the SSRIs except paroxetine were considered FDA category C agents under the now-superseded categorization, meaning that the risk of teratogenic effects cannot be ruled out because of insufficient evidence. In contrast, there are convincing data that valproate is associated with a variety of neural tube defects in the first trimester, including spina bifida, anencephaly, hydrocephalus, microcephaly, urogenital deficits, and fetal valproate syndrome (see Chapter 5, "Mood Stabilizers"). The rate of major congenital malformations associated with valproate is estimated at 6%–20% (Harden et al. 2009). Hydantoin and carbamazepine may be associated with similar defects. The fetal serum levels of the anticonvulsants are about 50%–80% of the maternal level. As a result, most of the anticonvulsants were category D agents. We know very little about lamotrigine, topiramate, and gabapentin in pregnancy, although these drugs were considered risk category C simply because data do not exist to define a risk. The available data suggest that lamotrigine and oxcarbazepine do carry some teratogenic risk, although much less than that of lithium, valproate, and carbamazepine. Lamotrigine may be associated with a high rate of cleft lip and palate (4–9/1,000), which appears to be at least 10 times the risk in the general population (Viguera et al. 2007).

In addition to being associated with neural tube defects, valproate use in pregnancy appears, with increasing evidence, to be associated with low IQs in children exposed in utero to the drug. Meador et al. (2009) examined the cognitive function of 309 children exposed to various antiepileptics in utero. At age 3 years, children who had been exposed to valproate had an IQ 9 points lower than that of children who had been exposed to lamotrigine and 6 points lower than that of children who had been exposed to carbamazepine. In addition, Meador and colleagues found an association between higher doses of maternal valproate and lower IQ in their offspring. This study supports earlier work suggesting an association of valproate with higher rates of intellectual deficits in exposed offspring (Thomas et al. 2008; Vinten et al. 2005). The growing evidence supporting an association of maternal valproate use with diminished cognitive function in their offspring suggests that valproate should not be used in pregnancy as a first-line agent in bipolar patients. Still, studies in Europe indicate there are probably too many women of childbearing potential still receiving valproate for epilepsy (Andrade 2018).

Second-generation antipsychotics (SGAs) (except clozapine) were listed in category C under the earlier pregnancy category system. Thus far, experience with the SGAs has not suggested that these agents are major teratogens (Damkier and Videbech 2018; Einarson et al. 2009). There may be a small increased risk associated with risperidone (Huybrechts et al. 2016). However, SGAs might carry other risks in pregnancy, including gestational diabetes and large-for-gestational-age infants. Interestingly, a study of more than 1,000 women taking an antipsychotic could find no significant differences in gestational birth weight, hypertensive disorders, or thromboembolism compared with an equal number of women not exposed to an antipsychotic in pregnancy (Vigod et al. 2015). The FDA issued a drug safety communication in 2011 about abnormal muscle movement and withdrawal symptoms in babies exposed to antipsychotics during pregnancy. This may be more an issue in third-trimester exposures to antipsychotics with short half-lives such as risperidone.

We are somewhat more confident about the first-generation antipsychotics (FGAs) in pregnancy because so many pregnant patients have been exposed to these agents since the 1950s. Many patients have been treated with phenothiazine-like agents for nausea during the first trimester, and there is no clear evidence of a teratogenic effect. Because psychosis, mania, or a severe depression can be such a hazard during pregnancy, the benefits of antipsychotics generally outweigh the risk. At this time, it is probably preferable to employ high-potency first-generation agents during pregnancy rather than either SGAs with metabolic risks or low-potency typical agents with significant anticholinergic properties. Haloperidol appears to have among the lowest placenta transfer rates to the fetus.

Benzodiazepines were traditionally considered to be contraindicated in pregnancy. Many benzodiazepines carried an FDA category X risk in pregnancy in the earlier system, indicating that the teratogenic risks of these agents generally outweigh the potential benefits, and are therefore contraindicated. The concern was that first-trimester exposure was associated with an increased risk of cleft lip and palate. However, the association of cleft palate with benzodiazepine exposure has been questioned in some studies (Dolovich et al. 1998; Eros et al. 2002). The risk of oral clefts with benzodiazepine exposure in pregnancy appears to be less than we once believed, but there does appear to be some increased risk.

The issue of behavioral teratogenicity of drugs taken during pregnancy is more difficult to assess. Cocaine and alcohol intake during pregnancy are sometimes associated with behavioral problems in child development, even if the child exhibits no physical deficits. Although physical anomalies are easy to quantify, behavioral effects may be more subtle. The best study to date could find no difference in language, temperament, activity level, or intelligence in 135 children exposed to fluoxetine or TCAs in utero compared with those who were not (Nulman et al. 1997, 2002). Another early study done by the Stanford group suggested that there may be mild motoric differences in children exposed to antidepressants in utero but no effects on mental development (Casper et al. 2003). A more recent study by Casper et al. (2011) found that greater length of prenatal exposure to SSRIs was associated with poorer scores in infancy on behavioral ratings on infant development scales. Delayed motor development has also been reported in a rat study of fluoxetine exposure in utero. However, in this same study, prenatal exposure to fluoxetine had an unexpected beneficial effect on subsequent cognitive ability in rat pups (Bairy et al. 2007). Children born to individuals taking FGAs also showed no significant differences in motor development, growth, or intellect up to age 4 years (Slone et al. 1977).

These studies, although important, have been insufficient to answer the question of whether in utero exposure to psychotropics has negative behavioral effects. Of greatest concern are two more recent studies on the relationship between in utero exposure to SSRIs and autism spectrum disorder. In an epidemiological study in Sweden, prenatal exposure to SSRIs was associated with a 3.36 times increased risk for autism without developmental disability (Rai et al. 2013), but this increased risk explained only 0.6% of the cases of autism. In another case-control study, prenatal exposure was found to increase risk of developing autism in boys (Harrington et al. 2014). These data do suggest that there could be behavioral effects due to exposure to SSRIs, although it is difficult to separate the effects of maternal mood and anxiety disorders on increasing risk. Our clinical experience, however, has not indicated any clear behavioral effects of antidepressant exposure during pregnancy, but further study is certainly warranted.

All known psychoactive drugs are secreted in breast milk. Although fetal serum levels of antidepressant may approach 50% of the maternal serum levels, less than 1% of the maternal dose is present in breast milk. In the absence of data on breast milk concentrations of a specific drug, it is hard to estimate the seriousness of this problem; generally, however, breast milk concentrations are much lower than drug levels in the blood, and the total dose ingested by the infant may be quite small (Berle et al. 2004). Studies have suggested that antidepressant serum levels are often undetectable in infants who breastfed while their mothers were taking antidepressants (Birnbaum et al. 1999; Gentile et al. 2007). Stowe et al. (1997) followed seven nursing women with severe postpartum depression who were taking sertraline and found that the maximum daily dose to which their infants were exposed was 0.026–0.044 mg/kg. In related work (Winn et al. 1995), nursing infants exposed to sertraline in breast milk were monitored by growth charts, number of illnesses, and developmental milestones; no adverse effects were noted as compared with controls. As with many risk-benefit situations in medicine, the suffering of the nursing parent must be weighed against the often unknown risk to the infant, as interpreted by the doctor, the patient, and the patient's family.

Treatment of Minority and Marginalized Populations

Many of the challenges faced by patients with serious mental health issues are even more prevalent in minoritized racial, ethnic, and LGBTQ+ communities (Ricci et al. 2023). Stigma is a barrier to seeking treatment for many psychiatric patients, and this may be particularly true for minority groups. Cultural norms, beliefs, and misconceptions about mental health often discourage individuals from seeking help before the illness has progressed to a more serious problem. In addition, experiences of historical trauma, discrimination, and racism have a lasting impact on mental health. Minority populations have often faced systemic discrimination, contributing to mental health disparities and reluctance to engage with mental health care systems. Language barriers may hinder effective communication between minority patients and mental health care providers. Access to qualified interpreters is often limited, impeding accurate diagnosis, treatment planning, and informed consent. In addition, minority populations may also encounter mental health care providers who are not adequately trained in culturally competent practices (Lok 2022). This mismatch can lead to misunderstandings, misdiagnoses, and inadequate treatment plans, resulting in suboptimal outcomes.

There are differences in the reported rates of various mental health conditions in minority communities in the United States. For example, African Americans and Hispanics tend to have lower rates of depression than do people of European descent, but depression may be more persistent in minority populations (Budhwani et al. 2015). PTSD and alcohol use disorder are more prevalent in Indigenous populations, including American Indians and Native Alaskans. People of European descent, particularly white males, have consistently had the highest suicide rate in the United States. LGBTQ+ youth are four times more likely than their peers to attempt suicide (Green et al. 2022). Although the rates of schizophrenia and bipolar disorder are probably fairly consistent across racial and ethnic groups, limited access to care may have contributed to somewhat lower rates reported in some minority groups.

Pharmacotherapy of specific racial and ethnic groups has been limited by the relative lack of participation of diverse racial and ethnic groups in clinical trials. Although there has been an attempt to diversify the populations in psychiatric drug trials since the 1990s, most participants in clinical trials still have been of European descent. Thus, tolerability and efficacy data from the average American clinical trial may not be generalizable to more diverse populations. Pharmacogenomic differences might contribute to differences in optimal dosing of medication across different racial ethnic groups. An example from the anticoagulant literature suggests racial differences in optimal dosing of warfarin. Warfarin is metabolized by cytochrone P450 (CYP) 2C9 and VKORC (Mak et al. 2019). Asian populations tend to be poorer metabolizers of warfarin and may require lower doses, whereas patients of African descent tend to be more efficient metabolizers and may require relatively higher doses to achieve therapeutic effects. Of course, there are significant pharmacogenomic variations among many different African and Asian populations (Bousman et al. 2021). For example, East Asian patients may be poorer metabolizers of CYP2C19 than patients from other Asian populations and thus may require lower doses of CYP2C19 substrates, including citalopram, diazepam, and some tricyclics. Patients of Han Chinese descent are more likely to have the HLA-B*1502 haplotype, which is known to increase the risk of Stevens-Johnsons syndrome when these patients are treated with carbamazepine.

Another factor that affects drug response in different racial and minority groups is the presence of specific comorbidities that could predispose patients to greater side effect burden and risk of drug interactions. Rates of obesity and diabetes are higher in the African American and Hispanic populations, particularly in lower socioeconomic groups, than in popuations of Asian or European descent. This may put them at greater risk for metabolic problems when taking antipsychotics. As many as half of Black and 25% of Hispanic gay males will be diagnosed with HIV illness in their lifetime (Mayer et al. 2021). About half of all HIV patients will also be treated with antidepressants at some point in their illness. Antiretrovirals and protease inhibitors are inhibitors of CYP2D6 and CYP3A4 and can substantially increase the levels of most SSRIs (Goodlet et al. 2019). HIV patients taking retonavir typically require lower doses of citalopram, sertraline, fluoxetine and paroxetine. Similarly, fluoxetine and fluvoxamine can significantly increase the risk of toxicity of some protease inhibitors.

Thus, the psychopharmacological treatment of racial, ethnic, and sexual minority patients requires consideration of many factors, including comorbidities, concurrent medications, and genetic factors, as is required in the treatment of other populations. In addition, effective treatment also requires an alliance that is facilitated by a cultural sensitivity and understanding of the unique history and stresses experienced by minority populations.

Pediatric Psychopharmacology

The decision to use a drug treatment for a psychiatrically ill child or young adolescent must be based on a clear clinical need. There are few data on the long-term consequences of psychiatric drug therapy in childhood for brain function, behavior, or physical health in adult life. The psychiatric disorder should pose significant danger to the child's development and well-being, and pharmacotherapy should be undertaken only after considered medical and psychiatric evaluation.

Prepubescent children have relatively efficient livers. This generally allows them to metabolize drugs rapidly and enables them to tolerate somewhat higher doses of psychiatric drugs per unit of weight than adults tolerate. After puberty, drug metabolism resembles that seen in young adults. The lesson here, of course, is not that 7-year-olds should be given huge doses of drugs, but that they should be started on very small doses and, if there is no response, the dose can be gradually increased to adult doses, adjusted for weight, without fear of unusual toxicity.

It should be noted that most standard psychiatric drugs have not received FDA approval for use in children or even in adolescents, mainly because the necessary studies have not been carried out. In the past 25 years, the FDA has begun to require that manufacturers of antidepressants do studies in children and adolescents.

Stimulants

The best studied and best validated drug therapy for psychiatrically ill children is the use of stimulants (D-amphetamine and methylphenidate) in ADHD (see Chapter 8, "Stimulants and the Treatment of ADHD"). More than 170 trials of stimulants in the treatment of ADHD involving 5,000 children attest to the benefits of these drugs. Since the early 1990s, the number of children taking stimulants has risen dramatically. Between 1990 and 1993, the number of outpatient visits devoted to ADHD increased from 1.6 million to 4.2 million per year, with 90% of children diagnosed with ADHD receiving a stimulant at some point in their treatment (Swanson et al. 1995). In 1996 alone, more than 10 million prescriptions for methylphenidate were written. By 2004, the rate of stimulant prescription (4.63/1,000) had doubled from the rate observed just 10 years earlier (Winterstein et al. 2008). It is unclear whether the marked increase in stimulant prescriptions is the result of better recognition of ADHD or overprescribing, but both factors are likely involved (Greenhill et al. 1999). However, the suggestion in some quarters that ADHD is simply an excuse to medicate annoying behavior in children or to sell more drugs does not appear sound.

Research regarding the effects of stimulants on various kinds of behavior suggests that the drug effects are complex. The dosage that controls overactivity best may be too high for optimal improvement in learning. The stimulants may cause a slight decrease in body growth, perhaps 1–3 cm in height over the entire developmental period, although one follow-up study showed no effect of stimulant exposure on adult height (Kramer et al. 2000). Children taking stimulants may show side effects such as anorexia, insomnia, dysphoria, and even tics.

Some children with ADHD receive marked benefits—generally more in behavior than in academic performance—whereas others receive only some benefit, and a few are not benefited or even become more agitated. Distractibility, overt aggression, and daily class performance are improved with stimulant use and worsen when the drug is stopped or a placebo is substituted. Most of the studies have been for 12 weeks or less. However, long-term trials with both stimulants and atomoxetine have confirmed that the benefits of pharmacotherapy in children treated for ADHD are sustained (Arnold et al. 1997; Barbaresi et al. 2006; Kratochvil et al. 2006). A number of long-acting or once-a-day stimulant preparations are currently available (see Chapter 8, Table 8–1).

Some children respond better to one of the two standard stimulants than to the other; this response is unpredictable. Dextroamphetamine is less expensive than branded Ritalin; most stimulant preparations now have generic equivalents. Methylphenidate (Ritalin) is usually started at 5 mg bid, and the dosage may be increased over time up to 20 mg tid. Dextroamphetamine is initiated at 2.5 mg bid, and the dosage is gradually increased to a maximum of

40 mg/day in two to four divided doses. The common clinical practice with the shorter-acting stimulants is to prescribe dosing twice a day, with the last dose around noontime to reduce the risk of insomnia. However, a report by Kent et al. (1995) suggested that adding a third dose in the late afternoon rarely disrupted sleep. Lunchtime doses are frequently a problem for school-children because they may forget to take a dose or because the medication has to be administered by an adult. The practice of giving a child with ADHD their medication only on school days may have the disadvantage of impairing the child's family and peer relationships as well as impairing learning outside school. Sustained-release preparations of D-amphetamine, methylphenidate, and methamphetamine are available, but their usefulness in children with ADHD is not well documented. These preparations can certainly be tried if once-a-day dosing is desired or needed. Whichever medication is used, the dosage may need to be adjusted up or down over time as the child grows and matures. Some children continue to benefit from stimulants into adolescence or even adulthood. In patients with a good stimulant response, drug holidays every few months to discover whether the drug is still needed are worth trying.

A number of other agents have proved useful in the treatment of ADHD. Studies have reported that bupropion may be effective for the behavioral and cognitive problems associated with ADHD (Casat et al. 1989) and in the treatment of adult ADHD (Wilens et al. 1995). In children, the bupropion dosage is 3–6 mg/kg/day in divided doses. One case report suggested that there may be a role for the SSRIs in the treatment of ADHD (Frankenburg and Kando 1994). Guanfacine (Tenex), an antihypertensive agent, has been used off-label in the treatment of ADHD over the years. In 2009, only the extended-release formulation of guanfacine (Intuniv) received an official indication for treatment of ADHD. The efficacy of guanfacine may be less than that of an antidepressant in the treatment of ADHD.

Finally, clonidine is often used in combination with stimulants to reduce side effects and enhance effects on hyperactivity and hyperkinesis. Clonidine at a dosage of 0.1 mg tid has been reported to reduce stimulant-induced insomnia as well as impulsivity. As a monotherapy of ADHD, however, clonidine appears to be inferior to desipramine (Singer et al. 1995). Clonidine was approved for the treatment of ADHD in 2009.

Two additional nonstimulant agents, atomoxetine and viloxazine, have been approved in the treatment of ADHD. Bothe atomoxetine and viloxazine inhibit the presynaptic norepinephrine transporter. Atomoxetine has been reported to be significantly more effective than placebo at dosages of 1.2 mg/kg/day and 1.8 mg/kg/day in children and adolescents with ADHD (Buitelaar et al. 2004; Kelsey et al. 2004). Most children are treated once a day, with the dosage in the range of 40–80 mg/day. Atomoxetine is well absorbed orally and has a half-life that averages about 4 hours. However, slow metabolizers of CYP2D6 metabolize the drug more slowly. We would anticipate that the combination of atomoxetine with SSRIs might increase toxicity. Thus, lower doses of atomoxetine may be needed when a patient is already taking fluoxetine or paroxetine.

Atomoxetine has the advantage over standard stimulants of not having a significant abuse potential. Thus, atomoxetine does not require a special prescription for controlled substances as do standard stimulants. On the other hand, atomoxetine shares with the stimulants a tendency to suppress weight and to increase heart rate and blood pressure. Both the anorexic and cardiovascular effects of atomoxetine appear to be dose related. Other reported side effects include rash, anxiety, somnolence, and, most recently, liver function test abnormalities. Atomoxetine also carries the same black box warning around suicidality that the antidepressants carry.

Several studies have evaluated the efficacy of atomoxetine compared with placebo or standard stimulants. In a randomized comparison of atomoxetine and methylphenidate in 228 children with ADHD, both drugs were equally effective (Kratochvil et al. 2002). In a placebo-controlled study of 297 children with ADHD, atomoxetine consistently beat placebo on measures of attention and hyperactivity (Michelson et al. 2001). In addition, atomoxetine also improved social and family functioning relative to placebo.

Viloxazine was approved by the FDA in 2022 for both children and adults with ADHD. It has a pharmacological profile very similar to that of generic atomoxetine. As another norepinephrine reuptake inhibitor, it does not have an abuse potential as do the stimulants. A number of trials have demonstrated the efficacy of viloxazine in a pediatric population. One randomized, double-blind, placebo-controlled trial involving 477 children with ADHD found that viloxazine was significantly more effective than placebo in reducing symptoms of ADHD, as measured by the ADHD Rating Scale IV. Adverse events were mild to moderate and included insomnia, headache, and decreased appetite (Nasser et al. 2020).

Another randomized, double-blind, placebo-controlled trial involving 324 children with ADHD found that viloxazine significantly improved symptoms of ADHD, as measured by the Conners' Parent Rating Scale—Revised Short Form, as compared with placebo (Prasad et al. 2019). Adverse events were similar to those reported in the Michelson et al. study. A third randomized placebo-controlled trial involving 417 children and adolescents with ADHD found that 400 mg/day but not 600 mg/day significantly improved symptoms on the ADHD rating scale (Nasser et al.. 2021b). Adverse events were mild to moderate and included decreased appetite, nausea, and vomiting.

The effect size and side-effect profile of the viloxazine studies appear comparable to those seen with atomoxetine. Because atomoxetine has been available generically for some time, viloxazine is clearly a much more expensive option without much clear advantage. However, one possible advantage gleaned from the trials outlined above is that viloxazine appears to separate from placebo at about week 1, which is about 2 weeks faster than is seen in atomoxetine studies. Head-to-head comparisons are not available, so it is not possible to say that viloxazine acts any faster than does atomoxetine.

The dosing of viloxazine for children ages 6–11 starts at a 100 mg capsule at week 1, then increases to 200 mg at week 2, 300 mg at week 3, and 400 mg at week 4. For adolescents ages 12–17, the dose starts at 200 mg at week 1 and jumps to the target dose of 400 mg at week 2. Most patients take the drug in the morning because it can be activating and can be taken with food. For children who have trouble swallowing capsules, the contents can be sprinkled over soft food.

Modafinil, which is FDA approved for the treatment of narcolepsy, has also been studied, but it has not been approved for the treatment of ADHD. Modafinil is a Drug Enforcement Administration schedule IV agent, and its abuse potential appears to be very low. In addition, it is better tolerated than amphetamines and is simple to dose.

Like atomoxetine, modafinil has been thought to not act on the dopaminergic system. It appears to act on excitatory histamine projections in very specific regions of the brain and lacks the generalized effects of stimulants. It may act on dopamine, as well as on the hypocretin/orexin system. As such, it is less likely than either amphetamine or atomoxetine to produce cardiovascular changes or weight gain. The most common side effect of modafinil has been headache, but the drug can also produce some mild gastrointestinal side effects.

CNS side effects such as anxiety or insomnia occur infrequently. Modafinil is an inducer of the CYP3A3/4 enzyme, so it can speed up the metabolism of oral contraceptives, steroids, and other 3A3/4-dependent compounds. Thus, patients taking birth control pills should be advised that there is a theoretical risk of contraceptive failure when modafinil is taken concurrently.

Modafinil has been studied in many conditions associated with producing fatigue, including shift work, sleep apnea, multiple sclerosis, fibromyalgia, Parkinson's disease, and depression (see Chapter 9, "Augmentation Strategies for Treatment-Resistant Disorders"). Preliminary results suggest that modafinil may have a role in the treatment of fatigue in many disorders without a significant downside.

The efficacy of modafinil in the treatment of ADHD has been evaluated in a number of trials. Studies of modafinil in the treatment of ADHD in children have suggested a benefit over placebo and effectiveness equal to that of dextroamphetamine (Rugino and Copley 2001; Taylor and Russo 2000). In a 4-week study of 248 children with ADHD, modafinil at a dosage of 300–400 mg/day was more effective than placebo in treating the symptoms of ADHD and was well tolerated (Biederman et al. 2006b). Likewise, in a 9-week double-blind trial of 194 children and adolescents with ADHD, 52% of patients randomly assigned to modafinil improved versus 18% of children randomly assigned to placebo (Greenhill et al. 2006). These data appeared to be sufficient to prompt an approval letter in 2005 for modafinil treatment of ADHD in children. However, there was a report of possible Stevens-Johnson syndrome in a child participating in one of the trials. The etiology of the rash was unclear but might have been related to the study drug. This report resulted in the FDA requesting additional safety information. The company decided to withdraw its application for modafinil in the treatment of ADHD, apparently because of the extensive safety studies that would be required for final approval. The *R*-enantiomer of modafinil is currently being investigated in the treatment of ADHD and other indications such as bipolar depression.

Antipsychotics

Historically, very few trials of FGAs were done with children who had schizophrenia. There has been a general impression that children benefit less from antipsychotics than do adults. However, with the limited data on drug therapy in childhood schizophrenia, it is difficult to make any generalizations. The first antipsychotic study showed a modest benefit of haloperidol and loxapine compared with placebo in 75 adolescents with schizophrenia (Pool et al. 1976). A later study showed that haloperidol was superior to placebo in the treatment of childhood schizophrenia (Spencer et al. 1992).

There are growing data on the efficacy and safety of SGAs in the treatment of childhood schizophrenia and bipolar disorder (Geller et al. 2012; Kumra et al. 2008). As of this writing, six SGAs are approved for various indications in children and adolescents: risperidone, paliperidone, asenapine, olanzapine, quetiapine, and aripiprazole. Olanzapine, risperidone, paliperidone, aripiprazole, and quetiapine are approved for the treatment of schizophrenia in adolescents. Asenapine, risperidone, aripiprazole, and quetiapine are approved for the treatment of bipolar mania in children ages 10–17. Olanzapine has an additional indication in the adjunctive treatment of bipolar depression for children ages 10–17. Aripiprazole and risperidone are approved to treat irritability in autism spectrum disorder in children ages 6–17.

Clozapine has been investigated in small pediatric studies. In one controlled trial, clozapine was compared with haloperidol in 21 patients over 6 weeks (Kumra et al. 1996). The average dosage of clozapine was 237 mg/day. The group that was randomly assigned to clozapine showed superior improvement in both positive and negative symptoms relative to the haloperidol-treated children. However, clozapine was poorly tolerated. Five of 10 clozapine-treated children had significant drops in their neutrophils. In addition, 2 of the 10 children experienced seizures. Another small randomized controlled trial found that olanzapine and risperidone were somewhat more effective than haloperidol in the treatment of childhood schizophrenia (Sikich et al. 2004). However, weight gain was significantly more problematic in the children treated with SGAs. In a Cochrane review, the SGAs were not found to be more effective than FGAs in adolescents with psychosis (Kumar et al. 2013). Side effects were viewed as more favorable with the SGAs, although olanzapine, clozapine, and risperidone were noted to be associated with weight gain.

SGAs can offer clear advantages in a population that may need to be treated for many years. The risk of extrapyramidal symptoms (EPS) with typical antipsychotics is substantial in children who need to be treated through adulthood. Although akathisia and dystonic reactions are seen in children treated with SGAs, the risk of tardive dyskinesia is apparently small (Correll et al. 2004). On the other hand, obesity may be a limiting factor for some SGAs.

Table 12–2. Antipsychotic dosages in children

Drug	Common pediatric therapeutic dosage
Chlorpromazine	0.25 mg/kg tid
Trifluoperazine	0.5–10 mg bid
Haloperidol	0.15–0.5 mg/kg/day (in divided doses [bid])
Aripiprazole	2–10 mg/day
Asenapine	2.5–10 mg bid
Olanzapine	2.5–5 mg qhs
Paliperidone	3–12 mg/day
Quetiapine	25–300 mg/day
Risperidone	1–2 mg/day

Low-dose risperidone (1–2 mg/day) appears to be effective for many without the weight gain associated with other SGAs (Ben Amor 2012), although one can see increases in weight as noted in a recent autism trial (Findling et al. 2014). Clozapine is a last resort in children in whom trials of both typical and atypical agents have failed.

Table 12–2 lists common pediatric therapeutic dosages of selected antipsychotics in children. In children with neurodevelopmental disorders such as autism, antipsychotics have a clearer utility. In fact, in 2006 risperidone became the first drug approved by the FDA for the treatment of some behavioral aspects of autism. Developmental disorders in children younger than age 15 rarely show marked improvement with antipsychotic treatment, although some decrease in overactive, disorganized behavior can occur. Among the best studies of the SGAs for any condition in childhood are studies of the use of risperidone in children with pervasive developmental disorders. For example, in a multisite study of 101 autistic children, risperidone was significantly more effective than placebo in controlling tantrums, aggression, and self-injurious behavior (McCracken et al. 2002). Additionally, the effects were sustained for at least 6 months. The drug has obtained FDA approval for irritability (e.g., aggressive behavior) in autism.

Psychosis associated with affective disorders in children is also helped by antipsychotics. There is no evidence that children are any less tolerant of these drugs than are adults, except perhaps for an even higher rate of dystonia early in treatment in adolescent males. However, the risk of tardive dyskinesia and the lower likelihood of marked improvement make it necessary for clinicians to use these agents cautiously, documenting carefully the clinical effects observed and periodically assessing the patient without the medication to make sure that the treatment is really useful as a maintenance therapy. In older adolescents, acute psychotic syndromes begin to resemble those seen in adults and may be treated in the same manner (see Chapter 4, "Antipsychotic Drugs").

Sedative FGAs (e.g., thioridazine, chlorpromazine) may interfere with learning. Of the nonsedative FGAs, haloperidol has been best studied in autistic children (children with DSM-IV pervasive developmental disorder) and has limited efficacy. Recent reports have discussed the utility of atypical antipsychotics such as risperidone and clozapine in treating children with psychosis. Earlier case reports attested to the utility of clozapine in child and adolescent patients with schizophrenia (Mozes et al. 1994).

Antipsychotics used at low dosages (e.g., 0.5–3 mg/day of haloperidol or 2–10 mg/day of pimozide) can also control the tics of Tourette's disorder. Although a number of antipsychotics probably can help symptoms of Tourette's disorder, aripiprazole is the only antipsychotic to receive a pediatric indication for children ages 6–17. It is typically started at 2 mg/day, and the therapeutic dosage range is 5–20 mg/day. Clonidine has also been reported to be helpful in severe cases of this disorder. Clonidine can suppress tics fairly well, but it may be more effective in patients with Tourette's disorder who have explosive violent behaviors. Clonidine causes dry mouth, sedation, constipation, and hypotension.

Antipsychotics have often been used to control the behavior of angry, impulsive children and adolescents without psychosis. This use is not well validated, but most clinicians use low doses of antipsychotics to control angry, violent behavior in child or adolescent inpatients. Some prefer haloperidol in low doses (e.g., 2 mg every hour until the patient is calm), whereas others use more sedative drugs such as chlorpromazine in 10- to 50-mg doses three or four times a day. Risperidone has been studied in the treatment of aggression associated with autism in adults and is clearly more effective than placebo (McDougle et al. 1998). Open studies and reports of risperidone in the treatment of aggression in children have also been positive at dosages of 1–2 mg/day (Horrigan and Barnhill 1997; Schreier 1998).

A well-controlled study comparing haloperidol (2–6 mg/day), lithium carbonate, and placebo in hospitalized nonpsychotic aggressive children with conduct disorder showed the two drug regimens to be more effective than placebo on various measures (Platt et al. 1984). The nursing staff judged the lithium responders to have done best. Sedation and dystonia were problems in patients taking haloperidol. The risks and benefits of this use are unclear. If antipsychotics are used to reduce aggression in children with conduct disorder and actually are effective, the continued use of these potentially harmful drugs to control deviant behavior must be strongly justified. For any individual patient, the drug must make a major and clinically important difference.

Another growing use of antipsychotics in children is for the treatment of anorexia. There are no known effective pharmacotherapies for anorexia nervosa. However, preliminary studies have reported that atypical antipsychotics may help with the agitation, obsessiveness, and disturbing cognitions associated with anorexia nervosa (Dennis et al. 2006; Mondraty et al. 2005). Olanzapine and quetiapine have been most investigated and, as expected, also may be associated with steady weight gain. Additional trials are clearly called for on the utility of antipsychotics in pediatric anorexia.

The side effects and risks of antipsychotics, including tardive dyskinesia with typical agents and weight gain with atypical agents, are similar in children and adults. However, the possibility of cognitive blunting with these drugs may be relatively more of a problem in children. An inert child who is not learning or functioning may be less trouble to others, but the child may develop more normally if medication is reduced or stopped. In addition, it appears that adolescent males are at much greater risk for dystonic reactions than are older adults (Rosenberg et al. 1994).

When antipsychotics are prescribed for children or adolescents, documented informed consent from the responsible parent or parents is mandatory. Even if the child or adolescent patient is too young to give informed consent, the risks and benefits of the drug should be explained to the patient, and their assent to the treatment should be obtained when possible (see Chapter 1, "General Principles of Psychopharmacological Treatment").

Antidepressants

The 2004 decision of an FDA advisory panel to put a black box warning on antidepressants used in children appeared to have had an effect on prescribing of these agents to children and adolescents. Although the FDA's review of 25 studies involving 4,600 children suggested an increased risk of suicidal thoughts or gestures by 3% in antidepressant-treated patients versus 1.5% in patients receiving placebo, the review did not adequately weigh the risks of no treatment at all. In addition, the increased suicidal activity did not result in any deaths. The black box warning resulted in a decrease in prescribing, particularly by pediatricians (Nemeroff et al. 2007). In the Netherlands, where there was a similar black box warning, an increase in suicide was also observed (Gibbons et al. 2007). After a period of 1–2 years, the drop in prescribing stabilized. Our view is that although some children appear to be at increased risk for worsening of suicidal thoughts while taking antidepressants, the benefit outweighs the risks. We suspect that pediatric depression is more likely to be associated with bipolar spectrum disorders, and those patients with treatment-emergent akathisia may be at greatest risk. However, this has not been borne out in studies. The slightly increased risk associated with antidepressants must be weighed against the clear risk of completed suicide in depressed children who are inadequately treated or not treated at all. Indeed, suicide risk in adolescents has been on the rise in recent years, particularly among young girls.

The SSRIs have been considered the pharmacotherapy of choice for depression in childhood and adolescence. Fluoxetine was the first antidepressant that was FDA approved in the treatment of childhood depression, followed by escitalopram in children ages 12 and older. Sertraline and fluvoxamine are approved for pediatric OCD. Duloxetine is approved for generalized anxiety disorder in children 7 years and older. The combination of olanzapine with fluoxetine is approved for bipolar depression in youth ages 10 and older. Clomipramine is approved for childhood OCD (ages 10 and older).

Although it was difficult to demonstrate that the TCAs or other antidepressants are more effective than placebo in the treatment of childhood depression, there are data regarding fluoxetine's and escitalopram's superiority to placebo in children. In addition, the safety and side-effect profiles of the SSRIs are superior to those of the TCAs. Emslie and colleagues (1997) randomly assigned 76 children (ages 7–17) to receive either fluoxetine 20 mg/day or placebo. Whereas 56% of the fluoxetine-treated patients responded in 8 weeks, only 33% of the placebo-treated patients responded. Nonetheless, remission was rare for both groups. A more recent study by Emslie and colleagues (2002) that included 219 children also found fluoxetine well tolerated and effective in the treatment of pediatric depression. In addition, fluoxetine maintenance treatment appears to be effective in preventing relapse in children (Emslie et al. 2004).

Fluoxetine's oral elixir is quite useful in children. Experience has shown that children are better off starting at lower dosages of fluoxetine. We tend to start at 5 mg/day and increase the dosage every 1–2 weeks to a maximum dosage of 60 mg/day. Wagner et al. (2006a) reported that escitalopram was significantly more effective than placebo in adolescents (ages 12–17) but not in children younger than age 12. A subsequent report by Emslie et al. (2009) confirmed this. The drug was well tolerated. The daily starting dosage is 10 mg, and the range is to 20 mg/day.

Studies on the efficacy of other SSRIs in pediatric depression have been less convincing. Two published trials of sertraline in the treatment of depression in childhood suggest a modest but statistically significant benefit of sertraline after 10 weeks of treatment (Wagner et al. 2003). One published study indicated a somewhat higher rate of remission in depressed children treated with paroxetine but little difference in mean depression scores at the end of 8 weeks (Keller et al. 2001). In another study, paroxetine (20–40 mg/day) and imipramine (200–300 mg/day) at their maximum did not separate from placebo in adolescent depression (Keller et al. 2001). In addition, two unpublished studies of paroxetine did not find benefit in adolescents. One study indicated that citalopram at an average dosage of about 23 mg/day was significantly more effective than placebo in childhood or adolescent depression (Wagner et al. 2001). However, response rates to both drug (36%) and placebo (24%) were relatively low. The drug was well tolerated.

The sum of published and unpublished studies suggests that the benefits of SSRIs appear most solid with fluoxetine in children and escitalopram in adolescents. Other SSRIs, including paroxetine, citalopram, and sertraline, do appear to have some benefits, but these benefits are more modest and are not established in controlled studies. Some investigators have concluded that when unpublished studies are considered and the risks of SSRIs are weighed against the benefits in children, the benefits are not overwhelming (Whittington et al. 2004). In contrast, a meta-analysis did reveal significant benefit for SSRIs overall compared with placebo in major depression, OCD, and anxiety disorders (Bridge et al. 2007). Moreover, as noted earlier, the FDA warning about the risk for suicidal behavior with the SSRIs did have a chilling effect on prescribing (Nemeroff et al. 2007) and, unfortunately, a resultant spike in the rates of suicides in adolescents (Gibbons et al. 2007). Given that only a relatively small handful of studies on the use of SSRIs in treating pediatric depression have been completed, we believe that it is too early to draw strong conclusions about the utility of many of the nonapproved SSRIs in children. There is obviously a need for clinicians to have access to previously unpublished studies. But there are children and adolescents who benefit from antidepressants, and they should be both treated and monitored carefully.

A recent review by Walkup (2017) questioned the methodology and validity of many of the industry-supported antidepressant trials in children and adolescents. He noted that the two National Institute of Mental Health–funded studies showed convincing data in support of antidepressant efficacy. In one now classic study, the Treatment for Adolescents With Depression Study, fluoxetine appeared more effective than placebo at 12 weeks (Kennard et al. 2009).

It has been even more difficult to demonstrate clear efficacy of TCAs and other antidepressants in controlled studies of childhood depression. For example, a meta-analysis of 12 randomized studies of TCAs in pediatric depression failed to demonstrate a significant difference relative to placebo (Hazell et al. 1995). However, some children who clearly meet criteria for major depressive disorder do appear to respond to TCAs. FDA guidelines recommend an upper dose limit of 2.5 mg/kg for imipramine; however, some studies report doses up to 5.0 mg/kg as often being necessary for clinical response (Table 12–3).

Monitoring of cardiac function is wise when TCAs are used in children: an electrocardiogram (ECG) should be done prior to starting therapy, again when the dose exceeds 3 mg/kg, and then every 2 weeks if the dose is being increased. Doses greater than 5 mg/kg should not be given without outside consultation. Significant slowing of cardiac conduction (PR interval >0.20 msec, QRS interval >0.12 msec) may require lowering the dose. Between 1986 and 1992, at least four cases of sudden death occurred in children taking desipramine. The cardiac long QT syndrome has been proposed as a mechanism of action in these sudden deaths. A more recent review of the topic (Biederman et al. 1995) failed to find a strong association between desipramine use and sudden death in children 5–14 years old.

TCAs are effective in the treatment of enuresis at doses of 0.3–1.0 mg/kg of imipramine or an equivalent drug, but behavioral treatments are generally preferred because they are also effective and may have a lower relapse rate.

Table 12–3.   Common antidepressant dosages in children

Drug	Dosage range	Serum level (ng/mL)
Imipramine	1–5 mg/kg/day	150–250
Desipramine	1–5 mg/kg/day	150–250
Nortriptyline	0.5–2 mg/kg/day	75–150
Phenelzine	0.25–1 mg/kg/day	NA
Fluoxetine	5–30 mg/day	NA
Bupropion	1–7 mg/kg/day	NA
Citalopram	10–20 mg/day	NA

Note.   NA=not applicable.

ADHD tends to respond in the same dosage range. It is interesting to note that TCAs improve enuresis within a few days, whereas response for ADHD or depression takes 1–4 weeks. Monoamine oxidase inhibitors (MAOIs) are also said to be effective in the treatment of both enuresis and ADHD, but their use has not been well studied. Clomipramine is available for the treatment of OCD; it has been shown to be effective in children and adolescents with this condition (see Chapter 6, "Antianxiety Agents," for additional discussion).

Side effects of antidepressants in children resemble those seen in adults. Blood level monitoring is about as useful as it is in adults. That is, it is useful for the TCAs but not for other antidepressants, except, perhaps, to test for compliance. Imipramine is the best-studied TCA, and positive correlations between blood level and improvement are often found in clinical trials. Our experience over the years suggests that depressive symptoms in adolescents rarely include major appetite changes or early morning awakening. Overly sound and lengthy sleep and dysphoria on awakening are more common. Physical symptoms, fatigue, irritability, anger, and retardation for the first few hours in the day may be present without subjective recognition of depression or sadness. Sex drive is decreased. These adolescents often have a family history of affective disorder. This pattern often responds to TCA therapy, although formal controlled studies have not been done. Panic disorder and agoraphobia can occur in adolescents and can be treated with antidepressants.

There are little published data on the use of serotonin$_2$ antagonists, selective serotonin-norepinephrine reuptake inhibitors (SNRIs), and bupropion in pediatric depression. One small, controlled trial of venlafaxine in pediatric depression showed no benefit (Mandoki et al. 1997). In addition, two unpublished trials did not show benefits for venlafaxine in pediatric depression. However, cautious trials with bupropion may be indicated if the patient has not responded to trials of SSRIs or TCAs. Bupropion has been used for ADHD at dosages of 3–7 mg/kg/day in divided doses. In addition, we (Killen et al. 2004) reported on a trial of sustained-release bupropion in combination with a nicotine patch in adolescent smoking cessation. The drug was well tolerated. In addition, open-label studies have suggested that there may be a role for bupropion in treating adolescents with depression and comorbid ADHD (Daviss et al. 2001; Solhkhah et al. 2005). Anorexia and the risk of seizures may be problems for some children, and, particularly in those cases, the dose should be titrated upward slowly. The few small studies of MAOIs in the treatment of children with depression and phobias have generally yielded positive findings, but the results are inconclusive.

Mood Stabilizers

Adolescents can show a typical bipolar picture that often responds to lithium therapy or treatment with an SGA. Preadolescent children rarely show mania, but they can show cyclic mood and behavior shifts with periods of impulsivity, hyperactivity, social intrusiveness, tantrums, mood lability, and nonpsychotic euphoria, with parallel shifts in vegetative symptoms, which sometimes respond to lithium. However, there are limited controlled studies with adequate sample size that have demonstrated the efficacy of lithium in childhood bipolar illness (Kafantaris 1995; Lopez-Larson and Frazier 2006). One of the better studies was a study in adolescents treated with lithium who had bipolar disorder with comorbid substance abuse (Geller et al. 1998). Lithium appeared to help both the bipolar disorder and the substance abuse. A randomized comparison of lithium and divalproex in the maintenance treatment of pediatric bipolar patients (average age 10.8 years) found that valproate was about as effective as lithium in the time it took to require an additional intervention (Findling et al. 2005).

Among the best studies to date was a randomized controlled 6-week trial comparing lithium at therapeutic serum levels to quetiapine at dosages of 400–600 mg/day in adolescents with mania or mixed symptoms (Patino et al. 2021). The response rate on a 50% reduction in the Young Mania Rating

Scale was 72% for the quetiapine group and 49% for the lithium group. However, there was no difference in remission rates between the two drugs. Quetiapine treatment was associated with more somnolence, weight gain, and dizziness than was lithium. Smaller open-label studies have suggested that lithium is effective and often well tolerated in treating adolescent bipolar depression (Patel et al. 2006) and in restabilizing bipolar disorder when combined with valproate in children (Findling et al. 2006). Geller et al. (2012) compared risperidone, lithium, and valproate in children and adolescents with bipolar I disorder. Risperidone was more effective than the other two drugs but had much greater metabolic side effects. On 18-month maintenance follow-up to an earlier study, lithium was equivalent to valproate in children who had originally been treated with the combination before randomization. Explosive, violent behavior in pediatric patients with conduct disorder, intellectual disability, and hyperactivity has also responded to lithium treatment in a number of studies (Campbell et al. 1984; Lopez-Larson and Frazier 2006; Vetró et al. 1985).

No one knows the long-term consequences of long-term maintenance lithium treatment begun in childhood or adolescence. Children have increased renal clearance relative to adults and may tolerate larger doses of lithium. For children older than 12 years, the lithium may often be dosed as it is for adults (Table 12–4). However, younger children under 25 kg are best started at 150–300 mg/day. The dosage may then be increased in 150- to 300-mg increments every 3–7 days in a thrice-daily regimen as tolerated. It is not unusual for children to require more than 2,100 mg/day in divided doses to maintain adequate serum levels. The serum levels should be monitored carefully and checked every 3–5 days after each increase in dosage. The side effects of lithium in children are the same as in adults.

Carbamazepine, oxcarbazepine, lamotrigine, and valproate appear to also have a role in pediatric psychiatric disorders. Controlled data demonstrate carbamazepine's efficacy in conduct disorder and intermittent explosive disorder in children and adolescents. There are also largely uncontrolled data suggesting that anticonvulsants may have utility in the treatment of bipolar disorder and other pediatric conditions. However, Wagner et al. (2009) reported no acute differences between valproate and placebo in a study of bipolar children and adolescents. Of note, Pavuluri et al. (2010) reported more rapid improvement with risperidone than with valproate, and Delbello et al. (2006) re-

Table 12–4. Common mood stabilizer dosages in children

Drug	Dosage range	Serum level
Lithium	300–2,400 mg/day	0.5–1.2 mEq/L
Valproate	15–60 mg/kg/day	50–100 μg/mL
Carbamazepine	10–50 mg/kg/day	8–12 μg/mL
Oxcarbazepine	5–30 mg/kg/day (150–1,200 mg/day)	NA
Lamotrigine	0.15–5.0 mg/kg/day (25–200 mg/day)	NA

Note.   NA = not applicable.

ported faster effects with quetiapine, similar to those noted by Geller et al. (2012) mentioned earlier regarding greater efficacy but higher side effects with SGAs as compared with valproate.

Oxcarbazepine may be somewhat easier to use in children, but the only double-blind study in a pediatric bipolar population failed to show a benefit of oxcarbazepine (Wagner et al. 2006b), and a later Cochrane review concurred (Vasudev et al. 2011). In Canadian studies, there is a suggestion that adolescents with bipolar disorder prefer valproate to lithium. Valproate has also been reported to help aggressive behavior in adolescents with or without mood disorders (Saxena et al. 2006; Steiner et al. 2003). Although there have been no controlled studies of lamotrigine in pediatric bipolar disorder, open-label studies have reported benefit in the treatment of bipolar depression (Chang et al. 2006).

Side effects of anticonvulsants in children parallel those in adults. However, very young children (younger than 2 years) appear at greatest risk for hepatic toxicity with valproate. As with lithium, children often require higher doses of carbamazepine or valproate on a mg/kg basis than do adults because of their more efficient hepatic and renal metabolism, as already mentioned. Children may be more at risk for rash while taking lamotrigine than are adults, and slow titration of the drug to therapeutic levels is prudent. The dosage range of carbamazepine in children is 10–50 mg/kg/day in divided doses; the dosage range of valproate is 15–60 mg/kg/day. One issue with valproate in girls is the risk of polycystic ovaries as they mature.

Antianxiety Drugs

Benzodiazepines are sometimes of use for short periods in treating pavor nocturnus or sleepwalking in children. Of course, benzodiazepines and nonbenzodiazepine hypnotics such as zolpidem also have been associated with somnambulism and amnesia in both children and adults. If used for daytime anxiety, they can increase activity and produce or aggravate behavior disorders, particularly in children with ADHD. Severe school phobia may be better treated with an antidepressant, although a single dose of a benzodiazepine may be used occasionally to allay anticipatory anxiety and help a child return to a feared situation for the first time. Alprazolam has been used successfully to treat panic disorder, generalized anxiety disorder, and avoidant personality disorder in children. Buspirone also appears to have some utility in childhood anxiety disorders (Siméon 1993). Sedative antihistamines are believed to have some antianxiety or hypnotic utility in children for short periods. Prolonged use may lead to anticholinergic side effects and cognitive impairment. Paroxetine has been reported to be highly effective in a large multicenter trial in children and adolescents with social phobia (Wagner et al. 2004). It is worth remembering that newer drugs are rarely studied in children or adolescents before marketing, and even the older drugs are often only partially studied in children and adolescents. Newer anticonvulsants, such as pregabalin, have not been studied in pediatric anxiety but could prove a useful alternative to benzodiazepines.

The place of drug therapy for children and adolescents is still controversial. Drugs should be reserved for clearly distressed or dysfunctional conditions for which psychosocial treatments either have failed or are likely to be only of short-term benefit. Drug therapy needs to be carefully monitored and requires close collaboration among the physician, the parents, and often school personnel or other caregivers. Prolonged maintenance drug therapy is sometimes justifiable, but there should be strong clinical evidence of benefit, and trials of withdrawal from medication are often indicated to make sure the drug is still making a useful difference.

Geriatric Psychopharmacology

Elderly psychiatric patients present a variety of potential problems for the psychiatrist considering prescribing psychoactive drugs. Elderly persons may have decreased ability to metabolize some drugs, although this has been documented only infrequently. These patients may have low serum protein levels, which could lead them to have relatively higher levels of free drug (not bound to protein) at any given blood level. Free drug is usually presumed to be more active and more likely to cross the blood-brain barrier. Elderly patients may be more sensitive to peripheral side effects (e.g., hypotension, constipation) than younger patients at the same dose or blood level. They may also be more prone to CNS side effects (e.g., delirium, tremor, tardive dyskinesia). None of these presumptions is well documented except for delirium and tardive dyskinesia, chiefly because no adequate studies have been done.

Elderly persons appear to have a reduced reserve of both brain function and cardiovascular competence, which leaves them more vulnerable to drug side effects. Decreased hepatic function and renal function also contribute to side effects in geriatric patients. In addition, the consequences of side effects—such as falls due to orthostatic hypotension, falls due to confusion, or ataxia or decubitus ulcers due to prolonged oversedation—are more likely to be serious in elderly persons. The situation is made worse by the higher likelihood of coexisting medical illness and the use of other drugs for these illnesses in elderly patients. In addition, there is a lack of clear criteria for predicting which elderly patients need very low, cautious dosage regimens of psychoactive drugs and which patients require (and tolerate) rather large dosages to attain adequate treatment response.

Moreover, the definition of geriatrics has changed over the years. The average 60-year-old of today is far more fit than their counterpart of 20 years ago and probably does not demonstrate any significant decrease in drug metabolism or tolerability. For the standard psychiatric conditions, such as depression, mania, chronic schizophrenia, and generalized anxiety disorder, the only safe and reasonable approach is to begin with a very low drug dosage and to increase the dosage cautiously after other organic etiologies are ruled out. As an example, 20 mg/day is a reasonable starting dosage of duloxetine for healthy patients older than 65, and perhaps even half of a 20-mg tablet for patients with concurrent medical problems such as liver disease or with evidence of dementia. In such patients, dosage increments should be scheduled for every week or so, so that the clinician has a chance to assess side effects before increasing the dosage.

Antidepressants

Most antidepressants and electroconvulsive therapy (ECT) have been used effectively in elderly patients with major depression. Transcranial magnetic stimulation also has been effective in older patients, although not as effective as ECT. In the past 30 years, SSRIs, particularly sertraline and escitalopram, have grown more popular in the first-line treatment of geriatric depression. Additionally, controlled trials of mirtazapine suggest that the sedating and weight-gain effects of the drug are useful in many elderly depressed patients. Furthermore, mirtazapine may be better tolerated in geriatric patients than some SSRIs with which it has been compared, such as paroxetine. The SSRI side-effect profile is superior to that of the TCAs in most geriatric patients. All TCAs, including the secondary amines, have the disadvantage of producing at least some anticholinergic side effects and orthostasis. However, for more serious depressive episodes in geriatric patients, many clinicians prefer an SNRI or nortriptyline to SSRIs. Some controversial data suggest that nortriptyline may be superior to fluoxetine in geriatric melancholic depression (see Chapter 3, "Antidepressants"). Our experience, confirmed by discussions with other geriatric psychiatrists and family practitioners, suggests that fluoxetine and other SSRIs are sometimes less useful than SNRIs or TCAs in hospitalized elderly depressed patients.

Five geriatric depression studies are worthy of comment. In one, venlafaxine, fluoxetine, and placebo were all of similar efficacy in depressed patients older than 65 years. The high response rate with placebo limits the inferences that can be drawn from this study. Both active drugs were well tolerated. ECG and blood pressure effects were minimal with both drugs (Schatzberg and Roose 2006). In contrast, a study involving frail nursing home patients reported higher rates, and perhaps less safety, with venlafaxine than with sertraline (Oslin et al. 2003). In another study, citalopram was not more effective than placebo in so-called old old patients (Roose et al. 2004). Again, a high placebo response was observed. In another, duloxetine was significantly more effective than placebo in depressed geriatric patients (Raskin et al. 2004). A composite cognition score was used as the primary outcome measure. In the last study, mirtazapine was significantly more effective than paroxetine in the first 6 weeks of an 8-week trial. Mirtazapine was associated with significantly fewer dropouts due to adverse events than was paroxetine. The average dosage in this study was approximately 30 mg/day for both (Schatzberg et al. 2002). Sertraline was associated with an increased risk of falls in one study (Flint et al. 2014) needs to be followed up on. Another study (Haddad et al. 2021) found about a 30% increase in fall risk among community-dwelling older patients who were taking SSRIs. Because there are many confounding risks in older patients taking SSRIs, including concomitant medications and comorbid health issues, it is difficult to ascertain how much of a fall risk the SSRIs pose.

Trazodone has been a somewhat effective antidepressant in elderly depressed patients and is an excellent hypnotic. It should not cause orthostatic hypotension except for a couple of hours after a bedtime dose. However, some patients in their 70s and 80s have daytime hypotension when treated with trazodone. Nefazodone is generally well tolerated in the elderly but is associated with orthostasis and dysphoric activation in some geriatric patients. The risk of hepatotoxicity has limited the use of nefazodone in the elderly, and it is now rarely used. Lower doses of both trazodone and nefazodone are often necessary in older patients, particularly when treatment is being started.

Bupropion appears to be well tolerated in the treatment of geriatric depression but is experienced as too activating by some patients. Dosages in the range of 100–300 mg/day appear to be adequate in many cases of geriatric depression.

ECT remains the major treatment for depressed elderly patients when drug therapy fails. ECT is often very effective. However, some patients with recurring depressions stop responding to ECT after the third to the tenth course of treatment in the same way that some patients may stop responding to some antidepressants.

Although stimulants are occasionally quite helpful in the treatment of recent-onset depression in elderly patients with medical problems, they often only induce agitation in treatment-resistant elderly depressed patients. We have seen some benefits in geriatric patients of adding 100–200 mg of modafinil (Provigil) to standard antidepressants in the morning. Alexopoulos et al. (2005) has suggested that some late-life depression that is characterized by problems with executive function and white matter changes might respond better to dopamine agonists and perhaps modafinil.

Another presumption in the treatment of elderly patients is that anticholinergic drugs increase the likelihood of delirium. On this basis, desipramine should be safer than amitriptyline, and fluphenazine should be safer than thioridazine. Our review of the literature on TCA use in elderly patients suggests, however, that delirium more often occurs in patients taking a TCA-antipsychotic combination and that this side effect can be transient and relatively easily managed. Again, there are no adequate controlled trials documenting this issue.

Hypnotics and Anxiolytics

Benzodiazepines can be problematic in elderly patients. If benzodiazepines are to be used as hypnotics or for daytime anxiety, again use the lowest dose first to observe whether this dose is adequate and to determine whether the drug is well tolerated. Elderly patients appear more likely than younger patients to experience cognitive side effects, falls, and impaired driving while taking benzodiazepines (Madhusoodanan and Bogunovic 2004). These are all very serious issues in a geriatric population. In general, 3-hydroxybenzodiazepines such as temazepam and lorazepam are the preferred agents for geriatric patients because of their lack of active metabolites and simpler metabolism. There is evidence that benzodiazepine metabolism is slowed in elderly persons, and there is a presumption that higher cumulative blood levels are associated with behavioral toxicity.

Occasionally, elderly (and young adult) patients complain of excessive morning sedation after taking slowly metabolized hypnotics such as flurazepam. However, there is a good deal of individual variability in the extent to which this consequence of slowed metabolism causes demonstrable clinical problems. Nonetheless, because of their long half-lives and tendency toward residual daytime drowsiness, the long-acting benzodiazepines such as flurazepam are not particularly good choices for the treatment of any insomnia. Temazepam is probably the best choice as a benzodiazepine hypnotic because of its shorter half-life and lack of active metabolites.

Zolpidem is still among the most widely used hypnotics in geriatric patients. Although a very effective agent, it may be less well tolerated than zaleplon, which is much shorter acting and may be as effective as zolpidem. Zaleplon has been well studied in geriatric patients and has the advantage of being able to be taken in the middle of the night, when some patients are most distressed about not being able to go back to sleep. A dose of 0.5 mg at night or on awakening is often sufficient. In 2014, the FDA lowered the recommended starting dose of eszopiclone, which may be dosed at 1–2 mg per night. The abuse potential appears low, and the chance of significant drug interactions or exacerbation of sleep apnea also appears low. As with benzodiazepines, Z-drugs have been associated with an increased risk of falls and cognitive problems in elderly patients.

Trazodone continues to be valuable as a hypnotic in the elderly. At higher doses in geriatric patients, the risk of orthostatic hypotension increases. Thus, we suggest checking orthostatic blood pressures at baseline and as the dose is titrated. The most common dosing is 50–100 mg 1–2 hours before bedtime. Mirtazapine is another fine agent to use as a sleeper. Like trazodone, it carries no risk of dependence and tends to be well tolerated. A dose of 7.5–15 mg at night works at least as well as trazodone without the risk of orthostatic hypotension. There are currently little controlled data on mirtazapine as a sedative hypnotic in the elderly.

Ramelteon may be worth trying before other hypnotics in geriatric patients. Unlike standard hypnotics, ramelteon is not likely to contribute to confusion or amnesia, nor is it associated with orthostatic hypotension as is trazodone. It appears to be somewhat less effective for maintaining sleep.

The use of benzodiazepines for the long-term management of anxiety is common but fraught with potential problems. Among the more serious risks associated with benzodiazepine use in the elderly is the risk of falls. Falls in the elderly are associated with significant morbidity and mortality, and there is little doubt that benzodiazepine effects on gait, motor coordination, and sedation can be a contributing factor. The risks of serious falls and hip fractures in older patients may be even greater when the patient is also taking a concurrent opioid (Machado-Duque et al. 2018). Given the additional risk of respiratory depression with the combination of opioids and benzodiazepine, this combination should be avoided when possible.

The negative effects of acute benzodiazepine use on cognition are well established, and these risks are greater in older patients. More debatable is whether long-term benzodiazepine use is associated with subsequent dementia. The studies of benzodiazepine use as a risk factor for dementia have been inconsistent, with some studies showing up to 50% increased risk of subsequent dementia in benzodiazepine users (e.g., Zhong et al. 2015), and other studies failing to find an association (e.g., Imfeld et al. 2015). Currently, the evidence seems to point to a greater risk of cognitive decline with chronic, higher-dose benzodiazepine use but not an increased risk of Alzheimer's or other dementias (Nafti et al. 2020). As with the teratogen association studies discussed earlier in the chapter, the benzodiazepine-dementia association studies often fail to take into account the impact of the underlying psychiatric illness on risk of dementia. For example, many patients chronically taking benzodiazepines suffer from insomnia and depression. Both chronic insomnia (Sindi et al. 2018) and depression (Kessing 2012) are independent risk factors for dementia. Thus, if there is an enhanced risk of dementia with benzodiazepine use, it is currently difficult to discern whether that association is related to the benzodiazepine or to the underlying psychiatric disorder. Nonetheless, there are enough other long- and short-term risks of benzodiazepine use in the elderly that caution is warranted. Other choices for managing anxiety in older patients include SSRIs, buspirone, and even low doses of SGAs such as quetiapine.

Mood Stabilizers

Lithium

Lithium excretion is, on the average, slowed in elderly patients as a consequence of an age-related decrease in kidney function. Therefore, this drug should be started at low dosages in older patients—300 mg/day in patients in their 60s and early 70s and 150 mg/day in older patients. Lithium levels and clinical signs of toxicity should be monitored scrupulously. It is our impression that elderly patients can slip from therapeutic to toxic blood levels more rapidly and insidiously than do young adult patients. In addition, elderly patients are often taking concurrent medications that may increase the risk of lithium toxicity, including nonsteroidal anti-inflammatory drugs, thiazide diuretics, and angiotensin-converting enzyme inhibitors. On the other hand, lithium can be as effective in some older bipolar patients as it is in younger ones, although some elderly patients whose condition is of late onset may have an underlying organic disorder that does not respond well to lithium.

Anticonvulsants

Valproate generally appears better tolerated than lithium in elderly patients. It often takes lower doses of valproate to achieve adequate serum levels in geriatric patients. We have seen dosages as low as 250 mg/day appear to result in adequate mood stabilization for some geriatric patients. However, many more patients will not achieve adequate serum levels with dosages below 750 mg/day.

Gabapentin is well tolerated in geriatric patients but is of no utility in the treatment of bipolar disorder. It may be as useful in geriatric agitation and anxiety states, as pregabalin appears to be.

Other anticonvulsant agents such as oxcarbazepine and lamotrigine have not been adequately studied in geriatric patients with bipolar disorder but are generally well tolerated. Carbamazepine, with its potential for interactions with so many medications, is often a poor choice in geriatric patients.

Antipsychotics

In older patients with chronic schizophrenia, there is a belief that lower antipsychotic dosages are needed than those used with younger adult patients. There is, again, little real evidence to support this belief, but there is some evidence that the same antipsychotic dose yields blood levels 1.5–2 times higher in elderly patients than in younger patients. Cautious attempts at gradually tapering dosage are indicated in schizophrenic patients older than 60 who are receiving maintenance neuroleptic treatment. When such patients have stopped their medication and become acutely psychotic, cautious low-dosage medication (e.g., 0.5–2.0 mg/day of haloperidol or risperidone or 1.25–5 mg/day of olanzapine) should be tried for the first week to see whether a clinical response can be obtained without resorting to high dosages. However, if the patient does not improve and has a history of requiring and tolerating a higher antipsychotic dosage, the dose can be gradually raised, again with monitoring of side effects. Quetiapine, even at higher doses, has a very low risk of EPS and is favored by some geriatric psychiatrists.

The use of antiparkinsonian drugs could cause delirium, but leaving the patient exposed to dystonia or pseudoparkinsonism is equally undesirable; clinicians are forced to feel their way, attempting to maximize benefit and to minimize adverse effects. This applies equally to the use of antipsychotics in younger adult patients, but in the elderly, the problems encountered in attempting to achieve the right balance of medications may be more frequent. Aripiprazole, olanzapine, risperidone, and quetiapine offer alternatives to standard antipsychotics. The orthostasis that may be secondary to use of these drugs has occasionally resulted in falls, with serious consequences. The anticholinergic properties of clozapine also tend to be poorly tolerated by geriatric patients. Olanzapine also has some anticholinergic properties. However, older patients are often able to tolerate and respond to lower doses of the atypical antipsychotics.

Tardive dyskinesia has been statistically more prevalent in elderly patients, especially women, who are taking maintenance antipsychotics, but in patients with chronic schizophrenia the dyskinesia usually has already been present for years and is not a contraindication to using antipsychotics to achieve relief of psychotic symptoms. Nonetheless, geriatric patients appear to be more vulnerable to developing some EPS, particularly pseudoparkinsonism, than do younger patients. In the rare older chronic patient showing new-onset dyskinesia, a trial of withdrawal from the antipsychotics is usually indicated. The concurrent presence of pseudoparkinsonism and dyskinesia in the same patient is more common in elderly patients than in other patients.

The use of SGAs in geriatric patients with dementia has been associated with increased mortality. In fact, all SGAs carry an FDA black box warning indicating a higher risk of mortality when these drugs are used in treating elderly patients with dementia. No SGA is approved in the treatment of dementia. Overall, it appears that there is a 1.6–1.7 times greater risk of mortality in geriatric patients with dementia who are treated with SGAs versus placebo. The risk of cerebrovascular accidents (CVAs) in controlled trials of olanzapine in the treatment of dementia was 1.3% versus 0.4% with placebo. Likewise, the risk of CVAs in controlled trials of risperidone was 4% versus 2% with placebo. However, a large observational study of 11,400 patients treated with antipsychotics in the Ontario Healthcare Database failed to find an increased risk of CVAs with either olanzapine or risperidone in patients older than age 66 (Herrmann et al. 2004). In fact, typical antipsychotics may be associated with the same mortality risks in elderly patients (Trifirò et al. 2007). In a Veterans Affairs study, no increased risk of mortality for SGAs was observed (Barnett et al. 2007). In the previous edition of this manual, we noted that when the potential for toxicity is considered along with the relative lack of benefit of antipsychotics as detailed in some carefully done studies such as the Clinical Antipsychotic Trials of Intervention Effectiveness (CATIE; Schneider et al. 2006), the routine use of antipsychotics in dementia populations should probably be avoided. In cases of behavioral dyscontrol in dementia patients, nonpharmacological interventions should be attempted first. If those interventions fail, a trial with an antipsychotic might be attempted, but the utility of such a trial should be reassessed on a regular basis. Of late, we have been using SGAs in elderly individuals with dementia when other methods have failed.

One antipsychotic, pimavanserin, is approved for treating hallucinations in patients with Parkinson's disease (see Chapter 4). Most patients with Parkinson's disease are elderly, and pimavanserin is the only antipsychotic currently approved that is specific for psychosis in an older population. Pimavanserin lacks the dopamine antagonism of most antipsychotics and so will not worsen the motor symptoms of Parkinson's disease. The most common side effect of pimavanserin is nausea, but other side effects, including peripheral edema and confusion, are reported. Although the recommended starting and maintenance dosage is 17 mg given twice daily, little is lost by starting at 17 mg/day and titrating up to 17 mg bid after a few days if tolerated.

Medications for Dementia

Most elderly patients with mild, moderate, or severe dementia have Alzheimer's disease, although some have multi-infarct dementia, a few have both, and some have neither. The best treatment for dementia is to diagnose a treatable, reversible cause such as vitamin deficiency, hypothyroidism, or congestive heart failure and to treat the underlying medical condition. The other confounding diagnosis is pseudodementia secondary to major depression. Some authors believe that depression can cause dementia in elderly persons, and depression can certainly aggravate mild, preexisting cognitive dysfunction. Depression probably unmasks some dementias. Thus, pseudodementias in geriatric patients tend to represent early progressive dementias if followed over time.

The evidence is clear that depression should be carefully and thoroughly treated when cognitive impairment and depression coexist. In recent years, greater attention has been paid to vascular depression, which may be associated with marked cognitive impairments. Optimal treatments have yet to be defined, although investigators in this area have suggested that calcium channel blockers and MAOIs might be useful, perhaps in combination. Data are not yet available as of this writing.

Antidepressants might be used in patients with strokes or organic mood lability, even if the depressive syndrome is only partially present. Results from at least 16 controlled trials confirm that antidepressants are effective in the treatment of poststroke depression and that the benefits extend beyond mood (Chen et al. 2006). Improvements in activities of daily living (ADLs), emotional incontinence, and general sense of well-being have been reported benefits of treating poststroke depression with SSRIs and other agents. The odds favor a substantial improvement over any worsening of organic deficit, although the dosage should be started low and raised cautiously. It is clear that patients with behavioral deficits due to strokes who show insomnia, weight loss, agitation, and inability to participate in rehabilitative programs can do well with TCAs and presumably with other antidepressants.

There are several favorable reports on the use of nortriptyline for poststroke depression. This strategy was undertaken because nortriptyline is less likely to produce orthostatic blood pressure changes at therapeutic blood levels than are other TCAs. In addition, a controlled trial showed fluoxetine to be superior to maprotiline in the treatment of poststroke depression (Dam et al. 1996). In another study (Robinson et al. 2000), nortriptyline was significantly more effective than fluoxetine or placebo in helping with mood and anxiety problems but not with cognitive function. Treatment should not be withheld just because a stroke patient's dysphoria seems appropriate to the disability: depression appears to be associated with high mortality in stroke patients.

It is unfortunate that there has been little progress in the past 30 years since tacrine, the first drug approved for treatment of Alzheimer's disease, became available in 1993. Despite billions of dollars invested, no drug that slows or alters the devastating and inexorable course of Alzheimer's disease has come to the market. However, in the past few years two drugs have been approved that appear to have an impact on the pathophysiology and perhaps the course of the illness. In June 2021, the FDA approved aducanumab, a monoclonal antibody that targets and removes amyloid-β plaques in the brain. The drug was tested in two Phase III clinical trials, ENGAGE and EMERGE, involving more than 3,000 patients with mild cognitive impairment or early Alzheimer's disease. The trials showed that the drug reduced the amount of amyloid-β plaques in the brain, although there was some controversy over the clinical significance of this effect. Nonetheless, the FDA granted accelerated approval of the drug on the basis of the reduction in amyloid-β plaques, with the condition that further studies are conducted to confirm the clinical benefit of the drug.

In 2023 a second anti-amyloid antibody, lecanemab, was approved by the FDA. This approval was less controversial than the approval of aducanumab because there appeared to be a slowing of cognitive decline in patients treated with the drug (van Dyck et al. 2023). The manufacturer reported on a trial of 1,795 adults with mild cognitive impairment or early Alzheimer's disease in whom amyloid pathology in the brain had been confirmed. Treatment consisted of lecanemab 10 mg/kg biweekly or matching placebo. After 18 months of treatment, lecanemab slowed cognitive decline by 27% compared with placebo, as measured by the Clinical Dementia Rating–Sum of Boxes (CDR-SB).

This was an absolute difference of 0.45 points (change from baseline: 1.21 for lecanemab vs. 1.66 with placebo; $P < 0.001$). Although a 0.45-point difference does not seem like much of a benefit, it does appear to be clinically meaningful. Thus, lecanemab may be the first drug available that actually modifies the course of Alzheimer's disease. Lecanemab is a very expensive drug, priced currently at $26,500 per year. It is not clear if the benefits accumulate, plateau, or decline after 18 months. The most common side effects of lecanemab given by infusion included flushing, chills, fever, and myalgias.

The amyloid-β antibodies are not likely to be used as first-line treatment of Alzheimer's disease because of their cost and the requirement of an infusion. Currently, the drug most commonly prescribed for the treatment of Alzheimer's disease is donepezil (Aricept). Although donepezil is considerably more benign than tacrine, it is probably no more effective. A number of studies have been completed that demonstrate a clear benefit of donepezil over placebo on such measures as the Alzheimer's Disease Assessment Scale (ADAS) or the Mini-Mental State Exam (Burns et al. 1999; Greenberg et al. 2000). Donepezil may improve cognitive function by 5%–10% and may improve, although modestly, the quality of life of some patients and their care providers. In addition to Alzheimer's disease, donepezil has also been shown to have mild efficacy in the treatment of other dementias, including Lewy body dementia and vascular dementias.

Donepezil tends to be well tolerated, with a dose-related increase in side effects. Dosages of 5 mg/day tend to be well tolerated; the most common side effects of the 10-mg dose are nausea, diarrhea, insomnia, fatigue, muscle cramps, and anorexia. Some adaptation to most of these side effects tends to occur over time.

Some anecdotal reports suggest that donepezil may help ameliorate depression but exacerbate mania (Benazzi and Rossi 1999). Some patients have reported improvement in cognition, even if they did not have dementia, and some reports suggest that donepezil can help with medication-induced memory problems (Jacobsen and Comas-Díaz 1999).

Another cholinesterase inhibitor, rivastigmine (Exelon), was approved in 2000 for the treatment of dementia. Rivastigmine produces a dose-dependent increase in acetylcholine and appears to bypass hepatic metabolism. Thus, it appears safe for hepatic function. Rivastigmine has a half-life of 10 hours and is more centrally active than peripheral in its effects on the cholinergic system, a feature that makes it reasonably well tolerated. Two large studies have demonstrated the superiority of a dosage of rivastigmine 6–12 mg/day over placebo in the treatment of Alzheimer's dementia (Jann 2000). It may be somewhat better tolerated than donepezil in some patients. Gastrointestinal upset is the most common side effect, although rivastigmine is reported to produce fewer and less severe gastrointestinal effects, including diarrhea, than donepezil. However, it does not appear to be any more effective than donepezil. In 2007, a transdermal form of rivastigmine was approved for use in Alzheimer's dementia. The transdermal administration of rivastigmine bypasses the gut and tends to be far better tolerated than the oral form.

Galantamine (Reminyl) was the next cholinesterase inhibitor, after rivastigmine, on the U.S. market. Galantamine's mechanism of action is a variation on the theme of acetylcholinesterase inhibitors. This agent is a competitive inhibitor of acetylcholinesterase and allosterically modulates nicotinic receptors to enhance cholinergic transmission. This mechanism may theoretically give galantamine some advantages over other acetylcholinesterase inhibitors, but none as yet have been demonstrated. What has been proven is that galantamine is more effective than placebo in treating the cognitive deficits of Alzheimer's disease and that these effects are sustained for at least 12 months. The drug seems to be reasonably well tolerated at dosages of 24–32 mg/day, with nausea occurring in up to 40% of treated patients and diarrhea in up to 19% of patients. No significant effects were seen on liver function or any other laboratory tests.

In 2003, memantine (Namenda) became the first drug approved for moderate to severe Alzheimer's disease. Memantine is a moderate N-methyl-D-aspartate (NMDA) antagonist that is thought to mitigate the toxic effects of increased calcium flow into neurons by blocking NMDA receptors. This blockade then reduces the neurodegenerative effects caused by lower glutamate levels and increased calcium influx in Alzheimer's disease. Memantine appears to improve cognition and ADLs significantly more than placebo in patients with moderate or more severe dementia (Reisberg et al. 2003). Importantly, memantine also appears to modestly reduce the amount of time caregivers must spend with an Alzheimer's patient. In addition, patients who are already taking a cholinesterase inhibitor, such as donepezil, appear to improve with the addition of memantine to the regimen (Tariot et al. 2004).

Memantine has been quickly adopted in clinical practice not because it is dramatically efficacious but rather because it is impressively benign. In clinical trials, the rate of side effects was not different from the rate with placebo. In fact, no side effect occurred at statistically different rates than with placebo in more than 5% of patients. The most commonly reported side effects were dizziness, confusion, headaches, and hallucinations.

The drug is not a potent inhibitor or dependent substrate of any CYP enzyme. As a result, it has few drug interactions. The only condition known to substantially affect serum levels of memantine is alkaline urine. A urine pH > 8, such as caused by urinary tract infections or carbonic anhydrase inhibitors, will substantially reduce the clearance of the drug and may be associated with increased side effects.

Memantine is usually started at 5 mg/day, with a target dosage of 20 mg/day. We have generally had no trouble increasing the dosage by 5 mg per week until the patient is taking 10 mg bid. Although many patients will tolerate a more rapid titration, it is unclear whether there are any advantages to more rapid titration.

It is nice for the clinician to have options, but it is unlikely that any acetylcholinesterase inhibitor, with or without memantine, will produce anything more than moderate benefits for the cognitive function and behavioral difficulties of most dementia patients. Donepezil is currently the first choice for most clinicians only because it is the best studied and there is no evidence yet that the newer agents are any more efficacious. Memantine appears to be an important additional option for patients. However, we appear to be a long way from having interventions that substantially affect the course of the disease or the quality of life of Alzheimer's patients. In the future, we may have more accessible, disease-modifying drugs that can be given earlier in the course of illness, but that future has not yet arrived.

Medications for Agitation

Patients with chronic dementia often show agitation, irascibility, night wandering, paranoid ideation, or hallucinations and become major management problems at home or in psychiatric hospitals or nursing homes. Behavioral dyscontrol represents one of the most common reasons geriatric patients are placed in nursing homes. Many of these patients were routinely treated with low-dose FGAs such as haloperidol, often with dubious benefit. A review of the few controlled studies in this area suggested that only a third of these patients clearly benefited from low-dose first-generation drugs (Cole 1990).

We have found low doses of SGAs (0.5–1 mg of risperidone or 2.5–5 mg of olanzapine) sometimes helpful in controlling the agitation and psychosis associated with dementia. These tend to produce few, if any, EPS at low doses. Although many SGAs have failed to demonstrate efficacy in the treatment of agitation in randomized controlled trials and all the SGAs carry a boxed warning around increased mortality in elderly dementia patients, many clinicians still find the SGAs more useful than other medication choices. In 2023, brexpiprazole became the first medication approved for treating agitation associated with Alzheimer's disease. Grossberg and colleagues (2020) found 2 mg of brexpiprazole was more effective than placebo in controlling agitation in Alzheimer's patients over 12 weeks of treatment. Brexpirazole was generally well tolerated, with headache and somnolence being the common medication-related side effects. The recommended starting dosage is 0.5 mg/day, with a maximum dosage of 3 mg/day. Because the boxed warning is a class warning, the warning remains in place for brexpirazole.

There are a number of other options for treating agitation in patients with dementia. First, treating the underlying dementia with an acetylcholinesterase inhibitor often helps with behavioral problems associated with dementia. Thus, the acetylcholinesterase inhibitors should be tried first. We had good success with treating some agitated depressed patients with moderate dosages of valproate (500–1,250 mg/day) (Schatzberg and DeBattista 1999). However, many geriatric patients do not tolerate higher doses of valproate. Tariot's group first reported that the maximum tolerated dosage in this population is about 800 mg/day, or 11.5 mg/kg/day (Profenno et al. 2005; Tariot et al. 2005). One multicenter trial involving 153 patients did not find valproate at a mean dosage of 800 mg/day to be significantly more effective than placebo in reducing agitation in nursing home patients (Tariot et al. 2005). A more recent study failed to observe that the drug was significantly more effective than placebo in preventing the emergence of agitation or psychosis in patients with dementia (Tariot et al. 2011). A number of studies have demonstrated the utility of carbamazepine in the treatment of agitated patients with dementia (Gleason and Schneider 1990). There is one controlled trial in which a modal dose of 300 mg of carbamazepine was significantly more effective than placebo in reducing agitation in patients with dementia (Tariot et al. 1998). We still tend to prefer valproate over carbamazepine because carbamazepine tends to be more poorly tolerated, has a lower therapeutic index, and has more drug interactions in these elderly patients, who tend to be taking multiple drugs.

Newer anticonvulsants, such as gabapentin and pregabalin, make intuitive sense for the treatment of agitation but are largely untested. As with benzodiazepines, it has been suggested that gabapentin can induce agitation in some brain-injured patients but can help agitation in patients with dementia (Buskova et al. 2011; Miller 2001). Some patients probably would respond to a benzodiazepine, preferably oxazepam, because of its simple metabolism and low abuse potential. This drug at least offers hope of an early response when the dose is adjusted properly. Many patients with dementia become confused while taking benzodiazepines, and we now tend to prefer SGAs and valproate over benzodiazepines, despite the limitations and risks of SGAs.

Another pharmacological approach to agitation in the elderly is the combination drug dextromethorphan 20 mg plus quinidine sulfate 10 mg (Nuedexta). The drug is approved for the treatment of pseudobulbar affect but is being increasingly used to treat agitation in nursing home patients. Prescriptions for the dextromethorphan + quinidine combination quadrupled between 2012 and 2017, and much of that increase appeared to be off-label use for the treatment of behavioral dyscontrol in nursing home patients. Given the risks of antipsychotics in these patients, clinicians have been eager to adopt other strategies, even if still unproven. As of this writing, there have been several case reports and one large placebo-controlled trial suggesting the benefit of dextromethorphan + quinidine for treating agitation and aggression in elderly nursing home patients. In the controlled study, 220 Alzheimer's patients were randomly assigned to receive dextromethorphan + quinidine or placebo for two consecutive 5-week periods (Cummings et al. 2015). Patients treated with the dextromethorphan + quinidine combination showed a significant reduction in agitation and aggression without a worsening of cognition or sedation. Additional studies are under way. Given the limited options for treating agitation in patients with dementia, dextromethorphan + quinidine is promising. The usual dosage is dextromethorphan 20 mg and quinidine 10 mg once daily for 7 days and then twice daily subsequently as tolerated. The most common side effects of the combination relative to placebo are gastrointestinal upset, dizziness, asthenia, and peripheral edema.

Other drugs have been the subject of individual case reports. Propranolol had been the most widely studied, but mainly for agitation and assaultiveness in nonelderly brain-injured patients (Greendyke and Kanter 1986; Greendyke et al. 1989; Weiler et al. 1988). Some case reports have suggested that agitation decreases as soon as the right dosage of propranolol is reached, but most studies report improvement after a month of taking the right dosage. In the hospitalized, agitated, restless, irascible patient with dementia, a month is a very long time, and propranolol carries the risk of orthostatic hypotension, with resulting falls. If it is to be tried in elderly patients, the starting dosage should be 10 mg bid, and dosage should be increased in increments of 10–20 mg every 2 days to 200 mg/day, stopping at a lower dosage if hypotension or other side effects occur. Propranolol can cause delirium. Glassman et al. (1979) showed that orthostatic hypotension due to TCAs is far worse in cardiac patients taking multiple cardiac medications than in medically healthy depressed patients. The same is likely with propranolol—it probably should not be tried in patients taking multiple cardiac or other medications.

There are a number of studies on the helpfulness of trazodone and buspirone in treating agitated elderly patients with dementia (Colenda 1988; Lebert et al. 1994; Pinner and Rich 1988; Sultzer et al. 2001). Buspirone is used quite commonly in some nursing home settings at dosages of 10–45 mg/day. More recently, controlled trials of SSRIs, such as citalopram at approximately 20 mg/day, have demonstrated benefits for controlling behavioral outbursts in patients with dementia (Peters et al. 2016).

Psychosocial measures may be more useful than drugs in treating agitation in elderly patients with dementia. Simple interventions such as keeping the patient oriented with a calendar and clock and keeping the lights on can substantially reduce agitation in patients with dementia. Also, looking for and treating concurrent medical problems such as a urinary tract infection will often do more than any pharmacological treatment for agitation. Better studies of more kinds of drug therapy in elderly patients are needed, but in their absence, clinicians have to cautiously try to do their best with available measures.

Intellectual Developmental Disorders

As with elderly patients with dementia, institutionalized patients with severe intellectual disabilities have been treated routinely for decades with antipsychotics, such as small doses of haloperidol or risperidone, for a wide range of behavioral disorders. Many patients with even mild intellectual deficits end up taking either antipsychotics or mood stabilizers at some point to control behavioral problems (Haw and Stubbs 2005). Court decisions have mandated evaluating such patients while they are not taking medications, and it now appears that only a fraction of patients receiving long-term antipsychotic medication are clinically better with them than without them.

Antipsychotic-responsive patients with intellectual developmental disorders have not been well characterized, but it seems probable that some show psychotic symptoms that would qualify for a diagnosis of schizophrenia. Since the mid-1990s, the SGAs have been increasingly employed for the management of behavioral dyscontrol in patients with intellectual developmental disorders or brain injury. The evidence has accumulated that agents such as risperidone and clozapine may be useful in both the acute and the long-term management of disruptive behavior, affective symptoms, or self-injurious behavior in patients with subaverage intelligence (Biederman et al. 2006a; Perry et al. 2018; Rohde et al. 2018).

A general principle in the treatment of patients with intellectual developmental disorders may be useful as a guideline. Such patients often show aberrant behaviors (e.g., disrobing, jumping, poking fingers in eyes) that can increase dramatically when they become psychiatrically upset. Counting (monitoring) these target behaviors can be a useful guide to treatment effect in often nonverbal patients. The real diagnosis may have to be inferred from changes in vegetative symptoms such as sleep, appetite, and motor activity or from family history of psychiatric disorders. All this gives a trial-and-error quality to the drug therapy of behaviorally disturbed patients with intellectual developmental disorders, reinforcing Sovner's (1989) practice of monitoring target behaviors or symptoms before and during trials. It may take a few weeks to be sure that any given drug is or is not useful.

Some articles have documented the existence of depressive and bipolar disorders that manifest somewhat atypically in relatively or completely nonverbal patients (Sovner and Hurley 1983). Such patients are appropriate candidates for treatment with standard antidepressants or mood stabilizers.

If one accepts that overactive, turbulent, and episodically violent behaviors toward others or self are usually not a manifestation of psychosis in patients with intellectual developmental disorders, or if it has been empirically determined that these are not antipsychotic responsive behaviors, what then? Candidate drugs include SGAs, SSRIs, valproate, lithium, buspirone, propranolol, gabapentin, and carbamazepine. None of these have been the subject of placebo-controlled clinical trials in disturbed patients with intellectual developmental disorders. However, all of the drugs have been the subject of small open trials with reported sustained, if often delayed, benefit in the patients described here.

In addition to the antipsychotics, lithium carbonate and valproate have among the best credentials as anti-anger drugs in a variety of psychiatric populations. If the patient has a seizure disorder, shifting to carbamazepine or valproate seems sensible. Nadolol is of theoretical interest because it is a β-blocker that does not cross the blood-brain barrier and because it is hypothesized to decrease episodic violence by peripheral action on muscles. Propranolol requires more titrating (30–480 mg/day) to determine an effective dosage, and it can cause hypotension, bradycardia, and delirium. The desirable monitoring of vital signs before each dosage greater than 120 mg/day may be impossible in some residential facilities.

Buspirone has been useful at dosages of 15–60 mg/day, but onset of clinical action appears to be delayed. Various experts inform us that buspirone is less useful in treating more violent patients with intellectual developmental disorder. Preliminary data show that the SSRIs may be effective in such patients. Further discussion of many of these drugs is found in Chapters 3, 4, and 5.

In patients with a seizure disorder, in the presence or absence of an intellectual developmental disorder, there is a worry that psychiatric drugs, including TCAs and neuroleptics, may lower the seizure threshold and increase the likelihood or frequency of convulsions. There is no firm evidence that this occurs. In our experience, maprotiline, imipramine, and amitriptyline have been more often connected with seizure occurrences in depressed patients, but these drugs were also the most commonly used TCAs in the McLean Hospital system at the time seizures were seen. Trazodone is least likely to affect seizure threshold. Bupropion and clomipramine have also been associated with seizures. There is a belief that among the typical antipsychotics, haloperidol and molindone are least likely to affect seizure occurrence. In our experience, chlorpromazine and loxapine are occasionally associated with seizures, and seizures are more of a problem with clozapine (see Chapter 4). In patients with a known seizure disorder that is adequately treated with anticonvulsants, it is relatively unlikely that any of the standard psychiatric drugs will make a clinically important difference in seizure frequency. In patients with intellectual disabilities taking phenytoin, phenobarbital, or primidone for seizure control, there is a real possibility that the seizure medication may be causing cognitive dysfunction. It may be worth shifting the patient to carbamazepine to determine whether the patient may function better with that relatively different medication.

Stimulants may also be worth a trial in hyperactive patients with intellectual developmental disorders who are under close clinical observation. Stimulants have the advantage of causing clear clinical effects (improvement or worsening) within a few hours or days of reaching an adequate dose; therefore, the trials of a stimulant may be completed in 1–2 weeks.

Medical Conditions

Some psychiatric syndromes are caused by or strongly associated with medical disorders. Others are commonly associated with medications used to treat medical or neurological conditions. On the other hand, some medical conditions and some drugs used to treat medical conditions complicate the use of standard psychoactive drugs to treat coexisting psychiatric disorders.

Psychiatric Disorders Resulting From Medical Illness

Psychiatric disorders, especially depression, can occur with (and are presumably caused by) thyroid or adrenal cortical dysfunction, uremia, cancer of the pancreas, and any metastatic carcinomatosis sufficiently often to make it worth ascertaining whether these conditions exist in depressed patients. Other, more obvious conditions, such as strokes, multiple sclerosis, lupus erythematosus, and Parkinson's disease, are often associated with depression, as well as with organic brain dysfunction.

Chronic pain syndromes, including headache and low back pain, are so confounded with depressive syndromes that primary antidepressant therapy is often indicated and effective. For some medical conditions such as hypothyroidism, treating the underlying condition is the first order of business. For others, the presence of an untreatable medical or neurological condition is not per se a contraindication to standard antidepressant therapy.

Hyperthyroidism, caffeinism, hypoglycemia, temporal lobe epilepsy, paroxysmal tachycardias, and pheochromocytoma can all mimic panic disorder and should be ruled out. A medical reevaluation is indicated if standard drug therapies fail. A review by Raj and Sheehan (1988) suggested some useful tips for making such key differential diagnoses. For example, attacks of paroxysmal atrial tachycardia generally begin and end more abruptly than do panic attacks and produce heart rates of 140–200 bpm. In contrast, heart rates in panic disorder rarely exceed 140 bpm. In pheochromocytoma, anxiety is only the fourth most common symptom, and many patients with this condition experience tachycardia and increased blood pressure without becoming unduly fearful; in this disorder there is often an increased familial prevalence of neurofibromatosis and café au lait spots.

Hyperthyroidism is associated with sleep disturbance, heat sensitivity, and a more enduring tremor, among other symptoms. Finally, temporal lobe epilepsy may represent a more difficult diagnostic dilemma. In almost 25% of patients with this disorder, anxiety occurs during the aura or interictally. However, such patients frequently also complain of other symptoms, such as perceptual distortions and lapses of concentration. In assessing patients with possible panic disorder, a routine medical history and physical examination should be obtained. Laboratory tests should be ordered as needed to rule out suspected conditions.

There have been many positive case reports on the use of stimulants—mainly methylphenidate at a dosage of 10 mg once or twice a day—in patients with serious medical or surgical illnesses on medical services. These patients were noted on psychiatric consultation to be depressed; developmentally delayed, even almost mute; losing weight; not eating; unable to cooperate in treatment; withdrawn; and hopeless. Stimulants can produce relief in a day or two and can often be discontinued in 2–4 weeks once the patient is generally improving. Of the many such case reports, none describe any serious side effects. By inference, elevated pulse or blood pressure is not a problem. Despite the appetite-reducing effect of stimulants in overweight subjects, these medically ill patients rapidly regain weight while taking methylphenidate. Sometimes stimulants are used because TCAs are contraindicated, but the results are positive enough for stimulants to be considered first-choice drugs in treating these patients. Standard antidepressants rarely improve mood or functioning in just a few days.

Depression following stroke has received some special study in recent years. It is clear that depression following CVAs occurs in about half the patients affected and can be relieved by antidepressants. In fact, the majority of studies of antidepressants in the treatment of poststroke depression have found significant benefits in mood and behavior and even improvement in ADLs (Chen et al. 2006; Gaete and Bogousslavsky 2008). Several controlled studies have been conducted: one of nortriptyline (Lipsey et al. 1984), one of trazodone (Reding et al. 1986), and one of fluoxetine (Dam et al. 1996). Nortriptyline was generally effective, but 3 of the 17 patients studied developed delirium (Lipsey et al. 1984). Patients treated with medication longer and those with plasma levels above 100 ng/mL did better. Trazodone was less effective relative to placebo, but significant positive effects were found in dexamethasone nonsuppressors and patients with higher levels of depressive symptoms (Reding et al. 1986). Slow, cautious dosage increases are best with both drugs to avoid adverse effects. In the study by Dam et al. (1996), fluoxetine (20 mg/day) appeared to substantially facilitate recovery in poststroke patients who were undergoing rehabilitation. In this study of 52 severely disabled hemiplegic patients, fluoxetine-treated patients showed significant improvements in depression, ADLs, and neurological deficits relative to both maprotiline-treated patients and patients receiving placebo. In fact, maprotiline seemed to hinder rehabilitation, whereas fluoxetine generally helped a variety of indices of recovery in these poststroke patients treated for 3 months. Fluoxetine may also help with the emotional incontinence that often occurs after a stroke (Choi-Kwon et al. 2006). ECT has also been reported to be effective in poststroke depression. Most patients with cognitive impairment before ECT were found to have improved cognitive functioning after ECT. In contrast, Robinson et al. (2000) reported that nortriptyline was more effective than fluoxetine or placebo in poststroke depression. As indicated earlier, sertraline can prevent poststroke depression.

Many psychiatric disorders may be seen in patients with AIDS, but the prevalence of these disorders is not higher than in carefully matched control subjects. Studies suggest that subsyndromal depression is the most common disorder seen in this population, and it is thought that the SSRIs may be useful in treating these patients. However, some psychiatric conditions can be a direct consequence of neurological involvement in HIV infection. HIV encephalitis occurs in most AIDS patients at some point in their illness. Mood and personality changes may occur early in the course of the encephalitis, and psychosis, mania, and dementia may occur later. Patients with other neurological consequences of HIV infection, including cerebral lymphoma and toxoplasmosis, often present with cognitive and psychiatric symptoms. These problems generally occur late in the progression of the disease.

Zidovudine (formerly azidothymidine, or AZT) is often helpful in reversing the psychopathology associated with HIV encephalopathy. Antidepressants, lithium, and high-potency antipsychotics may also help treat HIV-associated psychopathology. However, because AIDS patients tend to be quite sensitive to the side effects of psychotropic medications, caution must be exercised.

The introduction of the protease inhibitors has made a tremendous impact on the treatment of HIV-positive patients. All the current protease inhibitors are potent inhibitors of the CYP enzyme 3A3/4 and are themselves metabolized by this enzyme. Thus, some protease inhibitors can significantly raise the serum levels of concurrent clozapine as well as a number of benzodiazepines, such as diazepam, alprazolam, and triazolam. Conversely, carbamazepine is a potent CYP3A4 inducer and may render concurrent protease inhibitors less effective. Even St. John's wort has modest CYP3A4-inducing effects and has been associated with decreasing the effectiveness of protease inhibitors. In addition, one protease inhibitor, ritonavir (Norvir), also inhibits the CYP enzyme 2D6 and may raise the serum levels of TCAs and other drugs dependent on this enzyme.

Psychiatric Disorders Associated With Nonpsychiatric Drugs

A variety of older antihypertensive drugs (e.g., reserpine, methyldopa) were sometimes associated with depression. These drugs rarely are used in current clinical practice. However, propranolol is commonly used now and has sometimes been associated with major depression. In many instances, the β-blockers do not appear to be inducing depression. Rather, high doses of lipophilic β-blockers such as propranolol can induce a lethargy and indifference that is sometimes confused with depression. Shifting to a thiazide diuretic or to a different, non–centrally acting β-blocker (e.g., atenolol) can be helpful, or a TCA alone can sometimes adequately treat both depression and hypertension.

Diazepam has occasionally been associated with increased depression. Both benzodiazepines and barbiturates can aggravate ADHD. Benzodiazepines may produce memory problems, particularly in the elderly. Stimulants can aggravate schizophrenia or mania. Steroids and L-dopa can mimic almost any known psychiatric syndrome, including delirium, paranoid psychosis, mania, depression, and anxiety.

The whole range of drugs used in treating Parkinson's disease can cause hallucinosis and confusion. As described earlier in this chapter and in Chapter 4, pimavanserin is an option for treating psychotic symptoms without worsening the motor symptoms of Parkinson's. Sometimes anticholinergic drugs used in gastrointestinal disorders can also cause anticholinergic confusion and delirium, as can digitalis-like and cimetidine-like agents. It is impossible to list or predict all the drugs or drug combinations that at some doses in some patients can elicit or aggravate symptoms of a psychiatric disorder. In a patient receiving several drugs for medical conditions who presents with depression, anxiety, or psychosis appearing after the drugs were begun, a careful reevaluation of the patient's pharmacotherapies is necessary. When some medication is necessary, stopping the less obviously crucial medications and shifting to less centrally active alternative drugs are reasonable steps.

Psychiatric Disorders Complicated by Medical Disorders

Renal Disease

Many medical disorders could have reasonably predictable effects on the pharmacokinetics of standard psychiatric drugs, but the transition from theoretical data to practical application is often not exact. In the case of kidney failure and lithium therapy, the facts are clear. If renal clearance is decreased, lithium excretion will be decreased in a reasonably proportionate manner. In patients with substantially elevated serum creatinine and blood urea nitrogen who are not in acute renal failure, very small dosages of lithium (e.g., 150 mg/day) can be cautiously begun and titrated in the same way as in a healthy patient, but more cautiously and with smaller increments. In this situation, lithium citrate given in milliliter doses could give extra flexibility. Some patients on renal dialysis may be stabilized on lithium, with a single 300-mg dose after each episode of dialysis. This dose may maintain an adequate blood level until the next dialysis removes the lithium ions. Likewise, older patients experience a 30%–40% decrease in glomerular filtration and therefore require lower starting and maximum doses than do younger patients.

Like lithium, gabapentin and pregabalin do not undergo hepatic metabolism and are excreted by the kidneys. Thus, patients with renal insufficiency are more likely to experience toxicity with both drugs at higher doses. Patients with a creatinine clearance of < 15 mL/min probably should receive a maximum dosage of 300 mg/day of gabapentin and 75 mg/day of pregabalin. On the other hand, patients with a creatinine clearance in the higher range of 30–59 mL/min can be treated with dosages as high as 700 mg bid of gabapentin or 150 mg bid of pregabalin.

The hydroxylated metabolites of TCAs and other psychotropic agents may also be elevated in elderly patients and in those with advanced renal disease. This suggests that a more gentle titration of these medications is required in these two groups of patients.

Dehydration states are not uncommon, and they can increase the toxicity of lithium therapy. Furthermore, there is some evidence that dehydration is a risk factor in the development of neuroleptic malignant syndrome, although this association is somewhat tenuous. Finally, dehydration can exacerbate the orthostasis caused by risperidone, clozapine, TCAs, and MAOIs.

Urinary retention can be quite problematic in elderly patients, particularly in males with prostate difficulties. The most anticholinergic agents, including tertiary-amine TCAs (amitriptyline, imipramine), low-potency antipsychotics, and antiparkinsonian drugs such as benztropine, should be avoided if possible in elderly patients.

Liver Disease

When there is liver damage or decreased liver efficiency due to normal aging, the effects are more complicated. Most drugs are at least partially metabolized in the liver after absorption from the small intestine (the first-pass effect). When liver tissue is damaged, many drugs get into the general circulation at much higher levels. Usually, glucuronidation as a method of drug deactivation is well preserved, whereas demethylation and other metabolic processes are more readily impaired. This is why drugs that need to be demethylated, such as diazepam, cause much higher blood levels per unit dose in cirrhosis, whereas drugs that are only glucuronidated, such as lorazepam, are handled normally. Unfortunately, it is not always clear to even a skilled clinical pharmacologist exactly what the effect of chronic liver disease on the clinical actions of any particular drug will be.

It is likely that in patients with partial liver failure, TCAs such as amitriptyline and imipramine will be less readily converted to their desmethyl metabolites, nortriptyline and desipramine. The consequences of this shift—perhaps more sedation, confusion, or anticholinergic side effects—are less clear. The obvious lesson is to proceed very cautiously; to use blood level determinations, if available; and to assume that liver damage will markedly increase a drug's half-life, making gradual accumulation of higher and higher blood levels quite possible over a couple of weeks at a constant daily dose. Most psychiatrists find fluoxetine a safe drug to use in spite of its long half-life. Also, patients with active liver disease should not be started on nefazodone because baseline abnormalities may complicate monitoring of nefazodone-induced hepatotoxicity, albeit rarely. Lowered blood protein levels, common in liver disease, may also increase free-drug levels, unbound to protein, making a drug more potent at lower total blood levels measured in the conventional manner. This is less of a problem with venlafaxine, which demonstrates low protein binding.

An overly efficient liver can also pose problems. Some known drugs, including barbiturates, phenytoin, carbamazepine, and nicotine, induce hepatic enzymes and increase the rate at which some psychiatric drugs are metabolized, making higher dosages necessary in order to achieve clinical results (see Chapters 3, 5, and 9). It is also worth noting that even drug-free patients can show large degrees of biological variability in their natural rates of drug metabolism. As an example, in a classic study, Glassman et al. (1977) found imipramine levels to vary from 40 to 1,040 ng/mL in depressed patients receiving 2.5 mg/kg of imipramine (see discussion in Chapter 3). Again, the lesson is that patients taking other drugs for medical reasons may well have an altered response based on either increased or decreased hepatic metabolism of the psychiatric drug that has just been added (not to mention pharmacological interactions such as additive sedation or additive postural hypotension). It has also become evident that a number of psychotropic drugs may be associated with causing elevations in liver enzymes.

For example, in the likely absence of clear knowledge about the drug interactions in a particular patient of cimetidine, phenytoin, chlorothiazide, and isoniazid with imipramine, the clinician adding imipramine in a patient taking all these other drugs must be prepared to proceed cautiously but to use high dosages of imipramine if neither side effects nor clinical response occurs, if blood levels are low, and if ECG changes are not seen.

The SSRIs, the TCAs, carbamazepine, and valproate, among other medications, may be associated with increases in aspartate transaminase (formerly serum glutamic-oxaloacetic transaminase) and alanine transaminase (formerly serum glutamic-pyruvic transaminase). The clinical significance of these elevations remains unclear. However, persisting elevations to greater than twice the normal levels are of particular concern. There are rare reports of children younger than 2 years who are taking valproate and who have developed fulminant hepatic failure; the risk in adults appears to be minimal. There are also a few isolated reports of hepatic failure in children that was believed to be associated with TCA use. In general, it is prudent practice to obtain baseline liver function tests (LFTs) when initiating therapy with carbamazepine and valproate and to check LFTs every 6–12 months thereafter.

Several drugs pose less of a problem in patients with advanced liver disease because they are not appreciably metabolized by the liver. These include agents such as gabapentin, pregabalin, and lithium. Transdermal selegiline also bypasses the liver to a large extent and might be used in patients with advanced liver disease.

Cardiac Illness

There is substantial evidence that depression both is a risk factor for coronary artery disease and significantly increases the risk of mortality in patients who have suffered a myocardial infarction (MI). In fact, depression in the post-MI period is a stronger predictor of subsequent mortality than many more intuitive factors such as systolic ejection fraction, which is one measure of the extent of heart damage. The mechanism by which depression may increase the risk of an MI or subsequent risk of mortality after an MI is unknown. Current speculation is that depression may increase platelet binding and therefore clotting or that depression may decrease heart rate responsiveness. In any case, it would be helpful to know if antidepressant therapy in the post-MI period decreases mortality. It is evident that sertraline in the post-MI period is well tolerated and effective for concurrent depression (Glassman et al. 2002).

In cardiac patients, there has long been a fear that all TCAs are cardiotoxic and likely to cause disastrous arrhythmias. Although TCAs produce mild tachycardia (an increase of 10 bpm) in medically healthy depressed patients, their arrhythmogenic potential appears to occur primarily if the drugs are taken in overdose. The mechanism by which the TCAs and maprotiline affect cardiac function is a quinidine-like slowing of cardiac conduction. TCAs have an ability to decrease cardiac irritability and to suppress premature contractions. They are therefore not contraindicated at ordinary dosages in depressed patients with premature ventricular contractions, and they may well help both cardiac irritability and depression. Nortriptyline has been shown to be effective and generally well tolerated in cardiac patients with melancholic depression (Roose et al. 1994). Other studies indicate that paroxetine is as effective as nortriptyline in post-MI patients but is better tolerated frsom a cardiovascular perspective (Roose et al. 1998).

However, the TCAs should be used with caution in patients with preexisting conduction defects, such as bundle-branch block. Patients with first-degree block have a 9% rate of 2:1 atrioventricular block development when taking TCAs, compared with a 0.7% rate in patients without first-degree block. TCAs should not be given to patients with known intracardiac conduction delays. This is particularly true in patients already taking cardiac antiarrhythmic drugs, which act by slowing cardiac conduction, because additive effects on conduction could be harmful. Not all cardiologists are aware of the cardiac effects of TCAs, and psychiatrists who collaborate with cardiologists or primary care physicians may need to do some educating of their consultants.

The other antidepressants with a possible effect on cardiac irritability are trazodone and venlafaxine. Trazodone does not affect conduction, but it has occasionally (not regularly) been associated with an increase in premature ventricular contractions (PVCs) and should be avoided in patients with runs of PVCs or ventricular bigeminies. There has been concern that venlafaxine overdoses might be associated with a greater risk of mortality, mostly from cardiac events, than are the SSRIs. Venlafaxine overdoses, often in combination with other drugs or alcohol, have been associated with QT prolongation, bradycardia, ventricular tachycardia, and other arrhythmias. Thus, the package insert for venlafaxine was changed at the request of the FDA to reflect this evidence. The risks appear to be substantially less than with TCA overdoses and may be an artifact of more ill patients typically being treated with venlafaxine rather than with SSRIs. However, more careful monitoring is recommended. Venlafaxine, like the SSRIs, can produce a mild increase in heart rate. It can also increase diastolic blood pressure. Therefore, patients with current and advanced congestive heart failure may not be the best candidates for treatment with venlafaxine. Patients with a history of hypertension may also require increased vigilance when treatment with venlafaxine is being initiated. In one report, venlafaxine was poorly tolerated cardiovascularly in nursing home patients (Oslin et al. 2003). Because of these effects, and given the recent report of British regulators regarding lethality in overdose, the drug should be prescribed cautiously in vulnerable populations (e.g., elderly patients with cardiac disease).

The SSRIs appear to produce a mild (3 bpm) increase in heart rate in medically healthy depressed patients. Although these agents have not yet been widely studied in post-MI patients, their possible use in such patients is suggested by animal studies and by data available in cardiovascularly healthy depressed patients. In addition, these agents produce milder alterations in blood pressure than do other antidepressants. However, the SSRIs may slow the metabolism of a variety of cardiovascular medications, including digoxin, some β-blockers, and Class 1C antiarrhythmics. The SSRIs can raise the levels of these other medications by competitive inhibition of the CYP enzyme 2D6 and require close monitoring (Table 12–5).

Roose et al. (1994) reported that fluoxetine was less effective than nortriptyline in melancholic cardiac patients, although there are other data indicating that it does have efficacy and relative safety in cardiac patients with milder depression. Two major multicenter studies in the last decade have explored the effect of sertraline in cardiac patients. The drug appears to improve quality of life and may increase long-term survival while having less dramatic effects on mood per se (O'Connor et al. 2010; Swenson et al. 2003; Taylor et al. 2005).

Several antipsychotics prolong QTc intervals, but the clinical significance is often small (Beach et al. 2018). For example, haloperidol is known to increase QTc intervals but is rarely associated with clinically significant consequences, even with high-dose intravenous use. Among the SGAs, ziprasidone and iloperidone are somewhat more likely to cause QTc prolongation, but aripiprazole is less likely. Baseline ECGs are not the standard of care but might be useful in older patients and certainly in those with a history of arrhythmias.

Citalopram is the SSRI of most concern in patients at risk for an arrhythmia. Citalopram at a dosage of 60 mg/day has been shown to prolong QTc intervals by an average of 18.5 ms compared with 8.5 ms for 20 mg/day and 12.5 ms for 40 mg/day. Thus, there is a dose-related increase in the risk of ventricular arrhythmia, including torsades de pointes, and the maximum recommended dosage of citalopram has been lowered from 60 mg/day to 40 mg/

Table 12–5.   Interactions of commonly used psychoactive drugs with cardiovascular medications

Drug	TCA	SSRI	Antipsychotic	Lithium	Carbamazepine
Calcium channel blockers	Increase hypotension	NA	Increase hypotension	Raise or lower lithium levels, bradycardia	Increase carbamazepine levels
Thiazide diuretics	May increase hypotension	NA	Increase hypotension	Increase lithium levels	NA
β-Blockers	May increase hypotension	May increase β-blockers	Increase antipsychotic levels	NA	Decrease β-blocker levels
Reserpine, guanethidine	Antagonize antihypertensive agents	NA	Increase hypotension	NA	Unknown
Clonidine, prazosin	Increase hypotension	NA	Increase hypotension	NA	Unknown
1A antiarrhythmics	Prolong cardiac conduction	NA	Prolong cardiac conduction	Prolong sinus recovery time	May decrease antiarrhythmic levels
1C antiarrhythmics	Prolong cardiac conduction	Increase 1C levels	May prolong cardiac conduction	Prolong sinus recovery time	May decrease antiarrhythmic levels
Digitalis	Increases digoxin and TCA levels	May increase digoxin levels	May increase digoxin levels	Prolongs sinus recovery time	Unknown

Note.   NA=not applicable; SSRI=selective serotonin reuptake inhibitor; TCA=tricyclic antidepressant.

day. Older patients taking citalopram might be advised to get a baseline ECG and a follow-up ECG with dose increases. Escitalopram may also prolong QTc intervals, but to a lesser degree than citalopram does. A minority of patients who overdose on escitalopram have some evidence of QTc prolongation, but these arrhythmias have rarely been problematic. Even very high plasma levels of escitalopram have not been associated with increasing QTc interval (Carceller-Sindreu et al. 2017).

The more significant effect of TCAs and MAOIs is postural hypotension, which can be aggravated (potentiated) in patients already taking drugs that are likely to cause hypotension as well, such as propranolol. Although patients who have stable cardiac disease but are not in congestive failure probably tolerate antidepressants well, patients taking multiple cardiac drugs are particularly prone to postural hypotension and other cardiac side effects. For seriously ill cardiac patients with severe depression, ECT may be the treatment of choice.

Bupropion has been assessed in depressed patients with moderate cardiac disease and seems to be better tolerated than the TCAs. Even in overdose, bupropion does not typically have a major effect on cardiac function (Spiller et al. 1994).

Pulmonary Disorders

Patients with pulmonary disorders, including asthma, emphysema, and sleep apnea, are commonly encountered in psychiatric practice, and some psychotropic medications may present problems in this population. Benzodiazepines, for example, may be contraindicated in patients with sleep apnea; the benzodiazepines may relax the airway further and exacerbate already restricted airflow. Zolpidem may be less likely to produce this problem than the benzodiazepines. In addition, benzodiazepines reduce the hypoxic response to ventilation and therefore should be used with caution in patients with chronic obstructive pulmonary disease who retain CO_2. Furthermore, psychotropic medications with significant anticholinergic activity may decrease bronchial secretions and exacerbate pulmonary disorders. Thus, caution should be exercised in treating pulmonary patients with drugs such as amitriptyline or benztropine.

Many medications used to treat pulmonary problems are affected by concurrent use of some psychotropic agents. For example, fluvoxamine inhibits the metabolism of theophylline, which can lead to potentially toxic levels. Thus, theophylline levels should be checked frequently if fluvoxamine must be used concurrently. Conversely, theophylline-like drugs increase the excretion and lower the serum levels of lithium.

Seizure Disorders

Many psychotropic medications are known to lower the seizure threshold and, therefore, must be used with caution in patients with a history of a seizure disorder. Most antipsychotics have this potential, although molindone and thioridazine may be less problematic in patients with seizure disorders. Clozapine, among the antipsychotics, has perhaps the greatest potential for inducing seizures: up to 5% of patients develop seizures at dosages greater than 600 mg/day. The TCAs and tetracyclic agents all have some potential for lowering the seizure threshold; amitriptyline and maprotiline are among the more problematic offenders. Bupropion is probably contraindicated in patients with a known seizure disorder because of its dose-related potential for producing seizures. However, the SSRIs and venlafaxine appear relatively safe in this population.

The anticonvulsants are also associated with a variety of interactions. Carbamazepine is an enzyme inducer that lowers the serum levels of a variety of drugs, including TCAs, clonazepam, and most antipsychotics. Oxcarbazepine is a much weaker inducer of the CYP3A3 and CYP3A4 enzymes. SSRIs, on the other hand, may substantially increase carbamazepine levels. Other additive or antagonistic interactions certainly occur. Some of the better-documented ones are discussed in previous chapters focusing on specific drug classes.

Pain Disorders

Antidepressants and other psychotropic drugs have long been used in the treatment of a variety of pain syndromes, including trigeminal neuralgia, peripheral neuropathy, arthritis, myofascial pain, fibromyalgia, migraine prophylaxis, and the pain associated with some forms of cancer. Many placebo-controlled studies have reported that antidepressants are useful in the management of pain, independent of whether depression is a part of the clinical picture.

The TCAs have the longest track record and, along with the SNRIs, are among the most consistently efficacious group of psychotropic agents used in the treatment of pain conditions. Tertiary amine TCAs, particularly amitriptyline, imipramine, and doxepin, have been well studied and found to be effective for a variety of pain conditions. Initially, it was thought that the mechanism of action of these drugs was to increase the peripheral availability of serotonin, which in turn modulated the pain response. This explanation does not appear to be correct. Some TCAs, which are more noradrenergic than serotonergic, also appear to be useful in the treatment of pain, whereas the SSRIs, which efficiently increase the availability of peripheral serotonin, are sometimes less useful. For example, a study comparing amitriptyline with the SSRI citalopram in the prophylaxis of chronic tension headaches found that amitriptyline was efficacious, but citalopram was ineffective (Bendtsen et al. 1996). Dosages as low as 25–50 mg/day of amitriptyline or imipramine are frequently useful in the prophylaxis and treatment of pain problems. However, the analgesic effect of the TCAs appears to be dose related, so higher doses may be more effective than lower doses.

The SSRIs have been disappointing in the management of pain disorders, although there is some evidence that they may help with neuropathic pain. Some patients have reported benefit from the SSRIs for migraine prophylaxis, although many patients experience a worsening of their headaches at the initiation of treatment. The results of open-label studies of paroxetine 10–50 mg/day for chronic daily headaches have been encouraging (Foster and Bafaloukos 1994), whereas findings from double-blind studies have been less promising (Langemark and Olesen 1994).

The SNRIs, which have a mechanism of action that closely resembles that of the TCAs, have also been extensively studied in the treatment of chronic pain conditions. Two SNRIs, duloxetine and milnacipran, are FDA approved in the treatment of fibromyalgia. In 2004 duloxetine became the first drug approved for the treatment of pain associated with diabetic neuropathy. In 2009, duloxetine and milnacipran were approved for the treatment of fibromyalgia (Arnold et al. 2004). Then, in 2010, duloxetine received approval for chronic musculoskeletal pain, including back pain and pain from osteoarthritis. Both daytime and nighttime pain in the diabetic pain study were substantially reduced by duloxetine as early as the first week of treatment. The dosages proven effective for diabetic neuropathy in clinical trials were 60–120 mg/day. Duloxetine also appeared to reduce painful symptoms in depressed patients, including their myalgias and back pain. Thus, duloxetine is among the most commonly prescribed drugs in pain clinics. For the patient with chronic neuropathic pain who is also depressed, duloxetine appears to be a particularly good choice.

As reported in Chapter 5, gabapentin and pregabalin have been well studied in neuropathic pain. Gabapentin at dosages up to 3,600 mg/day is both effective and well tolerated for many pain patients. As a result, gabapentin has become a standard in most pain specialty clinics. Pregabalin was also approved for the treatment of diabetic neuropathic pain as well as trigeminal neuralgia. It was also the first drug approved for the treatment of fibromyalgia. The typical therapeutic dosage for pregabalin in pain conditions is 150–300 mg/day taken in two divided doses. Dosages up to 600 mg/day have been studied but are probably not much more effective than smaller dosages.

Haloperidol and chlorpromazine, in several open-label studies, have been found to be useful in the management of neuropathic pain. Carbamazepine has been efficacious in the treatment of peripheral neuropathies, and lithium is sometimes used in the treatment of cluster headaches.

A number of common agents used in the management of pain disorders might interact with common psychotropic medications. For example, tramadol, which is indicated for moderate to severe pain, is an SNRI. In addition, it is a CYP2D6 substrate. Thus, there is the potential for both pharmacokinetic and pharmacodynamic interactions with some SSRIs, and serotonin syndrome has been sporadically reported with the combination. Opioids combined with CNS depressants (including benzodiazepines) are sometimes associated with respiratory depression, particularly in overdose. Likewise, carisoprodol (Soma) may interact with other CNS depressants, including barbiturates and benzodiazepines, to contribute to sedation, dizziness, and, in overdose, respiratory depression. Meperidine (Demerol) has long been associated with inducing a serotonin syndrome in combination with MAOIs, and the combination is thus contraindicated. Although MAOIs have been used safely with other narcotics, the interaction with opioids such as fentanyl is somewhat unpredictable.

Conclusion

It would be helpful if our current knowledge of drug actions could be put to precise clinical use in assessing the effects of adding a new psychiatric drug to a preexisting mixture of medical and psychiatric drugs. Unfortunately, drugs do not work like sums in an algebraic equation. One would think, for example, that the action of D-amphetamine, an indirect dopamine agonist, would be opposed by haloperidol, a reasonably pure dopamine-blocking drug. In practice, however, some patients feel more lively and functional, without becoming more psychotic, when D-amphetamine is added to haloperidol. Drugs usually act on several receptors and on both pre- and postsynaptic receptors of a single type, leading to potentially complex effects and interactions. The clinician is often faced with treating schizophrenia, agoraphobia with panic, or depression in a patient with several medical problems. This kind of situation requires drug therapy for the medical problems that is likely to influence the metabolism or absorption of a psychiatric drug or to have additive, antagonistic, or (more likely) unknown effects in combination with the most appropriate psychiatric drug treatment.

All drug therapy consists of a series of empirical clinical trials; treatment of medically ill patients simply presents more complicated empirical trials. The psychiatrist can try to guess at the more probable ways in which the new drug will act or be affected by the patient's medical disease and ongoing drug therapies, but it is likely to be only guesswork. If there are semipredictable adverse interactions, one can either try to avoid them by choosing the psychiatric drug least likely to cause trouble or proceed cautiously, with close monitoring of the patient for predictable and unpredictable side effects, in collaboration with the physicians managing the patient's nonpsychiatric disorders. One worries that medically ill patients will be very fragile and easily become toxic while taking psychiatric drugs, but it is likely that this is not a general problem; some patients may develop problems, whereas others tolerate psychiatric drugs unusually well.

Suggested Readings

ACOG Committee on Practice Bulletins—Obstetrics: ACOG Practice Bulletin: clinical management guidelines for obstetrician-gynecologists number 92, April 2008 (replaces practice bulletin number 87, November 2007): use of psychiatric medications during pregnancy and lactation. Obstet Gynecol 111(4):1001–1020, 2008 18378767

Alessi N, Naylor MW, Ghaziuddin M, et al: Update on lithium carbonate therapy in children and adolescents. J Am Acad Child Adolesc Psychiatry 33(3):291–304, 1994 8169173

Altshuler LL, Szuba MP: Course of psychiatric disorders in pregnancy: dilemmas in pharmacologic management. Neurol Clin 12(3):613–635, 1994 7990794

Aman MG, De Smedt G, Derivan A, et al: Double-blind, placebo-controlled study of risperidone for the treatment of disruptive behaviors in children with subaverage intelligence. Am J Psychiatry 159(8):1337–1346, 2002 12153826

Aman MG, Gharabawi GM; Special Topic Advisory Panel on Transitioning to Risperidone Therapy in Patients With Mental Retardation and Developmental Disabilities: Treatment of behavior disorders in mental retardation: report on transitioning to atypical antipsychotics, with an emphasis on risperidone. J Clin Psychiatry 65(9):1197–1210, 2004 15367046

Asarnow JR, Tompson MC, Goldstein MJ: Childhood-onset schizophrenia: a follow-up study. Schizophr Bull 20(4):599–617, 1994 7701271

Barbarich NC, McConaha CW, Gaskill J, et al: An open trial of olanzapine in anorexia nervosa. J Clin Psychiatry 65(11):1480–1482, 2004 15554759

Barrickman LL, Perry PJ, Allen AJ, et al: Bupropion versus methylphenidate in the treatment of attention-deficit hyperactivity disorder. J Am Acad Child Adolesc Psychiatry 34(5):649–657, 1995 7775360

Bellantuono C, Migliarese G, Gentile S: Serotonin reuptake inhibitors in pregnancy and the risk of major malformations: a systematic review (erratum: Hum Psychopharmacol 22:413, 2007). Hum Psychopharmacol 22(3):121–128, 2007 17397101

Benazzi F: Mania associated with donepezil. Int J Geriatr Psychiatry 13(11):814–815, 1998 9850879

Briggs G, Bodendorfer T, Freeman R, et al: Drugs in Pregnancy and Lactation: A Reference Guide to Fetal and Neonatal Risk. Baltimore, MD, Williams & Wilkins, 1983

Bousman CA, Bengesser SA, Aitchison KJ, et al: Review and consensus on pharmacogenomic testing in psychiatry. Pharmacopsychiatry 54(1):5–17, 2021 33147643

Budhwani H, Hearld KR, Chavez-Yenter D: Depression in racial and ethnic minorities: the impact of nativity and discrimination. J Racial Ethn Health Disparities 2(1):34–42, 2015 26863239

Burt T, Sachs GS, Demopulos C: Donepezil in treatment-resistant bipolar disorder. Biol Psychiatry 45(8):959–964, 1999 10386177

Campbell M: Drug treatment of infantile autism: the past decade, in Psychopharmacology: The Third Generation of Progress. Edited by Meltzer HY. New York, Raven, 1987, pp 1225–1232

Campbell M, Spencer EK: Psychopharmacology in child and adolescent psychiatry: a review of the past five years. J Am Acad Child Adolesc Psychiatry 27(3):269–279, 1988 3288611

Campbell M, Adams PB, Small AM, et al: Lithium in hospitalized aggressive children with conduct disorder: a double-blind and placebo-controlled study. J Am Acad Child Adolesc Psychiatry 34(4):445–453, 1995 7751258

Chambers CD, Johnson KA, Dick LM, et al: Birth outcomes in pregnant women taking fluoxetine. N Engl J Med 335(14):1010–1015, 1996 8793924

Chambers CD, Anderson PO, Thomas RG, et al: Weight gain in infants breastfed by mothers who take fluoxetine. Pediatrics 104(5):e61, 1999 10545587

Chambers CD, Hernandez-Diaz S, Van Marter LJ, et al: Selective serotonin-reuptake inhibitors and risk of persistent pulmonary hypertension of the newborn. N Engl J Med 354(6):579–587, 2006 16467545

Chavez B, Chavez-Brown M, Rey JA: Role of risperidone in children with autism spectrum disorder. Ann Pharmacother 40(5):909–916, 2006 16684811

Chavez B, Sopko MA Jr, Ehret MJ, et al: An update on central nervous system stimulant formulations in children and adolescents with attention-deficit/hyperactivity disorder. Ann Pharmacother 43(6):1084–1095, 2009 19470858

Cohen BM, Sommer BR: Metabolism of thioridazine in the elderly. J Clin Psychopharmacol 8(5):336–339, 1988 3183071

Cohen DJ, Detlor J, Young JG, Shaywitz BA: Clonidine ameliorates Gilles de la Tourette syndrome. Arch Gen Psychiatry 37(12):1350–1357, 1980 6255888

Cohen LS, Rosenbaum JF: Birth outcomes in pregnant women taking fluoxetine. N Engl J Med 336(12):872, author reply 873, 1997 9072682

Cohen LS, Heller VL, Rosenbaum JF: Treatment guidelines for psychotropic drug use in pregnancy. Psychosomatics 30(1):25–33, 1989 2643809

Cole J, Hardy P, Marcel B, et al: Organic states, in Common Treatment Problems in Depression. Edited by Schatzberg AF. Washington, DC, American Psychiatric Press, 1985, pp 79–100

Courtney DB: Selective serotonin reuptake inhibitor and venlafaxine use in children and adolescents with major depressive disorder: a systematic review of published randomized controlled trials. Can J Psychiatry 49(8):557–563, 2004 15453105

Cumming RG, Le Couteur DG: Benzodiazepines and risk of hip fractures in older people: a review of the evidence. CNS Drugs 17(11):825–837, 2003 12921493

Dahlin M, Knutsson E, Nergårdh A: Treatment of spasticity in children with low dose benzodiazepine. J Neurol Sci 117(1–2):54–60, 1993 8410067

Davis KL, Thal LJ, Gamzu ER, et al: A double-blind, placebo-controlled multicenter study of tacrine for Alzheimer's disease. N Engl J Med 327(18):1253–1259, 1992 1406817

DeVane CL, Sallee FR: Serotonin selective reuptake inhibitors in child and adolescent psychopharmacology: a review of published experience. J Clin Psychiatry 57(2):55–66, 1996 8591970

Dietrich A, Mortensen ME, Wheller J: Cardiac toxicity in an adolescent following chronic lithium and imipramine therapy. J Adolesc Health 14(5):394–397, 1993 7691178

DiGiacomo J: The hypertensive or cardiac patient, in Common Treatment Problems in Depression. Edited by Schatzberg AF. Washington, DC, American Psychiatric Press, 1985, pp 29–56

Djulus J, Koren G, Einarson TR, et al: Exposure to mirtazapine during pregnancy: a prospective, comparative study of birth outcomes. J Clin Psychiatry 67(8):1280–1284, 2006 16965209

Dodd S, Berk M: The safety of medications for the treatment of bipolar disorder during pregnancy and the puerperium. Curr Drug Saf 1(1):25–33, 2006 18690912

Dopheide JA, Pliszka SR: Attention-deficit-hyperactivity disorder: an update. Pharmacotherapy 29(6):656–679, 2009 19476419

Einarson A, Boskovic R: Use and safety of antipsychotic drugs during pregnancy. J Psychiatr Pract 15(3):183–192, 2009 19461391

Eisendorfer C, Fann WE (eds): Psychopharmacology and Aging. New York, Plenum, 1973

Farlow M, Gracon SI, Hershey LA, et al: A controlled trial of tacrine in Alzheimer's disease. JAMA 268(18):2523–2529, 1992 1404819

Fedoroff JP, Robinson RG: Tricyclic antidepressants in the treatment of poststroke depression. J Clin Psychiatry 50(7)(Suppl):18–23, discussion 24–26, 1989 2661548

Field T: Breastfeeding and antidepressants. Infant Behav Dev 31(3):481–487, 2008 18272227

Findling RL, Aman MG, Eerdekens M, et al: Long-term, open-label study of risperidone in children with severe disruptive behaviors and below-average IQ. Am J Psychiatry 161(4):677–684, 2004 15056514

Findling RL, Cavuş I, Pappadopulos E, et al: Efficacy, long-term safety, and tolerability of ziprasidone in children and adolescents with bipolar disorder. J Child Adolesc Psychopharmacol 23(8):545–557, 2013 24111980

Friedel R: Pharmacokinetics in the geropsychiatric patient, in Psychopharmacology: A Generation of Progress. Edited by Lipton M, DiMascio A, Killam K. New York, Raven, 1978, pp 1499–1506

Geller DA, Hoog SL, Heiligenstein JH, et al: Fluoxetine treatment for obsessive-compulsive disorder in children and adolescents: a placebo-controlled clinical trial. J Am Acad Child Adolesc Psychiatry 40(7):773–779, 2001 11437015

Gentile S: Pregnancy exposure to serotonin reuptake inhibitors and the risk of spontaneous abortions. CNS Spectr 13(11):960–966, 2008 19037175

Gentile S: Antipsychotic therapy during early and late pregnancy: a systematic review. Schizophr Bull 36(3):518–544, 2010 18787227

Gentile S, Bellantuono C: Selective serotonin reuptake inhibitor exposure during early pregnancy and the risk of fetal major malformations: focus on paroxetine. J Clin Psychiatry 70(3):414–422, 2009 19254517

Georgotas A, McCue RE, Cooper TB: A placebo-controlled comparison of nortripty-line and phenelzine in maintenance therapy of elderly depressed patients. Arch Gen Psychiatry 46(9):783–786, 1989 2673129

Gibbons RD, Hur K, Bhaumik DK, et al: The relationship between antidepressant prescription rates and rate of early adolescent suicide. Am J Psychiatry 163(11):1898–1904, 2006 17074941

Glassman AH: The newer antidepressant drugs and their cardiovascular effects. Psychopharmacol Bull 20(2):272–279, 1984 6427837

Glassman AH, Walsh BT, Roose SP, et al: Factors related to orthostatic hypotension associated with tricyclic antidepressants. J Clin Psychiatry 43(5 Pt 2):35–38, 1982 7076637

Gold M, Estroff T, Pottash A: Substance-induced organic mental disorders, in Psychiatry Update: The American Psychiatric Association Annual Review, Vol 4. Edited by Hales RE, Frances AJ. Washington, DC, American Psychiatric Press, 1985, pp 227–240

Goldenberg G, Kahaner K, Basavaraju N, et al: Gabapentin for disruptive behaviour in an elderly demented patient (letter). Drugs Aging 13(2):183–184, 1998 9739506

Goldstein DJ, Corbin LA, Sundell KL: Effects of first-trimester fluoxetine exposure on the newborn. Obstet Gynecol 89(5 Pt 1):713–718, 1997 9166307

Goldstein DJ, Sundell KL, Corbin LA: Birth outcomes in pregnant women taking fluoxetine. N Engl J Med 336(12):872–873, author reply 873, 1997 9072683

Goodlet KJ, Zmarlicka MT, Peckham AM: Drug-drug interactions and clinical considerations with co-administration of antiretrovirals and psychotropic drugs. CNS Spectr 24(3):287–312, 2019 30295215

Gualtieri TC, Barnhill J, McGinsey J, et al: Tardive dyskinesia and other movement disorders in children treated with psychotropic drugs. J Am Acad Child Psychiatry 19(3):491–510, 1980 6106027

Guérin P, Barthélémy C, Garreau B, et al: The complexity of dopamine receptors and psychopharmacotherapy in children. Acta Paedopsychiatr 56(2):139–151, 1993 7510920

Gupta S, Ghaly N, Dewan M: Augmenting fluoxetine with dextroamphetamine to treat refractory depression. Hosp Community Psychiatry 43(3):281–283, 1992 1555827

Hechtman L: Multimodal treatment plus stimulants vs stimulant treatment alone in ADH: results from a collaborative 2-year comparative treatment study. Presented at the Annual Meeting of the American Academy of Child and Adolescent Psychiatry, New Orleans, October 1995

Hellings JA, Zarcone JR, Reese RM, et al: A crossover study of risperidone in children, adolescents and adults with mental retardation. J Autism Dev Disord 36(3):401–411, 2006 16596465

Helms PM: Efficacy of antipsychotics in the treatment of the behavioral complications of dementia: a review of the literature. J Am Geriatr Soc 33(3):206–209, 1985 2857741

Herrmann N, Mamdani M, Lanctôt KL: Atypical antipsychotics and risk of cerebrovascular accidents. Am J Psychiatry 161(6):1113–1115, 2004 15169702

Huessy HR, Ruoff PA: Towards a rational drug usage in a state institution for retarded individuals. Psychiatr J Univ Ott 9(2):56–58, 1984 6379717

Janowsky DS, Barnhill LJ, Shetty M, et al: Minimally effective doses of conventional antipsychotic medications used to treat aggression, self-injurious and destructive behaviors in mentally retarded adults. J Clin Psychopharmacol 25(1):19–25, 2005 15643096

Källén B, Olausson PO: Maternal use of selective serotonin re-uptake inhibitors and persistent pulmonary hypertension of the newborn. Pharmacoepidemiol Drug Saf 17(8):801–806, 2008 18314924

Kalra S, Born L, Sarkar M, et al: The safety of antidepressant use in pregnancy. Expert Opin Drug Saf 4(2):273–284, 2005 15794719

Kaplan CA: Depression in childhood 1: drugs may be useful. BMJ 300(6734):1260–1261, 1990 2191737

Kemp DE, Gao K, Ganocy SJ, et al: A 6-month, double-blind, maintenance trial of lithium monotherapy versus the combination of lithium and divalproex for rapid-cycling bipolar disorder and co-occurring substance abuse or dependence. J Clin Psychiatry 70(1):113–121, 2009 19192457

Knapp MJ, Knopman DS, Solomon PR, et al: A 30-week randomized controlled trial of high-dose tacrine in patients with Alzheimer's disease. JAMA 271(13):985–991, 1994 8139083

Koren G, Graham K, Feigenbaum A, et al: Evaluation and counseling of teratogenic risk: the Motherisk approach. J Clin Pharmacol 33(5):405–411, 1993 8331196

Lavenstein B: Neonatal signs after in utero exposure to selective serotonin reuptake inhibitors. JAMA 294(18):2300 [author reply: 2300–2301], 2005 16278356

Leonard HL, Swedo SE, Rapoport JL, et al: Treatment of obsessive-compulsive disorder with clomipramine and desipramine in children and adolescents: a double-blind crossover comparison. Arch Gen Psychiatry 46(12):1088–1092, 1989 2686576

MacMillan CM, Korndörfer SR, Rao S, et al: A comparison of divalproex and oxcarbazepine in aggressive youth with bipolar disorder. J Psychiatr Pract 12(4):214–222, 2006 16883146

Mak M, Lam C, Pineda SJ, et al: Pharmacogenetics of warfarin in a diverse patient population. J Cardiovasc Pharmacol Ther 24(6):521–533, 2019 31064211

March JS, Klee BJ, Kremer CM: Treatment benefit and the risk of suicidality in multicenter, randomized, controlled trials of sertraline in children and adolescents. J Child Adolesc Psychopharmacol 16(1–2):91–102, 2006 16553531

Marcus A, Bahro M, Sartoris J, et al: Acute exogenic psychosis following oral ingestion of 2 mg lormetazepam in an eleven-year-old boy. Pharmacopsychiatry 26(3):102–103, 1993 8105496

McClellan J, Werry J; American Academy of Child and Adolescent Psychiatry: Practice parameters for the assessment and treatment of children and adolescents with schizophrenia. J Am Acad Child Adolesc Psychiatry 33(5):616–635, 1994 8056725

McFarlane A, Kamath MV, Fallen EL, et al: Effect of sertraline on the recovery rate of cardiac autonomic function in depressed patients after acute myocardial infarction. Am Heart J 142(4):617–623, 2001 11579351

McGlashan TH, Zipursky RB, Perkins D, et al: The PRIME North America randomized double-blind clinical trial of olanzapine versus placebo in patients at risk of being prodromally symptomatic for psychosis I: study rationale and design. Schizophr Res 61(1):7–18, 2003 12648731

Mellow AM, Solano-Lopez C, Davis S: Sodium valproate in the treatment of behavioral disturbance in dementia. J Geriatr Psychiatry Neurol 6(4):205–209, 1993 8251047

Merlob P, Birk E, Sirota L, et al: Are selective serotonin reuptake inhibitors cardiac teratogens? Echocardiographic screening of newborns with persistent heart murmur. Birth Defects Res A Clin Mol Teratol 85(10):837–841, 2009 19691085

Morgan MH, Read AE: Antidepressants and liver disease. Gut 13(9):697–701, 1972 4639404

Morrison JL, Riggs KW, Rurak DW: Fluoxetine during pregnancy: impact on fetal development. Reprod Fertil Dev 17(6):641–650, 2005 16263070

Mosholder AD, Willy M: Suicidal adverse events in pediatric randomized, controlled clinical trials of antidepressant drugs are associated with active drug treatment: a meta-analysis. J Child Adolesc Psychopharmacol 16(1–2):25–32, 2006 16553526

Mozes T, Greenberg Y, Spivak B, et al: Olanzapine treatment in chronic drug-resistant childhood-onset schizophrenia: an open-label study. J Child Adolesc Psychopharmacol 13(3):311–317, 2003 14642019

Nafti M, Sirois C, Kröger E, et al: Is benzodiazepine use associated with the risk of dementia and cognitive impairment—not dementia in older persons? The Canadian Study of Health and Aging. Ann Pharmacother 54(3):219–225, 2020 31595772

Nulman I, Koren G: The safety of fluoxetine during pregnancy and lactation. Teratology 53(5):304–308, 1996 8879088

Nguyen HT, Sharma V, McIntyre RS: Teratogenesis associated with antibipolar agents. Adv Ther 26(3):281–294, 2009 19330496

Patino LR, Klein CC, Strawn JR, et al: A randomized, double-blind, controlled trial of lithium versus quetiapine for the treatment of acute mania in youth with early course bipolar disorder. J Child Adolesc Psychopharmacol 31(7):485–493, 2021 34520250

Pavuluri MN, Henry DB, Carbray JA, et al: Divalproex sodium for pediatric mixed mania: a 6-month prospective trial. Bipolar Disord 7(3):266–273, 2005 15898964

Paykel ES, Fleminger R, Watson JP: Psychiatric side effects of antihypertensive drugs other than reserpine. J Clin Psychopharmacol 2(1):14–39, 1982 6121825

Payne JL: Psychopharmacology in pregnancy and breastfeeding. Psychiatr Clin North Am 40(2):217–238, 2017 28477649

Payne JL: Psychiatric medication use in pregnancy and breastfeeding. Obstet Gynecol Clin North Am 48(1):131–149, 2021 33573783

Pliszka SR, Matthews TL, Braslow KJ, et al: Comparative effects of methylphenidate and mixed salts amphetamine on height and weight in children with attention-deficit/hyperactivity disorder. J Am Acad Child Adolesc Psychiatry 45(5):520–526, 2006 16670648

Pomp EF, Gedde-Dahl A: Fluoxetine—safe during pregnancy and breast feeding [in Norwegian]. Tidsskr Nor Laegeforen 121(9):1156–1157, 2001 11354903

Popper CW: Psychopharmacologic treatment of anxiety disorders in adolescents and children. J Clin Psychiatry 54(suppl):52–63, 1993 8099578

Prasad S, et al: Viloxazine in children and adolescents with attention-deficit/hyperactivity disorder: a randomized, placebo-controlled, phase IV study. Child Adolesc Psychiatry Ment Health 13:29, 2019

Prien RF: Chemotherapy in chronic organic brain syndrome: a review of the literature. Psychopharmacol Bull 9(4):5–20, 1973 4148528

Purdon SE, Lit W, Labelle A, et al: Risperidone in the treatment of pervasive developmental disorder. Can J Psychiatry 39(7):400–405, 1994 7527293

Raskin DE: Antipsychotic medication and the elderly. J Clin Psychiatry 46(5 Pt 2):36–40, 1985 2859280

Rasmussen A, Lunde M, Poulsen DL, et al: A double-blind, placebo-controlled study of sertraline in the prevention of depression in stroke patients. Psychosomatics 44(3):216–221, 2003 12724503

Ratey JJ, Sovner R, Mikkelsen E, et al: Buspirone therapy for maladaptive behavior and anxiety in developmentally disabled persons. J Clin Psychiatry 50(10):382–384, 1989 2793836

Ray WA, Griffin MR, Schaffner W, et al: Psychotropic drug use and the risk of hip fracture. N Engl J Med 316(7):363–369, 1987 2880292

Ray WA, Griffin MR, Downey W: Benzodiazepines of long and short elimination half-life and the risk of hip fracture. JAMA 262(23):3303–3307, 1989 2573741

Reisberg B, Ferris SH, Gershon S: An overview of pharmacologic treatment of cognitive decline in the aged. Am J Psychiatry 138(5):593–600, 1981 7015883

Reiter S, Kutcher S, Gardner D: Anxiety disorders in children and adolescents: clinical and related issues in pharmacological treatment. Can J Psychiatry 37(6):432–438, 1992 1394022

Ricci F, Torales J, Bener A, et al: Mental health of ethnic minorities: the role of racism. Int Rev Psychiatry 35(3–4):258–267, 2023 37267026

Richardson MA, Haugland G, Craig TJ: Neuroleptic use, parkinsonian symptoms, tardive dyskinesia, and associated factors in child and adolescent psychiatric patients. Am J Psychiatry 148(10):1322–1328, 1991 1680296

Richardson PH, de C Williams AC: Meta-analysis of antidepressant-induced analgesia in chronic pain: comment. Pain 52(2):247–249, 1993 8455971

Riddle MA, Geller B, Ryan N: Another sudden death in a child treated with desipramine. J Am Acad Child Adolesc Psychiatry 32(4):792–797, 1993 8340300

Rugino TA, Samsock TC: Modafinil in children with attention-deficit hyperactivity disorder. Pediatr Neurol 29(2):136–142, 2003 14580657

Ryan ND: The pharmacologic treatment of child and adolescent depression. Psychiatr Clin North Am 15(1):29–40, 1992 1549547

Ryan ND: Pharmacological treatment of child and adolescent major depression. Encephale 19(2):67–70, 1993 8275899

Salzman C: Practical considerations in the pharmacologic treatment of depression and anxiety in the elderly. J Clin Psychiatry 51(1)(suppl):40–43, 1990 2404003

Schaerf FW, Miller RR, Lipsey JR, et al: ECT for major depression in four patients infected with human immunodeficiency virus. Am J Psychiatry 146(6):782–784, 1989 2729429

Scheffer RE, Kowatch RA, Carmody T, et al: Randomized, placebo-controlled trial of mixed amphetamine salts for symptoms of comorbid ADHD in pediatric bipolar disorder after mood stabilization with divalproex sodium. Am J Psychiatry 162(1):58–64, 2005 15625202

Schvehla TJ, Mandoki MW, Sumner GS: Clonidine therapy for comorbid attention deficit hyperactivity disorder and conduct disorder: preliminary findings in a children's inpatient unit. South Med J 87(7):692–695, 1994 8023201

Shader RI (ed): Psychiatric Complications of Medical Drugs. New York, Raven, 1972

Shapiro AK, Shapiro E, Wayne H: Treatment of Tourette's syndrome with haloperidol, review of 34 cases. Arch Gen Psychiatry 28(1):92–97, 1973 4509400

Shea S, Turgay A, Carroll A, et al: Risperidone in the treatment of disruptive behavioral symptoms in children with autistic and other pervasive developmental disorders. Pediatrics 114(5):e634–e641, 2004 15492353

Sheehan DV, Raj AB, Sheehan KH, et al: The relative efficacy of buspirone, imipramine and placebo in panic disorder: a preliminary report. Pharmacol Biochem Behav 29(4):815–817, 1988 3413203

Shepard TH: The Catalogue of Teratogenic Agents, 4th Edition. Baltimore, MD, Johns Hopkins University Press, 1983

Sheikha SH, Wagner KD, Wagner RF Jr: Fluoxetine treatment of trichotillomania and depression in a prepubertal child. Cutis 51(1):50–52, 1993 8419112

Silver JM, Hales RE, Yudofsky SC: Psychopharmacology of depression in neurologic disorders. J Clin Psychiatry 51(1)(suppl):33–39, 1990 2404002

Sivojelezova A, Shuhaiber S, Sarkissian L, et al: Citalopram use in pregnancy: prospective comparative evaluation of pregnancy and fetal outcome. Am J Obstet Gynecol 193(6):2004–2009, 2005 16325604

Spencer TJ, Faraone SV, Biederman J, et al: Does prolonged therapy with a long-acting stimulant suppress growth in children with ADHD? J Am Acad Child Adolesc Psychiatry 45(5):527–537, 2006 16670649

Sullivan MJL, Reesor K, Mikail S, et al: The treatment of depression in chronic low back pain: review and recommendations. Pain 50(1):5–13, 1992 1387469

Summers WK, Majovski LV, Marsh GM, et al: Oral tetrahydroaminoacridine in long-term treatment of senile dementia, Alzheimer type. N Engl J Med 315(20):1241–1245, 1986 2430180

Tariot PN, Jakimovich LJ, Erb R, et al: Withdrawal from controlled carbamazepine therapy followed by further carbamazepine treatment in patients with dementia. J Clin Psychiatry 60(10):684–689, 1999 10549685

Thakur A, Jagadheesan K, Sinha VK: Lamotrigine add-on to valproate therapy for paediatric bipolar affective disorder. Aust N Z J Psychiatry 39(7):639, 2005 15996148

Thompson TL II, Moran MG, Nies AS: Psychotropic drug use in the elderly. N Engl J Med 308(4):194–199, 1983 6129574

Tinetti ME, Speechley M: Prevention of falls among the elderly. N Engl J Med 320(16):1055–1059, 1989 2648154

Troost PW, Lahuis BE, Steenhuis MP, et al: Long-term effects of risperidone in children with autism spectrum disorders: a placebo discontinuation study. J Am Acad Child Adolesc Psychiatry 44(11):1137–1144, 2005 16239862

Tsuang MM, Lu LM, Stotsky BA, Cole JO: Haloperidol versus thioridazine for hospitalized psychogeriatric patients: double-blind study. J Am Geriatr Soc 19(7):593–600, 1971 4937658

Turner DC, Clark L, Dowson J, et al: Modafinil improves cognition and response inhibition in adult attention-deficit/hyperactivity disorder. Biol Psychiatry 55(10):1031–1040, 2004 15121488

van Dyck CH, Swanson CJ, Aisen P, et al: Lecanemab in early Alzheimer's disease. N Engl J Med 388(1):9–21, 2023 36449413

Varkukla M, Viguera AC, Gonsalves L: Depression and pregnancy. Compr Ther 35(1):44–49, 2009 19351104

Vigod SN, Gomes T, Wilton AS, et al: Antipsychotic drug use in pregnancy: high dimensional, propensity matched, population based cohort study. BMJ 350:h2298, 2015 25972273

Viguera AC, McElheny SA, Caplin PS, et al: Risk of poor neonatal adaptation syndrome among infants exposed to second-generation atypical antipsychotics compared to antidepressants: results from the national pregnancy registry for psychiatric medications. J Clin Psychiatry 84(1):22m14492, 2023 36602927

Wagner KD, Fershtman M: Potential mechanism of desipramine-related sudden death in children. Psychosomatics 34(1):80–83, 1993 8426895

Weller EB, Weller RA, Fristad MA: Bipolar disorder in children: misdiagnosis, underdiagnosis, and future directions. J Am Acad Child Adolesc Psychiatry 34(6):709–714, 1995 7608043

Whitaker A, Rao U: Neuroleptics in pediatric psychiatry. Psychiatr Clin North Am 15(1):243–276, 1992 1347940

Wilens TE, Haight BR, Horrigan JP, et al: Bupropion XL in adults with attention-deficit/hyperactivity disorder: a randomized, placebo-controlled study. Biol Psychiatry 57(7):793–801, 2005 15820237

Wragg RE, Jeste DV: Neuroleptics and alternative treatments: management of behavioral symptoms and psychosis in Alzheimer's disease and related conditions. Psychiatr Clin North Am 11(1):195–213, 1988 2898133

Wragg RE, Jeste DV: Overview of depression and psychosis in Alzheimer's disease. Am J Psychiatry 146(5):577–587, 1989 2653053

Yacobi S, Ornoy A: Is lithium a real teratogen? What can we conclude from the prospective versus retrospective studies? A review. Isr J Psychiatry Relat Sci 45(2):95–106, 2008 18982835

Yudofsky SC, Silver JM, Schneider SE: The use of beta blockers in the treatment of aggression. Psychiatry Lett 6:15–23, 1988

References

Alexopoulos GS, Schultz SK, Lebowitz BD: Late-life depression: a model for medical classification. Biol Psychiatry 58(4):283–289, 2005 16026764

Andrade C: Valproate in pregnancy: recent research and regulatory responses. J Clin Psychiatry 79(3):18f12351, 2018 29873961

Arnold LE, Abikoff HB, Cantwell DP, et al: National Institute of Mental Health Collaborative Multimodal Treatment Study of Children with ADHD (the MTA): design challenges and choices. Arch Gen Psychiatry 54(9):865–870, 1997 9294378

Arnold LM, Lu Y, Crofford LJ, et al: A double-blind, multicenter trial comparing duloxetine with placebo in the treatment of fibromyalgia patients with or without major depressive disorder. Arthritis Rheum 50(9):2974–2984, 2004 15457467

Bairy KL, Madhyastha S, Ashok KP, et al: Developmental and behavioral consequences of prenatal fluoxetine. Pharmacology 79(1):1–11, 2007 17077648

Barbaresi WJ, Katusic SK, Colligan RC, et al: Long-term stimulant medication treatment of attention-deficit/hyperactivity disorder: results from a population-based study. J Dev Behav Pediatr 27(1):1–10, 2006 16511362

Barnett MJ, Wehring H, Perry PJ: Comparison of risk of cerebrovascular events in an elderly VA population with dementia between antipsychotic and nonantipsychotic users. J Clin Psychopharmacol 27(6):595–601, 2007 18004126

Beach SR, Celano CM, Sugrue AM, et al: QT prolongation, torsades de pointes, and psychotropic medications: a 5-year update. Psychosomatics 59(2):105–122, 2018 29275963

Ben Amor L: Antipsychotics in pediatric and adolescent patients: a review of comparative safety data. J Affect Disord 138(suppl):S22–S30, 2012 22405602

Benazzi F, Rossi E: Mania and donepezil. Can J Psychiatry 44(5):506–507, 1999 10389619

Bendtsen L, Jensen R, Olesen J: A non-selective (amitriptyline), but not a selective (citalopram), serotonin reuptake inhibitor is effective in the prophylactic treatment of chronic tension-type headache. J Neurol Neurosurg Psychiatry 61(3):285–290, 1996 8795600

Berle JO, Steen VM, Aamo TO, et al: Breastfeeding during maternal antidepressant treatment with serotonin reuptake inhibitors: infant exposure, clinical symptoms, and cytochrome p450 genotypes. J Clin Psychiatry 65(9):1228–1234, 2004 15367050

Biederman J, Thisted RA, Greenhill LL, et al: Estimation of the association between desipramine and the risk for sudden death in 5- to 14-year-old children. J Clin Psychiatry 56(3):87–93, 1995 7883735

Biederman J, Mick E, Faraone SV, et al: Risperidone for the treatment of affective symptoms in children with disruptive behavior disorder: a post hoc analysis of data from a 6-week, multicenter, randomized, double-blind, parallel-arm study. Clin Ther 28(5):794–800, 2006a 16861101

Biederman J, Swanson JM, Wigal SB, et al: A comparison of once-daily and divided doses of modafinil in children with attention-deficit/hyperactivity disorder: a randomized, double-blind, and placebo-controlled study. J Clin Psychiatry 67(5):727–735, 2006b 16841622

Birnbaum CS, Cohen LS, Bailey JW, et al: Serum concentrations of antidepressants and benzodiazepines in nursing infants: a case series. Pediatrics 104(1):e11, 1999 10390297

Boukhris T, Sheehy O, Mottron L, et al: Antidepressant use during pregnancy and the risk of autism spectrum disorder in children. JAMA Pediatr 170(2):117–124, 2016 26660917

Bousman CA, Bengesser SA, Aitchison KJ, et al: Review and consensus on pharmacogenomic testing in psychiatry. Pharmacopsychiatry 54(1):5–17, 2021 33147643

Bridge JA, Iyengar S, Salary CB, et al: Clinical response and risk for reported suicidal ideation and suicide attempts in pediatric antidepressant treatment: a meta-analysis of randomized controlled trials. JAMA 297(15):1683–1696, 2007 17440145

Budhwani H, Hearld KR, Chavez-Yenter D: Depression in racial and ethnic minorities: the impact of nativity and discrimination. J Racial Ethn Health Disparities 2(1):34–42, 2015 26863239

Buitelaar JK, Danckaerts M, Gillberg C, et al: A prospective, multicenter, open-label assessment of atomoxetine in non-North American children and adolescents with ADHD. Eur Child Adolesc Psychiatry 13(4):249–257, 2004 15365896

Burns A, Rossor M, Hecker J, et al: The effects of donepezil in Alzheimer's disease: results from a multinational trial. Dement Geriatr Cogn Disord 10(3):237–244, 1999 10325453

Buskova J, Busek P, Nevsimalova S: Gabapentin in the treatment of dementia-associated nocturnal agitation. Med Sci Monit 17(12):CS149–CS151, 2011 22129906

Campbell M, Small AM, Green WH, et al: Behavioral efficacy of haloperidol and lithium carbonate: a comparison in hospitalized aggressive children with conduct disorder. Arch Gen Psychiatry 41(7):650–656, 1984 6428371

Carceller-Sindreu M, de Diego-Adeliño J, Portella MJ, et al: Lack of relationship between plasma levels of escitalopram and QTc-interval length. Eur Arch Psychiatry Clin Neurosci 267(8):815–822, 2017 28116499

Casat CD, Pleasants DZ, Schroeder DH, et al: Bupropion in children with attention deficit disorder. Psychopharmacol Bull 25(2):198–201, 1989 2513592

Casper RC, Fleisher BE, Lee-Ancajas JC, et al: Follow-up of children of depressed mothers exposed or not exposed to antidepressant drugs during pregnancy. J Pediatr 142(4):402–408, 2003 12712058

Casper RC, Gilles AA, Fleisher BE, et al: Length of prenatal exposure to selective serotonin reuptake inhibitor (SSRI) antidepressants: effects on neonatal adaptation and psychomotor development. Psychopharmacology (Berl) 217(2):211–219, 2011 21499702

Chang K, Saxena K, Howe M: An open-label study of lamotrigine adjunct or monotherapy for the treatment of adolescents with bipolar depression. J Am Acad Child Adolesc Psychiatry 45(3):298–304, 2006 16540814

Chen Y, Guo JJ, Zhan S, et al: Treatment effects of antidepressants in patients with post-stroke depression: a meta-analysis. Ann Pharmacother 40(12):2115–2122, 2006 17119102

Choi-Kwon S, Han SW, Kwon SU, et al: Fluoxetine treatment in poststroke depression, emotional incontinence, and anger proneness: a double-blind, placebo-controlled study. Stroke 37(1):156–161, 2006 16306470

Cohen LS, Friedman JM, Jefferson JW, et al: A reevaluation of risk of in utero exposure to lithium (erratum: JAMA 271:1485, 1994; also see comments: 271:1828–1829, 1994). JAMA 271(2):146–150, 1994 8031346

Cole JO: Research issues, in Anxiety in the Elderly. Edited by Salzman C, Lebowitz BD. New York, Springer, 1990

Colenda CC III: Buspirone in treatment of agitated demented patient. Lancet 1(8595):1169, 1988 2896993

Correll CU, Leucht S, Kane JM: Lower risk for tardive dyskinesia associated with second-generation antipsychotics: a systematic review of 1-year studies. Am J Psychiatry 161(3):414–425, 2004 14992963

Cummings JL, Lyketsos CG, Peskind ER, et al: Effect of dextromethorphan-quinidine on agitation in patients with Alzheimer disease dementia: a randomized clinical trial. JAMA 314(12):1242–1254, 2015 26393847

Dam M, Tonin P, De Boni A, et al: Effects of fluoxetine and maprotiline on functional recovery in poststroke hemiplegic patients undergoing rehabilitation therapy. Stroke 27(7):1211–1214, 1996 8685930

Damkier P, Videbech P: The safety of second-generation antipsychotics during pregnancy: a clinically focused review. CNS Drugs 32(4):351–366, 2018 29637530

Daviss WB, Bentivoglio P, Racusin R, et al: Bupropion sustained release in adolescents with comorbid attention-deficit/hyperactivity disorder and depression. J Am Acad Child Adolesc Psychiatry 40(3):307–314, 2001 11288772

Delbello MP, Kowatch RA, Adler CM, et al: A double-blind randomized pilot study comparing quetiapine and divalproex for adolescent mania. J Am Acad Child Adolesc Psychiatry 45(3):305–313, 2006 16540815

Dennis K, Le Grange D, Bremer J: Olanzapine use in adolescent anorexia nervosa. Eat Weight Disord 11(2):e53–e56, 2006 16809970

Dolovich LR, Addis A, Vaillancourt JM, et al: Benzodiazepine use in pregnancy and major malformations or oral cleft: meta-analysis of cohort and case-control studies. BMJ 317(7162):839–843, 1998 9748174

Einarson A, Choi J, Einarson TR, et al: Incidence of major malformations in infants following antidepressant exposure in pregnancy: results of a large prospective cohort study. Can J Psychiatry 54(4):242–246, 2009 19321030

Emslie GJ, Rush AJ, Weinberg WA, et al: A double-blind, randomized, placebo-controlled trial of fluoxetine in children and adolescents with depression. Arch Gen Psychiatry 54(11):1031–1037, 1997 9366660

Emslie GJ, Heiligenstein JH, Wagner KD, et al: Fluoxetine for acute treatment of depression in children and adolescents: a placebo-controlled, randomized clinical trial. J Am Acad Child Adolesc Psychiatry 41(10):1205–1215, 2002 12364842

Emslie GJ, Heiligenstein JH, Hoog SL, et al: Fluoxetine treatment for prevention of relapse of depression in children and adolescents: a double-blind, placebo-controlled study. J Am Acad Child Adolesc Psychiatry 43(11):1397–1405, 2004 15502599

Emslie GJ, Ventura D, Korotzer A, et al: Escitalopram in the treatment of adolescent depression: a randomized placebo-controlled multisite trial. J Am Acad Child Adolesc Psychiatry 48(7):721–729, 2009 19465881

Eros E, Czeizel AE, Rockenbauer M, et al: A population-based case-control teratologic study of nitrazepam, medazepam, tofisopam, alprazolum and clonazepam treatment during pregnancy. Eur J Obstet Gynecol Reprod Biol 101(2):147–154, 2002 11858890

Findling RL, McNamara NK, Youngstrom EA, et al: Double-blind 18-month trial of lithium versus divalproex maintenance treatment in pediatric bipolar disorder. J Am Acad Child Adolesc Psychiatry 44(5):409–417, 2005 15843762

Findling RL, McNamara NK, Stansbrey R, et al: Combination lithium and divalproex sodium in pediatric bipolar symptom re-stabilization. J Am Acad Child Adolesc Psychiatry 45(2):142–148, 2006 16429084

Findling RL, Mankoski R, Timko K, et al: A randomized controlled trial investigating the safety and efficacy of aripiprazole in the long-term maintenance treatment of pediatric patients with irritability associated with autistic disorder. J Clin Psychiatry 75(1):22–30, 2014 24502859

Flint AJ, Iaboni A, Mulsant BH, et al: Effect of sertraline on risk of falling in older adults with psychotic depression on olanzapine: results of a randomized placebo-controlled trial. Am J Geriatr Psychiatry 22(4):332–336, 2014 23642462

Foster CA, Bafaloukos J: Paroxetine in the treatment of chronic daily headache. Headache 34(10):587–589, 1994 7843954

Frankenburg FR, Kando JC: Sertraline treatment of attention deficit hyperactivity disorder and Tourette's syndrome (letter). J Clin Psychopharmacol 14(5):359–360, 1994 7806695

Gaete JM, Bogousslavsky J: Post-stroke depression. Expert Rev Neurother 8(1):75–92, 2008 18088202

Geller B, Cooper TB, Sun K, et al: Double-blind and placebo-controlled study of lithium for adolescent bipolar disorders with secondary substance dependency. J Am Acad Child Adolesc Psychiatry 37(2):171–178, 1998 9473913

Geller B, Luby JL, Joshi P, et al: A randomized controlled trial of risperidone, lithium, or divalproex sodium for initial treatment of bipolar I disorder, manic or mixed phase, in children and adolescents. Arch Gen Psychiatry 69(5):515–528, 2012 22213771

Gentile S, Rossi A, Bellantuono C: SSRIs during breastfeeding: spotlight on milk-to-plasma ratio. Arch Women Ment Health 10(2):39–51, 2007 17294355

Gibbons RD, Brown CH, Hur K, et al: Early evidence on the effects of regulators' suicidality warnings on SSRI prescriptions and suicide in children and adolescents. Am J Psychiatry 164(9):1356–1363, 2007 17728420

Glassman AH, Perel JM, Shostak M, et al: Clinical implications of imipramine plasma levels for depressive illness. Arch Gen Psychiatry 34(2):197–204, 1977 843179

Glassman AH, Bigger JT Jr, Giardina EV, et al: Clinical characteristics of imipramine-induced orthostatic hypotension. Lancet 1(8114):468–472, 1979 85056

Glassman AH, O'Connor CM, Califf RM, et al: Sertraline treatment of major depression in patients with acute MI or unstable angina. JAMA 288(6):701–709, 2002 12169073

Gleason RP, Schneider LS: Carbamazepine treatment of agitation in Alzheimer's outpatients refractory to neuroleptics. J Clin Psychiatry 51(3):115–118, 1990 1968457

Goodlet KJ, Zmarlicka MT, Peckham AM: Drug-drug interactions and clinical considerations with co-administration of antiretrovirals and psychotropic drugs. CNS Spectr 24(3):287–312, 2019 30295215

Green AE, Price MN, Dorison SH: Cumulative minority stress and suicide risk among LGBTQ youth. Am J Community Psychol 69(1–2):157–168, 2022 34534356

Greenberg SM, Tennis MK, Brown LB, et al: Donepezil therapy in clinical practice: a randomized crossover study. Arch Neurol 57(1):94–99, 2000 10634454

Greendyke RM, Kanter DR: Therapeutic effects of pindolol on behavioral disturbances associated with organic brain disease: a double-blind study. J Clin Psychiatry 47(8):423–426, 1986 3525523

Greendyke RM, Berkner JP, Webster JC, et al: Treatment of behavioral problems with
pindolol. Psychosomatics 30(2):161–165, 1989 2652180

Greenhill LL, Halperin JM, Abikoff H: Stimulant medications. J Am Acad Child Adolesc Psychiatry 38(5):503–512, 1999 10230181

Greenhill LL, Biederman J, Boellner SW, et al: A randomized, double-blind, placebo-
controlled study of modafinil film-coated tablets in children and adolescents with
attention-deficit/hyperactivity disorder. J Am Acad Child Adolesc Psychiatry
45(5):503–511, 2006 16601402

Grossberg GT, Kohegyi E, Mergel V, et al: Efficacy and safety of brexpiprazole for the
treatment of agitation in Alzheimer's dementia: two 12-week, randomized, double-blind, placebo-controlled trials. Am J Geriatr Psychiatry 28(4):383–400,
2020 31708380

Haddad YK, Luo F, Bergen G, et al: Special report from the CDC antidepressant subclass use and fall risk in community-dwelling older Americans. J Safety Res
76:332–340, 2021 33653566

Harden CL, Meador KJ, Pennell PB, et al: Management issues for women with epilepsy—focus on pregnancy (an evidence-based review) II: teratogenesis and perinatal outcomes: report of the Quality Standards Subcommittee and Therapeutics
and Technology Subcommittee of the American Academy of Neurology and the
American Epilepsy Society. Epilepsia 50(5):1237–1246, 2009 19507301

Harrington RA, Lee LC, Crum RM, et al: Prenatal SSRI use and offspring with autism
spectrum disorder or developmental delay. Pediatrics 133(5):e1241–e1248,
2014 24733881

Haw C, Stubbs J: A survey of off-label prescribing for inpatients with mild intellectual
disability and mental illness. J Intellect Disabil Res 49(Pt 11):858–864, 2005
16207284

Hazell P, O'Connell D, Heathcote D, et al: Efficacy of tricyclic drugs in treating child
and adolescent depression: a meta-analysis. BMJ 310(6984):897–901, 1995
7719178

Hendrick V, Smith LM, Suri R, et al: Birth outcomes after prenatal exposure to antidepressant medication. Am J Obstet Gynecol 188(3):812–815, 2003 12634662

Herrmann N, Mamdani M, Lanctôt KL: Atypical antipsychotics and risk of cerebrovascular accidents. Am J Psychiatry 161(6):1113–1115, 2004 15169702

Horrigan JP, Barnhill LJ: Risperidone and explosive aggressive autism. J Autism Dev
Disord 27(3):313–323, 1997 9229261

Huybrechts KF, Hernández-Díaz S, Patorno E, et al: Antipsychotic use in pregnancy and the risk for congenital malformations. JAMA Psychiatry 73(9):938–946, 2016 27540849

Imfeld P, Bodmer M, Jick SS, et al: Benzodiazepine use and risk of developing Alzheimer's disease or vascular dementia: a case-control analysis. Drug Saf 38(10):909–919, 2015 26123874

Jacobsen FM, Comas-Díaz L: Donepezil for psychotropic-induced memory loss. J Clin Psychiatry 60(10):698–704, 1999 10549687

Jann MW: Rivastigmine, a new-generation cholinesterase inhibitor for the treatment of Alzheimer's disease. Pharmacotherapy 20(1):1–12, 2000 10641971

Kafantaris V: Treatment of bipolar disorder in children and adolescents. J Am Acad Child Adolesc Psychiatry 34(6):732–741, 1995 7608046

Keller MB, Ryan ND, Strober M, et al: Efficacy of paroxetine in the treatment of adolescent major depression: a randomized, controlled trial. J Am Acad Child Adolesc Psychiatry 40(7):762–772, 2001 11437014

Kelsey DK, Sumner CR, Casat CD, et al: Once-daily atomoxetine treatment for children with attention-deficit/hyperactivity disorder, including an assessment of evening and morning behavior: a double-blind, placebo-controlled trial. Pediatrics 114(1):e1–e8, 2004 15231966

Kennard BD, Silva SG, Mayes TL, et al: Assessment of safety and long-term outcomes of initial treatment with placebo in TADS. Am J Psychiatry 166(3):337–344, 2009 19147693

Kent JD, Blader JC, Koplewicz HS, et al: Effects of late-afternoon methylphenidate administration on behavior and sleep in attention-deficit hyperactivity disorder. Pediatrics 96(2 Pt 1):320–325, 1995 7630692

Kessing LV: Depression and the risk for dementia. Curr Opin Psychiatry 25(6):457–461, 2012 22801361

Killen JD, Robinson TN, Ammerman S, et al: Randomized clinical trial of the efficacy of bupropion combined with nicotine patch in the treatment of adolescent smokers. J Consult Clin Psychol 72(4):729–735, 2004 15301658

Kramer JR, Loney J, Ponto LB, et al: Predictors of adult height and weight in boys treated with methylphenidate for childhood behavior problems. J Am Acad Child Adolesc Psychiatry 39(4):517–524, 2000 10761355

Kratochvil CJ, Heiligenstein JH, Dittmann R, et al: Atomoxetine and methylphenidate treatment in children with ADHD: a prospective, randomized, open-label trial. J Am Acad Child Adolesc Psychiatry 41(7):776–784, 2002 12108801

Kratochvil CJ, Wilens TE, Greenhill LL, et al: Effects of long-term atomoxetine treatment for young children with attention-deficit/hyperactivity disorder. J Am Acad Child Adolesc Psychiatry 45(8):919–927, 2006 16865034

Kumar A, Datta SS, Wright SD, et al: Atypical antipsychotics for psychosis in adolescents. Cochrane Database Syst Rev 10(10):CD009582, 2013 24129841

Kumra S, Frazier JA, Jacobsen LK, et al: Childhood-onset schizophrenia: a double-blind clozapine-haloperidol comparison. Arch Gen Psychiatry 53(12):1090–1097, 1996 8956674

Kumra S, Oberstar JV, Sikich L, et al: Efficacy and tolerability of second-generation antipsychotics in children and adolescents with schizophrenia. Schizophr Bull 34(1):60–71, 2008 17923452

Langemark M, Olesen J: Sulpiride and paroxetine in the treatment of chronic tension-type headache: an explanatory double-blind trial. Headache 34(1):20–24, 1994 8132436

Lebert F, Pasquier F, Petit H: Behavioral effects of trazodone in Alzheimer's disease. J Clin Psychiatry 55(12):536–538, 1994 7814348

Lipsey JR, Robinson RG, Pearlson GD, et al: Nortriptyline treatment of post-stroke depression: a double-blind study. Lancet 1(8372):297–300, 1984 6141377

Lok P: Mental health: cultural competency is key to improving outcomes for ethnic minority patients, leaders say. BMJ 378:o1718, 2022 35820693

Lopez-Larson M, Frazier JA: Empirical evidence for the use of lithium and anticonvulsants in children with psychiatric disorders. Harv Rev Psychiatry 14(6):285–304, 2006 17162653

Machado-Duque ME, Castaño-Montoya JP, Medina-Morales DA, et al: Association between the use of benzodiazepines and opioids with the risk of falls and hip fractures in older adults. Int Psychogeriatr 30(7):941–946, 2018 29223172

Madhusoodanan S, Bogunovic OJ: Safety of benzodiazepines in the geriatric population. Expert Opin Drug Saf 3(5):485–493, 2004 15335303

Mak M, Lam C, Pineda SJ, et al: Pharmacogenetics of warfarin in a diverse patient population. J Cardiovasc Pharmacol Ther 24(6):521–533, 2019 31064211

Mandoki MW, Tapia MR, Tapia MA, et al: Venlafaxine in the treatment of children and adolescents with major depression. Psychopharmacol Bull 33(1):149–154, 1997 9133767

Mayer KH, Nelson L, Hightow-Weidman L, et al: The persistent and evolving HIV epidemic in American men who have sex with men. Lancet 397(10279):1116–1126, 2021 33617771

McCracken JT, McGough J, Shah B, et al: Risperidone in children with autism and serious behavioral problems. N Engl J Med 347(5):314–321, 2002 12151468

McDougle CJ, Holmes JP, Carlson DC, et al: A double-blind, placebo-controlled study of risperidone in adults with autistic disorder and other pervasive developmental disorders. Arch Gen Psychiatry 55(7):633–641, comment 643–644, 1998 9672054

Meador KJ, Baker GA, Browning N, et al: Cognitive function at 3 years of age after fetal exposure to antiepileptic drugs. N Engl J Med 360(16):1597–1605, 2009 19369666

Michelson D, Faries D, Wernicke J, et al: Atomoxetine in the treatment of children and adolescents with attention-deficit/hyperactivity disorder: a randomized, placebo-controlled, dose-response study. Pediatrics 108(5):E83, 2001 11694667

Miller LJ: Gabapentin for treatment of behavioral and psychological symptoms of dementia. Ann Pharmacother 35(4):427–431, 2001 11302405

Mondraty N, Birmingham CL, Touyz S, et al: Randomized controlled trial of olanzapine in the treatment of cognitions in anorexia nervosa. Australas Psychiatry 13(1):72–75, 2005 15777417

Moses-Kolko EL, Bogen D, Perel J, et al: Neonatal signs after late in utero exposure to serotonin reuptake inhibitors: literature review and implications for clinical applications. JAMA 293(19):2372–2383, 2005 15900008

Mozes T, Toren P, Chernauzan N, et al: Clozapine treatment in very early onset schizophrenia. J Am Acad Child Adolesc Psychiatry 33(1):65–70, 1994 8138523

Nafti M, Sirois C, Kröger E, et al: Is benzodiazepine use associated with the risk of dementia and cognitive impairment—not dementia in older persons? The Canadian Study of Health and Aging. Ann Pharmacother 54(3):219–225, 2020 31595772

Nasser A, Liranso T, Adewole T, et al: A Phase III, randomized, placebo-controlled trial to assess the efficacy and safety of once-daily SPN-812 (viloxazine extended-release) in the treatment of attention-deficit/hyperactivity disorder in school-age children. Clin Ther 42(8):1452–1466, 2020 32723670

Nasser A, Liranso T, Adewole T, et al: Once-daily SPN-812 200 and 400 mg in the treatment of ADHD in school-aged children: a Phase III randomized, controlled trial. Clin Ther 43(4):684–700, 2021a 33750646

Nasser A, Liranso T, Adewole T, et al: A Phase 3 placebo-controlled trial of once-daily 400-mg and 600-mg SPN-812 (viloxazine extended-release) in adolescents with ADHD. Psychopharmacol Bull 51(2):43–64, 2021b 34092822

Nemeroff CB, Kalali A, Keller MB, et al: Impact of publicity concerning pediatric suicidality data on physician practice patterns in the United States. Arch Gen Psychiatry 64(4):466–472, 2007 17404123

Newport DJ, Fernandez SV, Juric S, Stowe ZN: Psychopharmacology during pregnancy and lactation, in The American Psychiatric Publishing Textbook of Psychopharmacology, 4th Edition. Edited by Schatzberg AF, Nemeroff CB. Washington, DC, American Psychiatric Publishing, 2009, pp 1373–1412

Ng QX, Venkatanarayanan N, Ho CYX, et al: Selective serotonin reuptake inhibitors and persistent pulmonary hypertension of the newborn: an update meta-analysis. J Womens Health (Larchmt) 28(3):331–338, 2019 30407100

Nulman I, Rovet J, Stewart DE, et al: Neurodevelopment of children exposed in utero to antidepressant drugs. N Engl J Med 336(4):258–262, 1997 8995088

Nulman I, Rovet J, Stewart DE, et al: Child development following exposure to tricyclic antidepressants or fluoxetine throughout fetal life: a prospective, controlled study. Am J Psychiatry 159(11):1889–1895, 2002 12411224

O'Connor CM, Jiang W, Kuchibhatla M, et al: Safety and efficacy of sertraline for depression in patients with heart failure: results of the SADHART-CHF (Sertraline Against Depression and Heart Disease in Chronic Heart Failure) trial. J Am Coll Cardiol 56(9):692–699, 2010 20723799

Oslin DW, Ten Have TR, Streim JE, et al: Probing the safety of medications in the frail elderly: evidence from a randomized clinical trial of sertraline and venlafaxine in depressed nursing home residents. J Clin Psychiatry 64(8):875–882, 2003 12927001

Patel NC, Delbello MP, Bryan HS, et al: Open-label lithium for the treatment of adolescents with bipolar depression. J Am Acad Child Adolesc Psychiatry 45(3):289–297, 2006 16540813

Patino LR, Klein CC, Strawn JR, et al: A randomized, double-blind, controlled trial of lithium versus quetiapine for the treatment of acute mania in youth with early course bipolar disorder. J Child Adolesc Psychopharmacol 31(7):485–493, 2021 34520250

Patorno E, Huybrechts KF, Bateman BT, et al: Lithium use in pregnancy and the risk of cardiac malformations. N Engl J Med 376(23):2245–2254, 2017 28591541

Pavuluri MN, Henry DB, Findling RL, et al: Double-blind randomized trial of risperidone versus divalproex in pediatric bipolar disorder. Bipolar Disord 12(6):593–605, 2010 20868458

Payne JL: Psychiatric medication use in pregnancy and breastfeeding. Obstet Gynecol Clin North Am 48(1):131–149, 2021 33573783

Perry BI, Cooray SE, Mendis J, et al: Problem behaviours and psychotropic medication use in intellectual disability: a multinational cross-sectional survey. J Intellect Disabil Res 62(2):140–149, 2018 29349928

Peters ME, Vaidya V, Drye LT, et al; CitAD Research Group: Citalopram for the treatment of agitation in Alzheimer dementia: genetic influences. J Geriatr Psychiatry Neurol 29(2):59–64, 2016 26303700

Pinner E, Rich CL: Effects of trazodone on aggressive behavior in seven patients with organic mental disorders. Am J Psychiatry 145(10):1295–1296, 1988 3048122

Platt JE, Campbell M, Green WH, et al: Cognitive effects of lithium carbonate and haloperidol in treatment-resistant aggressive children. Arch Gen Psychiatry 41(7):657–662, 1984 6428372

Pool D, Mileke DH, Ronger JJ, et al: A controlled evaluation of Loxitane in 75 schizophrenic adolescents. Curr Res Ther 19:99–104, 1976 812671

Prasad S, et al: Viloxazine in children and adolescents with attention-deficit/hyperactivity disorder: a randomized, placebo-controlled, phase IV study. Child Adolesc Psychiatry Ment Health 13:29, 2019

Profenno LA, Jakimovich L, Holt CJ, et al: A randomized, double-blind, placebo-controlled pilot trial of safety and tolerability of two doses of divalproex sodium in outpatients with probable Alzheimer's disease. Curr Alzheimer Res 2(5):553–558, 2005 16375658

Rahimi R, Nikfar S, Abdollahi M: Pregnancy outcomes following exposure to serotonin reuptake inhibitors: a meta-analysis of clinical trials. Reprod Toxicol 22(4):571–575, 2006 16720091

Rai D, Lee BK, Dalman C, et al: Parental depression, maternal antidepressant use during pregnancy, and risk of autism spectrum disorders: population based case-control study. BMJ 346:f2059, 2013 23604083

Raj AB, Sheehan DV: Medical evaluation of the anxious patient. Psychiatr Ann 18:176–181, 1988

Raskin DE, et al: Presentation at the International College of Geriatric Psychopharmacology, Basel, Switzerland, 2004

Ray-Griffith SL, Newport DJ, Stowe ZN: Psychopharmacology during pregnancy and lactation, in The American Psychiatric Association Publishing Textbook of Psychopharmacology, 5th Edition. Edited by Schatzberg AF, Nemeroff CB. Washington, DC, American Psychiatric Association Publishing, 2017, pp 1543–1592

Reding MJ, Orto LA, Winter SW, et al: Antidepressant therapy after stroke: a double-blind trial. Arch Neurol 43(8):763–765, 1986 3729755

Reisberg B, Doody R, Stöffler A, et al: Memantine in moderate-to-severe Alzheimer's disease. N Engl J Med 348(14):1333–1341, 2003 12672860

Ricci F, Torales J, Bener A, et al: Mental health of ethnic minorities: the role of racism. Int Rev Psychiatry 35(3–4):258–267, 2023 37267026

Robinson RG, Schultz SK, Castillo C, et al: Nortriptyline versus fluoxetine in the treatment of depression and in short-term recovery after stroke: a placebo-controlled, double-blind study. Am J Psychiatry 157(3):351–359, 2000 10698809

Rohde C, Hilker R, Siskind D, et al: Real-world effectiveness of clozapine for intellectual disability: results from a mirror-image and a reverse-mirror-image study. J Psychopharmacol 32(11):1197–1203, 2018 29944071

Roose SP, Glassman AH, Attia E, et al: Selective serotonin reuptake inhibitor efficacy in melancholia and atypical depression. Paper presented at the 147th Annual Meeting of the American Psychiatric Association, Philadelphia, PA, May 21–26, 1994

Roose SP, Laghrissi-Thode F, Kennedy JS, et al: Comparison of paroxetine and nortriptyline in depressed patients with ischemic heart disease. JAMA 279(4):287–291, 1998 9450712

Roose SP, Sackeim HA, Krishnan KR, et al: Antidepressant pharmacotherapy in the treatment of depression in the very old: a randomized, placebo-controlled trial. Am J Psychiatry 161(11):2050–2059, 2004 15514406

Rosenberg DR, Holttum J, Gershon S: Textbook of Pharmacotherapy for Child and Adolescent Psychiatric Disorders. New York, Brunner/Mazel, 1994

Rugino TA, Copley TC: Effects of modafinil in children with attention-deficit/hyperactivity disorder: an open-label study. J Am Acad Child Adolesc Psychiatry 40(2):230–235, 2001 11211372

Saxena K, Howe M, Simeonova D, et al: Divalproex sodium reduces overall aggression in youth at high risk for bipolar disorder. J Child Adolesc Psychopharmacol 16(3):252–259, 2006 16768633

Schatzberg AF, DeBattista C: Phenomenology and treatment of agitation. J Clin Psychiatry 60(Suppl 15):17–20, 1999 10418809

Schatzberg A, Roose S: A double-blind, placebo-controlled study of venlafaxine and fluoxetine in geriatric outpatients with major depression. Am J Geriatr Psychiatry 14(4):361–370, 2006 16582045

Schatzberg AF, Kremer C, Rodrigues HE, et al: Double-blind, randomized comparison of mirtazapine and paroxetine in elderly depressed patients. Am J Geriatr Psychiatry 10(5):541–550, 2002 12213688

Schneider LS, Tariot PN, Dagerman KS, et al: Effectiveness of atypical antipsychotic drugs in patients with Alzheimer's disease. N Engl J Med 355(15):1525–1538, 2006 17035647

Schreier HA: Risperidone for young children with mood disorders and aggressive behavior. J Child Adolesc Psychopharmacol 8(1):49–59, 1998 9639079

Sikich L, Hamer RM, Bashford RA, et al: A pilot study of risperidone, olanzapine, and haloperidol in psychotic youth: a double-blind, randomized, 8-week trial. Neuropsychopharmacology 29(1):133–145, 2004 14583740

Siméon JG: Use of anxiolytics in children. Encephale 19(2):71–74, 1993 7903927

Simon GE, Cunningham ML, Davis RL: Outcomes of prenatal antidepressant exposure. Am J Psychiatry 159(12):2055–2061, 2002 12450956

Sindi S, Kåreholt I, Johansson L, et al: Sleep disturbances and dementia risk: a multicenter study. Alzheimers Dement 14(10):1235–1242, 2018 30030112

Singer HS, Brown J, Quaskey S, et al: The treatment of attention-deficit hyperactivity disorder in Tourette's syndrome: a double-blind placebo-controlled study with clonidine and desipramine. Pediatrics 95(1):74–81, 1995 7770313

Slone D, Siskind V, Heinonen OP, et al: Antenatal exposure to the phenothiazines in relation to congenital malformations, perinatal mortality rate, birth weight, and intelligence quotient score. Am J Obstet Gynecol 128(5):486–488, 1977 879206

Solhkhah R, Wilens TE, Daly J, et al: Bupropion SR for the treatment of substance-abusing outpatient adolescents with attention-deficit/hyperactivity disorder and mood disorders. J Child Adolesc Psychopharmacol 15(5):777–786, 2005 16262594

Sovner R: The use of valproate in the treatment of mentally retarded persons with typical and atypical bipolar disorders. J Clin Psychiatry 50(3)(suppl):40–43, 1989 2494159

Sovner R, Hurley AD: Do the mentally retarded suffer from affective illness? Arch Gen Psychiatry 40(1):61–67, 1983 6849621

Spencer EK, Kafantaris V, Padron-Gayol MV, et al: Haloperidol in schizophrenic children: early findings from a study in progress. Psychopharmacol Bull 28(2):183–186, 1992 1513922

Spiller HA, Ramoska EA, Krenzelok EP, et al: Bupropion overdose: a 3-year multicenter retrospective analysis. Am J Emerg Med 12(1):43–45, 1994 8285970

Steiner H, Petersen ML, Saxena K, et al: Divalproex sodium for the treatment of conduct disorder: a randomized controlled clinical trial. J Clin Psychiatry 64(10):1183–1191, 2003 14658966

Stowe ZN, Owens MJ, Landry JC, et al: Sertraline and desmethylsertraline in human breast milk and nursing infants. Am J Psychiatry 154(9):1255–1260, 1997 9286185

Sultzer DL, Gray KF, Gunay I, et al: Does behavioral improvement with haloperidol or trazodone treatment depend on psychosis or mood symptoms in patients with dementia? J Am Geriatr Soc 49(10):1294–1300, 2001 11890487

Swanson JM, Lerner M, Williams L: More frequent diagnosis of attention deficit-hyperactivity disorder (letter). N Engl J Med 333(14):944, 1995 7666894

Swenson JR, O'Connor CM, Barton D, et al: Influence of depression and effect of treatment with sertraline on quality of life after hospitalization for acute coronary syndrome. Am J Cardiol 92(11):1271–1276, 2003 14636902

Tariot PN, Erb R, Podgorski CA, et al: Efficacy and tolerability of carbamazepine for agitation and aggression in dementia. Am J Psychiatry 155(1):54–61, 1998 9433339

Tariot PN, Farlow MR, Grossberg GT, et al: Memantine treatment in patients with moderate to severe Alzheimer disease already receiving donepezil: a randomized controlled trial. JAMA 291(3):317–324, 2004 14734594

Tariot PN, Raman R, Jakimovich L, et al: Divalproex sodium in nursing home residents with possible or probable Alzheimer Disease complicated by agitation: a randomized, controlled trial. Am J Geriatr Psychiatry 13(11):942–949, 2005 16286437

Tariot PN, Schneider LS, Cummings J, et al: Chronic divalproex sodium to attenuate agitation and clinical progression of Alzheimer disease. Arch Gen Psychiatry 68(8):853–861, 2011 21810649

Taylor CB, Youngblood ME, Catellier D, et al: Effects of antidepressant medication on morbidity and mortality in depressed patients after myocardial infarction. Arch Gen Psychiatry 62(7):792–798, 2005 15997021

Taylor FB, Russo J: Efficacy of modafinil compared to dextroamphetamine for the treatment of attention deficit hyperactivity disorder in adults. J Child Adolesc Psychopharmacol 10(4):311–320, 2000 11191692

Thomas SV, Ajaykumar B, Sindhu K, et al: Motor and mental development of infants exposed to antiepileptic drugs in utero. Epilepsy Behav 13(1):229–236, 2008 18346940

Trifirò G, Verhamme KM, Ziere G, et al: All-cause mortality associated with atypical and typical antipsychotics in demented outpatients. Pharmacoepidemiol Drug Saf 16(5):538–544, 2007 17036366

van Dyck CH, Swanson CJ, Aisen P, et al: Lecanemab in early Alzheimer's disease. N Engl J Med 388(1):9–21, 2023 36449413

Vasudev A, Macritchie K, Vasudev K, et al: Oxcarbazepine for acute affective episodes in bipolar disorder. Cochrane Database Syst Rev 2011(12):CD004857, 2011 22161387

Vetró A, Szentistványi I, Pallag L, et al: Therapeutic experience with lithium in childhood aggressivity. Neuropsychobiology 14(3):121–127, 1985 3938528

Vigod SN, Gomes T, Wilton AS, et al: Antipsychotic drug use in pregnancy: high dimensional, propensity matched, population based cohort study. BMJ 350:h2298, 2015 25972273

Viguera AC, Koukopoulos A, Muzina DJ, et al: Teratogenicity and anticonvulsants: lessons from neurology to psychiatry. J Clin Psychiatry 68(suppl 9):29–33, 2007 17764382 (erratum: J Clin Psychiatry 68:1989, 2007)

Viguera AC, McElheny SA, Caplin PS, et al: Risk of poor neonatal adaptation syndrome among infants exposed to second-generation atypical antipsychotics compared to antidepressants: results from the national pregnancy registry for psychiatric medications. J Clin Psychiatry 84(1):22m14492, 2023 36602927

Vinten J, Adab N, Kini U, et al: Neuropsychological effects of exposure to anticonvulsant medication in utero. Neurology 64(6):949–954, 2005 15781806

Wagner KD, Robb AS, Findling R, et al: Citalopram is effective in the treatment of major depressive disorder in children and adolescents: results of a placebo-controlled trial. Presented at 40th Annual Meeting of the American College of Neuropsychopharmacology, Waikoloa, HI, 2001

Wagner KD, Ambrosini P, Rynn M, et al: Efficacy of sertraline in the treatment of children and adolescents with major depressive disorder: two randomized controlled trials. JAMA 290(8):1033–1041, 2003 12941675

Wagner KD, Berard R, Stein MB, et al: A multicenter, randomized, double-blind, placebo-controlled trial of paroxetine in children and adolescents with social anxiety disorder. Arch Gen Psychiatry 61(11):1153–1162, 2004 15520363

Wagner KD, Jonas J, Findling RL, et al: A double-blind, randomized, placebo-controlled trial of escitalopram in the treatment of pediatric depression. J Am Acad Child Adolesc Psychiatry 45(3):280–288, 2006a 16540812

Wagner KD, Kowatch RA, Emslie GJ, et al: A double-blind, randomized, placebo-controlled trial of oxcarbazepine in the treatment of bipolar disorder in children and adolescents. Am J Psychiatry 163(7):1179–1186, 2006b 16816222 (erratum: Am J Psychiatry 163(10):1843, 2006)

Wagner KD, Redden L, Kowatch RA, et al: A double-blind, randomized, placebo-controlled trial of divalproex extended-release in the treatment of bipolar disorder in children and adolescents. J Am Acad Child Adolesc Psychiatry 48(5):519–532, 2009 19325497

Walkup JT: Antidepressant efficacy for depression in children and adolescents: industry- and NIMH-funded studies. Am J Psychiatry 174(5):430–437, 2017 28253735

Weiler PG, Mungas D, Bernick C: Propranolol for the control of disruptive behavior in senile dementia. J Geriatr Psychiatry Neurol 1(4):226–230, 1988 3252890

Whittington CJ, Kendall T, Fonagy P, et al: Selective serotonin reuptake inhibitors in childhood depression: systematic review of published versus unpublished data. Lancet 363(9418):1341–1345, 2004 15110490

Wilens TE, Biederman J, Mick E, et al: A systematic assessment of tricyclic antidepressants in the treatment of adult attention-deficit hyperactivity disorder. J Nerv Ment Dis 183(1):48–50, 1995 7807071

Winn S, Stowe ZN, Landry JC, et al: Sertraline in breast milk and nursing infants, in 1995 New Research Program and Abstracts, American Psychiatric Association 148th Annual Meeting, Miami, FL, May 20–25, 1995. Washington, DC, American Psychiatric Association, 1995, p 73

Winterstein AG, Gerhard T, Shuster J, et al: Utilization of pharmacologic treatment in youths with attention deficit/hyperactivity disorder in Medicaid database. Ann Pharmacother 42(1):24–31, 2008 18042808

Yonkers KA, Wisner KL, Stewart DE, et al: The management of depression during pregnancy: a report from the American Psychiatric Association and the American College of Obstetricians and Gynecologists. Gen Hosp Psychiatry 31(5):403–413, 2009 19703633

Zhong G, Wang Y, Zhang Y, et al: Association between benzodiazepine use and dementia: a meta-analysis. PLoS One 10(5):e0127836, 2015 26016483

13

Laboratory-Guided Pharmacotherapy

Since around 2010, there has been a proliferation of laboratory tests that purport to improve treatment outcome. The promise of personalized medicine is that a laboratory test will help the clinician choose the right medication for the right patient. Currently, prescribing in psychiatry involves the clinician making an educated guess about which medication might be most useful for the patient on the basis of the presenting symptoms, concurrent medications, and comorbid conditions along with the pharmacological profile of the drug, including the known side effects. Psychiatrists lack the equivalent of the culture and sensitivity (so-called C&S) tests that the infectious disease specialist can employ to match an antibiotic to a specific bacterium. Similarly, we do not have genetic tests, such as those available to the oncologist, that characterize the genetic profile of a tumor so that the most effective medication can be chosen (e.g., human epidermal growth factor receptor 2 [*HER2*] sensitivity in breast cancer).

As of this writing, no laboratory test has proven consistently useful in the diagnosis or treatment of any psychiatric disorder. For example, the official position of the American Psychiatric Association (APA) Task Force on Gene Testing for Antidepressant Efficacy in 2018 is that the routine use of such tests is not supported by the available data to justify the current costs (Moran 2018). Likewise, the APA Work Group on Neuroimaging Markers of Psychiatric Disorders, formed in response to an action paper in 2009 calling for an APA position paper, concluded in 2012 that there was no empirical basis to support the clinical use of any neuroimaging modality in the diagnosis and treatment of psychiatric disorders (First et al. 2012). That being acknowledged, there are limited circumstances in which biomarkers may have a role in the management of several psychiatric conditions. In this chapter, we lay out the case for the restricted application of certain biomarkers of pharmacogenomics testing, cognitive testing, quantitative electroencephalography (qEEG), and neuroimaging in the selection of, predicting response to, and tolerability of psychotropic medications.

Pharmacogenomic Testing

As of this writing, there are many companies who market pharmacogenomic tests specifically to psychiatrists. Most of these tests purport to substantially improve clinical outcome relative to treatment as usual (TAU). However, those claims are based on very limited data. In fact, in some cases, there may simply be no data or clinical trials to back up the utility or reliability of the test in question. That has not prevented the aggressive promotion of some pharmacogenetic assays. Clinicians may be surprised that the requirements for the promotion of laboratory tests are not necessarily the same as those that guide the advertising and promotion of pharmaceuticals and devices.

The FDA has generally classified *laboratory developed tests* (LDTs) by degree of complexity and risk of harm to the patient. A Class I test is a simple test that uses a proven technology, such as glucose strips for testing blood sugar or in-office strep tests. These tests do not have to be formally approved before they are marketed but are registered with the FDA. A Class II LDT, such as an automated complete blood count device or tests for a comprehensive metabolic panel, might entail sophisticated technology and can pose a greater risk to a patient if inaccurate. These Class II LDTs typically require some reliability testing and postmarketing oversight. Finally, a Class III LDT is a test of high complexity that needs to be very reliable in order to prevent harm to the patient. Most of the genetic tests for mutations of cancer genes, such as *HER2*, fall in this class. These tests require the most validity testing and oversight.

In 2014, the FDA proposed guidance on LDTs that would provide more oversight on approval and marketing of laboratory tests (U.S. Food and Drug Administration 2014). It was clear that more careful monitoring of LDTs was needed because clinical decisions based on those tests could result in treatment that was unnecessary or even dangerous. In 2017, the FDA issued a "Discussion Paper on Laboratory-Developed Tests (LDTs)" that was based on feedback from the 2014 proposed guidance (U.S. Food and Drug Administration 2017). In that paper, the FDA proposed risk-based oversight of LDTs and the exemption or grandfathering of some tests that were already on the market.

Pharmacogenomic tests for psychiatric disorders, for the most part, have little oversight. Companies that market pharmacogenomic tests in psychiatry have not been required to demonstrate efficacy or validity. Neither the FDA nor other governmental agencies have claimed jurisdiction of psychiatric pharmacogenomic tests. That remains the case as of 2023 but may change under the proposed guidelines described in the previous paragraph.

The first pharmacogenomic test available to psychiatrists was the Roche AmpliChip, introduced in 2004 (Jain 2005). This first-generation test evaluated single polymorphisms for the cytochrome P450 (CYP) 2D6 and 2C19 enzymes. Because the corresponding genes code for the hepatic isoenzymes that metabolize most psychotropics, these polymorphisms were reasonable targets for a pharmacogenomic test. The test was neither a commercial nor a clinical success. Although the Roche test proposed to predict side effects of antidepressants and other drugs, it was not particularly useful in doing so (de Leon 2016). Indeed, our group early on reported that in a randomized clinical trial that compared mirtazapine and paroxetine in geriatric depression and that used the gene chip, CYP2D6 and CYP2C19 enzyme variation failed to predict side effects to either drug, particularly failing with paroxetine, which is an inhibitor and substrate for the enzyme (Murphy et al. 2003).

The next generation of pharmacogenomic tests used a combinatorial approach to assess the effects of multiple genes on drug response and tolerability. Almost all pharmacogenomic tests evaluate polymorphisms for CYP2D6 and CYP2C19, as did the original Roche AmpliChip. However, there has been an explosion of other pharmacokinetic enzymes added to the commercial tests, including those for CYP3A4, CYP1A2, CYP2B6, and several other genes. In addition, the current generations of tests sometimes include pharmacodynamic genotyping. In our studies on geriatric depression, we demonstrated that in white people, the short form in the promoter region of the serotonin transporter gene and the 102 T/C allele for the serotonin$_2$ (5-HT$_{2A}$) receptor were associated with intolerance to paroxetine (i.e., pharmacodynamic genes were more important for our new compounds) (Murphy et al. 2003, 2004). Some commercial algorithms include measures of the 5-HT transporter promoter polymorphism. Previous to our work, others had reported that the short form of the 5-HT transporter promoter predicted poor response to selective serotonin reuptake inhibitors (SSRIs); in our work, we observed a prediction of side effects rather than of response. The effect sizes of these alleles are often small by themselves, leading some people to argue that testing based on them is not cost-effective. However, there are relatively few data on the effect size of combination approaches.

To date, there have been a small number of randomized trials of commercial pharmacogenomic tests in patients with depression, and the results have been mixed. These trials have been funded predominantly by companies that perform the assays and apply the algorithms. Winner et al. (2013) randomly assigned 51 patients with major depressive disorder (MDD) to receive either gene-guided treatment (GeneSight) or TAU. After 10 weeks of treatment, there was a trend favoring the gene-guided treatment, but the separation did not reach statistical significance. In a 12-week double-blind randomized controlled trial, Singh and colleagues randomly assigned 152 patients with MDD to receive either gene-guided treatment (CNSDose) or TAU. In that study, 72% of patients in the gene-guided treatment group achieved remission versus only 28% in the TAU group (Singh 2015).

Three large randomized controlled trials have provided some support to the use of pharmacogenomic testing in depression. Psychiatrists may have a clear sense of what to prescribe based on training and clinical experience, but this may be less true for colleagues who see many depressed patients in obstetrics-gynecology, internal medicine, and family practice clinics. In one real-world study that included 685 patients with MDD from a variety of medical disciplines, patients were randomly assigned to receive 12 weeks of gene-guided treatment (NeuroIDgenetix) or TAU (Bradley et al. 2018). Patients in the gene-guided treatment group had significantly higher remission rates (36% vs. 13%) and response rates (73% vs. 36%) compared with the TAU group. One of the larger pharmacogenomic studies of a psychiatric disorder evaluated the GeneSight test in 1,167 patients with MDD (The Guided Trial; Greden et al. 2019). This study failed to show a significant difference between TAU and gene-guided treatment on the primary endpoint, which was overall symptom improvement. However, patients in the gene-guided treatment group were significantly more likely than patients receiving TAU to experience a remission (15% vs. 10%) or response (26% vs. 20%). Because many of the patients in the TAU group ended up taking medications that would have been chosen by the gene-guided treatment anyway, a separate analysis was done on patients who were prescribed and started taking a medication incongruent with gene-guided treatment. Those patients were significantly more likely to have a response or remission than patients who remained in the incongruent group. The largest randomized trial to date, the Precision Medicine in Mental Health Care (PRIME) trial, involved 1,944 patients with MDD at 22 Veterans Affairs Medical Centers (Oslin et al. 2022). Patients were randomly assigned to either gene-guided treatment or TAU for 24 weeks. Patients in the gene-guided treatment were significantly more likely than the TAU group to achieve remission at some point over the 24 weeks ($P=0.02$), but the difference was quite modest. Patients in the gene-guided treatment were only 2.8% more likely to achieve remission than the TAU patients at some point in the study, and there was no difference in the remission rate at week 24.

Meta-analyses of large and small randomized pharmacogenomic studies in patients with MDD have been generally consistent in concluding some benefit of these tests in improving the response and remission rates (Arnone et al. 2023; Bousman et al. 2019). However, there are problems with many of the studies done to date, including inadequate blinding, lack of transparency about the algorithms employed to determine medication choice, possible bias from having all the larger studies funded by the companies that market them, and lack of independent repeat studies.

The current pharmacogenomic tests may be better at predicting tolerability than efficacy. In fact, even the studies showing improved efficacy may do so in no small part because patients who tolerate a drug are more likely to continue taking it and thus improve. Among the pharmacokinetic markers, CYP2D6, CYP2C9, and CYP2C19 are probably the most useful. Because most tricyclic antidepressants (TCAs), SSRIs, and antipsychotics are CYP2D6 substrates, the pharmacogenomic tests may provide utility in avoiding certain risks. For example, because metabolism of TCAs is dependent on CYP2D6, identifying the 20% or so of the white population who are slow metabolizers may have clinical relevance. These slow metabolizers may be at greater risk of TCA-induced arrhythmias because poor metabolizers have higher serum TCA levels and are not be able to clear the drug effectively. Likewise, citalopram is associated with dose-related QTc prolongation and is a CYP2C19 substrate. Thus, patients who are slow metabolizers of CYP2C19 might not be ideal candidates for citalopram. It is debatable, however, whether the cost or predictive value of a pharmacogenomic test has advantages over getting an inexpensive electrocardiogram at baseline and when steady state of these drugs is achieved.

There are emerging tests that appear to predict antidepressant responses, but as of this writing they are available only in some European countries. A good example is a test of variants of the gene *ABCB1* (*MDR1*), which predicts responses to several commonly used agents. This gene encodes for a glycoprotein that transports many antidepressants out of the brain and as such controls neuronal exposure to specific agents. The original observations were made by Uhr et al. (2008) at the Max Planck Institute of Psychiatry in Munich, and our group has replicated some of their markers and reported on others (Sarginson et al. 2010; Schatzberg et al. 2015). Another positive predictor of response that has replication is the corticotropin-releasing hormone binding protein (O'Connell et al. 2018). Testing these single nucleotide polymorphisms could potentially provide a highly sensitive predictor of response to specific agents and lead to true personalized medicine for the depressed patient.

Given the small but significant benefit of pharmacogenomic testing in the treatment of MDD, it is probably not cost-effective to order testing for every patient. There are, however, a few situations where it is probably worthwhile to have pharmacogenomic testing done. One potential indication for pharmacogenomic testing is for individuals who have been intolerant of multiple medications. We see patients who have severe side effects with low doses of many medications. The failure to attain and maintain a therapeutic dose for a long enough duration all but assures the lack of a response. A trial-and-error process that results in many side effects but few benefits is often frustrating for patients and clinicians alike. Pharmacogenomic testing can, at the very least, provide some reassurance to patients that the medication being prescribed is not a complete shot in the dark.

Another potential indication is in more severely depressed individuals. Testing might modestly improve the chance of selecting a medication that a patient with more severe depression might tolerate and respond to. The risks and long-term prognosis of a severely depressed patient staying in a depressive episode might make an even modest chance of recovery worth the cost of testing.

A third possible indication is limiting the risk of a negative gene-related drug-drug interaction in a patient with a medical comorbidity that might put them at risk for such an interaction, such as a patient with a history of an arrythmia who is being considered for treatment with a TCA for pain or citalopram for depression. Knowing that the patient is a slow metabolizer of CYP2D6 or CYP2C19 could be useful in that case.

Among the pharmacodynamic markers, the only one that has clear empirical support for its use clinically is the HLA-B*1502 marker. The gene *LA-B*1502* substantially increases the risk of Stevens-Johnson syndrome in Han Chinese individuals who are being treated with carbamazepine. About 10%–15% of patients of Chinese descent carry the allele. In 2007 the FDA changed the label on carbamazepine to recommend pharmacogenomic testing in at-risk populations. Many psychiatric drugs have pharmacogenomic data included in the package insert, but carbamazepine is currently the only drug used by psychiatrists that has a clear recommendation for pharmacogenomic testing for the HLA allele. An *HLA-DQB1* assay was commercially available in the early 2000s for clozapine-induced agranulocytosis. Although specific, the test was only 21% sensitive. As a result, the test was neither commercially successful nor clinically useful. As far as we know, *HLA-DQB1* is not commonly included in the current pharmacogenomic tests. However, more sensitive HLA markers for clozapine-induced agranulocytosis are on the horizon and may show up in subsequent iterations of the pharmacogenomic tests geared to the psychiatrist.

Our recommendations for the limited circumstances in which pharmacogenomic testing may be indicated are summarized below. In the future, as the cost of pharmacogenomic testing falls and the empirical evidence supports the broader use of testing, the list of indications will surely grow and perhaps may result in more routine use of these assays.

The following are possible indications for pharmacogenomic testing:

- When the patient has a history of intolerance to multiple psychotropic drugs
- When the patient has more severe MDD

- When a potentially cardiotoxic drug (TCAs, citalopram) is being considered
- When carbamazepine is being considered in patients of Han Chinese descent

Neurocognitive Testing

Whereas pharmacogenomic tests currently are probably obtained too frequently on a cost-benefit basis, cognitive testing is probably not done frequently enough. Although simple cognitive tests do not inform about the side effects of a drug, they may be a better predictor of response or lack of response, at least in depression and schizophrenia, than is any genetic, imaging, or physiological test that we currently have available.

Cognitive deficits, including inattention and indecisiveness, are part of the core symptoms of major depressive disorder in DSM-5-TR (American Psychiatric Association 2022). It is estimated that 94% of patients with MDD demonstrate cognitive deficits in acute episodes, with 44% continuing to have deficits between episodes (Lam et al. 2014). The deficits in MDD, including inattention, slow processing speed, and executive dysfunction, may persist despite remission. Improvement in cognition in MDD may be a better predictor of return to premorbid functioning than other core symptoms, such as mood (McIntyre et al. 2013).

Cognitive deficits are also common in schizophrenia spectrum disorders (Bora et al. 2017). The types of deficits in schizophrenia include problems with social cognition, visual memory, executive function, processing speed, and attention. Greater deficits in cognition in schizophrenia are directly related to difficulties in both interpersonal and vocational functioning.

It has been known for some time that difficulties with specific types of cognition are predictive of response to both antipsychotics and antidepressants. In patients with schizophrenia, the better the baseline functioning in planning and reasoning, the more likely a patient will respond to both first- and second-generation antipsychotics in first-episode psychosis (Trampush et al. 2015). Similarly, Robinson et al. (1999) found that a simple measure of attention predicted positive symptom response over the first year after an initial psychotic break.

As with antipsychotics in schizophrenia, patients with MDD who have poorer cognitive functioning at baseline appear to have poorer outcomes with standard antidepressants. In the International Study to Predict Optimized Treatment in Depression (iSPOT-D) trial, patients with MDD who had more global cognitive deficits tended to do more poorly with standard antidepressants (Etkin et al. 2015). Early changes in some forms of cognitive dysfunction with antidepressant treatment, such as changes in facial emotion recognition in the first few weeks of treatment, tend to predict subsequent response to treatment (Park et al. 2018). Unfortunately, standard antidepressants do not seem to do much for the cognitive deficits in MDD.

The data suggesting that poorer cognition predicts poorer response to pharmacotherapy in both schizophrenia and MDD beg two questions: what are the alternatives to standard pharmacotherapy, and what tests should be used? Referral to our neuropsychologist colleagues is always an option and provides that most detailed testing and expert interpretation of those tests. However, the cost and time involved can be challenging for patients. A number of commercial computer-based (Cantab), touch screen (Brain Resource), online (General Cognitive Assessment Battery [CAB]), and even phone-based (Defense Automated Neurobehavioral Assessment [DANA]) tools are available to the clinician. The cost of these assessment tools varies considerably, but most test for memory, attention, and executive functioning, which appear predictive of response to antipsychotics and antidepressants. Some, such as the tests from Cantab and Brain Resource, are customized to a specific diagnosis such as MDD. All these assessments include interpretation of the results and comparison with normative databases.

The question about what the alternatives are if cognitive testing predicts poorer outcome to standard pharmacotherapy is less clear. In depression, adjunctive treatment with drugs that enhance attention might be beneficial to address cognitive symptoms. These include stimulants, modafinil/armodafinil, and atomoxetine. Vortioxetine has been demonstrated to improve performance on the Digit Symbol Substitution Test, which is a measure of sustained attention, response speed, and set shifting. In addition, transcranial magnetic stimulation may help with cognition in depression (Levkovitz et al. 2009).

The options for the patient with schizophrenia who demonstrates poor cognitive function at baseline are more limited. A second-generation antipsychotic is probably a better option than first-generation antipsychotics. Among the second-generation antipsychotics, those that are 5-HT$_{1A}$ agonists, including clozapine, aripiprazole, and cariprazine, might enhance neurogenesis and be somewhat more helpful than other antipsychotics in patients with poorer cognitive functioning (Schreiber and Newman-Tancredi 2014). Adjunctive strategies, including the use of cholinergic and glutamatergic medications, armodafinil, and SSRIs, have had modest and inconsistent benefits in schizophrenia (Choi et al. 2013). Results with novel adjunctive agents, such as the estrogen modulator raloxifene and oxytocin to address social and cognitive deficits, have also been mixed.

The most consistent way to address poor social and cognitive baseline performance in patients with schizophrenia is with some kind of psychosocial remediation. Although antipsychotics are still required to treat the positive symptoms, cognitive remediation and social remediation with a skilled therapist are often very helpful in the other domains (Grant et al. 2017). Cognitive remediation may involve practicing a cognitive skill repeatedly until greater mastery is achieved. Likewise, social cognitive training can improve interpersonal skills important to both vocational and social interactions.

Thus, baseline cognitive testing does appear to predict responsiveness to pharmacotherapy in depression and schizophrenia. Cognitive assessments are routinely done in disorders such as dementia, delirium, ADHD, and traumatic brain injury, and the case can certainly be made that cognitive testing in schizophrenia and major depression may inform the clinician about pharmacotherapy choices.

Quantitative Electroencephalography

There are a few commercially available qEEG tests that purport to predict response to psychiatric medications. The qEEG test is simply a method for quantifying the brain waveform on an electroencephalogram. The encephalogram reflects neuronal electrical activity and has been studied extensively in many psychiatric disorders. Among the disorders most extensively studied using qEEG are MDD and ADHD. As with pharmacogenomic testing, the marketing of qEEG for predicting drug response is not subject to extensive oversight by the FDA or other governmental agencies. It is relatively easy to perform a qEEG test in the office, and the test may be relatively inexpensive compared with modalities such as neuroimaging or even pharmacogenomics.

A major focus of electroencephalographic studies in depression and ADHD has been theta wave activity. Depression has been associated with elevated theta wave activity localized to the frontal areas and may also reflect increased theta-to-alpha activity in the anterior cingulate. Similarly, some, but certainly not all, studies in ADHD have reported an elevated theta-to-beta wave ratio (TBR). In fact, a high TBR has been proposed as diagnostic of ADHD but is neither sensitive nor specific. Other EEG findings include an elevated relative alpha wave asymmetry and changes in the loudness dependence of the auditory evoked potential in both depression and ADHD.

Antidepressants are known to have specific electroencephalographic effects, and there have been a number of studies that suggest that EEG biomarkers might predict antidepressant response. Several multicenter studies have suggested a possible role for qEEG in predicting antidepressant response. In one study, Leuchter et al. (2009) examined a frontal qEEG biomarker's ability to predict response to the SSRI escitalopram after 1 week of treatment. In this study, 375 patients with MDD were randomly assigned to either remain on treatment or be crossed over to alternative treatment. Seventy-five subjects continued to take escitalopram, and 52% responded to therapy after 49 days. The qEEG biomarker was able to predict responders to escitalopram with an accuracy of 72% on the basis of changes in the asymmetry composite EEG index between the baseline electroencephalogram and an electroencephalogram completed after 1 week of pharmacological treatment.

We examined a different type of qEEG, referenced EEG (rEEG), in predicting antidepressant response (DeBattista et al. 2011). In rEEg, the qEEG of a subject is referenced to a normative database of patients who either did or did not respond to a given antidepressant. In this study, 114 patients with MDD were randomly assigned to receive rEEG-guided treatment or TAU on the basis of options evaluated in the Sequenced Treatment Alternatives for Resistant Depression (STAR*D) trial. Patients in the rEEG group had greater overall symptom improvement relative to the control group.

The largest qEEG study to date was part of iSPOT-D (Arns et al. 2017). In this study, qEEG was obtained for 1,008 patients with MDD. Patients in the study were randomly assigned to receive treatment with escitalopram, sertraline, or extended-release venlafaxine. A type of baseline qEEG was designed to extract theta activity in the frontal cortex and rostral anterior cingulate cortex. High frontal and rostral anterior cingulate cortex activity was associated with less likelihood of response across all three treatments, particularly in patients who had not responded to multiple previous treatments.

Because all of the large studies used different types of qEEG with different designs, it is difficult to draw conclusions about the utility of qEEG in predicting antidepressant response. The ADHD literature parallels the MDD literature, in that less-than-clear conclusions can be drawn about qEEG efficacy in predicting response.

The commercial companies currently marketing qEEG for the prediction of medication response use different qEEG paradigms. One commonality of these commercial qEEG tests is that they produce detailed reports that outline medications to which the patient is predicted to respond. These reports do not necessarily predict tolerability in the way pharmacogenomic tests might and are not diagnostic in any way. These companies include working government agencies, such as the Department of Defense, and third-party payers attempting to evaluate whether qEEG is cost-effective by helping clinicians choose a medication that a patient may respond to earlier in the course of treatment.

At this time, there does not appear to be a basis for routinely using qEEG in the treatment of psychiatric patients. However, there probably is reason to think qEEG may be a useful tool in predicting medication response in the future.

Neuroimaging

Neuroimaging has proved to be invaluable as a research tool in psychiatry. Many important insights about schizophrenia, bipolar disorder, major depressive disorder, PTSD, and many other psychiatric conditions have been gained via neuroimaging modalities such as functional MRI (fMRI), PET, and SPECT. In addition, neuroimaging has been very important in drug development. Imaging has been useful in establishing the mechanism of novel drugs, providing new potential targets for drug development, and demonstrating the effects of a drug on brain function. However, neuroimaging has fallen short as a tool for helping clinicians establish a diagnosis or predict psychotropic drug response.

Preliminary studies suggested a role for functional neuroimaging in predicting medication response. A number of studies have suggested that hyperactivity in the amygdala and anterior cingulate cortex predicts response to antidepressants. Effective antidepressant treatment might increase functional connectivity between the frontal and limbic areas while decreasing activity in the default network. Likewise, baseline hypofrontality on fMRI may predict response to both first- and second-generation antipsychotics. None of these findings have been consistent or practical enough to be translated into clinical practice.

Neuroimaging is relatively expensive and cumbersome. Thus, the role of imaging is limited to a few situations in clinical practice, and it is still structural rather than functional imaging that is used clinically. The primary role of neuroimaging in clinical practice is to diagnose neurological disorders manifesting as psychiatric conditions (e.g., a frontal tumor manifesting as depression). The case can be made that neuroimaging is indicated in any elderly patient with new-onset psychosis or mania. Another indication is in diagnosing some subtypes of dementia. If a clinician is unsure of the type of dementia after observing the patient for, say, 2 years or more, a CT scan or MRI might be useful in distinguishing a more purely vascular dementia or Creutzfeldt-Jakob disease from dementia due to Alzheimer's disease.

Despite years of continued research on the clinical application of neuroimaging in psychiatry since the original APA action paper on neuroimaging markers of psychiatric disorders in 2009, translating those findings into a practical technology that helps clinicians choose a medication appears to be a long way off.

Suggested Readings

Day CV, Gatt JM, Etkin A, et al: Cognitive and emotional biomarkers of melancholic depression: an iSPOT-D report. J Affect Disord 176:141–150, 2015 25710095

de Leon J, Spina E: What is needed to incorporate clinical pharmacogenetic tests into the practice of psychopharmacotherapy? Expert Rev Clin Pharmacol 9(3):351–354, 2016 26580456

de Leon J, Arranz MJ, Ruaño G: Pharmacogenetic testing in psychiatry: a review of features and clinical realities. Clin Lab Med 28(4):599–617, 2008 19059065

Swen JJ, Nijenhuis M, de Boer A, et al: Pharmacogenetics: from bench to byte—an update of guidelines. Clin Pharmacol Ther 89(5):662–673, 2011 21412232

References

American Psychiatric Association: Diagnostic and Statistical Manual of Mental Disorders, 5th Edition, Text Revision. Washington, DC, American Psychiatric Association, 2022

Arnone D, Omar O, Arora T, et al: Effectiveness of pharmacogenomic tests including CYP2D6 and CYP2C19 genomic variants for guiding the treatment of depressive disorders: systematic review and meta-analysis of randomised controlled trials. Neurosci Biobehav Rev 144:104965, 2023 36463971

Arns M, Gordon E, Boutros NN: EEG abnormalities are associated with poorer depressive symptom outcomes with escitalopram and venlafaxine-XR, but not sertraline: results from the multicenter randomized iSPOT-D study. Clin EEG Neurosci 48(1):33–40, 2017 26674366

Bora E, Binnur Akdede B, Alptekin K: Neurocognitive impairment in deficit and nondeficit schizophrenia: a meta-analysis. Psychol Med 47(14):2401–2413, 2017 28468693

Bousman CA, Arandjelovic K, Mancuso SG, et al: Pharmacogenetic tests and depressive symptom remission: a meta-analysis of randomized controlled trials. Pharmacogenomics 20(1):37–47, 2019 30520364

Bradley P, Shiekh M, Mehra V, et al: Improved efficacy with targeted pharmacogenetic-guided treatment of patients with depression and anxiety: a randomized clinical trial demonstrating clinical utility. J Psychiatr Res 96:100–107, 2018 28992526

Choi KH, Wykes T, Kurtz MM: Adjunctive pharmacotherapy for cognitive deficits in schizophrenia: meta-analytical investigation of efficacy. Br J Psychiatry 203(3):172–178, 2013 23999481

DeBattista C, Kinrys G, Hoffman D, et al: The use of referenced-EEG (rEEG) in assisting medication selection for the treatment of depression. J Psychiatr Res 45(1):64–75, 2011 20598710

de Leon J: Pharmacogenetic tests in psychiatry: from fear to failure to hype. J Clin Psychopharmacol 36(4):299–304, 2016 27269957

Etkin A, Patenaude B, Song YJ, et al: A cognitive-emotional biomarker for predicting remission with antidepressant medications: a report from the iSPOT-D trial. Neuropsychopharmacology 40(6):1332–1342, 2015 25547711

First M, Botteron K, Carter C, et al; Work Group on Neuroimaging Markers of Psychiatric Disorders: Consensus Report of the APA Work Group on Neuroimaging Markers of Psychiatric Disorders. Arlington, VA, American Psychiatric Association, 2012

Grant N, Lawrence M, Preti A, et al: Social cognition interventions for people with schizophrenia: a systematic review focussing on methodological quality and intervention modality. Clin Psychol Rev 56:55–64, 2017 28688282

Greden JF, Parikh SV, Rothschild AJ, et al: Impact of pharmacogenomics on clinical outcomes in major depressive disorder in the GUIDED trial: a large, patient- and rater-blinded, randomized, controlled study. J Psychiatr Res 111:59–67, 2019 30677646

Jain KK: Applications of AmpliChip CYP450. Mol Diagn 9(3):119–127, 2005 16271013

Lam RW, Kennedy SH, McIntyre RS, Khullar A: Cognitive dysfunction in major depressive disorder: effects on psychosocial functioning and implications for treatment. Can J Psychiatry 59(12):649–654, 2014 25702365

Leuchter AF, Cook IA, Marangell LB, et al: Comparative effectiveness of biomarkers and clinical indicators for predicting outcomes of SSRI treatment in major depressive disorder: results of the BRITE-MD study. Psychiatry Res 169(2):124–131, 2009 19712979

Levkovitz Y, Harel EV, Roth Y, et al: Deep transcranial magnetic stimulation over the prefrontal cortex: evaluation of antidepressant and cognitive effects in depressive patients. Brain Stimul 2(4):188–200, 2009 20633419

McIntyre RS, Cha DS, Soczynska JK, et al: Cognitive deficits and functional outcomes in major depressive disorder: determinants, substrates, and treatment interventions. Depress Anxiety 30(6):515–527, 2013 23468126

Moran M: Task force on gene testing for antidepressant efficacy concludes tests not yet ready for widespread use. Psychiatr News July 19, 2018

Murphy GM Jr, Kremer C, Rodrigues HE, Schatzberg AF: Pharmacogenetics of antidepressant medication intolerance. Am J Psychiatry 160(10):1830–1835, 2003 14514498

Murphy GM Jr, Hollander SB, Rodrigues HE, et al: Effects of the serotonin transporter gene promoter polymorphism on mirtazapine and paroxetine efficacy and adverse events in geriatric major depression. Arch Gen Psychiatry 61(11):1163–1169, 2004 15520364

O'Connell CP, Goldstein-Piekarski AN, Nemeroff CB, et al: Antidepressant outcomes predicted by genetic variation in corticotropin-releasing hormone binding protein. Am J Psychiatry 175(3):251–261, 2018 29241359

Oslin DW, Lynch KG, Shih MC, et al: Effect of pharmacogenomic testing for drug-gene interactions on medication selection and remission of symptoms in major depressive disorder: the PRIME care randomized clinical trial. JAMA 328(2):151–161, 2022 35819423

Park C, Pan Z, Brietzke E, et al: Predicting antidepressant response using early changes in cognition: a systematic review. Behav Brain Res 353:154–160, 2018 30031025

Robinson DG, Woerner MG, Alvir JM, et al: Predictors of treatment response from a first episode of schizophrenia or schizoaffective disorder. Am J Psychiatry 156(4):544–549, 1999 10200732

Sarginson JE, Lazzeroni LC, Ryan HS, et al: ABCB1 (MDR1) polymorphisms and antidepressant response in geriatric depression. Pharmacogenet Genomics
20(8):467–475, 2010 20555295

Schatzberg AF, DeBattista C, Lazzeroni LC, et al: ABCB1 genetic effects on antidepressant outcomes: a report from the iSPOT-D trial. Am J Psychiatry
172(8):751–759, 2015 25815420

Schreiber R, Newman-Tancredi A: Improving cognition in schizophrenia with antipsychotics that elicit neurogenesis through 5-HT(1A) receptor activation. Neu-
robiol Learn Mem 110:72–80, 2014 24423786

Singh AB: Improved antidepressant remission in major depression via a pharmacokinetic pathway polygene pharmacogenetic report. Clin Psychopharmacol Neurosci 13(2):150–156, 2015 26243841

Trampush JW, Lencz T, DeRosse P, et al: Relationship of cognition to clinical response in first-episode schizophrenia spectrum disorders. Schizophr Bull
41(6):1237–1247, 2015 26409223

Uhr M, Tontsch A, Namendorf C, et al: Polymorphisms in the drug transporter gene
ABCB1 predict antidepressant treatment response in depression. Neuron
57(2):203–209, 2008 18215618

U.S. Food and Drug Administration: Framework for Regulatory Oversight of
Laboratory Developed Tests (LDTs): Draft Guidance for Industry, Food and
Drug Administration Staff, and Clinical Laboratories. Silver Spring, MD, U.S.
Food and Drug Administration, October 3, 2014. Available at: www.fda.gov/
downloads/medicaldevices/deviceregulationandguidance/guidancedocuments/
ucm416685.pdf. Accessed September 18 2018.

U.S. Food and Drug Administration: Discussion Paper on Laboratory Developed
Tests (LDTs). Silver Spring, MD, U.S. Food and Drug Administration, January
13, 2017. Available at: www.fda.gov/downloads/medicaldevices/
productsandmedicalprocedures/invitrodiagnostics/laboratorydevelopedtests/
ucm536965.pdf. Accessed September 18 2018.

Winner J, Allen JD, Altar CA, Spahic-Mihajlovic A: Psychiatric pharmacogenomics
predicts health resource utilization of outpatients with anxiety and depression.
Transl Psychiatry 3(3):e242, 2013 23511609

Index

Page numbers printed in **boldface** type refer to tables or figures.

SSRIs. *See* Selective serotonin reuptake inhibitors
Stabilization dose, of methadone, 667
Stanford Intelligent Accelerated Neuromodulation Therapy (SAINT), 646
Stanford University, 168
Starter kits of lamotrigine, 401
Steroids, and psychiatric syndromes, 752
Stevens-Johnson syndrome, 795
Stigma, and mental health care for minority populations, 710
Stimulants
    ADHD and, 551–553
    binge-eating disorder and, 559
    children and, 712–717
    depression and, 553–557
    drug combinations and, 559–560
    fatigue associated with chronic viral illness and, 557–559
    formulations and strengths of, 544–545
    geriatric patients and, 732
    hospital wards, use in, 559
    intellectual developmental disorders and, 748
    medical conditions and, 749
    overview of, 543, 546–549
    psychosis and, 560–561
    side effects of, 553
    substance abuse and, 552, 561–562, 687–689
    suggested readings on, 566–569
Stimulation, and MAOIs, 149
Stimulus control therapy, 512
Stress urinary incontinence, and duloxetine, 93
Study of Lemborexant in Subjects 55 Years and Older With Insomnia Disorder (SUNRISE), 526
Stupor, and emergency department, 654–655

Sublingual forms
    of antipsychotics, 649–650
    of asenapine, 277
    of benzodiazepines, 460
    of buprenorphine, 671
    of dexmedetomidine, 641–642
Substance dependence
    definition of, 38–39
    nonbenzodiazepine hypnotics and, 521–522
Substance-related and addictive disorders, diagnosis and classification of, 38–39
Substance use disorders. *See also* Alcohol and alcohol abuse/dependence; Opioids
    amphetamines and, 549–550
    benzodiazepines and, 465, 533–534
    cannabis and, 409, 664, 686
    definition of, 38
    drug testing and, 665–666
    hallucinogens and, 687
    ketamine and, 159–160, 162
    MDMA and, 478
    nicotine and, 685, **686**
    nonbenzodiazepine hypnotics and, 521–522
    overview of pharmacotherapy for, 663–665
    phencyclidine and, 689–690
    PTSD and, 476
    sedatives and hypnotics, 681–682
    stimulants and, 552, 561–562, 687–689
    suggested readings on, 690–693
Sudden death. *See also* Death; Mortality
    desipramine for children and, 724
    FGAs and, 288–289
Suicide and suicidal behavior
    antidepressant use in children or adolescents and, 10, 77, 722
    atomoxetine and, 563